Roger Narayan
Editor

Nanostructured Biomaterials and Their Applications

Springer

Editor
Roger Narayan
Department of Biomedical Engineering
North Carolina State University
Raleigh, NC, USA

ISBN 978-3-032-16315-8 ISBN 978-3-032-16316-5 (eBook)
https://doi.org/10.1007/978-3-032-16316-5

This Springer imprint is published by the registered company Springer Nature Switzerland AG
The registered company address is: Gewerbestrasse 11, 6330 Cham, Switzerland

Preface

Nanostructured materials are finding wider use for biomedical and biological applications. Based on their nanoscale features, nanostructured materials may exhibit specific interactions with viruses, proteins, and other small biological structures. In addition, nanostructured materials may enable the integration of multiple functions, an increase in performance, and a reduction in cost. This book brings together authors from a broad range of backgrounds to consider recent developments in nanostructured biomaterials, from fundamental concepts to translational applications. I would like to thank Dilruba Baykara, Sabereh Nouri, Hüseyin Berkay Ozarici, Omer Akgiray, Nazmi Ekren, Canan Dogan, and Oguzhan Gunduz for their contribution entitled "Historical Evolution of Nanobiomaterials," J. Randhari, P. K. Mallik, and S. K. Senapati for their contribution entitled "Functional Properties of Nanostructured Materials," Karolina Jurczyk, Mieczyslawa U. Jurczyk, and M. Jurczyk for their contribution entitled "Nanostructured Surfaces in Biomaterials," Otto Wilson, Awatef Alsheri, Jeff Morgan, Winston Anderson, and Ayelle Gugssa for their contribution entitled "Multifunctional Microtubule Nanocomposite Models in Medicine," Yiqiang Fan, Kexin Gao, Xueqin Chen, and Siyuan Ding for their contribution entitled "Microfluidic Synthesis of Nanoparticles for Biological Applications," Prem Chandra Pandey for his contribution entitled "Reactive Organic Functionality Linked to Trialkoxysilane in Designing Nanostructured Material with Exceptional Properties for Technological Applications," Govind Pandey, Tharuna Chandra Pandey, and Shivangi Pandey for their contribution entitled "Synthesis and Biomedical Applications of Cationic Polymer Coated Noble Metal Nanoparticles," Akiyoshi Osaka for his contribution entitled "Synthesis and Nano-Structure Control of Four Morphs of Calcium Carbonate," Antonia Ressler for her contribution entitled "Ion-Substituted Nano-Hydroxyapatite: A Multifunctional Biomaterial with Anticancer, Antibacterial, and Osteogenic Properties," Wencheng Zhu and Xujun Zheng for their contribution entitled "The Biological Activity of Iron Oxide Nanoparticles," Tharini Jeyapragasam, Sridhar Jayavel, Lakshmini Narayanan, Prathingara Subramanian, J. Meena Devi, and Rasu Ramachandran for their contribution entitled "Carbon Biomaterials for Sensing," Alejandra Garcia-Garcia, Huma Sadiq, and René Hernandez Delgadillo for their contribution entitled "Graphene-Based Heterostructures and Their Applications as Bionanomaterial," Natan Luis Nozella, João Vitor Paulin, João Victor Morais Lima, and Carlos Frederico de Oliveira Graeff for their contribution entitled "Eumelanin as a Key Material in Bioelectronic Interfaces and Eco-Friendly Technologies," Manuela Ciocca, Luisa Petti, Paolo Lugli, Antonella Camaioni, and Thomas M. Brown for their contribution entitled "Light Modulation of Biological/Semiconductor Interfaces for Affecting Cell Growth and for Advancing Artificial Retina Development," Madan L. Verma, Irfan Ahmad, John Jeslin, Sarita Devi, and Asim K. Jana for their contribution entitled "Nanocarriers Immobilized Enzymes and Their Potential Industrial Applications," Shangsi Chen, Xiaodie Chen, Jie Huang, and Min Wang for their contribution entitled "Materials, Technologies and Applications of 3D/4D Printing in Tissue Engineering," Zicheng Deng, Vladimir V. Kalinichenko, and Donglu Shi for their contribution entitled "Nanoparticle Designs for Specific Targeting in Precision Theranostics," Toshiki Miyazaki for his contribution entitled "Development of Hybrid Biomaterials Able to Achieve Both Hyperthermia and Bone Repair," and Vivek Aggarwal and Saranjit Singh Bhasin for their contribution entitled "Silver Nanoparticles in Dental Adhesives: Antibacterial Mechanisms, Incorporation Strategies, and Clinical Applications."

I am grateful to the many individuals at Springer Nature who made this book possible, including Michael Luby (Executive Editor for Physical Sciences and Engineering), Kaitlyn Olivia Bonomo (Editorial Assistant for Applied Sciences), Brian P. Halm (Project Coordinator for Group Book Production and Publishing Services), and Pradheepa Vijay (Production Editor). Their expertise was essential to bring this book to completion.

Raleigh, USA Roger Narayan

Contents

Historical Evolution of Nanobiomaterials

Dilruba Baykara, Sabereh Nouri, Hüseyin Berkay Ozarici, Omer Akgiray, Nazmi Ekren, Canan Dogan, and Oguzhan Gunduz

Abstract The terms nanobiomaterials, nanoscience and nanotechnology have become terms that are frequently used in scientific literature and have found their place in everyday life. Research in this field has origins that trace back to some of the earliest inquiries into the fundamental principles of nature. Many scientists and engineers around the world are working in this field and shaping the technologies of the future. Nanobiomaterials, which are between 1 and 100 nm in size, are used in many different fields thanks to their large surface-area-to-volume ratio and the ability to modify their surfaces easily. Nanobiomaterials offer breakthrough innovations in medicine, drug delivery, tissue engineering, diagnostics, personalised nanomedicine, biosensor technology, cancer therapy and many other fields, enabling the development of smaller, stronger and more efficient products. This improves the quality of our

D. Baykara (✉) · H. B. Ozarici · C. Dogan · O. Gunduz
Department of Metallurgical and Materials Engineering, Faculty of Technology, Marmara University, Istanbul, Turkey
e-mail: dilrubabaykara@marun.edu.tr

H. B. Ozarici
e-mail: huseyin.berkay@marun.edu.tr

C. Dogan
e-mail: canan.dogan@marmara.edu.tr

O. Gunduz
e-mail: oguzhan@marmara.edu.tr

S. Nouri
Department of Cell, Molecular Biology and Microbiology, Faculty of Biological Science and Technology, University of Isfahan, Isfahan, Iran
e-mail: sabere.nuri@yahoo.com

O. Akgiray
Department of Environmental Engineering, Faculty of Engineering, Marmara University, Istanbul, Turkey
e-mail: omer.akgiray@marmara.edu.tr

N. Ekren
Department of Electrical and Electronics Engineering, Faculty of Technology, Marmara University, 34854 Istanbul, Turkey
e-mail: nazmiekren@marmara.edu.tr

R. Narayan (ed.), *Nanostructured Biomaterials and Their Applications*,
https://doi.org/10.1007/978-3-032-16316-5_1

daily lives and shapes future technologies. Nanomaterials can be classified according to their origin, structural configuration and composition, number of dimensions and pore size. This classification helps us better understand nanotechnology's applications in various fields. This chapter gives an overview of the history and development of nanobiomaterials. It also describes the areas of application and the classification of nanomaterials with different properties.

Keywords Nanobiomaterials · Nanotechnology · History of nanobiomaterials · Classification

1 Introduction: An Overview of Nanobiomaterials

Nanobiomaterials, as they are named, are nano-sized materials that are compatible with biological tissues. This biomaterial technology has been developed and is still in the process of development by many different techniques. Nanobiomaterials are about 10^{-9} m in size and can be observed only by special tools like light microscopy or scanning electron microscopy.

1.1 Definition and Scope of Nanobiomaterials

Nanobiomaterials are nanoscale materials, typically ranging in size from 1 to 100 nm (1 nm = 10^{-9} m), that are biocompatible and can integrate seamlessly with biological tissues and organs. These materials are non-toxic and do not induce inflammatory responses, making them ideal for biomedical applications. Key fields utilising nanobiomaterials include pharmacology, biomaterials science, tissue engineering, and biosensor technology. Their roles in these areas range from diagnostics and drug delivery systems to regenerative medicine and cancer therapy (Sinha et al. 2022). The structural variety of nanobiomaterials, comprising fibres, particles, composites, and nanowires, allows for tailored applications in specific research objectives (Hashemi et al. 2024).

The convergence of nanotechnology and biomaterials science has revolutionised the manipulation, integration, and functionalisation of materials at the nanoscale. This integration facilitates advancements such as tissue-specific drug delivery systems and precision medicine approaches targeting cellular and molecular levels (Kyriakides et al. 2021).

Nanobiomaterials can be categorised based on composition, including carbon-based, organic/dendrimers, inorganic and composites. These materials are utilised for various purposes, such as antiviral and antimicrobial agents, biocompatible scaffolds, controlled drug release systems, and bioactive surfaces. Their selection depends on the specific requirements of the intended application (Kyriakides et al. 2021; Mekuye and Abera 2023).

1.2 Significance and Applications in Biomedicine

The significance of nanobiomaterials in biomedicine is evidenced by a growing body of research demonstrating their diverse applications. Examples include:

- Starch nanoparticles used in the production of edible films (Restu et al. 2021),
- Synthetic nano-hydroxyapatite for tooth enamel repair (Ince and Ermis 2021),
- Manganese oxide (MnO) and iron oxide (FeO) nanostructures for anticancer therapies (Smitha et al. 2022),
- Poly(lactic-co-glycolic acid) (PLGA) nanoparticles for cancer cell targeting and breast cancer research (He et al. 2023, 2024),
- Microporous and magnetic scaffolds for bone regeneration (Aghajanian et al. 2022).

Depending on the application, nanobiomaterials can be engineered to be either biodegradable or non-biodegradable. Biodegradable polymers, such as PLA, PLGA, and PCL, are often preferred for biomedical applications due to their ability to degrade within biological environments, minimising long-term risks. Non-degradable materials, while suitable for certain industrial applications, are less favoured in biomedicine due to potential biocompatibility concerns.

1.3 Historical Development and Evolution

The use of nanostructured materials dates back thousands of years. Ancient Egyptians, for instance, produced 'Egyptian blue', the first synthetic pigment composed of nano-sized glass particles and quartz. This pigment, a mixture of $CaCuSi_4O_{10}$ and SiO_2, exemplifies early nanomaterial innovation. Similarly, medieval artisans employed gold, copper, and silver nanoparticles to produce metallic alloys and decorative materials.

The modern era of nanotechnology began in the twentieth century with the synthesis of silica (SiO_2) nanoparticles for electronic applications. Commercial production expanded to include magnetically active nanoparticles, antibacterial agents, optical materials, and fillers for industrial uses (Jeevanandam et al. 2018). Over time, nanomaterials have evolved to address increasingly complex challenges, culminating in today's sophisticated nanobiomaterials for biomedical and tissue engineering applications.

Nanobiomaterials are poised to redefine the boundaries of medicine and materials science. As research continues to explore new combinations of materials and their interactions with biological systems, the possibilities for innovation appear boundless. The development of personalised nanomedicine, where treatments are tailored to an individual's genetic and cellular profile, exemplifies the transformative potential of this field. Furthermore, integrating nanobiomaterials with emerging technologies such as artificial intelligence and bioinformatics promises to accelerate discovery and application in previously unimaginable ways.

In essence, nanobiomaterials represent a confluence of science and engineering, merging the nanoscale manipulation of materials with the complexities of biological systems. Their ability to address challenges in drug delivery, tissue engineering, diagnostics, and beyond positions them as critical components in the advancement of modern healthcare. As the field evolves, it promises to improve existing therapies and pioneer entirely new paradigms in medicine and technology.

2 Fundamental Terms in Nanotechnology

Nanotechnology, with its ability to manipulate materials at the atomic and molecular scale, has revolutionised various fields, particularly biomedicine. To fully appreciate its transformative potential, it is essential to understand the fundamental terms and concepts that underpin this discipline. These terms provide the framework for describing the unique properties of nanoscale materials, their interactions with biological systems, and the techniques used to fabricate and manipulate them.

2.1 *Nanomaterials and Nanoscale*

As previously mentioned, nanomaterials, which are characterised by their dimensions on the nanometer scale (10^{-9} m), possess unique and distinctive features due to their physical and chemical properties. Attributes such as porosity, degradability, composite structure, inducibility, modulatory capacity, and ease of interaction contribute to their versatility and potential applications in various fields (Liu 2023; Liu et al. 2024; Park et al. 2024).

Nanomaterials including nanofibres, nanoparticles, nanocarriers, and nanobubbles—are widely used in biomedical research in both in vitro and in vivo studies. They are particularly significant in drug delivery and targeted therapeutic systems, enabling precise diagnostics and effective treatments within biological organisms. These advancements and their applications will be elaborated upon in subsequent sections.

2.2 *Surface-Area-to-Volume Ratio*

The surface-area-to-volume ratio (SA/V) is characterised by the amount of area exposed per unit of volume of a given body. The decrease of a particle to nanoscale works towards an increase in the unit SA/V ratio. This is because the surface area increases as the square of the radius while the volume scales as the cube of the radius. In nanotechnology, this characteristic is quite crucial since it enhances reactivity, interacts with biological systems, and enhances the functionalisation capacity.

In nanomaterials, a high SA/V ratio is associated with:

Increased Reactivity: More atoms or molecules are exposed on the surface, which enables faster and more efficient chemical reactions

Improved Drug Loading and Release: Nanoparticles in drug delivery can load more active molecules and may uncontrollably release them due to their large surface area.

Enhanced Cellular Interactions: In tissue engineering, the high SA/V ratio of nanofibres and scaffolds resembling the extracellular matrix enhances cell attachment and growth (Raja et al. 2021; Chen 2022; Yang et al. 2022).

One study demonstrated the production of PCL nanofibrous, and the investigation showed that high values of this ratio enabled sufficient cell adhesion and oxygen diffusion (Azari 2021).

2.3 *Modification and Bioactivity*

One significant advantage of nanobiomaterials is their ability to be easily modified and functionalised to meet specific application requirements. For instance, liposomes, nanocarriers composed of lipid bilayers, are designed to encapsulate and deliver active molecules. They are particularly effective in localised drug delivery and can be tailored for targeted applications. A notable example is bilosomes, which are liposomes modified with bile acids to enhance their resistance to harsh physiological conditions, such as stomach acidity (Cekuc et al. 2024). Through additional surface modifications, these nanocarriers can be engineered to attach to specific sites and release their payload in a controlled manner. This can be achieved by utilising environmental conditions such as pH, temperature, charge, or hydrophilic and hydrophobic interactions. Ultimately, functionalising nanomaterials enables the modulation of their bioactivity and physicochemical properties to suit diverse biomedical applications.

2.4 *Controlled Release*

Controlled release is a critical aspect of targeted drug delivery systems. Depending on the properties of the material used in the study, it can be localised and occur either immediately or gradually. Even rapidly degrading materials can be modified to extend their retention time through surface engineering. Retention time refers to the duration between the nanomaterial reaching the targeted site and its subsequent degradation, during which the encapsulated content, such as an enzyme, drug, or other desired molecule, is released and metabolised.

For instance, gelatin, a biological polymer commonly used in biomaterial applications, demonstrates rapid degradation upon interaction with biological fluids, leading to the immediate release of its payload. To optimise such systems, various physicochemical factors can be adjusted to influence the rate, mechanism, and duration of the drug release, collectively referred to as retention time. Another key concept in this context is release kinetics. Release kinetics is zero-order kinetics, in which a drug is eliminated constantly over time, regardless of the drug's concentration in the system (Adepu and Ramakrishna 2021).

3 The Advancements in Nanobiomaterials

3.1 Early Developments in Nanobiomaterials

Nanobiomaterials arose from the combination of nanotechnology and biomedical sciences, utilising the distinct features of nanoscale materials to address medical concerns. The use of nanotechnology in biomaterials dates back to the late twentieth century when scientists began investigating nanoparticles for medication delivery and biomolecular detection (Aguilar 2012). The historical timeline of nanoparticle discovery and development is shown in Fig. 1. These early experiments were critical in defining the fundamental principles of nanobiomaterials, including surface enhancement, controlled drug release, and increased bioavailability. In 1943, Hoar and Schulman first discovered and reported the nanoemulsion system (Souto et al. 2022). One of the first reported applications of nanoparticles in medicine was medication delivery, when researchers attempted to employ microscopic particles to improve drug delivery efficiency to target tissues. Liposomes, lipid-based nanoparticles, were produced in the 1960s and have since been extensively explored for drug delivery due to their capacity to encapsulate hydrophilic and hydrophobic pharmaceuticals (Beck and Tice 1983; Gandhi and Shastri 2024). These liposomal formulations paved the way for a better knowledge of nanoparticle interactions with biological systems, as well as new drug delivery applications. While the initial development of liposomes laid the foundation for drug delivery, their contemporary relevance is evident in the success of lipid nanoparticles in mRNA vaccine delivery, such as those used in the COVID-19[1] vaccine. These advancements highlight the enduring importance of early nanobiomaterial innovations.

Polymeric nanoparticles for drug delivery and tissue engineering were first developed in the 1980s by scientists. PLGA,[2] a biodegradable polymer, has been proposed as a useful nanomaterial for controlled drug delivery. It takes advantage of its ability to dissolve in the body over time, allowing for sustained release (Beck and Tice 1983). PLGA nanoparticles demonstrate the benefits of nanomaterials in terms of controlled release kinetics and reduced drug toxicity, both of which are important in clinical applications.

[1] Coronavirus disease 2019.

[2] Poly (lactic-co-glycolic acid).

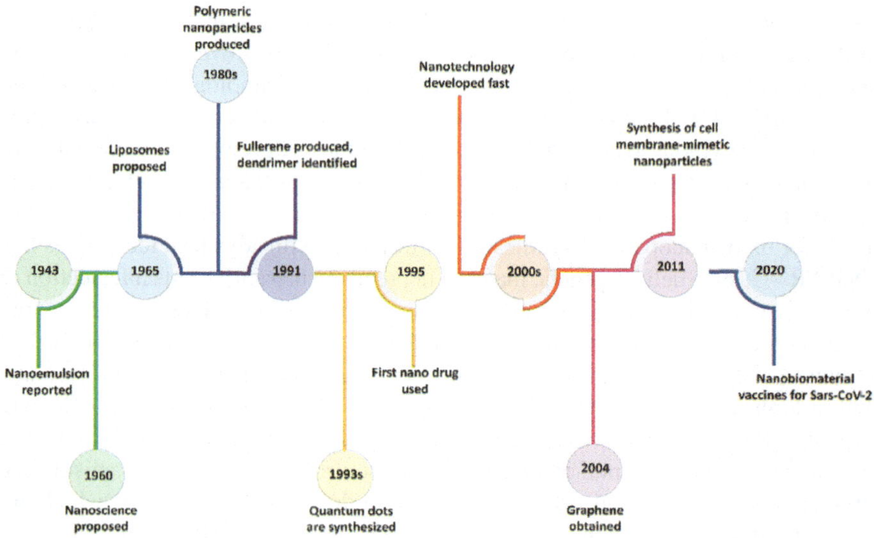

Fig. 1 Historical timeline of the nanoparticle discovery and development process

In 1985, carbon-based fullerenes were first discovered, while dendrimers were produced after they were identified by Tomalia (Xu et al. 2022). Furthermore, the emergence of nanoscale biomaterial coatings in the late 1990s led to a significant rise in implant compatibility. Researchers revealed that nanostructured surfaces can mimic the natural extracellular matrix, promoting more excellent cell adhesion, proliferation, and differentiation than conventional materials (Tabasum et al. 2017). This discovery was crucial for using nanostructured scaffolds in tissue engineering applications because their surface topography and chemistry resulted in better cell interactions. These early investigations laid a solid foundation for the study of nanobiomaterials. They demonstrated how nanoscale features, including large surface area, variable degradation rate, and surface functionalisation, might improve the performance of biomaterials in medical applications. This course's insights have continued to guide the formation of the next generation of nanobiomaterials for applications such as medication delivery, tissue engineering, and diagnostics.

The liposomal formulation of doxorubicin, approved by the Food and Drug Administration (FDA) in 1995, was the first approved nanoparticle formulation (Dominska and Dykxhoorn 2012).

3.2 Key Innovations in Nanomaterial Synthesis

The development of nanomaterial synthesis follows an evolution path of fundamental milestones and state-of-the-art developments, driven by increasingly high demands for tailored nanomaterials in various areas of applications, especially those on biomedicine. Early ones, like top-down approaches, including mechanical milling and lithography, gave the starting points of control over nanoparticle size and morphology. The successive use of bottom-up-type technologies, such as sol-gel processing and CVD,[3] allowed increased precision at the molecular scale to assemble nanostructures (Indiarto et al. 2021) as sol-gel synthesis developed as a crucial technique in obtaining oxide nanoparticles with homogeneous features for electronic and optical applications (Parashar et al. 2020). The sol-gel method, which gained prominence for oxide nanoparticle synthesis, is now paired with advanced techniques like CRISPR[4]-Cas9 to deliver genetic material in precision therapies. This intersection of old and new techniques is revolutionising drug delivery and gene therapy, showcasing the dynamic evolution of nanomaterials in clinical medicine (Kaur et al. 2024). The invention of colloidal synthesis in the late 1990s facilitated the ability to formulate, with a high degree of control, quantum dots and plasmonic nanoparticles having variable optical properties (Cortie and McDonagh 2011). Surfactants and stabilising agents became instrumental in morphological control to produce such anisotropic structures as nanorods and nanowires. Quantum dots nanobiomaterials, which are widely used in cancer diagnosis studies, were synthesised by Murray et al. in 1993 (Gil 2021; Ramburrun et al. 2022).

The twenty-first century, addressing environmental concerns, directed a shift towards green synthesis. The different approaches using plant extracts, bacteria, and fungi during nanoparticle fabrication have reduced ecological impact and resulted in biocompatible material for drug delivery and tissue engineering (Nouri et al. 2021). Recent progress was towards more scalability and precision. Microfluidics-assisted synthesis has allowed for high-throughput nanoparticle production with consistent properties required for both clinical and industrial use (Cai 2021). Atomic layer deposition these days offers unmatched control in nanoscale coatings and has enhanced the functionality of nanomaterials in catalysis and energy storage (Loiudice et al. 2020). Combining chemical and biological methods, hybrid synthesis approaches have further diversified functionality, enabling hierarchical nanostructures for regenerative medicine (Prasert et al. 2020). Computational modelling further complements these techniques by optimising reaction conditions and predicting outcomes, thus accelerating material development. These cumulative innovations continue to shape nanomaterial synthesis for advanced applications.

3.3 Advances in Nanobiomaterials for Tissue Engineering

Recent developments in nanobiomaterials have revolutionised tissue engineering and provide innovative solutions for regenerative medicine. Applications of nanobiomaterials in different fields are shown in Fig. 2. The development of nanofibres,

[3] Chemical vapor deposition.

[4] Clustered regularly interspaced palindromic repeats.

biocompatible scaffolds, and 3D printing enabled the fabrication of complex structures similar to native tissues (Phutane et al. 2023). The large surface-area-to-volume ratio of nanofibres is the main factor contributing to their advantages in properties that could be tuned for the processes involved in cell adhesion, growth, and differentiation. They can also mimic the extracellular matrix apart from enabling the controlled release of bioactive molecules into tissue regeneration(Yu et al. 2023). Scaffold technologies have now begun to use nanostructured materials to enhance mechanical strength, porosity, and bioactivity. The ability of these scaffolds to promote cell infiltration and vascularisation can help overcome some of the significant challenges in the repair of tissues (Fu 2022). All of that has changed dramatically with the concept of 3D printing, by means of which one can fabricate constructs with high precision, even in patients. To that end, customised scaffold fabrication enhances integration at the host tissue level, significantly resulting in better clinical outcomes upon application. Recent successes now bring to the forefront the transformative potential of nanobiomaterials in regenerative medicine and the dawn of the next generation of tissue engineering.

3.4 *Role of Nanobiomaterials in Drug Delivery Systems*

Nanobiomaterials have been one of the cornerstones in developing drug delivery systems that offer transformative solutions in controlled release, targeted therapy, and bioavailability enhancement. Their unique nanoscale properties and versatility allow precise drug delivery with fewer side effects and maximum therapeutic efficacy (Rahimnejad et al. 2021). One of the most significant advances indeed lies in the area of controlled drug release. These nanomaterials can be designed as liposomes, polymeric nanoparticles, and hydrogels; they release the drug in a manner pre-programmed to maintain predetermined therapeutic levels over time. Other benefits include reducing dosing frequency and thus increasing the compliance of patients with chronic conditions (Rahimnejad et al. 2021). Targeted therapy with nanobiomaterials looks very promising. Functionalised by ligands or antibodies, nanoparticles afford targeted drug delivery through recognition and binding to target cells or tissues. Most of the impact of targeted therapy is seen in oncology, where it improves the accumulation of chemotherapeutics in tumour sites, sparing healthy tissues from damage caused by drugs and thereby reducing systemic toxicity (Qin et al. 2022). Moreover, nanomaterials are effective in increasing the bioavailability of poorly water-soluble drugs. The enhancement in surface area of the drugs, improvement in their solubility, and protection of the active pharmaceutical ingredient from premature degradation by nanoscale carriers assure higher absorption rates and, therefore, guarantee better therapeutic outcomes in oral and transdermal drug delivery systems (Sharma and Saroha 2024). The advancement in nanobiomaterials as drug delivery systems continues to change the pharmaceutical landscape, rendering innovative solutions to the long-standing challenges in medicine and opening a way towards more effective, patient-centred treatments.

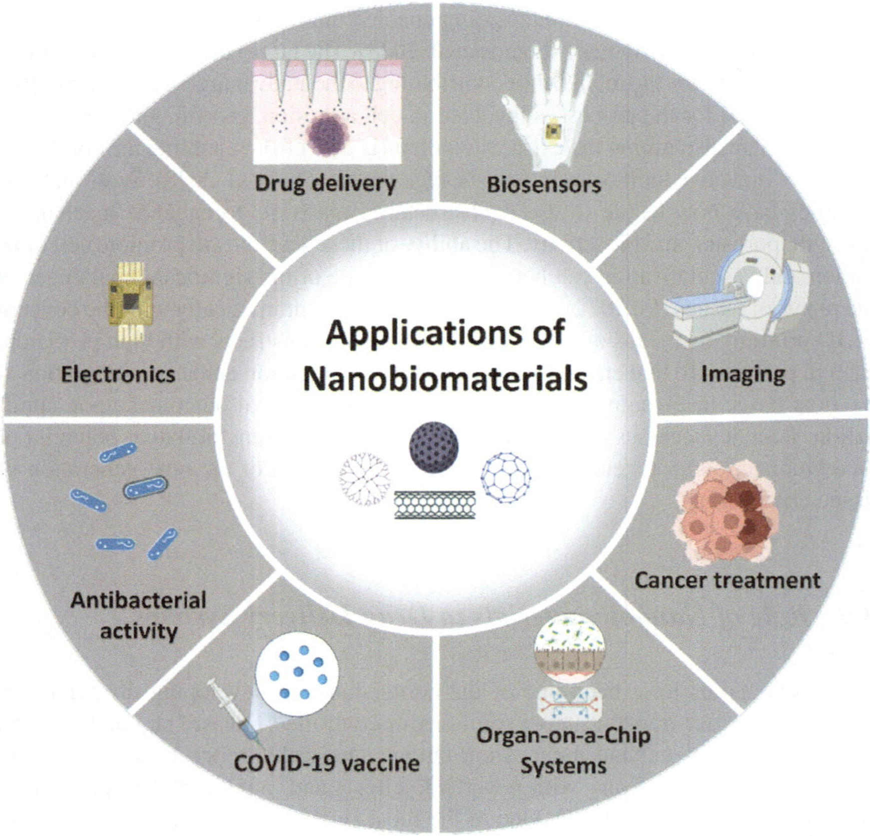

Fig. 2 Applications of nanobiomaterials in various fields

3.5 Role of Nanobiomaterials in Diagnostics and Imaging

Nanobiomaterials are revolutionising diagnostics and imaging applications with a level of specificity and sensitivity never experienced before, mostly in early disease detection and monitoring. Some of the innovations in the area of nanodiagnosis using special features of nanomaterials to enhance performances in diagnostic devices and biosensors are excellent. With their large surface-area-to-volume ratios and tailor-made functionalities, nanomaterials are one step ahead in fabricating biosensors with high sensitivity and specificity (Sood et al. 2024). In this respect, biosensors enable the detection of biomolecules, pathogens, and disease biomarkers at the molecular level—rapid and precise—such that early intervention and tailored medical interventions can be developed. Nanobiomaterials have greatly enhanced imaging technologies by improving contrast agents and allowing multimodal imaging. Integrating nanoparticles such as quantum dots and gold nanoparticles into systems increases resolution, giving high-precision visuals of biological structures and conditions (Zhang et al. 2023). All the enhancements mentioned above indicate the significant role of nanobiomaterials in modern medical diagnostics and imaging for disease detection and management.

3.6 Biomedical Nanomaterials in Smart Medical Devices: From Lab to Clinic

Integrating biomedical nanomaterials into smart medical devices represents a landmark for real-world applications in clinical practice. Following their development, nanotechnologies have made innovative biomaterials possible that respond to environmental stimuli and adapt to individual healthcare and real-time diagnostics. These improve functionality and effectiveness in the clinical performance of medical devices (Pothala et al. 2024). Due to their high surface area, biocompatibility, and responsiveness to triggers such as pH, temperature, or electrical fields, nanomaterials are increasingly being incorporated into wearable health devices and sensors. These devices could monitor physiological parameters in real time, offering critical data for detecting and managing diseases. Wearable sensors, coupled with nanomaterials, can now track vital signs such as glucose levels, heart rate, and oxygen levels in real time, providing feedback to the patient and healthcare providers (Yao et al. 2018). Their translation from the lab to clinical practice faces several challenges. The greatest obstacle persists: high regulatory hurdles—if nanomaterials are to be integrated into medical devices, then extensive safety and efficacy tests are usually demanded (Foulkes et al. 2020). The FDA requires such devices to meet hard-to-achieve standards through a long-drawn-out, complex procedure. Due to technological and logistical barriers, large-scale manufacturing of smart nanomaterial-based devices with uniform quality is yet to be achieved. The challenges notwithstanding, biomedical nanomaterials hold tremendous potential in innovative medical devices. Continuing the research and adapting regulations are going to transform these into huge game changers, with healthcare interventions made in a precise, timely, and personalised way.

3.7 Multidisciplinary Integration of Nanobiomaterials

Integrating multidisciplinary nanobiomaterials, nanotechnology, biology, chemistry, and engineering promotes the development and design of novel medical device applications. This kind of research will be crucial in offering appropriate solutions to complex issues concerning human health and will open new avenues for highly versatile and sophisticated devices with precision, versatility, and performance. Nanotechnology, at the atomic and molecular level of material manipulation, is a backbone for advanced biomedical applications. Combining it with biology lets researchers design nanomaterials that interact in a bio-friendly manner, enhancing their biocompatibility, cell interaction, and therapeutic efficiency (Ramesh et al. 2022). For example, biomolecular understanding can be used to develop nanomaterials that encourage cell adhesion or even the stimulation of cellular regeneration, thus helping repair and regenerate tissues in the clinic (Nouri et al. 2023a). Chemistry plays a decisive role in the chemical composition and the engineering of surface properties towards desired final nanomaterials' properties, allowing the very accurate tunability of its reactivity, stability, and even compatibility with either drugs or biological molecules. This plays a role in realising controlled release and targeted drug delivery approaches that minimise undesired drug side effects with concomitant improvement in therapeutic indices (Pinheiro et al. 2024). However, translating those inventions through engineering into working, scalable medical devices has been equally important. Advanced manufacturing techniques, such as microfabrication, 3D printing, and nano-patterning, lead to complicated device architectures that incorporate nanomaterials with ease. Such devices, which could be biosensors, diagnostic platforms, or wearable health monitors, are optimised for operation in the real world by realising high performance, precision, and ease of use that might be integrated into the workflows in patient care (Basu 2021). This collaborative approach not only drives the development of novel medical technologies but also accelerates the transition of these innovations from laboratory research to clinical application. By merging the strengths of nanotechnology, biology, chemistry, and engineering, the multidisciplinary integration of nanobiomaterials is paving the way for the next generation of medical devices that are smarter, more efficient, and more tailored to individual patient needs.

3.8 Ethical, Safety, and Future Perspectives of Nanobiomaterial Advances

Rapid advances in nanobiomaterials for medical use carry great promise but raise critical ethical and safety issues. The unique properties of nanomaterials, with large surface areas relative to mass and the capability to interface with biological systems at a cellular level, pose a great challenge regarding toxicity, biocompatibility, and long-term health effects (Dmytriv and Lushchak 2024). Key risks include cytotoxicity, immunogenicity, and unintended interactions with tissues; thorough preclinical testing is necessary to establish a safety profile. Besides, environmental impact-for example, the bioaccumulation and degradation of nanomaterials (Uddin et al. 2021)—emphasises strict environmental safety. On the bright side, near-future technologies such as nanomedicine, nanorobotics, and personalised medicine offer great promise for healthcare. Nanomedicine, in particular, offers excellent opportunities for targeted and controlled delivery of drugs with minimum side effects, especially for cancer diseases (Zhang et al. 2020). Nanorobotics will, for example, be able to enable very precise and minimally invasive surgical interventions, while personalised medicine will provide treatments adapted to the particular genetic and molecular profile (Noronha and Bhat 2024). In this setting, however, many ethical considerations on patient consent, data privacy, and access should be seriously addressed to make these technologies responsible and safe. As nanobiomaterials progress from basic research to clinical application, transdisciplinary collaboration and moving regulation targets would be required to minimise hazards but optimise their potential contribution towards health.

4 The Latest Developments in Nanobiomaterials

4.1 Sustainable and Advanced Nanobiomaterial Green Fabrication Techniques

Recent advances in the eco-friendly synthesis of nanobiomaterials have strongly emphasised various novel strategies in line with environmental and biocompatibility goals. These approaches emphasise toxic byproduct reduction, improved energy efficiency, and using renewable resources to produce scalable and functional nanomaterials (Nouri et al. 2021; El-Sayyad et al. 2024). Green synthesis techniques have recently received significant attention as an eco-friendly alternative to conventional chemical and physical fabrication methods. Utilising natural resources, such as plant extracts, enzymes, and microbial cultures, provides an environmentally friendly route for producing nanoparticles with desirable biological properties. For instance, biosynthesis using plant-based reducing agents has produced silver nanoparticles with good antimicrobial efficacy, which may be helpful for both medical and environmental applications (Saravanan et al. 2021).

Microbial processes represent a significant improvement in the production of nanobiomaterials. Bacteria, fungi, and other microorganisms can reduce metals to their nanoparticle forms through enzymatic reduction and pigment production. For example, species of *Lactobacillus* have been used to synthesise titanium dioxide nanoparticles, which show excellent photocatalytic activity and good biocompatibility. Likewise, species of Streptomyces synthesise gold and silver nanoparticles through nitrate reductase activity, thus enabling nanomaterials to be built for applications such as targeted cancer therapy and wound healing (Nouri et al. 2023b). The green synthesis of nanobiomaterials by probiotics such as *Bacillus subtilis* and *Bacillus coagulans* is an eco-friendly and biocompatible method to produce materials such as nano-hydroxyapatite and nano-calcite (Nouri et al. 2022). Hydroxyapatite obtained from probiotics has been shown to promote stem cell growth, induce osteogenic differentiation in SHED[5] cells, and promote osteogenic mineralisation and anticancer properties (Nouri et al. 2023a). Hydroxyapatite is a good prospect for tissue engineering, regenerative medicine, and cancer therapy (Nouri et al. 2024a.

[5] Stem Cells from Human Exfoliated Deciduous Teeth.

b). Moreover, it was discovered that scaffolds with hydroxyapatite produced from probiotics showed high biocompatibility, mechanical properties similar to that of trabecular bone, and enhanced proliferation of cells compared to other biological materials used (Nouri et al. 2024a, b).

Integrating biogenic processes in nanomaterial fabrication has opened new avenues in the fight against infectious diseases and cancer. Biosynthesised nanoparticles, such as selenium and silver nanoparticles, have shown potent antimicrobial and anticancer properties. Selenium nanoparticles synthesised by microbial systems inhibit the proliferation of cancer cells through the induction of oxidative stress and apoptosis. In contrast, silver nanoparticles offer broad-spectrum antimicrobial efficacy against drug-resistant pathogens (Nouri et al. 2023a). The sustainable approach with these advanced green fabrication techniques revolutionises the fabrication of nanobiomaterials towards their applications involving critical performances with the least environmental burdens. Further refinement in developing such approaches is likely to upscale the possibility and functionality of achieving wider utilisations for medical, industrial, and environmental sectors with nanobiomaterials.

4.2 Hybrid Nanobiomaterials for Multifunctional Applications

Hybrid nanobiomaterials with organic and inorganic constituents are advancing the field of multi-functionality in biomedical and industrial applications by improving mechanical strength, biocompatibility, and versatility. Organic materials, especially polymers, provide flexibility and biodegradability. At the same time, adding inorganic components, such as metal oxides or ceramics, confers strength, thermal stability, and specific properties related to antimicrobial activity (Park et al. 2020). For instance, both polymer-hydroxyapatite and collagen-silica composites are important components in bone tissue engineering with respect to cell adhesion and osteointegration (Bauso et al. 2024). These hybrids also have important roles in drug delivery, imaging, and regenerative medicine. Materials such as mesoporous silica, combined with natural polymers like chitosan, provide targeted drug delivery and sustained release, thus improving therapeutic efficacy (Mohammadi et al. 2017). Other emerging systems, such as graphene-polymer composites, have potential applications in bioelectronics and neural tissue engineering (Xu et al. 2021), while magnetic nanoparticle-biopolymer hybrids enhance drug delivery and cancer treatment (Constantino 2024). Hybrid nanobiomaterials also make their mark in environmental applications such as water purification and catalysis (Constantino 2024). Metal-organic frameworks combined with biopolymers have shown excellent pollutant adsorption and degradation properties, thus helping to meet sustainable development goals (Agamendran et al. 2023). Integrating organic and inorganic components offers immense potential to address challenges in medicine, industry, and environmental sustainability.

4.3 Bioinspired Nanomaterials

By biomimicking structures or processes, rationally designed bioinspired nanomaterials continue to be obtained from naturally abundant ones; these nanomaterials harness nature's ingenuity to fulfil the most complicated functionalities into novel applications within biomedicine and materials science, extending from diagnostics to environmental sustainability.

Nature-inspired design principles: The structural complexity and hierarchical organisation in biological systems, such as the nanoscale organisation in nacre or bone, have been used as templates in developing bioinspired nanomaterials. For example, by biomimicking the layered structure of nacre, it has been possible to produce tough, heat-resistant hybrid composites for applications related to implants and wear-resistant coatings (Wang et al. 2024). Similarly, the natural self-assembly of proteins and lipids inspires the fabrication of nanocarriers for targeted drug delivery (Hu et al. 2024).

Biomimetic functionalisation: Newer approaches aim at incorporating biomimetic strategies for value addition. Superhydrophobic surfaces inspired by lotus leaves have been applied to fabricate anti-fouling and self-cleaning coatings (Aslam et al. 2024). In contrast, bone-mimetic hydroxyapatite-based materials tailored for porosity and bioactivity are used in tissue engineering applications for cell adhesion and the induction of osteogenesis (Han et al. 2024).

Biologically innovative applications in biomedicine: Bioinspired nanomaterials play an increasingly important role in regenerative medicine, providing cell differentiation and tissue repair. Examples include silk-fibroin-based scaffolds for nerve regeneration and peptide amphiphile nanofibres that mimic extracellular matrix properties for wound healing (Li et al. 2024; Moradi 2024). Such materials ensure enhanced cell signalling, biocompatibility, and degradability.

The convergence of biology, chemistry, and engineering has driven the continuous development of bioinspired nanomaterials. Computational design and molecular modelling now enable the precise replication of biological architectures, allowing for innovative materials with adaptive and multifunctional capabilities. Such materials can advance personalised medicine, energy-efficient devices, and sustainable environmental technologies.

4.4 Stimuli-Responsive Nanobiomaterials

Stimuli-responsive nanobiomaterials, so-called smart materials, are designed to respond dynamically and adaptively to some environmental trigger, such as temperature, pH, light, magnetic field, or biochemical signal. These advanced materials will lead the way to precision in biomedical and industrial applications due to their controlled and localised functionality.

The mechanisms of stimuli-responsive nanobiomaterials include conformational changes, phase transitions, or alteration of surface properties. For instance, thermoresponsive polymers such as poly(N-isopropylacrylamide) (PNIPAM) have a phase transition near physiological temperature and, thus, are ideal for drug delivery systems that have temperature-controlled release (Zhang et al. 2024a, b). pH-sensitive hydrogels are also widely used in cancer therapy due to their capability of releasing therapeutic agents in the acidic microenvironment of tumours (Gomte et al. 2024).

These materials have revolutionised drug delivery by offering spatiotemporal control. Photo-activated nanoparticles, like gold nanorods, enable photothermal therapy through heat release by light exposure to selectively target cancerous cells (Zarepour et al. 2024). Magnetic-responsive nanomaterials are applied in hyperthermia-based therapies and magnetically guided drug delivery (Kesharwani et al. 2024). In regenerative medicine, the stimuli-responsive scaffolds modify their physical properties to support cell proliferation and differentiation under specific biological conditions (Zhang et al. 2024a, b).

In diagnostics, stimuli-responsive biosensors detect and quantify biomarkers with high specificity. For example, glucose-responsive hydrogels embedded in wearable devices provide real-time glucose monitoring for diabetes management. Similarly, photoresponsive systems enable controlled imaging in optogenetics (Zhang et al. 2024a, b).

Recent developments also include multicompetent stimuli-responsive nanobiomaterials responding to several triggers simultaneously. For instance, dual-responsive materials based on pH and temperature sensitivity can be used together in synergy for drug delivery and treatment purposes (Zhang et al. 2024a, b). Another developing platform involves self-healing nanomaterials that regenerate their structure after external stimulations; these have started finding applications in soft robotics and bioelectronics (Venkateswaran et al. 2024).

4.5 *Nanobiomaterials for Organ-on-a-Chip Systems*

Organ-on-a-chip systems represent the most advanced development in bioengineering, offering a means for realising functions at an organ level on microscales. Nanobiomaterials play a significant role in such systems due to their structure and functional elements, which enhance biomimicry, allowing advanced drug testing, disease modelling, and precision medicine.Nanobiomaterials improve the design of microfluidic platforms by improving structural integrity, permeability, and functional responsiveness (Venkateswaran et al. 2024). Integrating with nanoparticles, polymers such as PDMS[6] provide biocompatibility, transparency, and tunable mechanical properties for the biomimicry of organ-specific microenvironments. In addition, nanoscale coatings allow for selective permeability, mimicking transport dynamics of physiological barriers such as the blood-brain barrier or kidney membranes

[6] Polydimethylsiloxane.

(Thenuwara et al. 2024). Nanostructured scaffolds and hydrogels have biomimetic properties of the ECM,[7] promoting cell adhesion, proliferation, and differentiation (Xiao et al. 2024). For example, collagen-based nano scaffolds with embedded graphene oxide have enhanced electrical conductivity, which is relevant for cardiac and neural models (Sardari et al. 2024). Electrospun nanofiber networks mimic alveolar-capillary interfaces in lung-on-a-chip applications that model respiratory diseases such as COVID-19 and asthma (Ozdemir et al. 2024).

Nanobiomaterials enable the integration of biosensors and imaging agents in organ-on-a-chip systems. For example, quantum dots and gold nanoparticles allow real-time observations of cell behaviour and drug interaction at the nanoscale (Anjali Devi et al. 2024). This is particularly advantageous for high-throughput screening: it minimises animal tests and provides accurate human-relevant data. The examples include nanoparticle-based sensors for liver-on-a-chip hepatotoxicity screening and tumour-on-a-chip models for investigating nanoparticle-mediated cancer therapy.

Advances in nanotechnology now allow the fabrication of multi-organ-on-a-chip systems for studying interactions between organs, such as the metabolism of drugs from the liver to the kidney. Besides, hybrid nanobiomaterials, such as thermoresponsive hydrogels combined with magnetic nanoparticles, enable dynamic control over cellular microenvironments, thus opening routes for more precise disease modelling. Integrating nanobiomaterials with artificial intelligence and 3D bioprinting will likely change the face of organ-on-a-chip technology. These developments are towards improving personalisation and scalability to ensure wider acceptance for pharmacology and regenerative medicine. Furthermore, environmentally friendly methods for synthesising nanomaterials will eventually align these innovations with international environmental and ethical standards.

4.6 AI and Machine Learning in Nanobiomaterial Research

AI (Artificial Intelligence) and ML (Machine Learning) are two newer technologies enabling innovation in the nanobiomaterial area, mostly through prediction and optimisation, since they allow efficiency for material design, synthesis, and application. Computational methods grant access for researchers to move with complexity in nanoscale systems quickly. Machine learning algorithms interpret large amounts of data to predict nanobiomaterial properties, such as size, morphology, stability, and biocompatibility (Der and Ercetin 2024). Deep learning models have been further used for predicting the mechanical and thermal properties of polymer-nanoparticle composites for biomedical and industrial applications (Lu and Jayaraman 2024). Other AI simulations also allow one to get more accurate estimations concerning interactions between the nanobiomaterials and biological systems, like protein corona formation, for a drug delivery system's enhanced safety and efficacy (Gao et al. 2024).

[7] Extracellular matrix.

AI-powered techniques enable high-throughput virtual screening of nanomaterials' composition and structure, thus identifying the best candidates for specific applications. For example, in drug delivery, ML models predict modifications in the nanoparticle surface to optimise targeted delivery and controlled release (Mi et al. 2024). Quantum-mechanical simulations coupled with AI provide detailed insight into the electronic and optical properties of hybrid nanobiomaterials towards developing multifunctional systems for imaging and therapy (Singh and Sahani 2024). Among their applications, AI systems can optimise synthesis parameters by minimising experimental trial and error. For example, reinforcement learning identifies the optimum reaction conditions, such as temperature, pressure, and precursor concentrations in nanoparticle synthesis, in a way that increases reproducibility and moves in harmony with green chemistry principles to cut down on waste and energy consumption (Subeshan et al. 2024).

AI bridges nanobiomaterials with bioinformatics by predicting interactions at the molecular level, such as binding affinities in ligand-receptor systems. This integration is instrumental in designing nanocarriers for personalised medicine, where AI models predict patient-specific responses to therapeutic nanoparticles. Moreover, the combination of AI and nanobiomaterials is driving advancements in biosensing, with ML algorithms enhancing sensor sensitivity and selectivity for real-time diagnostics. Despite its potential, integrating AI in nanobiomaterial research faces challenges, including the need for more high-quality data and the interpretability of complex models. Future advancements depend on collaborative efforts to standardise datasets and integrate AI with experimental validation. Emerging fields, such as GANs[8] for material discovery and federated learning for decentralised data analysis, hold promise for overcoming these barriers.

4.7 Other Emerging Frontiers in Nanobiomaterials

Nanobiomaterials are the spark that sets off transformative innovations, meeting critical challenges in medicine, environmental sustainability, and more. The emergence of antibiotic-resistant pathogens has accelerated the formulation of antimicrobial agents at the nanoscale, which includes silver nanoparticles, zinc oxide, and carbon-based nanomaterials (Abdullah et al. 2024). These agents disrupt microbial cell membranes and inhibit biofilm formation, hence offering alternative treatments for multidrug-resistant infections. Hybrid approaches using nanoparticles in combination with conventional antibiotics result in enhanced efficacy and reduced development of resistance. Sustainability is another important focus in the field of nanotechnology. The development of new biodegradable polymers, like PLA[9] and PHA,[10] has reduced the ecological footprint of nanobiomaterials (Anjos et al. 2024).

---

[8] Generative adversarial networks.

[9] Polylactic acid.

[10] Polyhydroxyalkanoates.

Biological synthesis with plant extracts or microbial production techniques offers a green approach to nanoparticle production that falls under the global sustainable development policy. Neurological applications were also developed with nanocarriers to cross the blood-brain barrier in brain-targeted drug delivery (Zeynalzadeh et al. 2024). Other materials that have been used include liposomes, dendrimers, and polymeric nanoparticles to deliver therapeutics against neurodegenerative disorders such as Alzheimer's and Parkinson's disease (Hemdan et al. 2024; Ozceylan and Bayindir 2024). In addition, conductive nanobiomaterials can imitate extracellular matrix structures and promote neural regeneration. Nanobiomaterials hold an important place in planning treatments for individual profiles of patients. Targeted nanoparticles, which are designed for drug release at specific sites, thus minimising systemic side effects, are an excellent basis for personalised medicine. Quantum dots and magnetic nanoparticles are diagnostic nanoprobes that enable real-time monitoring of the disease progression and ensure precision in therapeutic interventions (Hemdan et al. 2024). In immunotherapy, nanobiomaterials improve immune modulation and cancer treatment. Nanoparticle-based vaccines improve antigen presentation, boosting immune response. For example, LNP[11] enabled the development of mRNA COVID-19 vaccines (Hemdan et al. 2024). Similarly, nanoscale immune checkpoint inhibitors are promising in combating cancers resistant to traditional therapies. These developments point to the enormous potential of nanobiomaterials, reflecting their role in solving current scientific and social challenges.

5 Types of Nanobiomaterials

The extraordinary properties of nanobiomaterials enable their use in many areas. Therefore, classifying these materials according to their different types is essential for their fields of application. Nanobiomaterials can be divided into four categories depending on their origin, structural configuration and composition, number of dimensions and pore size, as shown in Fig. 3 (Alkaç et al. 2021).

5.1 Nanobiomaterial Categorisation by Origin

Depending on their origin, nanobiomaterials are divided into natural and synthetic materials. Nanobiomaterials that occur in various forms in nature are classified as natural nanobiomaterials. Nanobiomaterials that are intentionally and precisely manufactured using multiple production techniques are called synthetic nanobiomaterials. Protein molecules, viruses, natural colloids and corals are examples of natural nanobiomaterials. Carbon nanotubes and quantum dots are examples of synthetic nanobiomaterials (Mekuye and Abera 2023).

[11] Lipid nanoparticles.

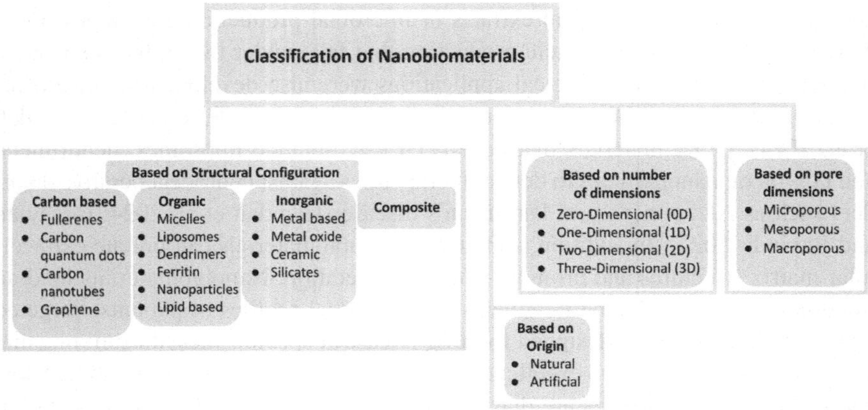

Fig. 3 Schematic overview of the classification of nanobiomaterials according to origin, composition, dimensionality and pore dimensions (Ramburrun et al. 2022)

5.2 Nanobiomaterial Categorisation by Structural Configuration and Composition

When nanomaterials are evaluated and classified according to their structure, they can be divided into four groups: carbon-based (fullerenes, carbon quantum dots, carbon nanotubes, graphene), organic (micelles, liposomes, dendrimer, ferritin, and nanoparticles), inorganic (metal-based, metal oxide, lipid-based, ceramic, and silicates), and composites (Mekuye and Abera 2023).

5.2.1 Carbon-Based Nanobiomaterials

This class consists of nanobiomaterials made entirely of carbon atoms. Due to their exceptional electrical and thermal conductivity, low toxicity, improved mechanical properties and high stability are used in various fields such as tissue engineering, biosensor applications and drug delivery systems. The best-known examples of this class include fullerenes, carbon quantum dots, carbon black and graphene (Holmannova et al. 2022).

5.2.2 Organic Nanobiomaterials

Organic compounds are converted into organic materials with a size of 100 nm or less (Qi and Zhang 2022). Commonly used organic structures include liposomes, dendrimers, micelles and ferritin. Organic nanobioparticles (NPs), which consist of non-covalent bonds, are very sensitive to forms of energy such as heat and light. This structural property makes them easily susceptible to environmental influences.

Micelles and liposomes, sensitive to external stimuli such as heat and light, are nanocapsules that can safely transport drug molecules with their hollow structure. The efficiency of drug delivery of these nanoparticles depends on factors such as size, composition and surface properties (Joudeh and Linke 2022).

In addition, organic polymeric nanobiomaterials, which can be produced from synthetic and natural polymers, are widely favoured materials for controlled and targeted drug delivery and tissue engineering studies. Polymers can be processed to make nanofibres, nanofilms, and nanocoatings. Synthetic polymers such as PLGA and PCL and natural polymers such as chitosan and silk are approved for applications such as tissue regeneration and drug delivery (Ramburrun et al. 2022).

5.2.3 Inorganic Nanobiomaterials

Inorganic nanobiomaterials are more stable and biocompatible compared to organic nanobiomaterials. Inorganic nanobiomaterials, which do not contain carbon in their structure, are of interest as drug and gene carriers due to their high cellular uptake capacity (Alshammari et al. 2023). The shape and size of metal oxides can vary depending on the different conditions in the production process. Nanoparticles with diameters below 20 nm can pass through these structures more efficiently, as they are close to the size of cell membranes and organelles. For this reason, iron oxide is often preferred for targeted drug delivery and medical imaging. The high biocompatibility and mechanical strength of titanium dioxide make it an ideal material for implants and prostheses (Bianchi 2022; Ramburrun et al. 2022).

Ceramics, which are characterised by their properties such as high biocompatibility, promoting bone formation and water retention, are among the materials that come closest to the natural structure of tooth and bone tissue and are, therefore, indispensable for bone engineering (John et al. 2023).

5.2.4 Composite Nanobiomaterials

Composite nanobiomaterials are hybrid structures formed by combining two or more different materials instead of nanobiomaterials consisting of a single material. This fusion takes place on the nanometer scale and the resulting new material can have other and better properties than the sum of its parts (Luo et al. 2014). This synergistic combination can significantly improve the intrinsic properties of materials (such as strength, flexibility, and heat resistance). Developing new functional materials offers excellent potential in tissue engineering and biomedical applications (Luo et al. 2015).

5.3 *Nanobiomaterial Categorisation by Number of Dimensions*

According to the classification of dimensions, nanobiomaterials are studied in four main categories: zero-dimensional (0D), one-dimensional (1D), two-dimensional (2D) and three-dimensional (3D) (Syduzzaman et al. 2023).

5.3.1 Zero-Dimensional (0D) Nanobiomaterials

Zero-dimensional nanobiomaterials with less than 100 nanometres are the most common nanobiomaterials. Materials with cubic and polygonal shapes on the nanoscale fall under this classification, whether in amorphous, monocrystalline or polycrystalline structure. 0D nanomaterials have more active sites per unit mass due to their small size and large surface area. Examples of 0D nanobiomaterials are carbon-based (carbon quantum dots, graphene quantum dots and fullerenes), inorganic (inorganic quantum dots), organic (Pnspots) and metallic (noble metal nanoparticle (Paras et al. 2022).

5.3.2 One-Dimensional (1D) Nanobiomaterials

Such nanobiomaterials have an aspect ratio of 1 to 100 nm in diameter. As an essential branch of nanobiomaterial systems, such nanobiomaterials have a high specific surface area and abundant exposed active points (Wang et al. 2021). An excellent crystal structure, homogeneous dispersion and simple synthesis methods also characterise them. These properties give these materials a large surface area, flexibility and a porous structure that provides a favourable environment for hydrogen storage. They can be made from different materials such as metals, ceramics and polymers and, therefore, have a wide range of applications (Paras et al. 2022).

5.3.3 Two-Dimensional (2D) Nanobiomaterials

These materials, which consist of single or multiple layers of atomic thickness, are classified as two-dimensional nanobiomaterials (Baig 2023). Put in other words, two of the three dimensions are of nanometer scale. They have a plate-like structure, and nanosheets, nanofilms and nanocoatings are examples of 2D nanomaterials (Jeevanandam et al. 2018). The fineness and strong bonding of 2D nanomaterials give them unique mechanical strength and flexibility. When subjected to mechanical stress, layered materials can transform into two-dimensional nanosheets and nanoplates. The unique topography, large surface area and directionally dependent chemical and physical properties of 2D nanomaterials make them ideal for many applications. Especially in areas where surface interactions are essential, the large and flat surfaces of these materials offer a significant advantage (Paras et al. 2022).

5.3.4 Three-Dimensional (3D) Nanobiomaterials

Three-dimensional nanobiomaterials are constructed by arranging tiny (nanoscale) structures within them. The three-dimensional structure formed by the arrangement of these particles gives the material unique properties. Compared to other dimensional nanobiomaterials, the 3D morphology increases mechanical stability. The pores enable mass transport within the structure. This allows a high loading capacity to transport functional components such as drugs and catalyst fragments (Verma et al. 2023). In recent years, three-dimensional nanobiomaterials have attracted the attention of scientists in various fields (Alshammari et al. 2023).

5.4 Nanomaterial Categorisation by Pore Dimensions

Nanoporous materials have recently become important in materials science research thanks to their excellent porous structure. According to the classification established by the International Union of Fundamental and Applied Chemistry (IUPAC), nanoporous materials are divided into three main categories depending on the pore diameter:

- Microporous (less than 2 nm).
- Mesoporous (between 2 and 50 nm).
- Macroporous (more than 50 nm) materials (Yuan et al. 2023).

6 Conclusions

This chapter is a journey from the origins of nanobiomaterials, which have become an integral part of today's technology, to the present day. The rapid developments in the field of nanotechnology have enabled nanobiomaterials to be used in a wide range of applications, from scientific research to industrial applications. In addition, the classification of nanobiomaterials according to different properties and the use of these materials in various sectors are studied in detail. Nanobiomaterials facilitate our daily lives and shape future technologies by enabling the development of smaller, stronger, more efficient and smarter products in many fields, such as medicine, drug delivery, tissue engineering, diagnostics, personalised nanomedicine, biosensor technology and cancer therapy. To increase efficiency, reduce costs and improve the usability of objects and processes, nanotechnology is being studied intensively by researchers from various disciplines, and new application areas are being discovered. Nanobiomaterials, in particular, have the potential to revolutionise drug delivery. Thanks to these tiny carrier materials, drugs can be delivered to the desired sites with high accuracy, maximising treatment efficacy and minimising side effects. These unique properties of nanobiomaterials open up new horizons in the treatment of many diseases and offer great promise for the future in many areas.

References

J. Abdullah et al., Recent advances in the development of metal/metal oxide nanoparticle and antibiotic conjugates (MNP–antibiotics) to address antibiotic resistance: review and perspective. Int. J. Mol. Sci. **25**(16), 8915 (2024)

S. Adepu, S. Ramakrishna, Controlled drug delivery systems: current status and future directions. Molecules **26**(19), 5905 (2021)

N. Agamendran et al., Nanoarchitectonics design strategy of metal-organic framework and bio-metal-organic framework composites for advanced wastewater treatment through adsorption. Langmuir (2023)

A.H. Aghajanian et al., A 3D macroporous and magnetic Mg_2SiO_4-$CuFe_2O_4$ scaffold for bone tissue regeneration: Surface modification, in vitro and in vivo studies. Biomater. Adv. **137**, 212809 (2022)

Z.P. Aguilar, *Nanomaterials for Medical Applications* (2012), pp. 1–461

İ.M. Alkaç et al., Nanomaterials and their classification, in *Nanomaterials for Direct Alcohol Fuel Cells: Characterization, Design, and Electrocatalysis*, pp. 17–33 (2021)

B.H. Alshammari et al., Organic and inorganic nanomaterials: Fabrication, properties and applications. RSC Adv. **13**(20), 13735–13785 (2023)

J.S. Anjali Devi et al., Luminescent carbon dots versus quantum dots and gold nanoclusters as sensors. Nanoscale Horiz. **9**(10), 1683–1702 (2024)

E.G.R. Anjos et al., Biodegradation behavior and life cycle assessment of PLA/PHBV/carbonaceous materials hybrid nanocomposites for antimicrobial multifunctional packaging. J. Polym. Environ. **32**(10), 5098–5114 (2024)

R. Aslam et al., Mimicking nature: advancements in self-cleaning coatings, in *Smart Biomimetic Coatings: Design, Properties, and Biomedical Applications*, pp. 129–145 (2024)

A. Azari, Electrospun polycaprolactone nanofibers: current research and applications in biomedical application. Adv. Pharm. Bull. **12**(4), 658 (2021)

N. Baig, Two-dimensional nanomaterials: A critical review of recent progress, properties, applications, and future directions. Compos. A: Appl. Sci. Manuf. **165**, 107362 (2023)

A. Basu, MEMS applications in biology and healthcare (2021)

L.V. Bauso et al., Bone tissue engineering and nanotechnology: a promising combination for bone regeneration. Biology **13**(4), 237 (2024)

L.R. Beck, T.R. Tice, *Poly Net Contraceptive System* (1983), p. 116

E. Bianchi, Inorganic nanomaterials in tissue engineering. Pharmaceutics **14**(6), 1127 (2022)

Z. Cai, From colloidal particles to photonic crystals: advances in self-assembly and their emerging applications. Chem. Soc. Rev. **50**(10), 5898–5951 (2021)

M.S. Cekuc et al., Functionalized bilosomes for cancer therapy, in *Functionalized Nanomaterials for Cancer Research: Applications in Treatments, Tools and Devices*, pp. 197–217 (2024)

Y. Chen, Recent advancements on three-dimensional electrospun nanofiber scaffolds for tissue engineering. Adv. Fiber Mater. **4**(5), 959–986 (2022)

J.S.F. Constantino, Antiviral and nontoxic dermal iron oxide nanoparticle/biopolymer coatings for cotton fabric. ACS Appl. Nano Mater. **7**(12), 13991–14004 (2024)

M.B. Cortie, A.M. McDonagh, Synthesis and optical properties of hybrid and alloy plasmonic nanoparticles. Chem. Rev. **111**(6), 3713–3735 (2011)

O. Der, A. Ercetin (2024) Advancing nanomaterial characterization: a machine learning approach to assessing h-BN mechanical properties
T.R. Dmytriv, V.I. Lushchak, Potential biosafety of Mxenes: stability, biodegradability, toxicity and biocompatibility. Chemical Record (New York, N.Y.) **24**(4) (2024)
M. Dominska, D.M. Dykxhoorn, RNAi as new class of nanomedicines, in *Handbook of Harnessing Biomaterials in Nanomedicine*, pp. 163–197 (2012)
G.S. El-Sayyad et al., Eco-friendly strategies for biological synthesis of green nanoparticles with promising applications. BioNanoScience **14**(3), 3617–3659 (2024)
R. Foulkes et al., The regulation of nanomaterials and nanomedicines for clinical application: current and future perspectives. Biomater. Sci. **8**(17), 4653–4664 (2020)
J.N. Fu, Scaffold-based tissue engineering strategies for osteochondral repair. Front. Bioeng. Biotechnol. **9**, 812383 (2022)
S. Gandhi, D.H. Shastri, Lipid-based nanoparticles as drug delivery system for modern therapeutics. Pharm. Nanotechnol. **13** (2024)
X.J. Gao et al., Toward the integration of machine learning and molecular modeling for designing drug delivery nanocarriers. Adv. Mater. **36**(45), 2407793 (2024)
H.M. Gil, NIR-quantum dots in biomedical imaging and their future. iScience **24**(3), 102189 (2021)
S.S. Gomte et al., Exploring the potential of pH-sensitive polymers in targeted drug delivery. J. Biomater. Sci. Polym. Ed. **35**(2), 228–268 (2024)
D. Han et al., Collagen-hydroxyapatite based scaffolds for bone trauma and regeneration: recent trends and future perspectives. Nanomedicine (Lond.) **19**(18–20), 1689–1709 (2024)
A. Hashemi et al., Functionalized nanobiomaterials for cancer-targeted therapy: an overview, in *Functionalized Nanomaterials for Cancer Research: Applications in Treatments, Tools and Devices*, pp. 63–80 (2024)
Y. He et al., Effective breast cancer therapy based on palmitic acid-loaded PLGA nanoparticles. Biomater. Adv. **145**, 213270 (2023)
Y. He et al., Application of doxorubicin-loaded PLGA nanoparticles targeting both tumor cells and cancer-associated fibroblasts on 3D human skin equivalents mimicking melanoma and cutaneous squamous cell carcinoma. Biomater. Adv. **160**, 213831 (2024)
M. Hemdan et al., Innovations in biosensor technologies for healthcare diagnostics and therapeutic drug monitoring: applications, recent progress, and future research challenges. Sensors **24**(16), 5143 (2024)
D. Holmannova et al., Carbon nanoparticles and their biomedical applications. Appl. Sci. **12**(15), 7865 (2022)
L. Hu et al., Self-assembly of polymers and their applications in the fields of biomedicine and materials. Polymers **16**(15), 2097 (2024)
S.G. Ince, B.R. Ermis, The in situ potential of synthetic nano-hydroxyapatite for tooth enamel repair. Bioinspired, Biomimetic and Nanobiomaterials **10**(3), 78–86 (2021)
R. Indiarto et al., Bottom–up nanoparticle synthesis: a review of techniques, polyphenol-based core materials, and their properties. Eur. Food Res. Technol. **248**(1), 1–24 (2021)
J. Jeevanandam et al., Review on nanoparticles and nanostructured materials: History, sources, toxicity and regulations. Beilstein J. Nanotechnol. **9**(1), 1050 (2018)
A. John et al., Ceramic nanomaterials: preparation and applications in osteoporosis and bone tissue regeneration. J. Mater. Res. **38**(17), 4023–4041 (2023)
N. Joudeh, D. Linke, Nanoparticle classification, physicochemical properties, characterization, and applications: a comprehensive review for biologists. J. Nanobiotechnol. **20**(1), 1–29 (2022)
G. Kaur et al., Nanotechnology and CRISPR/Cas-mediated gene therapy strategies: Potential role for treating genetic disorders. Mol. Biotechnol., 1–23 (2024)
P. Kesharwani et al., Functionalized magnetic nanoparticles for chemotherapy applications, in *Functionalized Magnetic Nanoparticles for Theranostic Applications*, pp. 377–416 (2024)
T.R. Kyriakides et al., Biocompatibility of nanomaterials and their immunological properties. Biomed. Mater. (Bristol, England) **16**(4) (2021). https://doi.org/10.1088/1748-605X/abe5fa

W. Li et al., Design and applications of supramolecular peptide hydrogel as artificial extracellular matrix. Biomacromolecules **25**, 6967 (2024)
T. Liu, Nanomaterials and nanomaterials-based drug delivery to promote cutaneous wound healing. Adv. Drug Deliv. Rev. **193**, 114670 (2023)
S. Liu et al., Porous nanomaterials for biosensing and related biological application in in vitro/vivo usability. Mater. Adv. **5**(2), 453–474 (2024)
A. Loiudice et al., Atomic control in multicomponent nanomaterials: When colloidal chemistry meets atomic layer deposition. ACS Mater. Lett. **2**(9), 1182–1202 (2020)
S. Lu, A. Jayaraman, Machine learning for analyses and automation of structural characterization of polymer materials. Prog. Polym. Sci. **153**, 101828 (2024)
G. Luo et al., Composite nanoparticles, in *Encyclopedia of Microfluidics and Nanofluidics*, pp. 1–9 (2014)
G. Luo et al., Composite nanoparticles, in *Encyclopedia of Microfluidics and Nanofluidics*, pp. 453–460 (2015)
B. Mekuye, B. Abera, Nanomaterials: an overview of synthesis, classification, characterization, and applications. Nano Select **4**(8), 486–501 (2023)
K. Mi et al., Predicting tissue distribution and tumor delivery of nanoparticles in mice using machine learning models. J. Control. Release **374**, 219–229 (2024)
M.R. Mohammadi et al., Nanomaterials engineering for drug delivery: a hybridization approach. J. Mater. Chem. B **5**(22), 3995–4018 (2017)
A. Moradi, On-demand release of fucoidan from 3D-printed cardiac scaffolds based on chitosan/silk fibroin/polyaniline. Mater. Lett. **373**, 137178 (2024)
Q.W. Noronha, R. Bhat, Harnessing nanorobotic technology for precision cancer treatment: a comprehensive review. Int. J. Pharm. Healthc. Innov., 2584–2781 (2024)
S. Nouri et al., Review on biological synthesis of nano-hydroxyapatite and its application in nanomedicine. Iran. J. Med. Microbiol. **15**(4), 369–383 (2021)
S. Nouri et al., Biosynthesis of nano-calcite and nano-hydroxyapatite by the probiotic bacteria of *Bacillus subtilis* and *Bacillus coagulans*. Appl. Food Biotechnol. **9**(4), 275–286 (2022)
S. Nouri et al., Osteoblastic differentiation of stem cells from human exfoliated deciduous teeth by probiotic hydroxyapatite. Cell J. **25**(11), 753–763 (2023a)
S. Nouri et al., Microbial synthesis of nano-selenium and nano-titanium dioxide: mechanisms of selenite respiration. Bioinspired, Biomimetic and Nanobiomaterials **11**(4), 128–140 (2023b)
S. Nouri et al., Advanced 3D printed bone scaffolds with sodium alginate/tri-calcium phosphate/probiotic bacterial hydroxyapatite: enhanced mechanical and biocompatible properties for bone tissue engineering. Polymer **311**, 127523 (2024a)
S. Nouri et al., The efficacy of probiotic mediated hydroxyapatite in mammalian cell culture: promotion of MG-63 and L-929, anti-MCF7 breast cancer cells activities, and cytokine production of PBMC. Emerg. Mater., 1–11 (2024b)
O. Ozceylan, S.Z. Bayindir, Current overview on the use of nanosized drug delivery systems in the treatment of neurodegenerative diseases. ACS Omega **9**(33), 35223–35242 (2024)
N.S. Ozdemir et al., Advances in in vitro blood-air barrier models and the use of nanoparticles in COVID-19 research. Tissue Eng. Part B Rev. **30**(1), 82–96 (2024)
K. Paras Yadav et al., A review on low-dimensional nanomaterials: nanofabrication, characterization and applications. Nanomaterials **13**(1), 160 (2022)
M. Parashar et al., Metal oxides nanoparticles via sol–gel method: A review on synthesis, characterization and applications. J. Mater. Sci. Mater. Electron. **31**(5), 3729–3749 (2020)
W. Park et al., Advanced hybrid nanomaterials for biomedical applications. Prog. Mater. Sci. **114**, 100686 (2020)
J. Park et al., Cytoskeleton-modulating nanomaterials and their therapeutic potentials. Adv. Drug Deliv. Rev. **211**, 115362 (2024)
P. Phutane et al., Biofunctionalization and applications of polymeric nanofibers in tissue engineering and regenerative medicine. Polymers **15**(5), 1202 (2023)

M.J. Pinheiro et al., Advances in engine efficiency: nanomaterials, surface engineering, and quantum-based propulsion. Magnetochemistry **10**(3), 17 (2024)

R.S.R. Pothala et al., Review on next-gen healthcare: the role of MEMS and nanomaterials in enhancing diagnostic and therapeutic outcomes. Biomater. Connect **1**(1) (2024)

A. Prasert et al., Polypropylene/ZnO nanocomposites: mechanical properties, photocatalytic dye degradation, and antibacterial property. Materials **13**(4), 914 (2020)

H. Qi, C. Zhang, Organic nanoparticles for electrogenerated chemiluminescence assay. Curr. Opin. Electrochem. **34**, 101023 (2022)

X. Qin et al., Robust strategies in nuclear-targeted cancer therapy based on functional nanomaterials. Mater. Des. **221**, 110999 (2022)

M. Rahimnejad et al., Emerging phospholipid nanobiomaterials for biomedical applications to lab-on-a-chip, drug delivery, and cellular engineering. ACS Appl. Bio Mater. **4**(12), 8110–8128 (2021)

I.S. Raja et al., Polyphenols-loaded electrospun nanofibers in bone tissue engineering and regeneration. Biomater. Res. **25**(1), 1–16 (2021)

P. Ramburrun et al., Design, preparation, and functionalization of nanobiomaterials for enhanced efficacy in current and future biomedical applications. Nanotechnol. Rev. **11**(1), 1802–1826 (2022)

M. Ramesh et al., Nanotechnology-enabled biosensors: a review of fundamentals, design principles, materials, and applications. Biosensors **13**(1), 40 (2022)

W.K. Restu et al., Preparation and characterization of edible films from starch nanoparticles and chitosan. Bioinspired, Biomimetic and Nanobiomaterials **10**(1), 1–7 (2021)

A. Saravanan et al., A review on biosynthesis of metal nanoparticles and its environmental applications. Chemosphere **264**, 128580 (2021)

S. Sardari et al., Nanotechnology in tissue engineering: expanding possibilities with nanoparticles. Nanotechnology **35**(39), 392002 (2024)

U. Sharma, K. Saroha, A review of hydrotropic solubilization techniques for enhancing the bioavailability of poorly soluble drugs. Int. J. Toxicol. **43**(1), 63–71 (2024)

S. Singh, H. Sahani, Current advancement and future prospects: biomedical nanoengineering. Curr. Radiopharm. **17**(2), 120–137 (2024)

A. Sinha et al., The translational paradigm of nanobiomaterials: biological chemistry to modern applications. Mater. Today Bio **17**(October), 100463 (2022)

S. Smitha et al., Cytotoxic and anticancer activity of mixed metal oxide FeO: MnO nanostructures. Mater. Today Proc. **66**, 2245–2250 (2022)

A. Sood et al., Cancer detection: nanodevices at the forefront of early diagnosis, in *Nanoparticles in Cancer Theranostics: Current Progress in Cancer Management*, pp. 153–169 (2024)

E.B. Souto et al., Microemulsions and nanoemulsions in skin drug delivery. Bioengineering **9**(4), 158 (2022)

B. Subeshan et al., Machine learning applications for electrospun nanofibers: a review. J. Mater. Sci. **59**(31), 14095–14140 (2024)

M. Syduzzaman et al., Nanotechnology for high-performance textiles: a promising frontier for innovation. ChemNanoMat **9**(9) (2023)

S. Tabasum et al., Glycoproteins functionalized natural and synthetic polymers for prospective biomedical applications: a review. Int. J. Biol. Macromol. **98**, 748–776 (2017)

G. Thenuwara et al., Biosensor-enhanced organ-on-a-chip models for investigating glioblastoma tumor microenvironment dynamics. Sensors **24**(9), 2865 (2024)

M.N. Uddin et al., Review of bioaccumulation, biomagnification, and biotransformation of engineered nanomaterials, in *Nanotoxicology and Nanoecotoxicology Vol. 2*, pp. 133–164 (2021)

M.R. Venkateswaran et al., Self-healing materials in biomedicine and the circular economy. Environ. Sci. Nano **11**(7), 2771–2802 (2024)

C. Verma et al., 3D nanomaterials: the future of industrial, biological, and environmental applications. Inorg. Chem. Commun. **156**, 111163 (2023)

Z. Wang et al., One-dimensional nanomaterials in resistive gas sensor: from material design to application. Chemosensors **9**(8), 198 (2021)

Q. Wang et al., Expanding from materials to biology inspired by biomineralization. Interdiscip. Mater. **3**(2), 165–188 (2024)

Y. Xiao et al., Nanoscale morphologies on the surface of substrates/scaffolds enhance chondrogenic differentiation of stem cells: a systematic review of the literature. Int. J. Nanomedicine **19**, 12743–12768 (2024)

B. Xu et al., Graphene and graphene-related materials as brain electrodes. J. Mater. Chem. B **9**(46), 9485–9496 (2021)

H. Xu et al., Nanoparticles in the diagnosis and treatment of vascular aging and related diseases. Signal Transduct. Target. Ther. **7**(1), 231 (2022)

Y. Yang et al., Structural and functional design of electrospun nanofibers for hemostasis and wound healing. Adv. Fiber Mater. **4**(5), 1027–1057 (2022)

S. Yao et al., Nanomaterial-enabled wearable sensors for healthcare. Adv. Healthc. Mater. **7**(1), 1700889 (2018)

H. Yu et al., Multifunctional porous poly (L-lactic acid) nanofiber membranes with enhanced anti-inflammation, angiogenesis and antibacterial properties for diabetic wound healing. J. Nanobiotechnol. **21**(1) (2023)

N. Yuan et al., Synthesis and environmental applications of Nanoporous materials derived from coal Fly ash. Sustainability **15**(24), 16851 (2023)

A. Zarepour et al., Innovative approaches for cancer treatment: Graphene quantum dots for photodynamic and photothermal therapies. J. Mater. Chem. B **12**(18), 4307–4334 (2024)

E. Zeynalzadeh et al., Navigating the neurological frontier: macromolecular marvels in overcoming blood-brain barrier challenges for advanced drug delivery. Heliyon **10**(15), e35562 (2024)

C. Zhang et al., Progress, challenges, and future of nanomedicine. Nano Today **35**, 101008 (2020)

H. Zhang et al., Advances in magnetic nanoparticle-based magnetic resonance imaging contrast agents. Nano Res. **16**(11), 12531–12542 (2023)

J. Zhang et al., Smart stimuli-responsive strategies for titanium implant functionalization in bone regeneration and therapeutics. Mater. Horiz. **11**(1), 12–36 (2024a)

X. Zhang et al., Antidehydration and stable mechanical properties during the phase transition of the PNIPAM-based hydrogel for body-temperature-monitoring sensors. ACS Appl. Mater. Interfaces **16**, 62776 (2024b)

Functional Properties of Nanostructured Materials

J. Randhari, P. K. Mallik, and S. K. Senapati

Abstract This paper highlights the synthesis and processing of alumina-calcium titanate (Al2O3-CaTiO3) composite for multifunctional applications in the biomedical industry. In this work, the Al2O3-CaTiO3 composite was synthesized via the Sol-Gel method. Calcium oxide, aluminum isopropoxide, titanium isopropoxide, ethanol, and nitric acid were used as precursors, solvents, stabilizers, and catalysts, respectively. The powder was calcined at 800 °C for 1 hour. The densification and sintering behavior of uniaxially pressed calcined powder were evaluated using a pressureless sintering electric furnace at 1400 °C for 2 hours. XRD and SEM analyses were used to determine the phases and morphology of powders and the sintered composite. The impedance analysis was used to investigate the electrical properties of the sintered composite. As a result, the phases and morphology of Al2O3 and CaTiO3 were confirmed by XRD, SEM, and HR-TEM analysis. Impedance analysis indicates that the dielectric constant and AC conductivity of the sintered sample increase with temperature and frequency. Finally, it can be concluded that both phases are biocompatible and can be fabricated and used in biomedical applications as functional biomaterials.

Keywords Alumina · Calcium titanate · Sol-Gel synthesis · Nanocomposite · Pressurless sintering · Dielectri analysis

J. Randhari
Department of Mechanical Engineering, IGIT, Sarang, BPUT, Rourkela, Dhenkanal, India

P. K. Mallik (✉)
Department of Metallurgical and Materials Engineering, IGIT, Sarang, Dhenkanal, India

S. K. Senapati
Department of Mechanical Engineering, IGIT, Sarang, Dhenkanal, India

R. Narayan (ed.), *Nanostructured Biomaterials and Their Applications*,
https://doi.org/10.1007/978-3-032-16316-5_2

1 Introduction

Bone is a natural nanostructured composite of organic (collagen) and inorganic minerals (nano-apatite), a calcium phosphate (CaP) ceramic dispersion in the collagen matrix (Minardi et al. 2015). Several bioceramics containing calcium and phosphorous have been used clinically for decades (Hench et al. 2014; Jones et al. 2016; Szpalski 2002; Campana et al. 2014), both for load- and non-load-bearing applications (Fernandez de Grado et al. 2018; Roberts and Rosenbaum 2012). However, conventional bioceramics had poor mechanical properties, unfavorable biodegradability, and porosity (Fielding and Bose 2013; Wen et al. 2017). The latest generation of bioceramics is structured at the nanoscale and has significantly improved bioactivity, biodegradation, and mechanical properties and proven superior at enhancing bone regeneration due to their multifunctional properties (e.g., physical, chemical, mechanical, magnetic, and electrical) (Perez et al. 2013; Wang et al. 2016). Natural bone, cartilage, and tendons are piezoelectric materials in-vivo under the applied dynamic body stress, generating the electric potential to help bone formation and growth (Teng et al. 2001; Perez et al. 2015; Ribeiro et al. 2015; Zhang et al. 2016). With this approach, nanotechnology offers and manipulates the electrical stimuli, which has emerged as a promising strategy to enhance bone regeneration (control growth and the remodeling process). The impact of nanotechnology on the development and rational design of Al_2O_3-$CaTiO_3$ nanocomposite is reviewed below.

This approach selected aluminum oxide powder as the primary matrix material. Varying proportions (0–20%) of the $CaTiO_3$ sol were added to Al_2O_3 sol by sol-gel synthesis to produce calcined Al_2O_3-$CaTiO_3$ nanocomposite powders and compacted in a hydraulic press to form disk-shaped green pellets that were conventionally sintered in an electrical resistance furnace. The sintered composites were characterized by density, dielectric constant, and AC conductivity as a function of the material composition, sintering parameters, frequency, and temperature. The experimental data were systematically recorded and analyzed to evaluate the functional behavior of the sintered Al_2O_3-$CaTiO_3$ nanocomposite materials.

2 Densification and Microstructural Analysis

Figure 1 shows the XRD results of sintered Al_2O_3, monolith $CaTiO_3$, A1OCT, and A20CT nanocomposites. The figure shows that all the phases are crystalline, and no secondary phase was detected. By the addition of $CaTiO_3$ in a matrix of nano-Al_2O_3 which varies from 10 to 20 wt.%, the absence of secondary phases after pressureless sintering 1400 °C for 2 h in air was detected in A10CT and A20CT nanocomposite. The absence of secondary phases in the XRD pattern is because of the presence of $CaTiO_3$ at the grain boundaries in the matrix of nano Al_2O_3, which tends to act as a sintered aid to enhance the densification of nanocomposites as compared to the monolith as shown in Table 1.

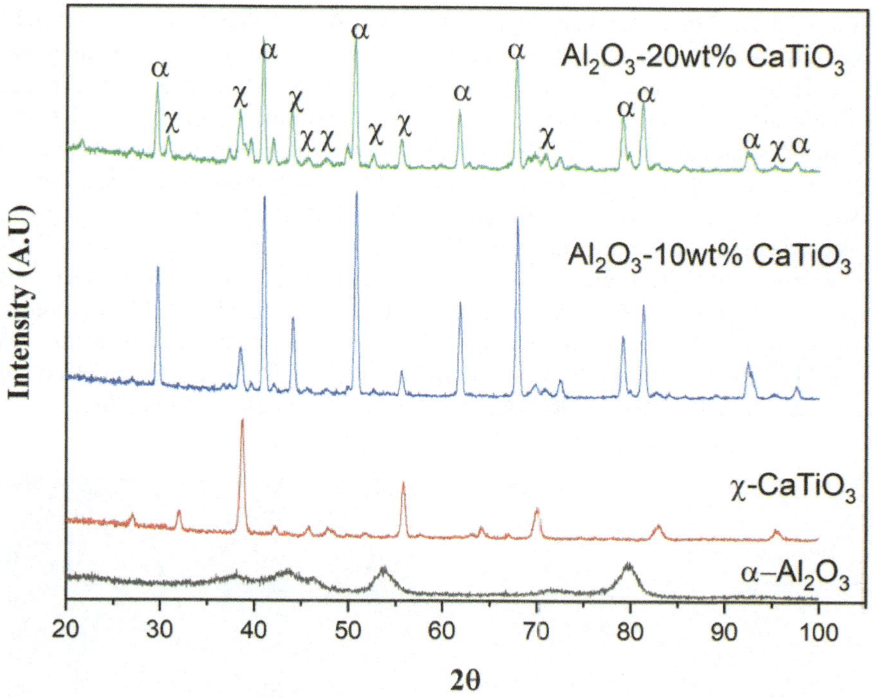

Fig. 1 XRD analysis of ACT composites monolithic Al_2O_3 and CT

Table 1 Designation and densities of sintered samples

S.No.	Composition	Sample designation	Bulk density (g/cm^3)	$\rho_{theoretical}$ (%)
1	Monolithic Al_2O_3	A	2.55 ± 0.58	64.67
2	Monolithic $CaTiO_3$	CT	1.99 ± 0.03	80.15
3	Al_2O_3—10 wt.% $CaTiO_3$	A10CT	3.15 ± 0.72	90.8
4	Al_2O_3—20 wt.% $CaTiO_3$	A20CT	3.58 ± 0.01	88.1

As a result, it will influence the nanocomposites' dielectric properties and AC conductivity, which will be discussed in detail later. Further, when the wt.% of $CaTiO_3$ increases, the peak intensity gradually increases while the peak intensity of Al_2O_3 decreases. The reduction of the peak intensity of Al_2O_3 is due to oxygen vacancy formation and a decrease in the structure factor of crystallographic planes.

In Fig. 2a, the TEM bright-field image shows calcined powder grains with regular shapes; the average grain size was 10–20 nm. Figure 2b, the HR-TEM image, shows the atomic planes and lattice fringes that confirm the crystalline nature of calcined powders. Figure 2c and d shows the influence of wt. percentage of $CaTiO_3$

on morphology and grain size of the A10CT and A20CT nanocomposites. It indicates that A10CT and A20CT nanocomposites are relatively dense and homogenous. The Al_2O_3 grain having less than 1 μm distributes well in microstructure, and the nanostructure well remained the same after pressureless sintering at 1400 °C. However, some abnormal $CaTiO_3$ grain is observed in microstructure A20CT in Fig. 2d compared to A10CT nanocomposite in Fig. 2c because of the increase for addition from 10 to 20 wt. %, and the grain size of $CaTiO_3$ increased from 1 to 2.5 μm. It is considered that the presence of $CaTiO_3$ rich in the grain boundary region leads to the growth of $CaTiO_3$ grain. As a result, the relative density of A20CT decreases compared to A10CT. From the microstructure, it is expected that the addition of $CaTiO_3$ in nano Al_2O_3 has a significant influence on grain size and densification, as shown in Table 1, and will have a substantial effect on the dielectric and electrical properties of A10CT and A20CT nanocomposites as compared to monolithic.

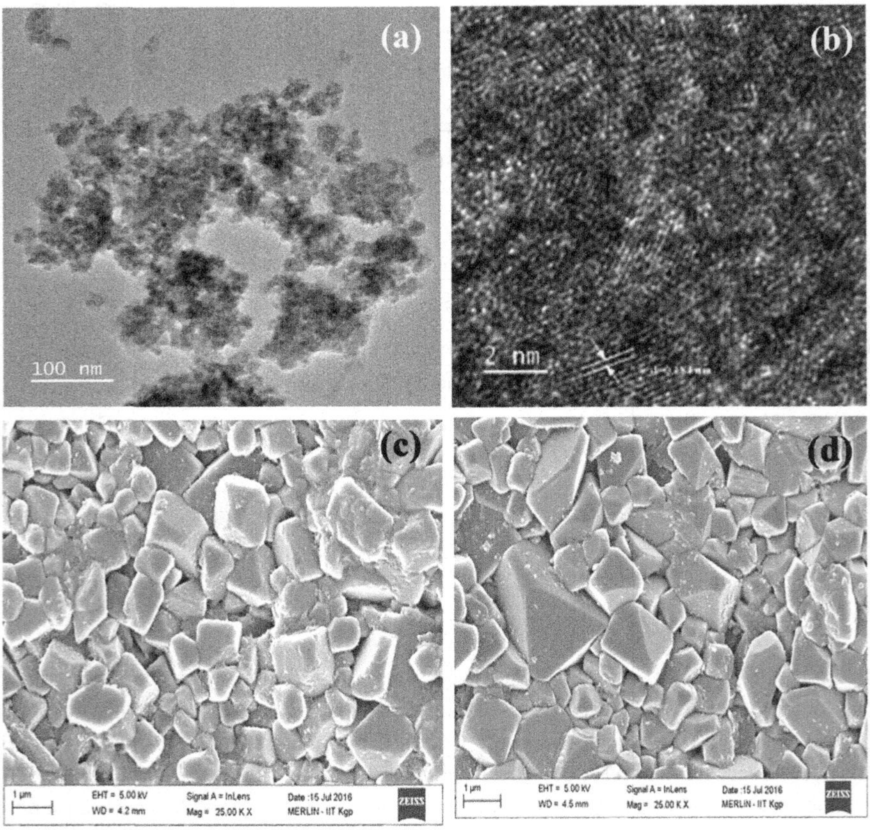

Fig. 2 **a** TEM bright-field image of the nanocomposite powders, **b** HR-TEM images of nanocomposite powders images of **c** A10CT, **d** A20 CT polished surfaces of Al_2O_3–$CaTiO_3$ nanocomposites

3 Dielectric Property's Analysis

3.1 Frequency-Temperature Dependence of Dielectric Constant

Figure 3a–d, respectively, shows the variation of dielectric constant with frequency ranging from 100 Hz to 1 MHz at different temperatures. The variation of dielectric constants with frequency can be observed at various temperatures. The dielectric dispersion appears at low temperatures of monolith Al_2O_3 and extends to the higher values due to the bulk effect of charge carriers in the monolith Al_2O_3. At high temperatures, the decrease in the dielectric constant of monolith Al_2O_3 occurs because of the activity of lattice vibration or phonons that restricts the motion of charge carriers or no longer follows the charge carriers the frequency of alternating signal. A less pronounced dispersion of the dielectric constant can be seen even at high temperatures. Because the change in frequency is too rapid for the charge carriers to follow the electric signal, their contribution to the total polarization becomes negligible. Since monolith $CaTiO_3$ is composed of Ca^{2+} ions and TiO_6 octahedra, which are so distorted that the position of central Ti^{4+} ions deviates from the center of gravity of the surrounding six oxygen ions, polarization appears [17]. Therefore, all the samples' dielectric constant decreases with increasing frequency at varying temperatures. The higher value of the dielectric constant at the lower frequency region is due to the various polarization effects in the composite A10CT and A20CT, as shown in Fig. 3c and d. The dielectric constant at high temperatures behaves linearly, as shown in Fig. 3a–d. Overall, increasing the amount of $CaTiO_3$ addition increases the dielectric of monolith Al_2O_3, respectively, in the function of frequency at varying temperatures.

Figure 4a–d, respectively, shows the variation of dielectric constant (ε) with temperature from 30 to 200 °C at different frequencies. Figure 4c indicates that the dielectric constant increases with an increase in temperature for A10CT and is dependent on frequency. The monolithic, Al_2O_3, and A20CT (Fig. 4a and d) indicate that dielectric constant values increase with increasing temperature up to 40 °C and decrease with increasing frequencies, respectively. After 60 °C, it remains constant In Fig. 4b, the dielectric constant of monolithic CT increases up to 40 °C and then gradually decreases with an increase in temperature. Because of the depolarization of space charge, lattice vibration increases, generating phonons.

Figure 4c shows that the dielectric constant of the A10CT value is monotonically increasing with the function of temperature at a particular frequency and decreasing the dielectric value with increasing frequencies. This is due to the combined effect of temperature and frequency depolarization of space charge and no longer response of charge carriers to the applied electric field frequency. Figure 4d shows that the dielectric value is initially higher at a particular frequency of 100 Hz in the low-temperature region up to 70 °C and then remains almost constant independent of temperature. As increasing the frequency from 100 kHz to 1 MHz, dielectric values gradually increase to the maximum value at 50 °C and then decrease up to 70 °C.

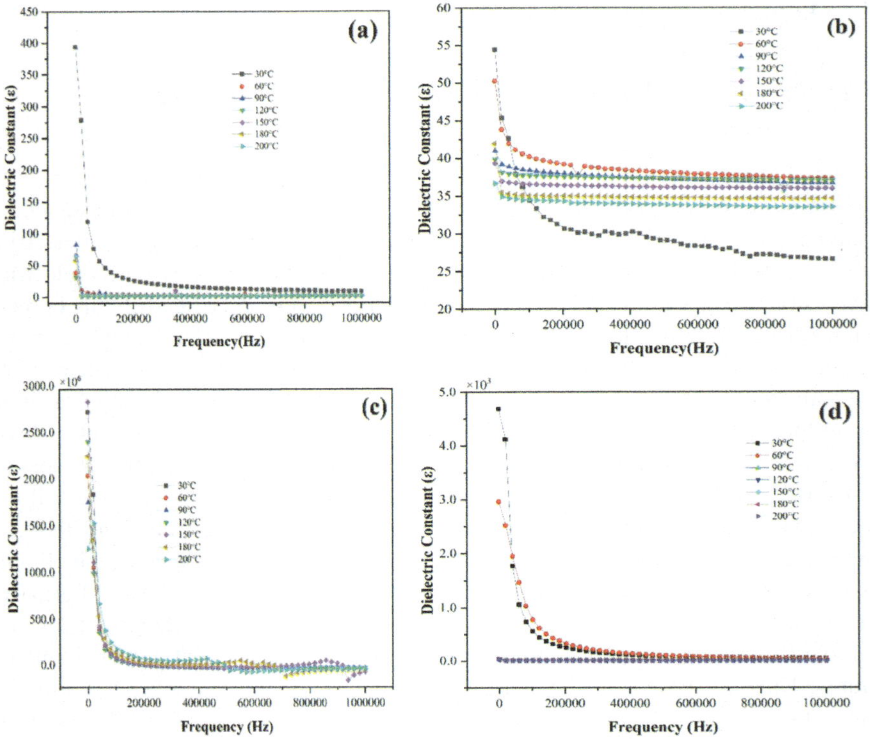

Fig. 3 **a** Dielectric constant of monolithic Al_2O_3; **b** the dielectric constant of monolithic $CaTiO_3$; **c** the dielectric constant of A10CT; **d** the dielectric constant of A20CT as a function of frequency at various temperatures, respectively

After 70 °C, follow the similar trend of constant value at all frequencies. This is due to the contribution of dipolar molecules, space charge effect, and active polarization mechanism at low temperatures toward increasing the dielectric maximum values. Then, it decreases in dielectric value up to temperature 70 °C and remains constant in dielectric values independent of temperature with varying frequencies. In other words, few active polarization mechanisms, such as electronics, operate at higher temperature regions.

Figure 5a and b represents the variation of the dielectric constant (log ε) with temperature ranging from 30C to 200 °C at different frequencies (100 kHz, 300 kHz, 600 kHz, 1 MHz) for different sintered samples. The comparison showed that the dielectric constant of monolith Al_2O_3, A20CT, and monolith $CaTiO_3$ sample initially increases and, after 60 °C, remains constant with increases in temperature and dependency of frequency. However, for the A10CT sample, the dielectric constant increases with an increase in temperature and maximum at 100 kHz. At lower frequencies, the dielectric of A10CT is higher than at higher frequencies. This is due to adding 10 wt. % of $CaTiO_3$, Ca^{2+}, and Ti^{4+} ions, increasing charger carrier concentration. Because

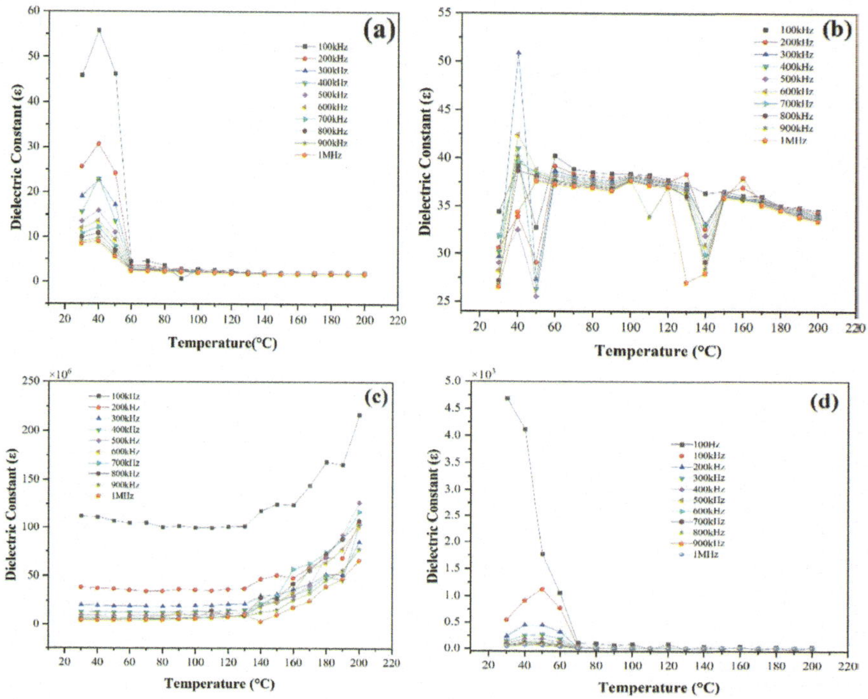

Fig. 4 **a** Dielectric constant of monolith Al_2O_3; **b** the dielectric constant of monolith $CaTiO_3$; **c** the dielectric constant of A10CT; **d** the dielectric constant of A20CT as a function of temperature at various frequencies, respectively

ionic and electronic polarization are not temperature-dependent mechanisms. As the $CaTiO_3$ increases from 10 to 20 wt. %, dielectric constant decreases to almost 80% reduction, with 20 wt. % of $CaTiO_3$; initially, the dielectric value increases in the low-temperature region from 30 to 60 °C, then remains constant independent of temperature. This is due to water molecules in $CaTiO_3$ grains that are polarized into OH^- and H^+ ions under the influence of temperature and frequency. In other words, with the addition of 20 wt. % of $CaTiO_3$, $CaTiO_3$ grain size became more extensive, and Al_2O_3 grain size remained the same, decreasing the dielectric constant. This is due to the decrease in the surface charge of $CaTiO_3$ grains [18].

3.2 Frequency-Temperature Dependence of Dielectric Loss

Dielectric loss is the electrical energy lost in the form of heat in the polarization process under an applied alternative electric field [19]. Figure 5a–d, respectively, shows the variation of the dielectric loss with frequencies ranging from 100 Hz to 1 MHz at different temperatures. At low frequencies, a higher value of dielectric loss

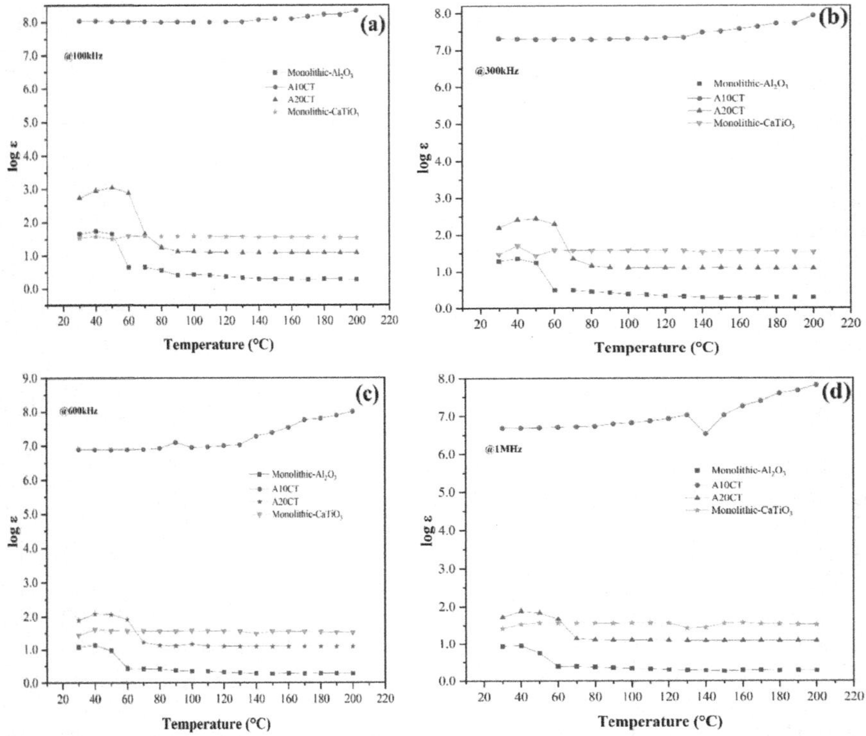

Fig. 5 **a** Dielectric constant monolithic Al_2O_3; **b** dielectric constant of monolithic $CaTiO_3$; **c** dielectric constant of A10CT; **d** dielectric constant of A20CT as a function of temperature at different frequency (100 kHz, 300 k Hz, 600 kHz, 1 MHz), respectively

is observed due to the higher resistance offered by the grain boundaries, as more energy is required for the motion of charge carriers. The rapid increase in dielectric loss at lower temperature regions for lower frequencies is likely due to the space charge polarization of monolith Al_2O_3 and $CaTiO_3$. Similarly, grains offer low resistance and the absence of space charge polarization at high frequency, resulting in a lower value of dielectric loss. The results show that dielectric loss decreases gradually at lower temperatures when frequency increases, but at higher temperatures, dielectric loss decreases parallel with the rise in frequency. This indicates that dielectric losses are due to the interaction of lattice vibration or phonons with the motion of charge carriers (Ca^{2+} and Ti^{4+} ions) with increasing frequency and temperature.

From Fig. 6c and d, it can be observed that dielectric loss values are higher than the monolith Al_2O_3 and $CaTiO_3$. The dielectric loss value of A10CT is 10^3 compared to A20CT nanocomposites. Decreasing grain size and increasing porosity lead to an increase of dipolar and space charge polarizations in the lower frequency region. As a result, electrical energy is highly absorbed in the form of heat due to the interaction between the dipole moment with space charge and charge carriers. Further, decreasing dielectric loss continues at a particular higher frequency and temperature.

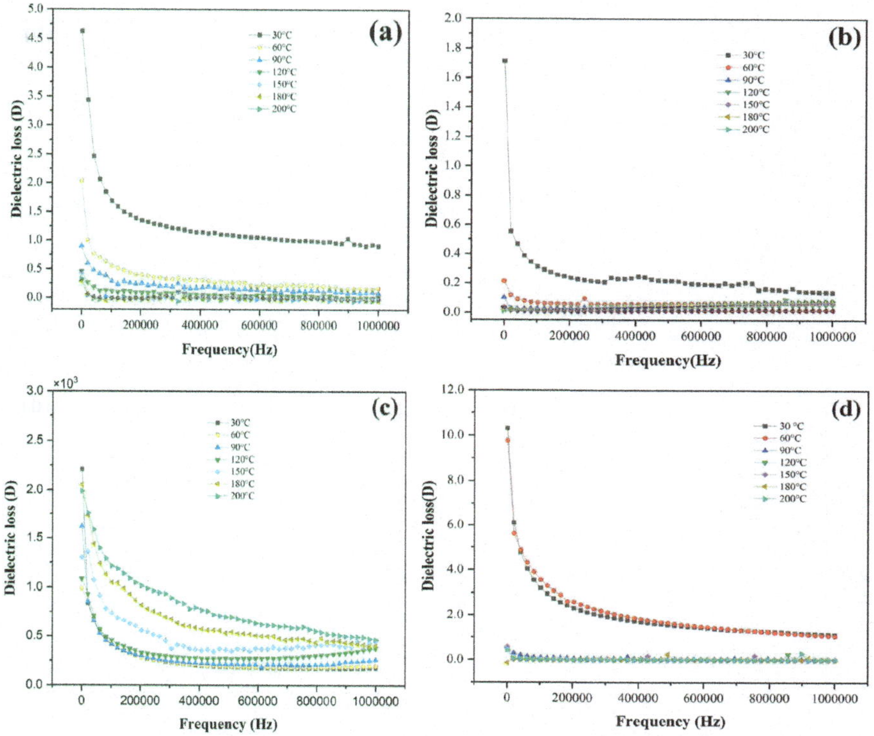

Fig. 6 **a** Dielectric loss of monolithic Al_2O_3; **b** dielectric loss of monolith $CaTiO_3$; **c** dielectric loss of A10CT; **d** dielectric loss of A20CT as a function of frequency at varying temperatures, respectively

Figure 7a–d shows the variation of dielectric loss as a function of temperature at different frequencies for each sample. From Fig. 7a of the monolith, Al_2O_3 observed that as the temperature increases from 30 to 200 °C, the dielectric loss rises to 40 °C and gradually decreases. This indicates the thermally activated nature of the dielectric loss of the A10CT nanocomposite.

The variation of dielectric loss with a function of temperature range 30–200 °C is shown in Fig. 8a–d at different frequencies for sintered samples. The comparison shows that monolithic Al_2O_3, monolithic $CaTiO_3$, and A20CT samples indicate lower dielectric loss values and remain constant, independent of temperature. For sample A10CT, the dielectric loss increases with increasing temperature and reaches maximum value at 160 °C and 150 °C for 600 kHz and 1 MHz frequency, respectively. Because of the high frequency and high-temperature region, the dielectric loss depends on electronic polarization only. As a result, dielectric loss is decreasing. In other words, at this frequency range, the polarization of the grain is more active than the grain boundary region, which shows a decreasing trend of dielectric loss. However, at lower frequencies of 100 kHz and 300 kHz, dielectric loss increases with increasing temperature from 30° to 200 °C, as shown in Fig. 5a and b.

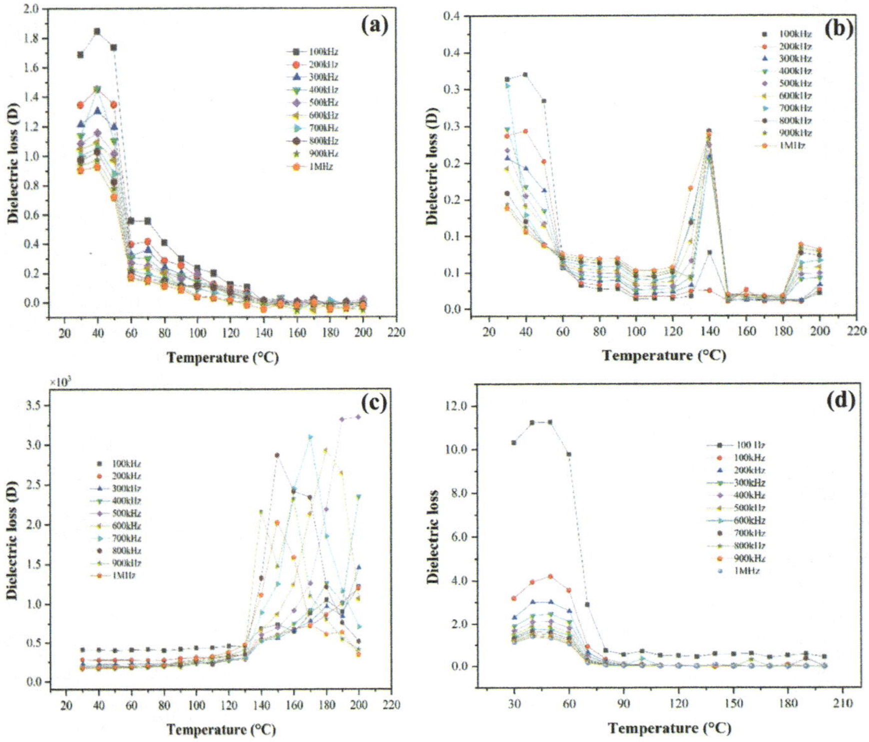

Fig. 7 **a** Dielectric loss of monolithic Al_2O_3; **b** dielectric loss of monolithic $CaTiO_3$; **c** dielectric loss of A10CT; **d** dielectric loss of A20CT as a function of temperature at varying frequency, respectively

It is to be noted that dielectric loss is temperature-dependent and increases with increasing temperature. This is due to the active polarization of the grain boundary region, which is supposed to be $CaTiO_3$ grains and porosity. This indicates the hopping of charge carriers (Ti^{4+}, Ca^{2+}, and O^{2-}), and vacancies are thermally activated in the grain boundary region compared to the grain interior. As a result, the dielectric loss increases with increasing temperature for the A10CT nanocomposite.

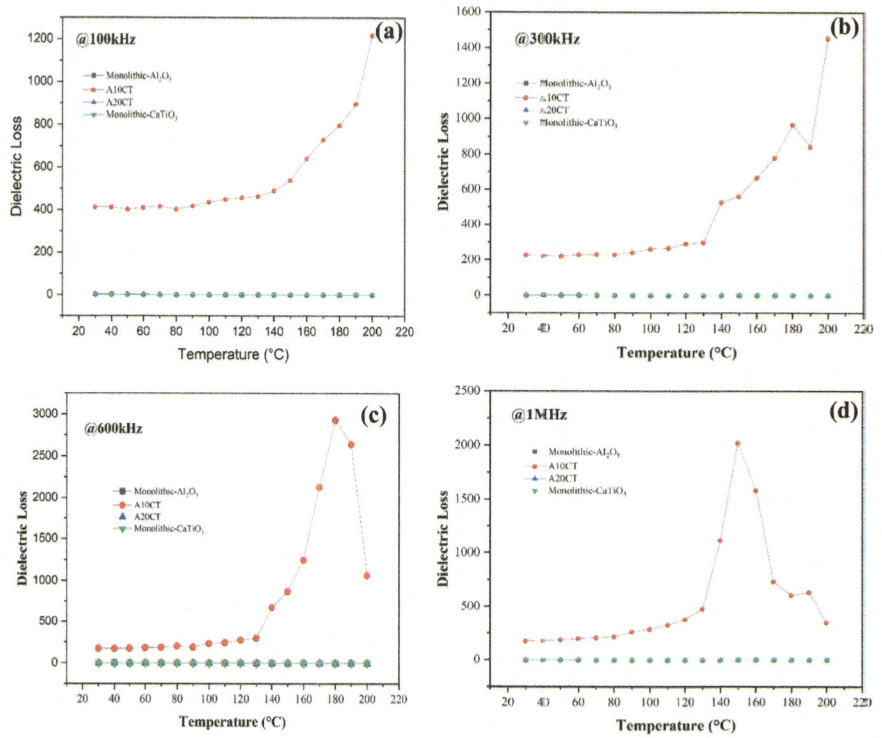

Fig. 8 **a** Dielectric loss of monolithic Al_2O_3; **b** dielectric loss of monolithic $CaTiO_3$; **c** dielectric loss of A10CT; **d** dielectric loss of A20CT as a function of temperature at different frequencies (100 kHz, 300 kHz, 600 kHz, 1 MHz), respectively

4 Conductivity Analysis

4.1 Frequency-Temperature Dependence of A.C. Conductivity

From the above results, it can be noted that the high values of dielectric constant and dielectric loss in lower frequency regions do not generally correspond to the bulk effect of monolithic Al_2O_3, $CaTiO_3$, and A20CT nanocomposite. Instead, it is attributed to the space charge build-up at the grain interface of Al_2O_3, $CaTiO_3$, and dipole of polar molecules, which can be explained by interfacial Maxwell–Wagner polarization [22]. Figure 9a–d shows the frequency-dependent AC conductivity at various temperatures plotted for monolithic Al_2O_3, A20CT monolithic $CaTiO_3$, A10CT, and A20CT samples. It is entirely fitted with the frequency-dependent a.c. The relation in Eq. 3 gives conductivity.

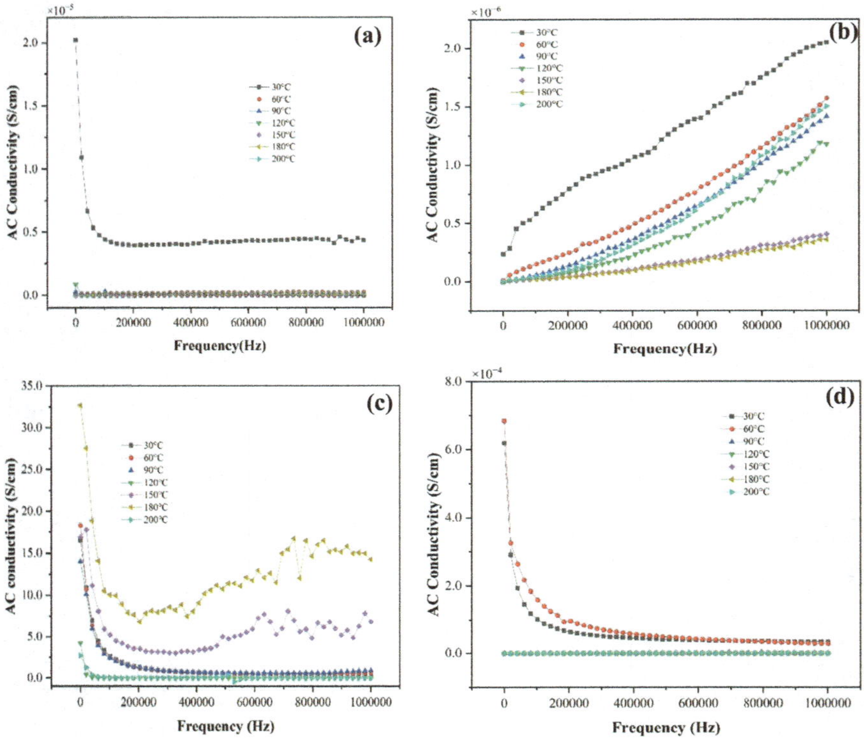

Fig. 9 **a** AC conductivity of monolithic Al_2O_3; **b** AC conductivity of monolithic $CaTiO_3$; **c** AC conductivity of A10CT; **d** AC conductivity of A20CT as a function of frequency at different temperatures, respectively

Figure 9a, c, and d shows that monolithic Al_2O_3, A10CT, and A20CT samples' AC conductivity is independent of increasing frequencies and temperature. At very low frequencies and high temperatures, this increase in AC conductivity correlates quite well with the increase in dielectric constant, as shown in Fig. 3a–d. However, from Fig. 9b, the values of AC conductivity obtained increase with increasing frequency. This indicates that a linear variation of σ_{ac} over a wide temperature range supports the existence of thermally activated polarization mechanisms following Arrhenius law given by

$$\sigma_{ac} = \sigma_0 \exp\left(\frac{-E_a}{K_B T}\right), \quad (1)$$

where σ_0 is the pre-exponential factor, E_a is the activation energy, and K_B is the Boltzmann constant. It was observed from Fig. 9b that the conductivity increases with an increase in frequency. Because of increasing frequency, the $CaTiO_3$ grain is more active by promoting the hopping frequency of charge carriers ($Ca^{2+,}$ Ti^{4+} ions). Thus, AC conductivity increases with increasing frequency.

The effect of temperature on the AC conductivity of monolithic ceramic samples and nanocomposites was studied in the range of 303 to 473 K. The variation of electrical conductivity (σ_{ac}) with 1000/T at different frequencies for different compositions was shown in Fig. 10a–d. In Fig. 10a and d, the AC conductivity remains constant with increases in temperature from 473 K to 343 K at different frequencies. However, with a decrease in temperature from 303 to 333 K, the AC conductivity increases with different frequencies. The variation is maximum with initial frequency. In Fig. 10c, there is a dispersion of increase in AC conductivity with a rise in temperature from 413 to 473 K with increasing frequencies. Still, after that, it remains independent with an increase in temperature in response to different frequencies. This indicates that the AC conductivity behavior of A10CT nanocomposite is thermally activated following the Arrhenius law at high temperatures and frequencies.

However, it is exceptionally different in monolithic Al_2O_3 and A20CT nanocomposite samples, as shown in Fig. 10a–d. The increase in a.c conductivity is observed at lower temperature regions due to the activity of all polarization mechanisms and

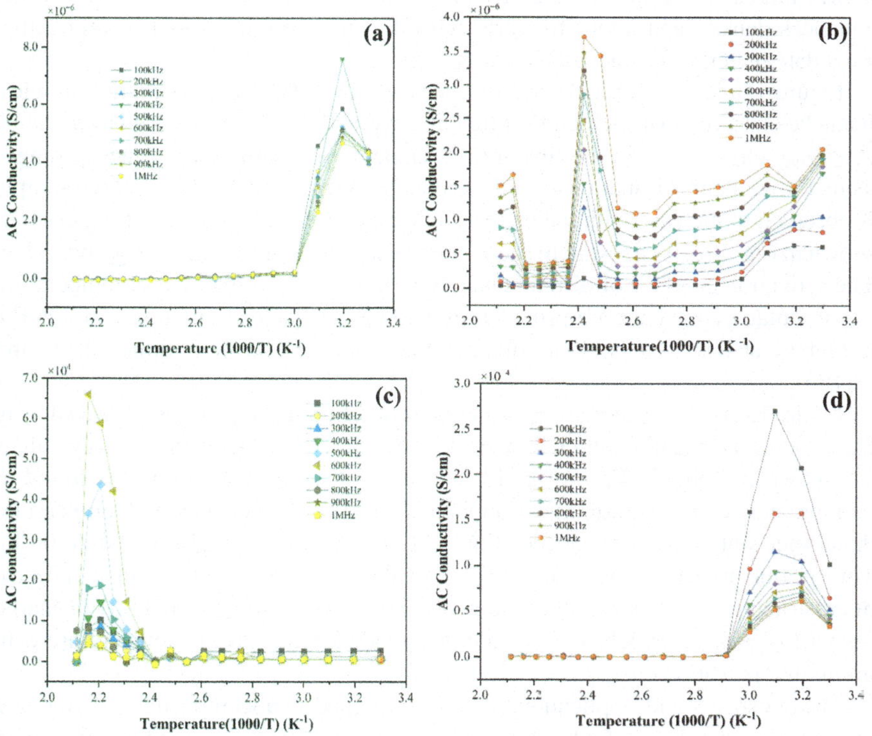

Fig. 10 **a** AC conductivity of monolithic Al_2O_3; **b** AC conductivity of monolithic $CaTiO_3$; **c** AC conductivity of A10CT; **d** AC conductivity of A20CT as a function of temperature (1000/T) at varying frequency, respectively

porosity, similar to the dielectric constant, as shown in Fig. 3. Then, the a.c conductivity remains independent with increasing frequency and temperature. This indicates that there is no polarization mechanism, such as the hopping of charge carriers, which ceases to follow the frequency of the alternative current. Therefore, the AC conductivity of monolithic Al_2O_3 and A20CT nanocomposite samples is observed independent of temperature and frequencies. Figure 10b shows that AC conductivity curves are divided into regions from lower to high temperatures at different frequencies. Each region of AC conductivity is quite well distinct from the other areas due to the activity of different polarization mechanisms. Overall, the AC conductivity of monolithic $CaTiO_3$ decreases with increasing temperature and frequencies, which is thermally active conductivity due to the hopping of charge carriers.

The comparison of log scale AC conductivity variation with temperature from 30 to 200 °C is shown in Fig. 11a–d. It was observed that electrical conductivity for all sintered ceramics decreases with temperature increases at different frequencies. The higher value of AC conductivity of the A10CT sample was observed at various frequencies. This indicates that the optimal addition of $CaTiO_3$ to the nano alumina matrix increases the dielectric constant, dielectric loss, and AC conductivity, and enhances density and microstructure. A10CT nanocomposite could be a potential candidate material for microwave resonators.

Figure 12a–d shows log AC conductivity versus 1000/T of all sintered samples. It can be observed that each plot is fitted linearly, and the slope was used to calculate activation energy (E_a) in the function of temperature at different frequency ranges using the Arrhenius Equation 4[20] The ac conductivity of the A10CT sintered sample is observed to increase with the increase in temperature at a particular frequency, as shown in Fig. 12c. As a result, the activation energy is found to have a negative value. The activation energies of different sintered samples in the function of temperature at particular frequencies are provided in Table 2. The activation energy of A20CT is highest at low frequency and temperature compared to monolithic Al_2O_3 and $CaTiO_3$.

Figure 13 compares the activation energies of different sintered samples at varying frequencies over temperatures from 30 to 200 °C, and the activation energy values are shown in Table 2. From Fig. 13, it can be observed that A10CT is found to be more active polarization under applied electric field frequency and temperature than other sintered samples (monolithic Al_2O_3, monolithic $CaTiO_3$, and A20CT). This is due to nanoscale grains and high densification, resulting in a uniform microstructure compared to other sintered samples. As a result, the mobility of charge carrier frequency is synchronized under the applied frequency and temperature with minimum activation energy.

The prospects and applications of the developed nanocomposite materials are summarized as follows. SiO_2-based (BioMEMES) devices such as biosensors and lab on the chip have been implanted in vivo for biomedical applications [21, 22]. However, SiO_2 has excellent insulating properties with a dielectric constant value of 3.9; these devices have a biocompatibility issue in vivo. Moreover, alumina possesses excellent biocompatibility and insulating properties with a dielectric constant of 9 [23]. Therefore, the developed monolithic and nanocomposite materials possess

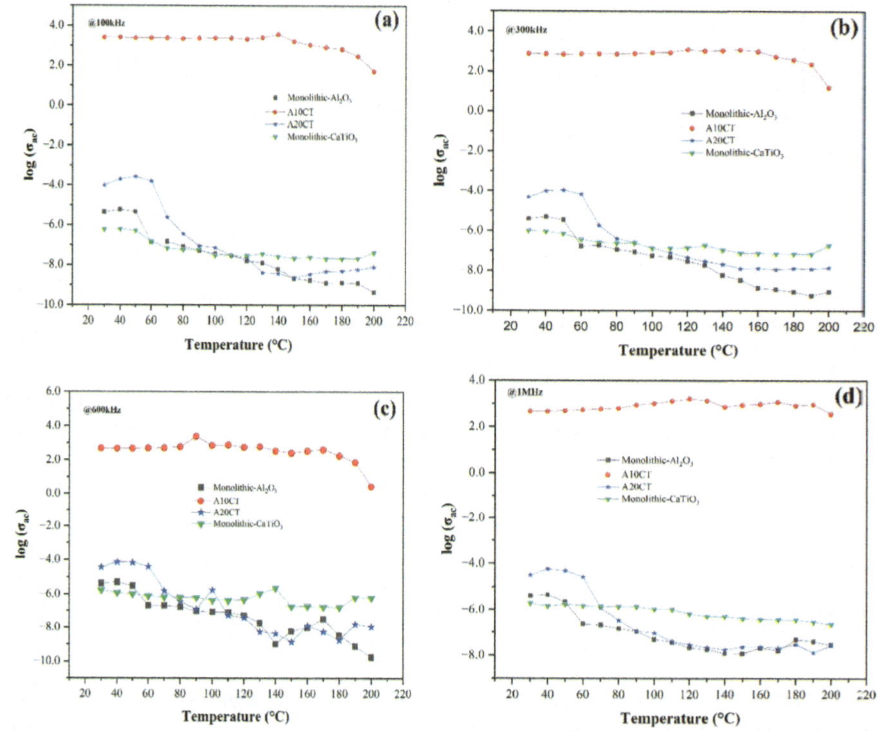

Fig. 11 **a** AC conductivity of monolithic Al_2O_3; **b** AC conductivity of monolithic $CaTiO_3$; **c** AC conductivity of A10CT; **d** AC conductivity of A20CT as a function of temperature at different frequencies (100 kHz, 300 kHz, 600 kHz, 1 MHz), respectively

better dielectric properties and biocompatibility compared to the reported dielectric values of SiO_2 and Al_2O_3, as shown in Table 3. As a result, it is suggested that the developed monolithic and nanocomposites have been studied extensively to replace SiO_2-based in future bioelectric devices.

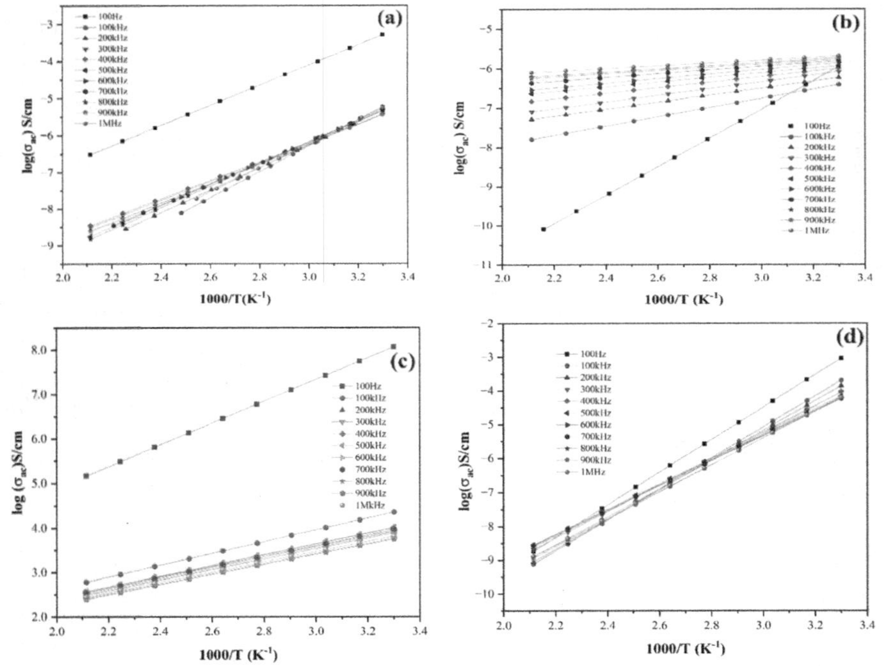

Fig. 12 **a** Log AC conductivity of monolithic Al_2O_3; **b** log AC conductivity of monolithic $CaTiO_3$; **c** log AC conductivity of A10CT; **d** log AC conductivity of A20CT as a function of temperature at different frequencies, respectively

Table 2 Activation energy of sintered samples at different frequency in the temperature from 30–200 °C

Frequency	Activation energy (E_a) eV			
	Monolithic Al_2O_3	Monolithic $CaTiO_3$	A10CT	A20CT
100 Hz	2.7 ± 0.4	3.6 ± 0.9	−0.1 ± 0.1	4.8 ± 0.5
100 kHz	3.5 ± 0.4	1.2 ± 0.2	−0.5 ± 0.1	4.6 ± 0.4
200 kHz	3.1 ± 0.3	0.9 ± 0.2	−0.6 ± 0.1	4.4 ± 0.4
300 kHz	2.6 ± 0.2	0.9 ± 0.2	−0.9 ± 0.1	3.9 ± 0.4
400 kHz	2.5 ± 0.2	0.7 ± 0.2	−1.2 ± 0.2	4.1 ± 0.4
500 kHz	2.9 ± 0.1	0.6 ± 0.2	−1.8 ± 0.3	3.7 ± 0.3
600 kHz	2.9 ± 0.3	0.6 ± 0.2	−1.9 ± 0.3	3.7 ± 0.3
700 kHz	2.8 ± 0.2	0.5 ± 0.2	−1.6 ± 0.2	3.7 ± 0.3
800 kHz	3.0 ± 0.1	0.4 ± 0.2	−1.1 ± 0.1	3.7 ± 0.3
900 kHz	2.7 ± 0.1	0.4 ± 0.2	−0.9 ± 0.1	4.0 ± 0.3
1 MHz	3.3 ± 0.3	0.3 ± 0.2	−1.0 ± 0.1	3.9 ± 0.3

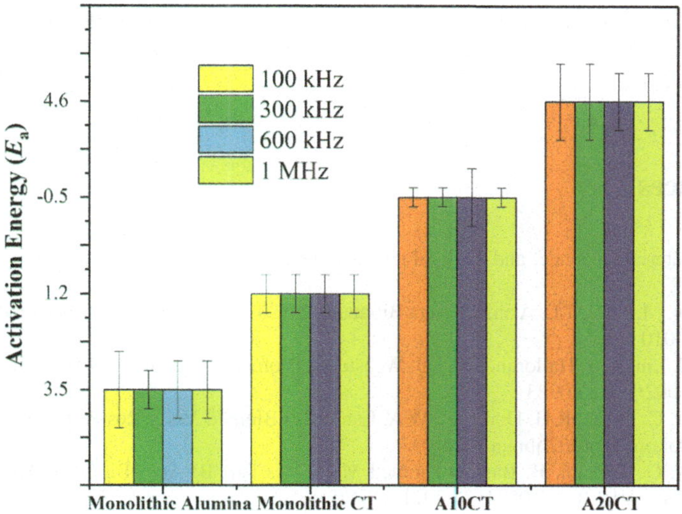

Fig. 13 Activation energy of monolith Al_2O_3 and $CaTiO_3$, A10CT, and A20CT at different frequencies (100 kHz, 300 kHz, 600 k Hz, 1 MHz), respectively

Table 3 Dielectric materials and their properties

S.No.	Composition	Experimental dielectric constant	Reported dielectric constant
1	Monolithic Al_2O_3	33	9
2	Monolithic $CaTiO_3$	30	160
3	A10CT	13×10^6	–
4	A20CT	337	–
5	SiO_2	–	3.9
6	TiO_2	–	80

5 Conclusion

Al_2O_3-$CaTiO_3$ nanocomposites were successfully prepared by the sol-gel method and pressureless sintering with varying wt.% of calcium titanate (A10CT, A20CT), resulting in better densification and microstructure compared to monolithic samples, as confirmed by XRD and SEM analysis. The high dielectric constant and AC conductivity obtained increased frequency and temperature for A10CT sintered nanocomposite compared to A20CT. Finally, Al_2O_3-$CaTiO_3$ composite could be a dielectric material for bioelectronics devices such as biochips and biosensors for biomedical applications.

Acknowledgments The authors acknowledge the financial support of the Science and Engineering Research Board (SERB), Department of Science and Technology (DST), Ministry of Science and

Technology, Government of India. Thanks to Dr. S.K. Sahoo, Professor, MME, NIT, Rourkela, for helpful discussions and the Director, IGIT, Sarang, for providing the facility.

References

P. Zeng, Materials Science, and Technology. **24**(2008) 5505. https://doi.org/10.1179/174328408X287682

A. H. Rajabi, M. Jaffe, T.L. Arinzeh, Acta Biomater. **24**(2015) 12. https://doi.org/10.1016/j.actbio.2015.07.010

C. Ergun, H. Liu, J. W. Halloran, and T. J. Webster, J. Biomed. Mater. Res. **990** (2006). https://doi.org/10.1002/jbm.a.30923

T.J. Webster, C. Ergun, R.H. Doremus, W.A. Lanford, J Biomed Mater Res Part A, **67**(2003) 975. https://doi.org/10.1002/jbm.a.10160

A.K. Dubey, G. Tripathi, B. Basu, J Biomed Mater Res Part B: Appl Biomater, **95**(2010) 320. https://doi.org/10.1080/10584587.2011.616425

T. Greeshma, P.K. Mallik, B. Basu, Biomaterials, **34**(2013) 7073. https://doi.org/10.1016/j.biomaterials.2013.05.076

P.K. Mallik, B. Basu, J Biomed Mater Res A, **102**(2014) 842. https://doi.org/10.1002/jbm.a.34752

C. Han, J. Liu, W. Yang, Q. Wu, H. Yang, X. Xue, J. Sol. Gel Sci. Technol. **81**(2017) 806, https://doi.org/10.1007/s10971-016-4261-3

G. Pfaff, Chem. Mater. **6**(1994) 58. https://doi.org/10.1021/cm00037a013

S. Holliday, A. Stanishevsky, Surface & Coatings Technology 188–189 **741**(2004). https://doi.org/10.1016/j.surfcoat.2004.07.044

S. Saha, J Sol-Gel Sci Technol, **3**(1994)117. https://doi.org/10.1007/BF00486718

B.M. Patil, R.S. Srinivasa, S.R. Dharwadkar, Bull. Mater. Sci., **30**(2007) 225. https://doi.org/10.1007/s12034-007-0040-7

K. C. Patil, S. T. Aruna, T. Mimani, Solid state material science, **6**(2002)507. https://doi.org/10.1016/S1359-0286(02)00123-7

A. Gedanken, Ultrasonic sonochemistry, **11**(2004)47. https://doi.org/10.1016/j.ultsonch.2004.01.037

W. Feng, L. Mu-sen, L. Yu-peng, Q. Yong-xin, Mater. Lett. **59**(2005) 916. https://doi.org/10.1016/j.matlet.2004.08.041

L. Liu, H. Fan, P. Fang, X. Chen, Mater. Res. Bull., **43**(2008) 1800. https://doi.org/10.1016/j.materresbull.2007.07.012

Ogura, S., Sato, K., Inoue, Y., Phys. Chem. Chem. Phys. **2**(2000) 2449. https://doi.org/10.1039/b000187m

K. Okazaki, K. Nagata, J. Am. Ceram. Soc. **56** (1973) 82. https://doi.org/10.1111/j.1151-2916.1973.tb12363.x

Dev K. Mahato Alok Dutta T.P.Sinha. Physica B **406** (2011) 2703, https://doi.org/10.1016/j.physb.2011.04.012

A. Kyritsis, P. Pissis, J. Grammatikakis, J. Polym. Sci. Polym. Phys. **33** (1995) 1737, https://doi.org/10.1002/polb.1995.090331205

G. Kotzar et al., Biomaterials **23** (2002) 2737–2750, https://doi.org/10.1016/S0142-9612(02)00007-8

G. Voskerician et al. Biomaterials **24** (2003) 1959–1967, https://doi.org/10.1016/S0142-9612(02)00565-3

J. Robertson, Eur. Phys. J. Appl. Phys. **28**, 265–291 (2004), https://doi.org/10.1051/epjap:2004206

Nanostructured Surfaces in Biomaterials

K. Jurczyk and M. U. Jurczyk

Abstract In 1959, Richard Feynman, a Physics Nobel laureate, presented his famous theory on nanostructure materials production (Feynman in Eng Sci 23:22–26, 1960). He stated: "The principles of physics, as far as I can see, do not speak against the possibility of maneuvering things atom by atom." Feynman proceeded to describe a building with atomic precision and outlined a pathway involving a series of increasingly smaller machines. Nanostructures represent key building blocks for nanoscale science and technology.

Keywords Biocompatibility · Dental implants · Nanostructured materials · Osseointegration · Surface modification · Titanium

Abbreviations

ASTM	American Society for Testing and Materials
Ca-P	Calcium phosphate
CVD	Chemical vapor deposition
cp Ti	Commercial purity titanium
ECAP	Equal channel angular pressing
EFD	Electrophoretic deposition
FA	Fluoroapatite
hTNTs	Hexagonal titanium dioxide nanotubes
HA	Hydroxyapatite ($Ca_{10}(PO_4)_6(OH)_2$)
HCA	Hydroxycarbonate apatite
HPT	High-pressure torsion
IBAD	Ion-bean-assisted deposition

K. Jurczyk (✉)
Pure Clinic, Centre dentaire de Sion, Sion, Switzerland
e-mail: karolajur@gmail.com

M. U. Jurczyk
Division of Mother's and Child's Health, Poznań University of Medical Sciences, Poznań, Poland

R. Narayan (ed.), *Nanostructured Biomaterials and Their Applications*,
https://doi.org/10.1007/978-3-032-16316-5_3

MAO	Micro-arc oxidation
MMC	Metal matrix composites
NHOst	Normal human osteoblast cell
PVD	Physical vapor deposition
R_a	Arithmetic mean roughness
R_t	Maximum height of the profile
R_z	Ten-point mean roughness
ROS	Reactive oxygen species
SEM	Scanning electron microscopy
SPD	Severe plastic deformation
TMP	Thermomechanical pressing
45S5 Bioglass	(45% SiO_2, 24.5% Na_2O, 24.5 CaO, 6% P_2O_5)

1 Introduction

In 1959, Richard Feynman, a Physics Nobel laureate, presented his famous theory on nanostructure materials production (Feynman 1960). He stated: "The principles of physics, as far as I can see, do not speak against the possibility of maneuvering things atom by atom." Feynman proceeded to describe a building with atomic precision and outlined a pathway involving a series of increasingly smaller machines. Nanostructures represent key building blocks for nanoscale science and technology.

There are two key approaches (top down and bottom up) in nanotechnology for creating smaller or better materials and the use of smaller constituents in more complex assembling (Khurshid et al. 2015; Zhang and Webster 2009; Ozak and Ozkan 2013). A top-down approach is based on solid-state processing of materials. Regardless of the defects produced by this approach, they will continue to play an important role in the synthesis of nanostructures. The top-down approaches such as chemical vapor deposition (CVD), monolithic processing, wet and plasma etching are used to fabricate functional structures at micro and nanoscales. These methods are successfully used for coatings of medical implants and stents using CVD technology to enhance blood flow and biocompatibility.

Over the past 20 years, nanomaterials have become very popular in dental applications (Webster et al. 2001; Valiev et al. 2009; Jurczyk 2012; Tulinski et al. 2025; Webster and Ejiofor 2004; Jakubowicz et al. 2015; Baker 2005; Bugunia-Kubik and Susisaga 2002; Bayne 2007; Lindhe et al. 2003). Nanomaterials can exhibit enhanced mechanical, biological, and chemical properties compared with their conventional microcrystalline counterparts (Sul 2003; Oh et al. 2008; Jakubowicz 2008; Koper and Jakubowicz 2015). In recent years, the enhancement of bone formation at the bone-implant interface has been achieved through the modulation of osteoblast adhesion and spreading, induced by modifications at the nanoscale level on the implant surfaces (Valiev et al. 2009; Webster and Ejiofor 2004; Bressan et al. 2013; Long and Rack 1998).

The branches in dentistry where nanotechnology has become popular, apart from implantology, are tooth regeneration, periodontal therapy, soft and hard tissue reconstruction, bone repair, plaque control, caries diagnostics, and caries treatments (Table 1) (Khurshid et al. 2015).

Titanium and titanium alloys are preferred materials in the production of implants (Long and Rack 1998). Titanium appears in two different allotropic forms. At low temperatures, it has a closed-packed hexagonal crystal structure (space group: $P6_3/$ mmc–hcp), which is known as α, whereas above 882 ± 2 °C, it has a body-centered cubic structure (space group: Im-3 m-bcc) termed β. The alloying elements, such as N, O, and Al, tend to stabilize the α phase, whereas elements V, Cr, Nb, and Mo stabilize the β phase, at room temperature.

Currently, titanium and its alloys are used for dentistry devices such as implants, crowns, bridges, overdentures, and dental implant prosthesis components (screws and abutments). There are currently four cp Ti grades and one titanium alloy specially made for dental implant applications. These metals are specified according to the American Society for Testing and Materials (ASTM) as Grades 1–5. Grades 1–4 are unalloyed, while Grade 5, with 6% aluminum and 4% vanadium, is the strongest. However, for permanent implant applications, the Ti–6Al–4V alloy has a possible toxic effect resulting from released vanadium and aluminum (Matusiewicz 2014; Guehennec et al. 2007).

By the elimination of toxic elements, it is possible to prepare Ti-type alloys with excellent biocompatibility. Ti–6Al–7Nb, which has been developed for surgical implants, is also attractive for dental applications (Kobayashi et al. 1995). Ti–Nb–Zr alloys are one of the other substitutes, too (Mohsin et al. 2014; Wang et al. 2016; Marczewski et al. 2018, 2020a, b, c). It is due to the fact of their chemical composition the phase (β-type titanium alloys) structure, and mechanical properties stay

Table 1 Application of nanomaterials in dentistry (Khurshid et al. 2015)

Specialty of dentistry	Materials
Restorative dentistry	Ketac™, Ketac N100; Nano-ionomers, Filtek Supreme XT, Fuji IX GP, Nano-primer, Premise™, Adper™ single bond plus adhesive, Ceram X™
Regenerative dentistry and tissue engineering	Ostim®, VITOSSO™, Nano-bone®
Periodontics	Arestin®, Nanogen®
Preventive dentistry	NanoCare® gold
Orthodontics	Ketac™ N100 light curing Nano-ionomers, Filtek supreme plus universal
Prosthodontics	Nanotech elite H-D plus, GC OPTIGLAZE color®
Oral implantology	Nanotite™ Nano-coated implant, SLA®, SLAactive®, Roxolid®, TiUnite®
Endodontic	AH plus™, Epiphany, Guttaflow®

attractive in the biomedical field of application. The alloyed cubic titanium structure allows making the Young modulus much lower even 50 GPa. The above relation minimizes the risk of mechanical unfit between the bone tissue and the implant. The problems of bone resorption and loosening of the implants due to of stress-shielding effect could be in the above manner significantly reduced (Mohsin et al. 2014).

Recently, ternary Ti–Zr–Nb alloys with β and pseudo-β structures were synthesized (Marczewski et al. 2018, 2020a, b, c). The produced alloys were modified by composite formation and electrochemical surface modification. Zr and Nb as β-stabilizer have been proven to form a single-phase structure in the right composition range and process conditions. Moreover, the use of mechanical alloying has led to ultrafine-grained structure formation. The composites with 45S5 Bioglass addition have lower Young modulus and better corrosion properties than the base material. The addition of silver can additionally improve corrosion properties. One wt. % of silver, copper, and zinc addition has revealed high antibacterial activity against *Streptococcus mutans*. Surface modification with the calcium hydroxide and hydroxyapatite coating deposition has led to corrosion properties and wettability improvement, which should further impact the bone tissue growth on the materials' surface. The proliferation of the bone cells (both osteoblasts and fibroblasts) of all the produced materials was equal to or even better than that of commercially pure titanium Grade 2.

Many attempts were made to create other low modulus β Ti biomaterials (Lin et al. 2007; Ho et al. 1999; Zhang et al. 2015; Murray 1981). Molybdenum is less toxic than aluminum and vanadium. The solubility limit of alloying Mo metal in Ti is 8 wt% (Murray 1981). The phase constitutions, hardness, and Young modulus are different for different contents of molybdenum in Ti–Mo system (Zhang et al. 2015). The latest research has shown that the addition of Mo forms β-phase in Ti-base alloy, and finally, increases the hardness, decreases the Young modulus as well as improves the corrosion resistance and biocompatibility (Lin et al. 2007).

The effect of molybdenum content was investigated (10–35 at. %) on phase transformations and mechanical properties of alloys obtained in the processes of mechanical synthesis and powder metallurgy (both cold and hot approaches) (Sochacka et al. 2019a, b, 2020, 2021). Molybdenum as a Ti (β) phase stabilizer allowed for obtaining single-phase alloys by applying the hot pressing process or pseudo-β alloys by the cold pressing and sintering process. The application of the mechanical synthesis process leads to nano-scale size object formation. The lowest Young's modulus was obtained for composites (95 GPa, 4%) or alloys with high porosity (Ti31Mo 55 GPa, 29%).

Proposed surface treatment procedures led to the formation of apatite layers on selected alloys (Sochacka et al. 2021). Fluorapatite was deposited on the oxidized surface (MAO) of the Ti23Mo alloy by the application electrophoretic deposition method. After hydrothermal treatment of Ti31Mo alloy, the surface layer mostly consists of Ca_{10} $(PO_4)_6(OH)_2$ with $CaHPO_4{\cdot}2H_2O$. The Ti31Mo alloy was also modified by introducing hydroxyapatite and selected antibacterial additives.

The modification of the surface layer caused an improvement in the alloys' corrosion resistance and the surface's wettability, thus improving the proliferation of bone cells. The viability of osteoblasts and fibroblasts was higher or similar for composites compared to microcrystalline titanium. Moreover, for biomaterials containing silver or cerium (IV) oxide, the reduction factor for *Staphylococcus aureus* bacteria was over 97% (Sochacka et al. 2020).

Recent studies proved clearly that nanostructuring of titanium can improve considerably not only the mechanical properties but also the biocompatibility (Webster et al. 2001; Valiev et al. 2009; Tulinski et al. 2025; Webster and Ejiofor 2004; Bugunia-Kubik and Susisaga 2002; Bressan et al. 2013). This approach also enhances the biological response of the cp titanium (cp Ti) surface (Webster et al. 2001). For providing fast osseointegration and long-term usage in the human body, the implant surface should be modified; that is, it should be rough or porous, oxidized, and covered by biocompatible coating including calcium phosphate compounds (Tulinski et al. 2025; Webster and Ejiofor 2004; Sul 2003; Oh et al. 2008). Surfaces showing micro- and nano-irregularities are useful in biocompatibility improvements (Webster et al. 2001).

The application of new materials such as biomaterials and implants increases steadily. However, not all replacement systems have provided trouble-free service. In dental implants, the rate of success is 98.6% after 5 years post-loading (Beschnidt et al. 2018). None of the failed implants presented the regular surface composition and depth profile of the TiO_2 overlayer; foreign elements (Ca, Na, P, Si, Cl, Zn, Pb, and Al) were observed on some implants (Arys et al. 1998). Fibrosis, lymphocytic and plasmocytic infiltrates, and granulomatous lesions were detected in the surrounding tissues. An appropriate surface modification would prevent their transfer into nearby tissues. The absence of debris particle generation is crucial for the prevention of implant malfunction.

This chapter provides an overview of the most common manufacturing techniques and the related cell-surface interactions and modulation. The discussion includes a range of different types of available nanoproducts and their potential in dentistry.

2 Surface Modification Methods of Titanium

To overcome the poor tribological properties of Ti and its alloys and to obtain significant property improvements in mechanical and medical aspects, there is a need for compositional modification. A generally known classification distinguishes bulk and surface modification approaches. The first approach is based on a change in the bulk microstructure simultaneously with grain size modification. Metal matrix composites (MMC) are an example of a proper engineering approach for the improvement of properties in the bulk stage. The second approach leads to the same property improvements, but only at the surface scale.

Different surface modifications are available. For example, electrochemical treatments, thermochemical surface treatments (such as boriding, oxidizing, carburization, and nitriding (Jakubowicz 2008; Koper and Jakubowicz 2015; Sarma and Chandran 2011; He et al. 2006; Jakubowicz et al. 2009)), physical vapor deposition (PVD), and chemical vapor deposition (CVD) methods could also be assisted by plasma. Different plasma modification techniques are commonly applied to functionalize the biomaterials (Wang et al. 2008; Miklaszewski et al. 2013). Those methods provide an in situ process for chemically tailored surfaces, without compromising the inherent, favorable bulk properties of the biomaterials. Robust progress seems to be implied by energy beam surface modification techniques like electron beam alloying or laser and plasma techniques such as cladding, particle injection, and surface alloying (Miklaszewski et al. 2013, 2011).

Nanoscale modification can alter the chemistry and/or topography of the implant surface (Jakubowicz 2008; Koper and Jakubowicz 2015; Jakubowicz et al. 2009; Jakubowicz and Adamek 2009). Many methods are available for imparting nanoscale features to the implant surface (Table 2) (Mendonça et al. 2008). Surface modification methods for titanium and titanium alloys include the physical, chemical, and mechanical methods used for morphological modifications (roughness) and for obtaining different coatings on the surface of the implants (hydroxyapatite (HA), biomimetic calcium phosphate, and biomolecule functionalized coatings) as well as a mixture of morphological changes and coatings for a combined synergistic effect. The final goals are to improve the wear and corrosion resistance of titanium and titanium alloys as well as biocompatibility for different medical applications.

Several of these methods have already been used to modify implants available commercially (Mendonça et al. 2008; Stanford 2008). Such changes alter the implant surface interaction with ions, biomolecules, and cells. These interactions can favorably influence molecular and cellular activities and alter the process of osseointegration.

Nanoscale surfaces possess high surface energy, leading to increased initial protein adsorption, which is very important in regulating the cellular interactions on the implant surface. Surface properties also have an impact on adhesion, together with charge distribution and the chemistry of the material (Webster et al. 2001; Valiev et al. 2009; Bressan et al. 2013; Sarma and Chandran 2011). It was recently observed that the roughness of titanium nanostructures alone influences the adhesion of osteoblast cells and their spreading and proliferation (Mendonça et al. 2008).

To date, a few nanoscale surface topography modifications have been used to enhance bone responses at clinical dental implants (Davarpanah et al. 2002; Coelho and Suzuki 2005; Valiev et al. 2007; Valiev et al. 2008; Cao and Hench 1966; Hench 1991). For example, the OsseoSpeed surface (Astra Tech AB, Molndal, Sweden) possesses nanostructured features created by TiO_2 blasting followed by a proprietary hydrofluoric acid treatment (Rocci et al. 2008). The Astra Tech TiOblast is the precursor of the OsseoSpeed surface. This surface was grit blasted with titanium dioxide particles to achieve an isotropic, moderately roughened surface. OsseoSpeed was launched in the fall of 2004 and was a further development of the moderately roughened (grit blasted with titanium dioxide particles) titanium surface TiOblast. OsseoSpeed gains its additional surface characteristics via a chemical (fluoride) treatment and a slight topographic modification of the TiOblast surface (Ellingsen 2005).

Table 2 Overview of methods used for creating nanofeatures on cp titanium implants

Method	Modified layer	Objective
Physical		
Plasma spray	Coatings such as HA, bioglass, and boron-surface-modified layer	Improve wear-resistance, corrosion-resistance, and biological properties
Physical vapor deposition	TiN, TiC, TiCN, and thin film HA coating	Improve wear-resistance, corrosion-resistance, and biological properties
Ion implantation and deposition	Surface modification, layer, and thin film	Surface composition modification—improve wear-resistance, corrosion-resistance, and biological properties
Chemical		
Sol-gel	Thin films of calcium	Improve wear-resistance, corrosion-resistance, and biological properties
Chemical vapor deposition	Phosphate, TiO_2, and silica TiN, TiC, TiCN, and thin film HA coating	Improve wear-resistance, corrosion-resistance, and biological properties
Anodic oxidation	TiO_2 layers with specific surface topographies	Improve wear-resistance, corrosion-resistance, and biological properties
Cathodic deposition	Ca–P deposition	Improve corrosion-resistance and biological properties
Chemical treatments such as acidic, alkaline, and with hydrogen peroxide	Oxide layers, Sodium Titanate gel	Remove oxides and contaminations; improve biocompatibility
Biochemical methods	Coating deposition	Induce specific cell and tissue
Mechanical		
Severe plastic deformation mechanical alloying and powder metallurgy	Bulk ultrafine grain metals/alloys Alloys with nanostructure and nanocomposites	Improve mechanical and biological properties Improve mechanical properties, corrosion-resistance, and biological properties

Another nanoscale surface implant presently available in the clinical marketplace involves a Ca-P nanoparticle modification of a minimally rough titanium alloy implant (Rocci et al. 2008). The NanoTite implant starts with the industry-proven OSSEOTITE surface at the core. Next, discrete nanometer-scale crystals of calcium phosphate (Ca-P) are deposited onto the OSSEOTITE surface substrate. The nanoscale Ca-P surface created by DCD (NanoTite, 3i) was evaluated (Rocci et al. 2008). The histologic evaluation of clinical implants revealed bone-to-implant contact of 19% ± 14.2% and 32.2% ± 18.5% for the OSSEOTITE (3i) control and the NanoTite (3i) experimental implants, respectively.

Recently, the ion beam-assisted deposition (IBAD) process, which provides increased integration with the implant surface, known as high-energy sputter deposition, has been used to create a commercially available dental implant surface (Coelho and Suzuki 2005). In the NanoTite process, a high-energy ion beam source aims at a beam of ions at the surface of a target treated with HA. These high-energy ions eject the basic chemical elements of the HA from the target/substrate and create a molecular cloud whose molecules bond with the surface of the bicon Integra-Ti implant.

3 Bulk Nanostructured Titanium

Prostheses on osseointegrated dental implants have become a standard of care in the management of edentulous and partially edentulous patients. Titanium and titanium alloys have been the preferred materials in the production of fixed substitutes for roots of lost teeth (Long and Rack 1998; Wang 1996).

To date, several severe plastic deformations (SPDs) methods for producing bulk ultrafine grain metals/alloys have been developed (Valiev et al. 2009, 2007, 2008). Valiev and coworkers applied a process known as equal channel angular pressing (ECAP), which is a viable pro cessing route to grain refinement and property improvement (Valiev et al. 2007). Nanostructuring was performed using SPD by ECAP with subsequent thermomechanical processing (TMP), which made it possible to manufacture rod semi-products with a length of 3 m and a diameter of 7 mm. This processing resulted in a significant reduction in grain size, from the 25-μm-equiaxed grain structure of the initial titanium rods to 150 nm after combined SPD and TMT processing. Mechanical properties of conventionally processed and nanostructured cp Grade 4 titanium are summarized in Table 3. The strength of the nanostructured titanium is nearly twice that of conventional cp Ti. Additionally, the fatigue strength of nanostructured cp Ti in 10^6 cycles is almost twice that of microcrystalline Ti and surpasses that of Ti–6Al–4V alloy.

Cytocompatibility tests utilizing fibroblast mice cells L929 were carried out. After nanostructuring, fibroblast colonization of the cp Grade 4 titanium surface dramatically increases. For example, the surface cell occupation for conventional cp Ti was 53.0% after 72 h in contrast to 87.2% for nanostructured cp Grade 4. Compared to conventional titanium, a high osteointegration rate should be expected with nanostructured cp Grade 4 titanium.

The certified system of Timplant manufactured according to standard EN ISO 13485:2003 was used during the development of the Nano implant (Valiev et al. 2007, 2008). Nanostructuring of titanium by SPD processing has made the material's mechanical performance significantly superior to that of conventional cp Grade 4 titanium and Ti–6Al–4V alloy.

Table 3 Mechanical properties of conventionally processed and nanostructured cp Grade 4 Ti (Valiev et al. 2008)

Processing/ treatment conditions	UTS (MPa)	YS (MPa)	Elongation (%)	Reduction area (%)	Fatigue strength at 10^6 cycles
Conventional Ti (as received)	700	530	25	52	340
*n*Ti ECAP + TMT	1240	1200	12	42	620
Ti-6Al-4 V ELI annealed	940	840	16	45	530

A satisfactory clinical outcome depends on the capability of the implant to bear loads, which is obtained by primary stability immediately following implantation. However, long-term outcomes are the result of solid osseointegration of the implant into the host bone. The characteristics of the implant surface itself are of critical importance for the progression toward osseointegration (Mendonça et al. 2008; Albrektsson et al. 1981; Ehrenfest et al. 2010). Cell biological as well as biomechanical properties of the biomaterial play a crucial role in the initial formation of the bone-implant system. An open-porous structure and adequate pore sizes are the determinants for bone ingrowth (Ehrenfest et al. 2010; Brånemark 1983; Miklaszewski et al. 2017).

4 Bulk Titanium-Bioceramic Nanocomposites

One method that allows the change of mechanical, chemical, and biological properties of Ti and Ti-based alloys is to produce a nanocomposite, which will exhibit the favorable mechanical properties of titanium and the excellent biocompatibility and bioactivity properties of ceramics (Zhang and Webster 2009; Jurczyk 2012). The main ceramics used in medicine are HA (Ca_{10} $(PO_4)_6(OH)_2$) and 45S5 Bioglass (Jurczyk 2012; Marczewski et al. 2020c; Sochacka et al. 2020; Cao and Hench 1966; Hench 1991).

In 2011, mechanical alloying and powder metallurgy processes for the fabrication of titanium-45S5 Bioglass nanocomposites with a unique microstructure, higher hardness, and better corrosion resistance were developed (Table 4) (Jakubowicz et al. 2009; Jurczyk et al. 2011a; b, c). Microhardness tests showed that the obtained material exhibits Vickers microhardness as high as 770 $HV_{0.2}$ for Ti-20 wt% 45S5 Bioglass, which is more than three times higher than that of conventional microcrystalline titanium. Additionally, titanium-10 wt% of 45S5 Bioglass nanocomposites ($i_c = 1.20 \times 10^{-7}$A/cm^2, $E_c = ^-0.42$ V vs. SCE) were more corrosion resistant than microcrystalline titanium.

Table 4 Microhardness, mean values of corrosion current densities, and corrosion potentials of studied Ti-10 wt% 45S5 Bioglass nanocomposite scaffolds with different porosities in comparison with bulk Ti-10 wt% 45S5 Bioglass nanocomposite and microcrystalline titanium (Jurczyk et al. 2011a)

Sample	$HV_{0.2}$	i_C [A cm^{-2}]	E_C versus SCE (V)
Ti-10 wt% 45S5 with a porosity of 48%	–	3.63×10^{-6}	– 0.51
Ti-10 wt% 45S5 with a porosity of 67%	–	4.23×10^{-6}	– 0.49
Ti-10 wt% 45S5 with a porosity of 72%	–	4.71×10^{-6}	– 0.56
Bulk Ti-10 wt% 45S5 bioglass	620	1.20×10^{-7}	– 0.42
Ti (microcrystalline, grade 2)	225	2.27×10^{-6}	– 0.36

Young's modulus of the sintered Ti-10 wt% 45S5 Bioglass composite was found to be 110 GPa. The measured value of Young's modulus for microcrystalline titanium is about 150 GPa. From the point of view of future application for hard tissue replacement implants, a biomaterial with low elastic modulus is anticipated because the elastic modulus of natural bone is low (7–25 GPa). Implants with high elastic modulus can lead to severe stress concentration, namely load shielding from a natural bone, therefore destroying the implant/bone surface as well as the bone.

Nanograined materials due to a very high number of atoms on the surface possess high surface energy. Thus, they exhibit entirely different behavior than the micron-sized grains. The bone-forming cells generally attach themselves to the surface whose roughness is of nanometer range. It has been shown that composition, roughness, and surface energy affect the initial adhesion and spreading of cells (Miklaszewski et al. 2017).

In vitro, biocompatibility of these materials was evaluated and compared with conventional microcrystalline titanium, where normal human osteoblast (NHOst) cells from Cambrex (CC-2538) were cultured on the disks of the materials, and cell growth was examined (Fig. 1). The morphology of the cell cultures obtained on Ti-10 wt% 45S5 Bioglass nanocomposite was similar to those obtained on the microcrystalline titanium. On the other hand, on a porous scaffold, the cells adhered with their whole surface to the insert penetrating the porous structure, while on the polished surface, more spherical cells were observed with a smaller surface of adhesion.

Numerous reports demonstrate that the surface roughness of titanium implants affects the rate of osseointegration and biomechanical fixation (Mendonça et al. 2008). Surface roughness can be divided into three levels depending on the scale of the features: macrosized, microsized, and nanosized topologies. The macro level is defined for topographical features as being in the range of millimeters to tens of microns. The microtopographic profile of dental implants is defined for surface roughness as being in the range of 1–10 μm. This range of roughness maximizes the interlocking between mineralized bone and the surface of the implant. Surface profiles in the nanometer range play an important role in the adsorption of proteins and

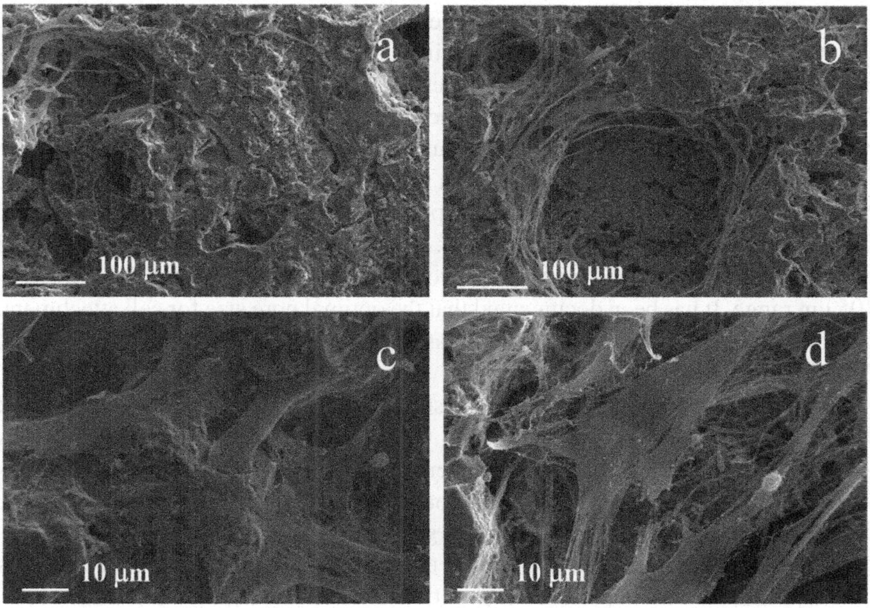

Fig. 1 Scanning electron micrographs of osteoblasts cultured on Ti-10 wt% 45S5 Bioglass scaffolds with 67% porosity after 1 day (**a**) and after 5 days (**b**); original magnification 5000×

the adhesion of osteoblastic cells, and thus in the rate of osseointegration (Webster et al. 2001; Valiev et al. 2009; Bressan et al. 2013; Guehennec et al. 2007).

The commercial Ti dental implant produced by mechanical cutting has a surface roughness R_a ranging from about 0.08 to 1.3 μm (Godarzi et al. 2008). Recent studies demonstrate that surface roughness affects cell spreading and proliferation, but not cell attachment, of human osteoblast-like cells (Rocci et al. 2008; Williams 1987). These findings indicate that modification of surface roughness might provide a more suitable microenvironment for early osteoblast response to implant materials (Krivoruchko et al. 2010). Cultures of human osteoblast-like cells revealed no significant difference in initial cell attachment among the various surfaces with surface roughness ($R_a = 0.0374$, 0.0911, and 0.2435 μm); however, cell spread was greater on rough surfaces than on glass slides and smoother surfaces. In addition, cell proliferation and Ki-67 expression were increased when cells were cultured on rough surfaces. These results suggest that a greater Ti–6Al–7Nb surface roughness supports the initial spread and proliferation of human osteoblast-like cells. Thus, modification of the surface roughness of dental implants might hasten osseointegration.

The process of osseointegration takes place in vitro as well as in vivo in four stages (Godarzi et al. 2008; Mendonça et al. 2008). In the first stage, stem cells and osteoblast precursor cells migrate to the implant and adhere to it by the formation of foot-like migration processes. In the second stage, the cells begin to be anchored onto the substrate wall with the help of matrix proteins and produce a dense network of matrix proteins at the implant. The mineralization of the extracellular matrix occurs in stage three and is dependent on the differentiation of osteoblasts. In the last stage, the network of extracellular matrix proteins and osteoblasts reorganizes and forms lamellar bone (Lee et al. 2007; Lefebvre et al. 2007).

The surface roughness parameters such as R_a, R_t, and R_z of the different Ti-based substrates are shown in Table 5 (Jurczyk et al. 2011a). The microcrystalline titanium presents a smooth surface with very low values of R_a, R_t, and R_z. The bulk Ti-10 wt% 45S5 Bioglass nanocomposite has R_a, R_t, and R_z values of around 0.91, 12.99, and 10.21 μm, respectively. The Ti-10 wt% 45S5 Bioglass scaffold with 67% porosity has average surface roughness, with R_a, R_t, and R_z in the 54–405 μm range. It has been documented that the optimal pore size for cell attachment, differentiation, and ingrowth of osteoblasts and vascularization is approximately 200–500 μm (Mendonça et al. 2008).

Surface characteristics of materials, such as their topography, chemistry, and surface energy, play an essential part in osteoblast adhesion to biomaterials (Mendonça et al. 2008). Studies have demonstrated that nanostructured materials with cell-favorable surface properties may promote greater amounts of specific protein interactions to stimulate new bone growth as compared to conventional materials (Williams 1987; Li et al. 2004). This may be one of the underlying mechanisms making nanomaterials superior to conventional materials for tissue growth.

In vitro cytocompatibility of bulk Ti-10 wt% 45S5 Bioglass nanocomposites and their scaffolds were also investigated independently (Figs. 2 and 3) (Kaczmarek et al. 2014). During the studies, an established cell line of human fibroblasts CCD-39Lu was cultured in the presence of tested materials, and its survival rate and proliferation activity were examined. There were no cytotoxic properties of the tested materials against cells from CCD-39Lu cell line. An evaluation of the survival rate demonstrated that the growth of CCD-39Lu fibroblasts cultured in the presence of both nanocrystalline and microcrystalline materials depends on the quantity of suspended material. The viability of cells in the culture decreased simultaneously with the increase of the tested material in the culture. Fibroblasts' survival rate at 24 and 48 h of culture was more intensively inhibited in the presence of a microcrystalline Ti compared to the nanocrystalline Ti-10 wt% 45S5 Bioglass powder. CCD-39Lu fibroblasts cultured in the presence of Ti-45S5 Bioglass nanocomposite in an amount of 0.005 mg/mL showed a higher survival rate as compared to the control population (Fig. 2).

Table 5 Roughness values R_a, R_t, and R_z (DIN) of the three surfaces used for culturing NHOst cells (the values are mean ± SD) (Jurczyk et al. 2011a)

	R_a (μm)	R_t (μm)	R_z (DIN) (μm)
Microcrystalline Ti (grade 2)[a]	0.21 ± 0.06	4.92 ± 0.61	3.61 ± 0.29
Bulk Ti-10 wt% 45S5[a]	0.91 ± 0.09	12.99 ± 0.75	10.21 ± 0.63
Ti-10 wt% 45S5 with porosity of 67%	54 ± 5	405 ± 25	392 ± 20

R_a, arithmetic mean roughness; R_t, maximum height of the profile; R_z, ten-point mean roughness.
[a]Polished surface

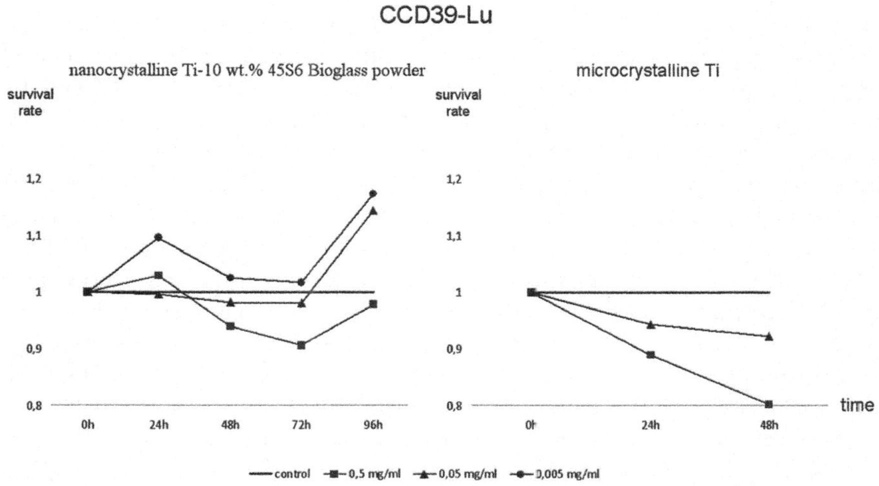

Fig. 2 MTT test results. Survival rate of CCD39-Lu cell line cultured in the presence of Ti–10 wt % 45S5 Bioglass nanocomposite and microcrystalline Ti, both in powder form

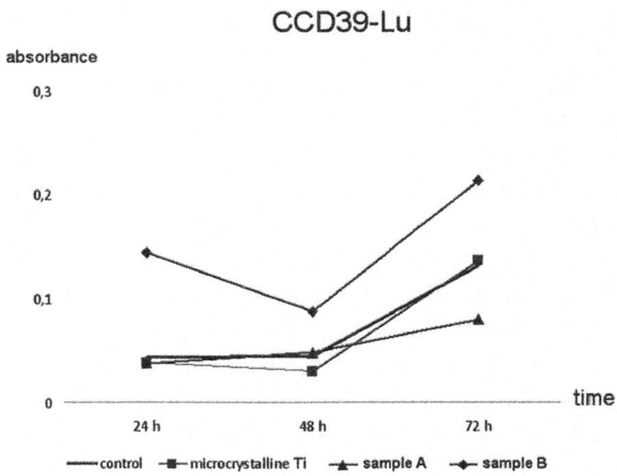

Fig. 3 MTT test results. Survival rate of CCD39-Lu cell line cultured in the presence of Ti-10 wt.% 45S5 Bioglass nanocomposite (sample A) and their scaffold (sample B), and microcrystalline Ti, both in the form of a disk

The study indicated that the nanocrystalline Ti-10 wt% 45S5 Bioglass scaffold showing the porous structure potentiated the survival rate of CCD-39Lu fibroblasts. Nanocrystalline scaffold material (sample B) in the form of a disk affects the survival rate of treated cells similarly as in the powder form—that is, intensifies the survival rate of CCD-39Lu fibroblasts (Fig. 3). In vitro biocompatibility studies showed that regardless of the type of material tested (nanocrystalline or microcrystalline), Ti-10 wt% 45S5 Bioglass samples did not show cytotoxic properties against cultured cells. Despite this, the intensity of cell growth on the surface is dependent on the surface structure of the sample. The obtained results suggest that the nanocrystalline sample displays good cytocompatibility compared to microcrystalline titanium. The survival rate of CCD-39Lu fibroblasts was higher in the presence of the nanocrystalline material as compared with microcrystalline material in the same concentrations of the same intervals. On the other hand, the survival rate of CCD-39Lu fibroblasts increased proportionally to the decrease on the amount of nanocrystalline material in powder form in the sample. Most likely, the quantity of the powdered tested material presented in the sample is crucial to the process of cell adhesion to the background. The barrier formed from tested material and the lack of physical contact of cells with the surface limit their ability to start subdivision processes. The proliferative activity of CCD-39Lu fibroblasts cultured in the presence of a nanocrystalline material correlates with the viability of these cells in the culture and is dependent on the quantity of associated material. The percentage of replicating cells increases simultaneously with a decreasing amount of tested material in the culture. However, note that a lack of cytotoxicity is not yet cell integrity.

An independent study showed that nanocrystalline Ti-10 wt% 45S5 Bioglass materials (scaffold and bulk) regardless of the form (powder or disk) do not affect the viability of *Candida albicans* and do not inhibit the growth of yeast on direct or indirect contact (Kaczmarek et al. 2014). Although tested nanomaterials do not have a negative influence on yeast, their structure and/or surface limits the growth of tested *Candida* yeast. Knowledge of the interaction of fungal cells and materials, from which dental implants are produced, is still poor and requires further detailed studies at a molecular level.

The best surface of the implant, from the viewpoint of cell biology, provides adequate adhesion and initiation of the cell subdivision process. However, these processes should be performed without an excessive growth rate, which could lead to cells escaping from the surveillance agents and exceeding the barriers of carcinogenesis. It still seems very important to develop such materials or composites for the production of dental implants that will demonstrate a reduced susceptibility to colonization and that upon implantation in the oral cavity will not cause pathogenic effects. Because the shape of the surface is often critical to tissue function, it seems that the nanocrystalline Ti-10 wt% 45S5 Bioglass scaffold may be an important step toward the production of such a structure, because it can support the process of adaptation of the implant by the host organism. Scaffold Ti-10 wt% 45S5 Bioglass nanocomposite would offer new structural and functional properties for innovative products in dental applications. An in vitro biocompatibility evaluation demonstrated that Ti-10 wt% 45S5 Bioglass nanocomposites display better cytocompatibility compared to that of microcrystalline titanium (Kaczmarek et al. 2014).

5 Nanostructured Surfaces

Among the many surface treatment technologies applied for Ti, the electrochemical one is very useful, giving surface roughening and new chemical and phase composition that improves surface biocompatibility (Jakubowicz 2008). Anodic oxidation results in the formation of rough titanium oxide, which improves osseointegration.

The oxidation process can be done in standard conditions and can be supported by a spark-discharge process in the plasma electrolytic oxidation (PEO), done at high voltages (Huang et al. 2005). As a result, the formation of different-sized pores or cavities as well as nanotubes is possible (Jakubowicz et al. 2015). Anodically oxidized titanium-based dental implants are commonly available (Guehennec et al. 2007). By carefully choosing the oxidation conditions, it is possible to control the oxide thickness, which is correlated with its color (Yang et al. 2006).

During and after implantation, there is a risk of bacterial attack in the wound tissue. To avoid this undesirable postoperative effect, introducing an antibacterial agent into the implant surface layer is possible and highly recommended. The commonly known antibacterial agents are silver ions; however, it should be noted that too many silver ions will act against osseointegration. Cytotoxicity of silver nanoparticles at a concentration of 8 μg/cm^2 to *Escherichia coli* was reported (Rai et al. 2009). The large surface area to volume ratio of silver nanoparticles allows for good antibacterial behavior (Chen and Schleusener 2008).

The surface, which is oxidized and has a porous topography, is an excellent template for the controlled introduction of silver ions. The preferential deposition mechanism of silver nano dendrites, which are deposited inside the pits in the oxide layer, has been observed (Koper and Jakubowicz 2015). So, the surface pits have a positive effect on both osteoblast cells and antibacterial nanoparticle attachment.

In 2016, biocompatibility in vitro of the Ti, which was anodically oxidized at high voltages with additionally deposited Ag in the form of nano dendrites, was studied (Kaczmarek et al. 2016). Biocompatibility of the tested material was referred to as established cell lines of human osteoblasts and gingival fibroblasts. Both osteoblasts and gingival fibroblasts are the major cellular elements that determine the osseointegration and the acceptance of implants in the oral cavity. During the studies, an established cell line of human gingival fibroblasts (HGF) and osteoblasts was cultured in the presence of tested materials, and its survival rate and proliferation activity were examined. Titanium samples modified with silver had a higher degree of biocompatibility in comparison with the unmodified reference material. Cells in contact with the studied material showed a higher relative viability potential, a stable level of proliferation activity, and a lower rate of mortality. Biocompatibility tests carried out indicated that the anodically oxidized titanium at high voltages with additionally deposited nanosilver may be a possible candidate for dental implants and other medicinal applications.

Current studies are focused on the synthesis of β-type titanium nanocrystalline alloys and composites (Sochacka et al. 2019a, 2021; Jurczyk et al. 2015, 2016; Jakubowicz et al. 2012). For example, the β type Ti23Mo-x wt% 45S5 Bioglass ($x =$ 0, 3, and 10) nanocomposites were synthesized by mechanical alloying and powder metallurgy methods (Jurczyk et al. 2016). The crystallization of the amorphous material upon annealing led to the formation of a nanostructured β type Ti23Mo alloy with a grain size of approximately 40 nm. With the increase of the 45S5 Bioglass contents in Ti23Mo, a nanocomposite increase of the α-phase was noticeable. The surface improvement was achieved by electrochemical treatment, which comprised two stages: anodic oxidation and Ca–P deposition. The porous surface was produced by anodic oxidation in 1 M H_3PO_4 + 2%HF electrolyte at 10 V for 30 min. Next, the Ca-P layer was deposited onto the formed porous surface, using cathodic potential − 5 V kept for 60 min in 0.042 M $Ca(NO_3)_2$ + 0.025 M $(NH_4)_2HPO_4$ + 0.1 M HCl electrolyte. The deposited Ca-P layer is anchored in the pores. Corrosion resistance potentiodynamic testing in a Ringer solution at 37 °C showed a positive effect of porosity and Ca–P deposition on nanostructured Ti23Mo 3 wt% 45S5 Bioglass nanocomposite. The contact angles of glycerol on the nanostructured Ti23Mo alloy were determined and showed a visible decrease for bulk Ti23Mo 3 wt% 45S5 Bioglass and etched Ti23Mo 3 wt% 45S5 Bioglass nanocomposites. In vitro tests of normal human osteoblast (NHOst) cells showed very good cell proliferation, colonization, and multilayering (Fig. 4). It has been shown that surfaces with appropriate chemical composition and topography, after combined electrochemical anodic and cathodic surface treatments, support osteoblast adhesion and proliferation.

Recently, ternary Ti–Zr–Nb alloys with β and pseudo-β structures by the mechanical alloying approach were synthesized (Marczewski et al. 2018, 2020a, b, c). Zr and Nb as β-stabilizer have been proven to form a single-phase structure in the right composition range and process conditions. Moreover, the use of mechanical alloying has led to ultrafine-grained structure formation. The composites with 45S5 Bioglass addition have lower Young modulus and better corrosion properties than the base material. The addition of silver can additionally improve corrosion properties. One

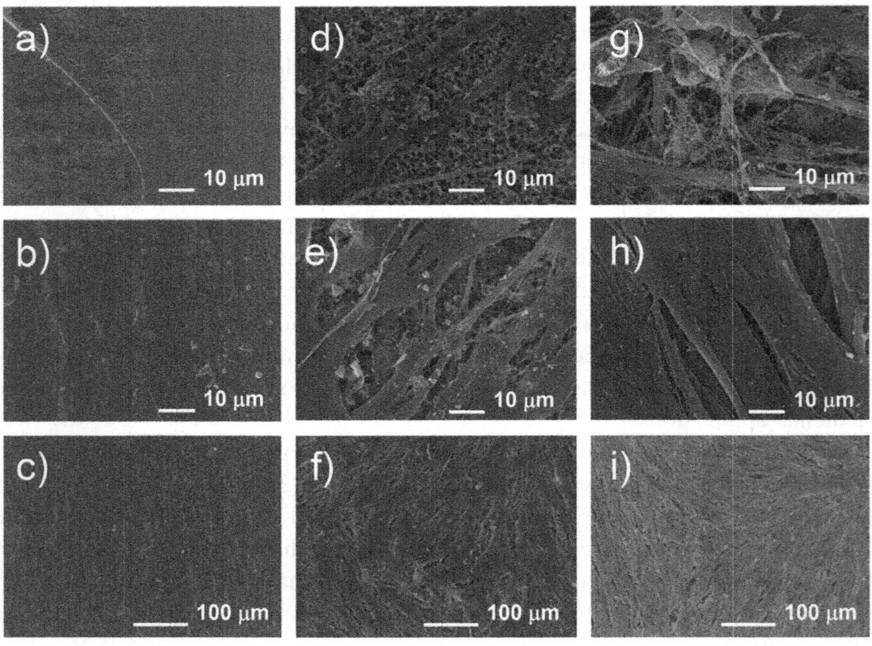

Fig. 4 Osteoblast culture on the surface of the Ti23Mo-3 wt% 45S5 Bioglass nanocomposite before etching (**a–c**), after etching (**d–f**), after etching with additional Ca–P deposition (**g–i**), after the first day (**a**, **d**, **g**), and after fifth day ((**b**, **c**), (**e**, **f**), and (**h**, **i**)), with different magnifications

wt. % of silver, copper, and zinc addition has revealed high antibacterial activity against *S. mutans*. Surface modification with the calcium hydroxide and hydroxyapatite coating deposition has led to corrosion properties and wettability improvement, which should further impact the bone tissue growth on the materials' surface. The proliferation of the bone cells (both osteoblasts and fibroblasts) of all the produced materials was equal to or even better than that of commercially pure titanium Grade 2.

The crystal structure, microstructure, mechanical, and corrosion properties of bulk Ti31MoxHA composites ($x = 0$, 2.5, 5, and 10 wt %) were investigated (Sochacka et al. 2019a, b, 2020, 2021). All these composites have elastic modulus lower than CP microcrystalline a-Ti, and their hardness is two times higher. The ultrafine Ti31Mo5HA composite was more corrosion-resistant in the Ringer solution than the bulk Ti31Mo alloy. Surface wettability measurements revealed the higher surface hydrophilicity of the bulk ultrafine-grained Ti31Mo10HA sample in comparison to the microcrystalline Ti sample. Ti31Mo5HA composites with the addition of 1 wt % Ag, 2 wt % Ta_2O_5, or 2 wt % CeO_2 were synthesized, too. The antibacterial activity of Ti31Mo5HA composite containing silver (Ag), tantalum (V) oxide (Ta_2O_5), or cerium (IV) oxide (CeO_2) against *S. aureus* was studied. In vitro bacterial adhesion studies indicated a significantly reduced number of *S. aureus* on the bulk ultrafine-grained Ti31Mo5HA-Ag (CeO_2) plate surfaces compared to microcrystalline Ti plate surfaces. Ultrafine-grained Ti31Mo5HA-Ag or Ti31Mo5HA-CeO_2 biomaterials can be considered the future generation of medical implants.

Additionally, for the Ti23Mo alloy, the micro-arc oxidation (MAO) and electrophoretic deposition (EPD) approaches were applied and led to the formation of apatite and fluorapatite (FA) layers, which improved analyzed surface properties compared to the base sample (Sochacka et al. 2019b). The structural analysis of obtained modified surfaces confirms, besides strong Ti(β)substrate reflexes for MAO, a complex composition based on the oxides-Ti_6O (01-073-1118)/$CaTiO_3$ (01-075-0437), hydroxides-$Ca(OH)_2$ (04-014-7726), and apatite-$Ca_3(PO_4)_2$ (00-048-0488) mixture, as for EPD a fluorapatite layer (FA 01-071-0881). The morphological view of the samples revealed on SEM microphotographs allows the characterization of the obtained surfaces as highly developed ones, with a specific formation. The EPD process fully obscures the MAO procedure, however, what remains important and confirmed in FA layer formation (Kazek-Kesik et al. 2014; Bai et al. 2016; Erakovi'c et al. 2013) is the influence of the substrate relation.

To improve the surface properties of titanium and expand titanium clinical application, boride microplasma surface alloying has been applied to modify titanium sur face, as well (Miklaszewski et al. 2013; Miklaszewski et al. 2011). Plasma surface alloying provides a wide range of layer thicknesses, which is controlled by the amount of the powder and process parameters. In our recent work, nano precursors with 2 and 10 wt% boron content were deposited onto microcrys talline titanium substrate by microplasma alloying. The formation of TiB phase precipitation was confirmed. The Vicker's microhardness was significantly improved from 180 HV for the original titanium substrate to 900 HV in the composite layer structure obtained, with a smooth hardness reduction in the cross-section profile. Strong heat penetration from a microplasma melt-in technique led to substrate dissolution with the formation of a stable TiB phase dispersed in the α-Ti matrix. The electrochemical treatment in phosphoric acid electrolyte resulted in a developed surface formation, attractive for tissue fixing and growth. The results of the in vitro test suggest that the TiB phase dispersed in the α-Ti matrix displays good cytocompatibility compared to that of microcrystalline titanium. Additionally, the SEM observation reveals a significant difference in the morphological characteristics of cells on developed and polished material, after only one day of cell culture. It can be concluded that plasma alloying is an effective method for producing TiB phase dispersed in α-Ti matrix with high hardness, and good cytocompatibility, which makes it a potential candidate for biomedical applications.

Plasma boriding of titanium is a promising method for improving the properties of this metal. The in vitro biocompatibility results of this study can be summarized as follows: (i) samples of titanium modified by boron showed satisfactory properties in terms of effects on survival and proliferative activity of HGF and osteoblasts and (ii) nano precursors with 2 wt% boron affected the more intense proliferative activity of fibroblasts and osteoblasts, while nano precursors with 10 wt% boron affected more stable growth.

Recently, much attention has been paid to the TiO_2 nanotube preparation on dense titanium implants using anodization (Goodarzi and Moztarzadeh 2016; Arkusz et al. 2018; Singhatanadgit et al. 2018; Voltrova et al. 2019; Arkusz et al. 2020; Nycz et al. 2020). Anodizing titanium foil is the most favorable method for the synthesis of self-ordered TiO_2 nanotube arrays because of its unique advantages. This technique is a simple, controllable, and repeatable process, and allows to regulate of the thickness and pore diameter (Arkusz et al. 2018). TiO_2 nanotubes can promote the differentiation and proliferation of bone marrow mesenchymal stem cells, osteoblasts, and chondrocytes, and greatly improve the ability to integrate the implant surface and surrounding bone tissue. Porous Ti mimics the morphology of the external cellular membranes of the osteoblasts that surround the implant. It causes nanosurface mechanisms to increase the rate of initial osseointegration between the Ti nanotube and the surrounding tissue, greatly increasing the strength of the bond between implant and bone. In addition, the physical and mechanical properties of titanium dioxide nanotubes as an implantable material depend on their geometric dimensions, which can be controlled by the selection of anodizing process parameters such as current density, voltage, time, electrolyte temperature, composition, and pH even by electrolyte aging. As shown in previous studies (Arkusz et al. 2020; Nycz et al. 2020), TiO_2 nanotubes with a diameter of about 15 nm strongly promote adhesion, proliferation, and differentiation of stem cells, and a diameter of about 100 nm turned out to be harmful because they induced programmed cell death (apoptosis). Voltrova et al. (2019) showed that nanotubes with a diameter ranging from 70 to 100 nm not only promote the adhesion of stem cells but also their differentiation to osteoblasts. Not only mesenchymal stem cells but also hematopoietic stem cells and endothelial cells show this selective response to TiO_2 nanotubes with different diameters.

The electrolyte composition and oxidation condition affect the surface state and finally result in the formation of a continuous oxide layer or a layer that consists of pits, pores, or nanotubes enlarging the surface roughness, which differentiates and enhances its biocompatibility (Arkusz et al. 2020; Nycz et al. 2020). Previous attempts at nanotubular layer formation on Ti6Al4V ELI foil, as well as on cervical screws, allow for the production of a layer of regular nanotubes (Arkusz et al. 2020). But these were nonhomogeneous and cracked. There are still numerous research gaps that prevent their successful shift to clinical testing and the commercial market.

The electrochemical and mechanical properties of hexagonal titanium dioxide nanotubes (hTNTs) have been studied recently (Arkusz et al. 2024). The fabrication process involved sonoelectrochemical anodization of titanium foil in various electrolytes to obtain titanium oxide layers with different morphologies. Scanning electron microscopy revealed the formation of well-ordered hexagonal TNTs with diagonals in the range of 30–95 nm and heights in the range of 3500–4000 nm. Electrochemical measurements performed in 3.5% NaCl and Ringer's solution confirmed a more positive open-circuit potential, lower impedance, higher electrical conductivity, and higher corrosion rate of hTNTs compared to compact TiO_2. Nanoindentation tests revealed that the mechanical properties of the hTNTs were influenced by their diagonal size, with decreasing hardness and Young's modulus observed with increasing diagonal size of the hTNTs, accompanied by increased plastic deformation. Overall, these findings suggest that hTNTs exhibit promising structural and electrochemical properties, making them potential candidates for various applications including biosensor platforms.

6 Antibacterial Activity of Nanostructured Ti-Based Composites

Nanostructuring is one of the options in the creation of Ti-based biomaterials with advanced properties. The purpose of our recent study was to develop Ti-10 wt% 45S5 Bioglass nanocomposites by nanosilver addition to improve their antibacterial function for medical applications (Jurczyk et al. 2016). The activity of silver and 45S5 Bioglass (45% SiO_2, 24.5% Na_2O, 24.5% CaO, and 6% P_2O_5) against the *S. mutans* and *S. aureus* was evaluated. In vitro bacterial adhesion study indicated a significantly reduced number of *S. mutans* and *S. aureus* on Ti-10 wt% 45S5 Bioglass-1.5 wt% Ag. When Ti-10 wt% 45S5 Bioglass-1.5 wt% Ag material is immersed in body fluid, the metallic Ag particles at the surface of the Ti-10 wt% 45S5 Bioglass-1.5 wt% Ag may react with the body fluid and release ionized Ag into the surrounding fluid. A steady and prolonged release of the silver biocide in a concentration level (0.1 ppb) is capable of rendering antibacterial efficacy (Kumar and Münstedt 2005). When there are enough Ag ions in the fluid, the Ti-10 wt% 45S5 Bioglass-1.5 wt% Ag nanocomposite can exhibit antibacterial activity against bacteria. The mechanism for bacterial toxicity of tested Ti-based nanocomposites may include free metal ion toxicity arising from the dissolution of metals from the surface of the silver particles (e.g., Ag+ from Ag) (Kim et al. 2007) or oxidative stress via the generation of reactive oxygen species (ROS) on crystal surfaces of some nanoparticles (e.g., anatase forms of TiO_2, silica (SiO_2), 45S5 Bioglass) (Wong et al. 2006). The latter mechanism may be important for TiO_2, where the TiO_2 surface reacts by photocatalysis with water to release the hydroxyl radical with the subsequent formation of superoxide (Linsebigler et al. 1995). *Streptococcus mutans* were killed not only by Ag particles but also by SiO_2 particles. Silica has been found to inhibit bacterial adherence to oral biofilms (Benesis et al. 2014). The silica induces an unfavorable change in the biofilm to reduce the adhesion, and therefore the proliferation of bacteria.

Silver particles had the highest antibacterial effect with a minimal inhibition concentration and a minimal bactericidal concentration of 4.86 ± 2.71 μg/mL and 6.25 μg/ mL, respectively (Hernández-Sierra et al. 2008). It was demonstrated that iron nanoparticles in the lower concentration (0.001 and 0.01 mg/mL) had a stimulating effect on bacterial growth, while in the higher concentration (0.1 and 1 mg/ mL), they had an inhibitory effect on clinical isolates of *S. aureus* (Babushkina et al. 2010).

Recently, the antibacterial activity of Ti31Mo5HA composite containing silver (Ag), tantalum (V) oxide (Ta_2O_5), or cerium (IV) oxide (CeO_2) against *S. aureus* was studied (Sochacka et al. 2020). In vitro bacterial adhesion, the study indicated a significantly reduced number of *S. aureus* on the bulk ultrafine-grained Ti31Mo5HA-Ag (Ce_2O_3) plate surfaces in comparison to microcrystalline Ti plate surfaces. On the other hand, the antibacterial activity of Ti23Zr25Nb-based composites containing silver, copper, or zinc against reference strain *S. mutans* ATCC 25175 was studied (Marczewski et al. 2020c). In vitro bacterial adhesion indicated a significantly reduced number of *S. mutans* on the bulk Ti23Zr25Nb-BG-Ag (or Cu, Zn) plate surfaces in comparison to the microcrystalline Ti plate surface.

Ultrafine-grained Ti31Mo5HA-Ag or CeO_2 and Ti23Zr25Nb-BG-Ag (or Cu, Zn) biomaterials can be considered to be the next generation of dental implants (Marczewski et al. 2020c; Sochacka et al. 2020).

7 Conclusion

Nanotechnology is foreseen to change medicine and dentistry fundamentally. Current trends in clinical dental implant therapy include the use of endosseous dental implant surfaces embellished with nanoscale topographies. It has been shown that implant surface character is one implant design factor affecting the rate and extent of osseointegration. Nanostructured surfaces possess unique properties that alter cell adhesion by direct (cell-surface interactions) and indirect (affecting protein-surface interactions) mechanisms. Surface nano topography appears to affect cell interactions at surfaces and to alter cell behavior when compared to conventional size topography. There is still little evidence to date of the long-term benefits of nanofeatures, as the promising results achieved in vitro and animals are not yet confirmed in humans.

The development of many new nanostructured Ti-based alloys has been noticed over the years, and in vivo tests as well as clinical trials have shown their success.

Nevertheless, products on the market are sparse. Enhancement of both short and long-term tissue integration of nano-titanium implants can be accomplished by increasing protein adsorption and cell adhesion through surface roughness modification at the nanoscale level, or by improving osteoconductivity through biomimetic calcium phosphate coatings, or by facilitating the bone healing process in the bone-implant area through adjunction of biological drugs.

The development of new strategies can be achieved by a better understanding of the interactions between proteins, cells, tissues, and implant material. The ideal implant will be based on a surface with a controlled and custom-made topography and chemistry. The local release of bone-stimulating drugs may help in advanced and complex clinical situations with poor bone quality and quantity. Reduction of osseointegration time for immediate loading cases will allow patients to have a shorter and safer rehabilitation treatment.

Adequate adhesion and initiation of the cell subdivision process is the desired property of the implant's surface. However, these processes should be stable to avoid uncontrolled growth rates which could lead to the escape of cells from the surveillant agents, thus exceeding barriers of carcinogenesis. It still seems very important to develop such titanium-type alloys for the production of dental implants, which will demonstrate a reduced susceptibility to bacterial colonization, and will not elicit pathogenic effects. It seems that the nanocrystalline Ti-type implants may be tailored to the production of structures, which support the process of continuous adaptation to the implant by the host organism.

References

T. Albrektsson, P.-I. Brånemark, H.A. Hansson, J. Lindstrom, Osseointegrated titanium implants. Requirements for ensuring a long lasting, direct bone-to-implant anchorage in man. Acta Orthop. Scand. **52**, 155–170 (1981)

K. Arkusz, E. Paradowska, M. Nycz, E. Krasicka-Cydzik, Influence of thermal modification and morphology of TiO_2 nanotubes on their electrochemical properties for biosensors applications. J. Nanosci. Nanotechnol. **18**, 1–9 (2018)

K. Arkusz, M. Nycz, E. Paradowska, Electrochemical evaluation of the compact and Nanotubular oxide layer destruction under ex vivo Ti6Al4V ELI Transpedicular Screw implantation. Materials **13**, 176 (2020)

K. Arkusz, A. Jedrzejewska, P. Siwak, M. Jurczyk, Electrochemical and mechanical properties of hexagonal titanium dioxide nanotubes formed by sonoelectrochemical anodization. Materials **17**, 2138 (2024)

A. Arys, C. Philippart, N. Dourov, Y. He, Q.T. Le, J.J. Pireaux, Analysis of titanium dental implants after failure of osseointegration: combined histological, electron microscopy and X-ray photoelectron spectroscopy approach. J. Biomed. Mater. Res. **43**, 300–312 (1998)

I.V. Babushkina, V.B. Borodulin, G.V. Korshunov, D.M. Puchinjan, Comparative study of antibacterial action of iron and copper nanoparticles on clinical *Staphylococcus aureus* strains. Saratov J. Med. Sci. Res. **6**, 11–14 (2010)

Y. Bai, J. Gao, C. Wang, W. Ma, M.H. Lee, Effect of solvent composition on the bioactive coating fabricated by micro-arc oxidation combined with electrophoretic deposition. Mater. Res. Innov. **20**, 451–457 (2016)

J.R. Baker Jr., What is nanomedicine? Nanomed. Nanotechnol. Biol. Med. **1**, 243 (2005)
S.C. Bayne, Dental restorations for oral rehabilitation—testing of laboratory properties versus clinical performance for clinical decision making. J. Oral Rehab. **34**, 921–932 (2007)
A. Benesis, T. De Peralta, R.D. Handy, The antibacterial effects of silver, titanium dioxide and silica dioxide nanoparticles compared to the dental disinfectant chlorhexidine on *Streptococcus mutans* using a suite of bioassays. Nanotoxicology **8**, 1–16 (2014)
S.M. Beschnidt, C. Cacaci, K. Dedeoglu, D. Hildebrand, H. Hulla, G. Iglhaut, G. Krennmair, M. Schlee, P. Sipos, A. Stricker, K.L. Ackermann, Implant success and survival rates in daily dental practice: 5-year results of a non-interventional study using CAMLOG SCREW-LINE implants with or without platform-switching abutments. Int. J. Implant Dent. **4**, 33–46 (2018)
P.I. Brånemark, Osseointegration and its experimental background. J. Prosthet. Dent. **50**, 399–410 (1983)
E. Bressan, L. Sbricoli, R. Guazzo, I. Tocco, M. Roman, V. Vindigni, E. Stellini, C. Gardin, L. Ferroni, S. Sivolella, B. Zavan, Nanostructured surfaces of dental implants, Int. J. Mol. Sci. **14**, 1918–1931 (2013)
K. Bugunia-Kubik, M. Susisaga, From molecular biology to nanotechnology and nanomedicine. J. Biosyst. **65**, 123–138 (2002)
W.P. Cao, L. Hench, Bioactive materials. Ceram. Int. **22**, 493–507 (1966)
X. Chen, H.J. Schleusener, Nanosilver: a nanoproduct in medical application. Toxicol. Lett. **176**, 1–12 (2008)
P.G. Coelho, M. Suzuki, Evaluation of an IBAD thin-film process as an alternative method for surface incorporation of bioceramics on dental implants. J. Appl. Oral Sci. **13**, 87–92 (2005)
M. Davarpanah, H. Martinez, D. Etienne, I. Zabalegui, P. Mattout, F. Chiche, J. Michel, A prospective multicenter evaluation of 1,538 BIOMET 3i implants: one to five year data, Int. J. Oral Maxillofac. Implants **17**, 820–828 (2002)
D.M.D. Ehrenfest, P.G. Coelho, B.S. Kang, Y.T. Sul, T. Albrektsson, Classification of osseointegrated implant surfaces: Materials, chemistry and topography—review. Trends Biotechnol. **28**, 198–206 (2010)
J.E. Ellingsen, Pre-treatment of titanium implants with fluoride improves their retention in bone. J. Mater. Sci. Mater. Med. **6**, 749–753 (2005)
S. Erakovi'c, A. Jankovi'c, D. Veljovi'c, E. Palcevskis, M. Mitri'c, T. Stevanovi'c, D. Jana'ckovi'c, V. Miškovi'c-Stankovi'c, Corrosion stability and bioactivity in simulated body fluid of silver/hydroxyapatite and silver/hydroxyapatite/lignin coatings on titanium obtained by electrophoretic deposition. J. Phys. Chem. B **117**, 1633–1643 (2013)
R.P. Feynman, There's plenty of room at the bottom. Eng. Sci. **23**, 22–26 (1960)
R. Godarzi, L. Rasmusson, A. Dasmah, T. Albrektsson, Effects of implant design and surface on osseointegration. An experimental study in the dog mandible. Appl. Osseointegration Res. **7**, 58–60 (2008)
G. Goodarzi, M. Moztarzadeh, Titanium dioxide nanotube arrays: a novel approach into periodontal tissue regeneration on the surface of titanium implants. Adv. Mater. Lett. **7**, 209–215 (2016)
L. Guehennec, A. Souedan, P. Layrolle, Y. Amouriq, Surface treatments of titanium dental implants for rapid osseointegration. Dent. Mater. **23**, 844–854 (2007)
L. He, X. Zhang, C. Tong, Surface modification of pure titanium treated with B_4C, Surf. Coat. Technol. **200**, 3016–3020 (2006)
L.L. Hench, Bioceramics: from concept to clinic. J. Am. Ceram. Soc. **74**, 1487–1510 (1991)
J.F. Hernández-Sierra, F. Ruiz, D.C. Pena, F. Matrtinez-Gutiérrez, A.E. Martinez, J.G. Ade, H. Tapia-Pérez, G.M. Castañón, The antimicrobial sensitivity of *Streptococcus mutans* to nanoparticles of silver, zinc oxide, and gold. Nanomedicine **4**, 237–240 (2008)
W.F. Ho, C.P. Ju, J.H. Chern Lin, Structure and properties of cast binary Ti-Mo alloys. Biomaterials **20**, 2115–2122 (1999)
P. Huang, K.-W. Xu, Y. Han, Preparation and apatite layer formation of plasma electrolytic oxidation film on titanium for biomedical application. Mater. Lett. **59**, 185–189 (2005)

J. Jakubowicz, Formation of porous TiO_x biomaterias in H_3PO_4 electrolytes, Electrochem. Commun. **10**, 735–739 (2008)
J. Jakubowicz, G. Adamek, Preparation and properties of mechanically alloyed and electrochemically etched porous Ti–6Al–4V. Electrochem. Commun. **11**, 1772–1775 (2009)
J. Jakubowicz, K. Jurczyk, K. Niespodziana, M. Jurczyk, Mechanoelectrochemical synthesis of porous Ti-based nanocomposite biomaterial. Electrochem. Commun. **11**, 461–465 (2009)
J. Jakubowicz, G. Adamek, M.U. Jurczyk, M. Jurczyk, 3D surface topography study of the biofunctionalized nanocrystalline Ti-6Zr-4Nb/ca-P. Mater Charact. **70**, 55–62 (2012)
J. Jakubowicz, J.K. Koper, G. Adamek, M. Połomska, J. Wolak, Silver nano-trees deposited in the pores of anodically oxidized titanium and Ti scaffold. Int. J. Electrochem. Sci. **10**, 4165–4172 (2015)
M. Jurczyk (ed.), *Bionanomaterials for Dental Applications* (Pan Stanford, Boca Raton, FL, 2012) ISBN: 9789814303835
M.U. Jurczyk, K. Jurczyk, A. Miklaszewski, M. Jurczyk, Nanostructured titanium-45S5 bioglass scaffold composites for medical applications. Mater. Des. **32**, 4882–4889 (2011a)
K. Jurczyk, K. Niespodziana, M.U. Jurczyk, M. Jurczyk, Synthesis and characterization of titanium-45S5 bioglass nanocomposites. Mater. Des. **32**, 2554–2560 (2011b)
K. Jurczyk, K. Niespodziana, U.U. Jurczyk, J. Jakubowicz, M. Jurczyk, Titanium-10wt% 45S5 bioglass nanocomposite for biomedical applications. Mater. Chem. Phys. **131**, 540–546 (2011c)
K. Jurczyk, A. Miklaszewski, M.U. Jurczyk, M. Jurczyk, Development of β type Ti23Mo- 45S5 Bioglass nanocomposites for dental applications. Materials **8**, 8032–8046 (2015)
K. Jurczyk, M.M. Kubicka, M. Ratajczak, M.U. Jurczyk, K. Niespodziana, D.M. Nowak, M. Gajecka, M. Jurczyk, Antibacterial activity of nanostructured Ti-45S5 Bioglass-Ag composite against *Streptococcus mutans* and *Staphylococcus aureus*. Trans. Nonferrous Metals Soc. China **26**, 118–125 (2016)
M. Kaczmarek, M.U. Jurczyk, B. Rubis, A. Banaszak, A. Kolecka, A. Paszel, K. Jurczyk, M. Murias, J. Sikora, M. Jurczyk, *In vitro* biocompatibility of Ti-45S5 bioglass nanocom posites and their scaffolds. J. Biomed. Mater. Res. A **102**, 1316–1324 (2014)
M. Kaczmarek, K. Jurczyk, J.J. Koper, A. Paszel-Jaworska, A. Romaniuk, N. Lipinska, J. Zurawski, P. Urbaniak, J. Jakubowicz, M.M. Jurczyk, In vitro biocompatibility of anodized titanium with deposited silver nanodendrites. J. Mater. Sci. **51**, 5259–5270 (2016)
A. Kazek-Kesik, G. Dercz, I. Kalemba, K. Suchanek, A. Kukharenko, D. Korotin, J. Michalska, A. Krzakała, J. Piotrowski, E. Kurmaev, et al., Surface characterisation of Ti–15Mo alloy modified by a PEO process in various suspensions. Mater. Sci. Eng. C **39**, 259–272 (2014)
Z. Khurshid, M. Zafar, S. Qasim, S. Shahab, M. Naseem, A. Abu Reqaiba, Advances in nanotechnology for restorative dentistry, review. Materials **8**, 717–731 (2015)
J.S. Kim, E. Kuk, K.N. Yu, J.H. Kim, S.J. Park, H.J. Lee, S H. Kim, Y.K. Park, Y.H. Park, C.Y. Hwang, Y.K. Kim, Y.S. Lee, D.H. Jeong, M.H. Cho, Antimicrobial effects of silver nanoparticles, Nanomedicine **3**, 95–101 (2007)
E. Kobayashi, H. Doi, M. Takahashi, T. Nakano, T. Yoneyama, H. Hamanaka, Castability and mechanical properties of Ti–6Al–7Nb alloy dental-cast. J. Jpn. Soc. Dent. Mater. Devices **14**, 406–413 (1995)
J.K. Koper, J. Jakubowicz, Corrosion resistance of porous titanium surface prepared at moderate and high potentials in H_3PO_4/HF electrolytes. Prot. Met. Phys. Chem. Surf. **51**, 295–303 (2015)
M. Krivoruchko, J. Allen, Birdsall, M., *Bioresorbable Stent*. United States Patent 7651527 (2010)
R. Kumar, H. Münstedt, Silver ion release from antimicrobial polyamide/silver composites. Biomaterials **26**, 2081–2088 (2005)
S.H. Lee, H.E. Kim, H.W. Kim, Nano-sized hydroxyapatite coatings on Ti substrate with TiO_2 buffer layer by e-beam deposition. J. Am. Ceram. Soc. **90**, 50–56 (2007)
L. Lefebvre, J. Chevalier, L. Gremillard, R. Zenati, G. Thollet, D. Bernache-Assolant, A. Govin, Structural transformations of bioactive glass 45S5 with thermal treatments, Acta Mater. **55**, 3305–3313 (2007)

L.H. Li, Y.M. Kong, H.W. Kim, Y.W. Kim, H.E. Kim, S.J. Heo, J.Y. Koak, Improved biological performance of Ti implants due to surface modification by micro-arc oxidation. Biomaterials **25**, 2867–2875 (2004)

D.J. Lin, C.C. Chuang, J.H. Chern Lin, J.W. Lee, C.P. Ju, H.S. Yin, Bone formation at the surface of low modulus tie 7.5Mo implants in rabbit femur. Biomaterials **28**, 2582–2589 (2007)

J. Lindhe, T. Karring, N.P. Lang, *Clinical Periodontology and Implant Dentistry* (Blackwell Munksgaard, Oxford, 2003)

A.L. Linsebigler, G. Lu, J.T. Yates, Photocatalysis on TiO_2 surfaces: principles, mechanisms, and selected results. Chem. Rev. **95**, 735–758 (1995)

M. Long, H.J. Rack, Titanium alloys in total joint replacement - a materials science perspective. Biomaterials **19**, 1621–1638 (1998)

M. Marczewski, A. Miklaszewski, M. Jurczyk, Structure evolution analysis in ultrafine-grained Zr and Nb-based beta titanium alloys. J. Alloys Compd. **765**, 459–469 (2018). https://doi.org/10.1016/j.jallcom.2018.06.224

M. Marczewski, A. Miklaszewski, X. Maeder, M. Jurczyk, Crystal structure evolution, microstructure formation, and properties of mechanically alloyed ultrafine-grained Ti-ZrNb alloys at $36 \leq Ti \leq 70$ (at. %), Materials (Basel) **13** (2020a). https://doi.org/10.3390/ma13030587

M. Marczewski, M.U. Jurczyk, K. Kowalski, A. Miklaszewski, P.K. Wirstlein, M. Jurczyk, Composite and surface functionalization of ultrafine-grained Ti23Zr25Nb alloy for medical applications. Materials (Basel). **13** (2020b). https://doi.org/10.3390/ma13225252

M. Marczewski, M. Jurczyk, P. Pecyna, M. Ratajczak, M. Gajecka, M.U. Jurczyk, The effect of 45S5 bioglass and Ag, Cu, or Zn addition on the crystal structure, properties, and antibacterial effect of bulk Ti23Zr25Nb biocomposites. Metals (Basel). **10** (2020c). https://doi.org/10.3390/met10091115

H. Matusiewicz, Potential release of in vivo trace metals from metallic medical implants in the human body: from ions to nanoparticles—a systematic analytical review. Acta Biomater. **10**, 2379–2403 (2014)

G. Mendonça, D.B.S. Mendonça, F.J.L. Araga˜o, L.F. Cooper, Advancing dental implant surface technology—from micron to nanotopography—review. Biomaterials **29**, 3822–3835 (2008)

A. Miklaszewski, M.U. Jurczyk, K. Jurczyk, M. Jurczyk, Plasma surface modification of titanium by TiB precipitation for biomedical applications. Surf. Coat. Technol. **206**, 330–337 (2011)

A. Miklaszewski, M.U. Jurczyk, M. Jurczyk, Microstructural development of Ti-B alloyed layer for hard tissue applications. Mater. Sci. Technol. **29**, 565–572 (2013)

A. Miklaszewski, M.U. Jurczyk, M. Kaczmarek, A. Paszel-Jaworska, A. Romaniuk, N. Lipinska, J. Zurawski, P. Urbaniak, M. Jurczyk, Nanoscale size effect in in situ titanium based composites with cell viability and cytocompatibility studies. Mater. Sci. Eng. C **73**, 525–536 (2017)

T.M. Mohsin, A.K. Zahid, N.S. Arshad, Beta titanium alloys: the lowest elastic modulus for biomedical applications: a review. Int. J. Chem. Mol. Nucl. Mater. Metall. Eng. **8**, 726–731 (2014)

J.L. Murray, The Mo-Ti (molybdenum-titanium) system. Bull. Alloy Phase Diagr. **2**, 185–192 (1981)

M. Nycz, E. Paradowska, K. Arkusz, D.G. Pijanowska, Influence of geometry and annealing temperature in argon atmosphere of TiO_2 nanotubes on their electrochemical properties. Acta Bioeng. Biomech. **22**, 165–177 (2020)

H.-J. Oh, J.-H. Lee, Y.-J. Kim, S.-J. Suh, J.-H. Lee, C.-S. Chi, Surface characteristics of porous anodic TiO_2 layer for biomedical applications. Mater. Chem. Phys. **109**, 10–14 (2008)

S.T. Ozak, P. Ozkan, Nanotechnology and dentistry. Eur. J. Dent. **7**, 145–151 (2013)

M. Rai, A. Yadav, A. Gade, Silver nanoparticles as a new generation of antimicrobials. Biotechnol. Adv. **27**, 76–83 (2009)

M. Rocci, A. Rocci, M. Martignoni, T. Albrektsson, A comparative study of TiOblast and OsseoSpeed implants retrieved from humans. Appl. Osseointegration Res. **7**, 26–30 (2008)

B. Sarma, K.S.R. Chandran, Recent advances in surface hardening of titanium. JOM **63**, 85–92 (2011)

W. Singhatanadgit, M. Toso, B. Pratheepsawangwong, A. Pimpin, W. Srituravanich, Titanium dioxide nanotubes of defined diameter enhance mesenchymal stem cell proliferation via JNK- and ERK dependent up-regulation of fibroblast growth factor-2 by T lymphocytes. J. Biomater. Appl. **33**, 997–1010 (2018)

P. Sochacka, A. Miklaszewski, M. Jurczyk, Development of β-type Ti-x at. % Mo alloys by mechanical alloying and powder metallurgy: Phase evolution and mechanical properties ($10 \leq x \leq 35$). J. Alloys Compd. **776**, 370–378 (2019a)

P. Sochacka, A. Miklaszewski, K. Kowalski, M. Jurczyk, Influence of the processing method on the properties of Ti-23 at.% Mo alloy. Meta **9**, 931 (2019b)

P. Sochacka, A. Miklaszewski, M. Jurczyk, P. Pecyna, M. Ratajczak, M. Gajecka, M.U. Jurczyk, Effect of hydroxyapatite and ag, Ta_2O_5 or CeO_2 addition on the properties of ultrafine-grained Ti31Mo alloy. J. Alloys Compd. **823**, 153749 (2020)

P. Sochacka, M.U. Jurczyk, K. Kowalski, P.K. Wildstein, M. Jurczyk, Ultrafine-grained Ti-31Mo-type composites with HA and Ag, Ta_2O_5 or CeO_2 addition for implant applications. Materials **14**, 644 (2021)

C.M. Stanford, Surface modifications of dental implants. Aust. Dent. J. **53**, 26–33 (2008)

Y.T. Sul, The significance of the surface properties of oxidized titanium to the bone response: special emphasis on potential biochemical bonding of oxidized titanium implant, Biomaterials **24**, 3893–3907 (2003)

M. Tulinski, M.U. Jurczyk, K. Arkusz, M. Nowak, M. Jurczyk, Nanotechnology for biomedical applications: Synthesis and properties of Ti-based nanocomposites. Nanomaterials **15**, 1417 (2025)

R.Z. Valiev, M.J. Zehetbauer, Y. Estrin, H.W. Höppel, Y. Ivanisenko, H. Hahn, G. Wilde, H.J. Roven, X. Sauvage, T.G. Langdon, The innovation potential of bulk nanostructured materials, Adv. Eng. Mater. **9**, 527–533 (2007)

R.Z. Valiev, I.P. Semenova, V.V. Latysh, A.V. Shcherbakov, E.B. Yakushina, Nanostructured titanium for biomedical applications: new developments and challenges for commercialization. Nanotechnol. Russ. **3**, 593–601 (2008)

R.Z. Valiev, I.P. Semenova, V.V. Latysh, H. Rack, T.C. Lowe, J. Petruzelka, L. Dluhos, D. Hrusak, J. Sochova, Nanostructured titanium for biomedical applications, Adv. Eng. Mater. **10**, B15–B17 (2009)

B. Voltrova, V. Hybasek, V. Blahnova, J. Sepitka, V. Lukasova, K. Vocetkova, V, Sovkova, R. Matejka, J. Fojt, L. Joska, M. Daniel, E. Filova, Different diameters of titanium dioxide nanotubes modulate Saos-2 osteoblast-like cell adhesion and osteogenic differentiation and nanomechanical properties of the surface. RSC Adv., 9 (2019) 11341–11355.

K. Wang, The use of titanium for medical applications in the USA. Mater. Sci. Eng. A **213**, 134–137 (1996)

G. Wang, X. Liu, C. Ding, Phase composition and *in-vitro* bioactivity of plasma sprayed calcia stabilized zirconia coatings. Surf. Coat. Technol. **202**, 5824–5831 (2008)

X. Wang, L. Zhang, Z. Guo, Y. Jiang, X. Tao, L. Liu, Study of low-modulus biomedical β Ti–Nb–Zr alloys based on single-crystal elastic constants modeling. J. Mech. Behav. Biomed. Mater. **62**, 310–318 (2016)

T.J. Webster, J.U. Ejiofor, Increased osteoblast adhesion on nanophase metals: Ti, Ti_6Al_4V, and CoCrMo. Biomaterials **25**, 4731–4739 (2004)

T.J. Webster, R.W. Siegel, R. Bizios, Nanoceramic surface roughness enhances osteoblast and osteoclast functions for improved orthopaedic/dental implant efficacy. Scr. Mater. **44**, 1639–1642 (2001)

D.F. Williams, Review: tissue-biomaterial interactions. J. Mater. Sci. **22**, 3421–3445 (1987)

M.S. Wong, W.C. Chu, D.S. Sun, H.S. Huang, J.H. Chen, P.J. Tsai, N.T. Lin, M.S. Yu, S.F. Hsu, S. Wang, H.H. Chang, Visible-light-induced bactericidal activity of a nitrogen-doped titanium photocatalyst against human pathogens. Appl. Environ. Microbiol. **72**, 6111–6116 (2006)

Ch.-L. Yang, F.-L. Chen, S.-W. Chen, Anodization of the dental arch wires. Mater. Chem. Phys. **100**, 268–274 (2006)

L. Zhang, T.J. Webster, Nanotechnology and nanomaterials: promises for improved tissue regeneration. Nano Today **4**, 66–80 (2009)

W.-D. Zhang, Y. Liu, H. Wu, M. Song, T.-Y. Zhang, X.-D. Lan, T.-H. Yao, Elastic modulus of phases in Ti-Mo alloys. Mater. Char. **106**, 302–307 (2015)

Multifunctional Microtubule Nanocomposite Models in Medicine

Otto C Wilson Jr, Awatef Alsheri, Jeffrey J Morgan, Winston A Anderson, and Ayelle Gugssa

Abstract Microtubules polymer nanocomposite is Microtubules (MTs) are the most unique protein-based polymer nanocomposite in living systems, possessing an astonishing variety of properties that make them one of the most elegant multifunctional biomaterials in existence. The importance of MTs arguably matches that of DNA due to their presence in all eukaryotic cells and the multifaceted role that they play in every conceivable process that contributes to life, from events preceding the moment of conception through all stages of cell development and functioning. Tubulin dimers are the building blocks of MTs which allow growth and shrinkage through self-assembly and disassembly, respectively. MTs serve as critically important structural elements within cells to influence cell morphology and mobility, provide a dynamic intracellular transportation network for dynein and kinesin motor proteins to move proteins, organelles, and signaling molecules within the cell, and play key roles in cell division. MTs can serve as a multidimensional model system to help address key questions in health, technology and learning, and brain function. MTs hold the key to understanding a host of pathological conditions and can be a foundation for developing effective therapeutic interventions and strategic cures for a multitude of cellular diseases including cancer, metabolic conditions like diabetes, and neurodegenerative diseases. Novel aspects of MTs related to learning and cognition will serve as a foundation to investigate roles for MTs in quantum biology and human consciousness. MTs serve as an important link between the neurons and axons in our brain and quantum computing.

O. C. Wilson Jr (✉) · J. J. Morgan
Department of Biomedical Engineering, The Catholic University of America, Washington, DC, USA
e-mail: wilsono@cua.edu

A. Alsheri
Department of Nanomedicine, King Abdullah International Medical Research Center (KAIMRC), Riyadh, Saudi Arabia

W. A. Anderson · A. Gugssa
Biology Department, Howard University, Washington, DC, USA

R. Narayan (ed.), *Nanostructured Biomaterials and Their Applications*,
https://doi.org/10.1007/978-3-032-16316-5_4

1 Introduction

Microtubules (MTs) are the most unique protein-based polymer nanocomposite in living systems. At first glance, MTs seem deceptively simple, but they possess an astonishing variety of properties that make them one of the most elegant multifunctional biomaterials in existence. The importance of MTs arguably matches that of DNA due to the multifaceted role that they play in every conceivable process that contributes to life. MTs serve as critically important structural elements within cells to influence cell morphology and mobility, provide one system or multiple to move proteins, organelles, and signaling molecules within the cell, and play key roles in cell division. MTs dynamically reconfigure via self-assembly and disassembly processes that are self-powered via interconversion of guanosine triphosphate (GTP) and guanosine diphosphate (GDP). MTs undergo modifications by incorporating proteins from a wide variety of MT-associated proteins (MAPs) that can fine-tune MT properties to achieve a wide array of capabilities and functionalities. MTs hold the key to unraveling many foundational mysteries related to healthy cell and tissue function that can be used to enhance overall global health.

MTs exhibit a wide range of chemical and physical properties that encompass unique electromagnetic, piezoelectric, and resonance behaviors where they can generate, transmit and receive signals. These unique biological-based properties can also be modeled to develop enhanced materials for various technological applications. MT properties can be adapted to develop a host of advanced material systems and devices that bridge between the biological world of the cell and advanced sensor, microelectronic and quantum-computing-based systems and devices. The ability to send and receive signals is especially relevant in neurons (Kelliher et al. 2019). This unique aspect of MTs opens up many possibilities for advancing our understanding of how our brains work and the nature of consciousness. MTs are truly remarkable nanocomposites that can serve as a multidimensional model system to help address key questions in health, technology and learning, and brain function.

In this chapter, MTs will be highlighted as an ideal model polymer nanocomposite system. A selective approach will be used because the amazing structure, properties, and functionality of MTs can easily fill a multi-volume series of books. In Sect. 2, an overview of the important role of models in advancing our understanding of the cell and its basic molecular building blocks will be presented with a focus on the unique structural adaptations of MTs. Key aspects of the structure of MTs will be highlighted by addressing questions such as "What are the fundamental building blocks for MTs?", "What are the advantages of forming a tubular structure?" and "What unique features of MTs make them a candidate for the title of ultimate functional model nanocomposite?". Section 3 will focus on the properties, present functionalities, and future potential uses for MTs based on the unique properties that they exhibit. Section 4 will present selected features of MT functions which provide cells with unique abilities. Health challenges and pathologies which are associated with MTs will be described with MT-targeting strategies that can help restore health and recover function for a number of chronic conditions. Metabolic challenges including diabetes, cognitive decline, and cancer will serve as the focus. In Sect. 5, novel aspects of MTs related to learning and cognition will serve as a foundation to investigate roles for MTs in quantum biology and human consciousness. MTs serve as an important link between the neurons and axons in our brain and quantum computing.

2 MT Structure

2.1 MT Overview from DNA to Models for Enhanced Health

Biomolecules are a special class of polymer nanocomposites that have revolutionized many areas of medicine and healthcare. Current developments in biomedical engineering and biotechnology are paving the way for a much brighter and healthier future for people across the globe as we gain more information and insight about the unique ways that the basic building blocks of life interact. Polymer nanocomposites are very important due to their functional role in orchestrating the wonderful symphony of life that is continuously playing within our cells, tissues and organs. Our cells are composed of polymer nanocomposite building blocks that are classified as lipids, polysaccharides, nucleic acids, and proteins. Lipids serve as smart barriers to provide boundaries for the cells and organelles, which reside within cells. Polysaccharides play important structural support roles in animals and plants as well as serve as a storage depot and vital source of energy. While lipids and polysaccharides serve very important roles in cellular processes and are worthy of a more detailed description, this chapter will focus on nucleic acids and proteins with a specific focus on the tubulin protein family. Tubulin is the main building block for MTs which play a role in every conceivable cellular process from events preceding the moment of conception through all stages of cell development and functioning. MTs even hold the key to understanding a host of pathological conditions and serve as a foundation for developing effective therapeutic interventions and strategic cures for a multitude of diseases including cancer, metabolic conditions like diabetes, and neurodegenerative diseases.

The nucleic acids deoxyribonucleic acid (DNA) and ribonucleic acid (RNA) fulfill important roles in storing and activating the code of life via transcription and translation of the information encoded within the DNA templates. The long chains of DNA are wrapped compactly around histone proteins and stored in chromosomes within the nucleus of all eukaryotic cells. At the proper time in the cell cycle, the DNA is unraveled and transcribed to create a messenger RNA (mRNA)-based copy of the original DNA template. The modified information in mRNA is then translated by ribosomes to synthesize proteins (Jeffery et al. 1983; Lawrence and Singer 1986; Das et al. 2021). Ribosomes are fascinating molecular machines that are composed of ribosomal RNA (rRNA) and special proteins that form a molecular structure that reads the specific sequence of nucleotide base pairs as it moves along the mRNA backbone. Proteins are assembled from specific arrangements of amino acids. The specific amino acid sequence is encoded in the mRNA and deciphered via frame-by-frame reading of the three-base-pair nucleotide codon which is interpreted as a specific amino acid. Transfer RNA (tRNA) locates the specific amino acid within the pool of amino acids in the cell cytoplasm and transports it for incorporation into the growing polypeptide chain. Amino acids are assembled in a precise order to make polypeptide chains. This polypeptide chain is destined to become a specific protein after structural fine tuning to make secondary, tertiary, and even quaternary protein structures which are modified into functionally activated shapes. Some of the final protein activation stages include post-translational modifications that occur in the Golgi apparatus and endoplasmic reticulum followed by origami-like folding processes to develop geometries for optimum functionality to participate in key life processes. When these basic building blocks for life unite to form supramolecular complexes, these elements of the "machinery of life" take on a life of their own. All the proteins that are synthesized within our bodies have very specific roles to play in maintaining health whether it is hemoglobin for transporting oxygen or insulin for glucose signaling and metabolism.

The current picture that we have about the intricate processes which play a role in orchestrating life has been assembled over time, one model at a time. Many inquisitive pioneers and scholars asked simple and elegant questions and worked diligently to find answers and develop models to explain new phenomena and uncover new mysteries to explore. There have been many models which have expanded our view of the cell and helped us to investigate what may be the ultimate question, "What is Life?" This question has been asked countless times across the span of history but it received a new level of attention when posed by Erwin Schrödinger in a series of lectures delivered in Dublin in 1943. The important lecture series was subsequently compiled into a book entitled "What is Life?" (Schrödinger 1944). This fundamental question served as a bridge to connect great ideas in cell biology with the quantum realm of atoms and molecules, and can be attributed as the foundation of modern molecular biology.

The question served as a catalyst to -pique the curiosity of great minds, including Watson, to explore the role- of biomolecular molecules in life. The classic physical model for the DNA double helix is a direct result of inspiration derived from Schrödinger's question. Unlocking the structure of DNA came from a collaborative effort that coupled the X-ray diffraction data of Dr. Rosalind Franklin with the insight of Crick and Watson to help crack the code which revealed the hidden secrets of the DNA molecule (Watson and Crick 1953). Contemporary models for the proposed structure of DNA such as Pauling and Corey's "Triple Helix" DNA Model which reversed the relative positions of the phosphate and nucleotide bases were cited in the classic paper (Pauling and Corey 1953a, b). However, the double helix model of Crick and Watson withstood the test of time and was instrumental in subsequent breakthrough findings and additional models which opened the field of genetic engineering.

2.2 Importance of Models in Advancing Learning

Models can be thought of as multidimensional analogs that help our minds to better understand complex concepts that we cannot always see clearly with our eyes. The simple elemental "building blocks" of models can be manipulated in real time and space to build our conceptual understanding of how system components come together and function in the natural world. Models play a very important role in helping people to understand multiscale phenomena in the world through inquiry and play. Children love to build things and ask many questions and want to learn as much as possible about their environment. They explore by taking things apart to see what makes them tick. Building blocks play a very important part of early childhood development and some of the most treasured toys from a child's formative years are alphanumeric building blocks. As children gain more advanced cognitive and motor skills, the building blocks increase in sophistication to include Erector Sets, Lincoln logs, Legos, Kinex and a host of other model-building toys and tools. This nostalgia and connection with blocks is perpetuated in popular computer games such as Minecraft and Roblox which reflect our move from physical objects to more computer and mixed reality-based interaction modes. A very high level of creative power can be unleashed through playing with model based building sets. Erector Sets played a prominent role in the design and building of one of the first heart pumps in 1949 that kept a dog's heart perfused for over an hour (Watson 2002). More recently, a Lego Mindstorm set was used to build a 3D bioprinter that uses bioink to print tissue engineering scaffolds with living cells (Moukachar et al. 2003).

2.3 Important Characteristics of Models

Key questions related to the extent to which physical components of the system that is being modeled come together and function can be illustrated and addressed in properly designed models. Some of the most important characteristics which lead to models that withstand the test of time are shown in Fig. 1. Models that are simple and elegant are highly valued. Einstein is often credited with the saying "Everything should be made as simple as possible, but not simpler." The accuracy of this statement being attributed to him has been called into question. However, the following is a verified quote from Einstein:

> It can scarcely be denied that the supreme goal of all theory is to make the irreducible basic elements as simple and as few as possible without having to surrender the adequate representation of a single datum of experience. (Einstein as quoted in Calaprice (2010))

The incorporation of adjustable parameters within models instills adaptability to cover the broadest range of situations that can be encountered. A reductionist viewpoint allows one to start from the simplest, most basic fundamental elements and build layers of complexity into the model as our understanding of the system deepens and our predictive capabilities increase. Timeliness adds an important element to

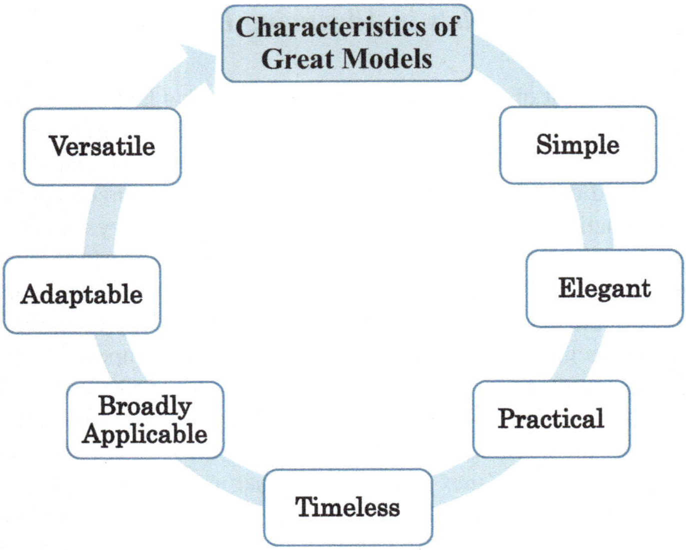

Fig. 1 Characteristics of great models

models. The battle with the COVID-19 pandemic (2020–2022) highlights the extreme urgency which some situations engender. A timely model fits the context of the current situation that gives birth to its need and can be adapted to fit future needs that are exposed by new discoveries and insights. Models may not always be popular. Some models start off as the subject of ridicule and scorn, especially when they challenge long-ingrained views. However, the best models withstand the test of time and emerge tried-and-true beacons to illuminate our pathway to greater truths regarding the foundations of life and the universe. After taking root in good soil, the seeds of a great model can sprout, take root, grow and in time produce a harvest of fruit that yield even better models. The newer models spark even more inspiration, a deeper understanding of our world, and a deeper vision for what can be achieved. The cascade of new discoveries that we are experiencing now as new tools of discovery are being developed and utilized to explore deeper and uncover fundamental mechanisms will lead to improved models and understanding in health and medicine.

2.4 Introduction to MT Structure

When we consider the vast number and amount of proteins that are synthesized within our bodies, which protein is the most strategically important? Hidden within each cell in your body exists a simple protein known as tubulin. Tubulin exists in multiple isoforms, but α and β are the most pervasively utilized types. α and β tubulin bond together to form a twin dimer that self-assembles into nanocomposite microtubes with an outer diameter of 25 nm and an inner diameter of 15 nm. It can easily be said that MTs play a key role in every process in life from conception throughout every stage of living. MTs are there at the moment of conception when the sperm cell unites with the egg and play a role in orchestrating the wonderful cascade of events that make this miracle happen. MTs provide a vital bridge to link the genetic code stored within the chromosomes in the new life growing within the Mother's womb and the vital proteins that will be fashioned from the encoded sequences within DNA in chromosomes. MTs play a key role in the process of transcription from DNA to messenger RNA and translation into polypeptide chains and post-translational modification to achieve the final protein conformation and functionality. MTs provide the raw materials for building and maintaining the intercellular network of tracks that transport proteins on their journey from creation to playing its specific role in promoting health and healing within the body. MTs are there at each step of the process. MTs also transport organelles and vesicles within the cell, play key roles in cell division, cell signaling, and hence, play key roles in monitoring overall health. Pathological conditions in MTs are linked with disease processes involved in cancer, Alzheimer's and neurodegenerative diseases, diabetes and other associated metabolic health conditions. How can one such seemingly simple protein have such a wide impact on life? Studies on MTs reveal that this is just the tip of the iceberg because the deceptively simple structure of MTs allows for the development of protein-based nanocomposites that possess an amazing range of properties and functionalities which allow it to function as nanowires, memristors, resonance cavities, and quantum computers. MTs even play a role in consciousness based on studies of the mechanism of how anesthesia agents bring about a state of unconsciousness. While the exact mechanism has not been fully elucidated, there is a growing body of evidence that the breaking apart of neural MTs plays a role in inducing an unconscious state (Craddock et al. 2012; Kelz and Mashour 2019; Zadeh-Haghighi and Simon 2022). This is a potential link that supports theories that attribute MTs as an important component of our consciousness and how we learn.

2.5 *Historical Overview of MTs*

MTs are one of the most overlooked structural proteins in our cells that has been hidden in plain sight since the beginning of life as we know it. They have faithfully conducted their important work within the cell as the anchor providing structural support, a vital cell-wide transportation network, and contributing important roles in cell division. However, this is just the tip of the iceberg in terms of the fascinating multifunctional roles that MTs play in the life of the cell. Our understanding of the roles that MTs play in treating chronic health issues is expanding exponentially as we elucidate key roles and mechanisms that contribute to MT functional diversity. It has only been within the last century that we have been able to properly utilize the tools of discovery to unravel key aspects of the fascinating protein which serves as the building block for MTs. While they were observed indirectly since the 1800s, it was not until the 1950s and early 1960s that MTs were specifically identified via direct observation with electron microscopy. The name MTs was assigned to these ubiquitous structures within cells in 1963 (Slautterback 1963; Ledbetter and Porter 1963). The name tubulin was assigned to the protein building blocks that produce MTs by Mohri (1968). Some of the earliest work to uncover the mechanism by which molecules interacted with MTs and inhibited mitosis was conducted by Taylor et al. using colchicine (Borisy and Taylor 1967a, b; Shelanski and Taylor 1967; Weisenberg et al. 1968). MT functions encompass specific roles within the approximately 10^{12} innate cells in your body and the approximately 10^{12} cells within your gut microbiome. MTs function within all eukaryotic cells on earth and even play a role in how our animal and plant-based foods are produced by orchestrating vital processes within the cells of food producers and consumers.

MTs are one of the most critically important structural elements in the body and, along with the additional cytoskeletal elements actin and intermediate filaments, form the foundation for the cytoskeletal network of all cells. The cell cytoskeleton is an elaborate network of actin and MT structural protein building blocks that serves as the nanoscale "skeletal" framework of the cell. There are a remarkable number of synergistic links among the cytoskeletal elements which are being uncovered. Hints of interactions were postulated in the late 1970s based on viscosity changes caused by gel formation dynamics when actin, MTs, and MAPs were mixed together Griffith and Pollard (1978). Recent studies highlight the advances in developing models to enhance our understanding of the ways that actin and MTs interact and communicate Dogterom and Koenderink (2019); Pimm and Henty-Ridilla (2021). Hohmann and Dehghani (2019) provide a thorough treatment of the cell cytoskeleton with detailed descriptions for the actin, MT, and intermediate filament contributions to the overall structure and function of this important network within our cells.

Bundles of proteins are packaged for shipment to intercellular and/or extracellular destinations, and these bundles are transported by dynein and kinesin motor proteins along the MT backbone. Specific organelles that need to be relocated to other regions within the cell are transported either along MTs or via facilitated interactions with MTs. The transport of mitochondria along MT tracks to help distressed cardiomyocytes escape apoptosis is an example of organelle transport along MTs (Shen et al. 2018). In addition, MTs regulate key aspects of cell division and are even the key elements that facilitate sperm morphology and the propulsion of the sperm cell on its journey to fertilize the egg cell (O'Donnell and O'Bryan 2014). Some researchers proposed the idea that MTs played a role in establishing the morphology of the sperm head during spermiogenesis. While this idea is reasonable based on established roles for MTs in cell morphology, the specific role of MTs in the shape of the sperm head has been questioned (Fawcett et al. 1971).

2.6 Key Features of MT Structure

The tubulin protein family consists of different isoforms named α, β, γ, δ, ε, and ϕ which play various roles across different species. α and β tubulin are the most abundant monomer units and they each possess multiple isotypes with at least 9 for each of these tubulin monomers. The multiple variations are based on C-terminal amino acid sequence and post-translational modifications which are referred to as the "tubulin code" (Verhey and Gaertig 2007; Ferreira et al. 2018; Maliekal et al. 2022). α and β are the primary units that bind together to form the α/β tubulin heterodimer units which are the fundamental building blocks of MTs. Schematic model diagrams that illustrate various aspects of the dynamics of MT formation are shown in Fig. 2. The tubulin heterodimer units assemble and disassemble in a dynamic fashion to coordinate important cell processes related to cell motility, intercellular transport of proteins, and cell division. Variations in the specific tubulin isotypes that assemble give rise to a wide variety of tailored functionalities for facilitating MT function.

The MT structure is based on the templated action of the γ tubulin ring complex (γ-TuRC) which facilitates the registered assembly of the α–β tubulin dimer units. MTs typically consist of 13 parallel linear protofilaments that are joined to form a hollow tube that is polar with seams that are visible using standard electron microscopy imaging techniques. Each of the 13 protofilaments consists of alternating α and β subunits. For 12 of the 13 connections between adjacent protofilaments, the α and β subunits align with the adjacent α and β subunits, respectively. For the remaining connection, at the seam, the α subunit connects to the β subunit, and the resulting offset gives the MT a helical form. It should be noted that MTs consisting of 15 or 16 protofilaments are connected with bonds between the α and β subunits, but there is still an offset that generates a helical form. The MTs grow or shrink by adding or losing tubulin dimer units. Along the MT, the alternating pattern of α and β subunits leads to the polar structure that has exposed β-tubulin at the fast-growing plus end and exposed α-tubulin at the slow-growing minus end. MTs exhibit dynamic instability where they undergo periods of growth (polymerization) followed by periods of shortening (depolymerization), primarily at the plus end. The minus end can be "capped" by MAPs to prevent depolymerization (and polymerization) from occurring. The minus end is usually embedded in the MT Organizing Center (MTOC). In radially organized cells, such as fibroblasts, the MTOC is centrally located (at the centrosome) and the fast-growing plus end is oriented toward the cell boundary. The MT array in vertebrate polarized epithelial cells exhibits a parallel, longitudinal orientation (Toya and Takeichi 2016; Toya et al. 2016). Transitions from growth to shortening through disassembly are known as "catastrophes" while transitions from disassembly to growth are known as "rescues." Assembly is driven by hydrophobic effects and disassembly is driven by nucleotide hydrolysis. MT-binding proteins (MTBPs) include stabilizers, destabilizers, capping proteins, bundlers, cross-linkers, motors that use MTs as tracks, and cytoskeletal integrators (Goodson and Jonasson 2018).

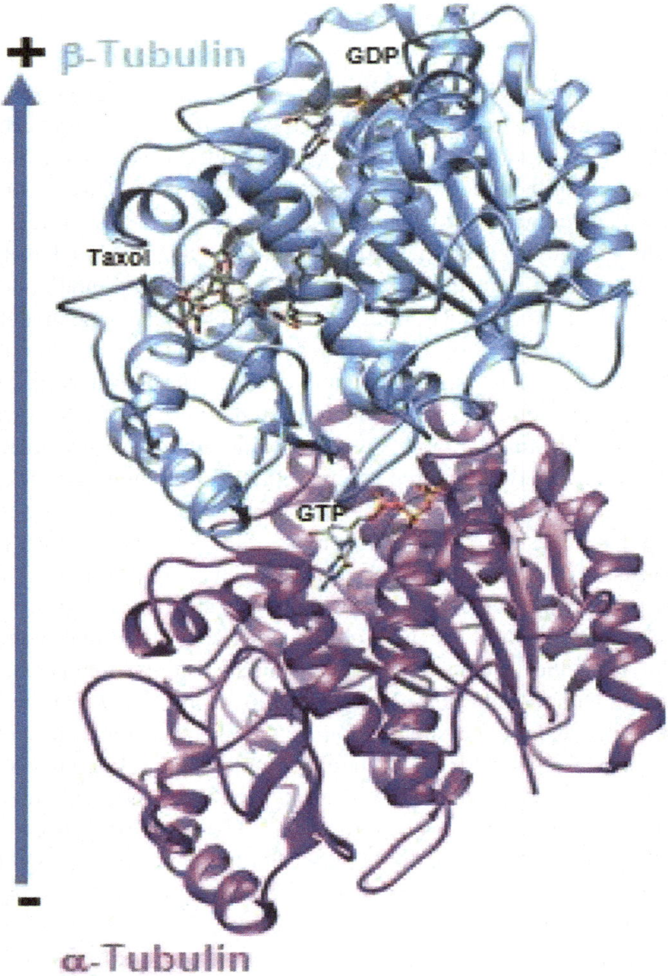

Fig. 2 Molecular-level depiction of the protein ribbon structure model for the ab tubulin heterodimer (used with permission from Cytoskeleton, Inc.)

There are many questions which can be asked as we explore the structure of MTs. How do α and β tubulin monomer units bond together to make the $\alpha\beta$ tubulin heterodimer and how do $\alpha\beta$ tubulin heterodimer units bond together? Computer simulations performed by Guo et al. (2023) showed that electrostatic interactions between the positively-charged β tubulin and the negatively-charged α tubulin were responsible for bonding the two discrete tubulin units together. Hydrogen bonding played a role as well. In the study, it was noted that $\alpha\beta$ interactions were the strongest while $\alpha\alpha$ interactions were the weakest. Schematic model diagrams that illustrate various aspects of the dynamics of MT formation are shown in Fig. 3. Assembly of the individual tubulin monomer units to form the $\alpha\beta$ heterodimer molecular building

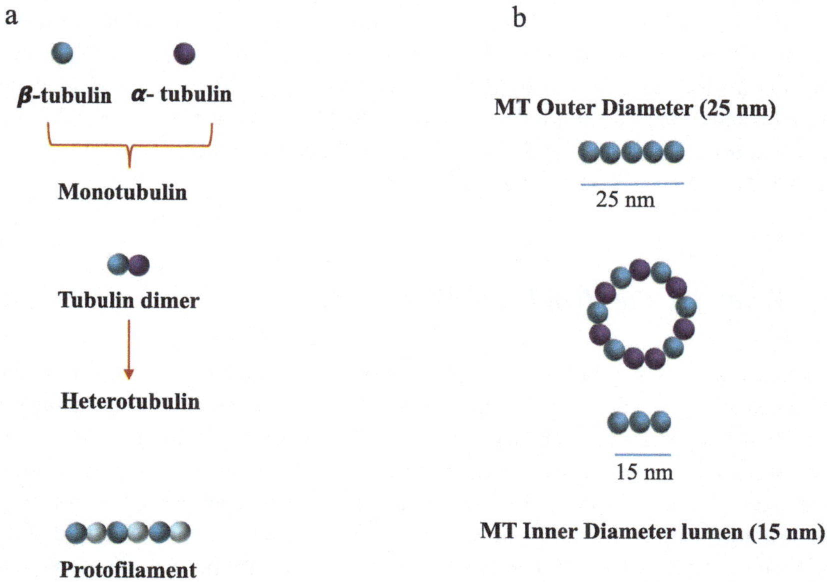

Fig. 3 Schematic diagrams that illustrate various aspects of the dynamics of MT formation. **a** Progression from individual tubulin monomers to tubulin protofilament. **b** Tubulin ring structure showing the dimensions of the inner and outer diameter

block base unit for the MT protofilament is shown in Fig. 3a. A cross-section showing the array of 13 protofilaments in the structure of MTs is shown in Fig. 3b. The "molecular footprint" of the $\alpha\beta$ tubulin heterodimer is about 5 nm in diameter while the height is approximately 8 nm. This size registry is reflected in the reported inner and outer diameter of the MT which is 25 nm for the outer diameter and approximately 15 nm for the diameter of the inner lumen. As a consequence of their well-defined dimensions, MTs are being developed for use as a measurement standard in expansion microscopy (Chowdhury et al. 2025).

2.7 MTs: The Ultimate Model Nanocomposite

From a Materials Science point of view, MTs can be considered a model for the "Ultimate Nanocomposite." MTs present an example of a nanocomposite that more or less exhibits completely ordered mixing. This is due to the alternating pattern of the structural units that are built into the primary heterodimer building blocks. In addition, the overall assembly of MTs is a thermodynamically driven process with order/disorder entropy transitions and additional mixing rule considerations. The versatility of the controlled self-assembly of the MT structure is further expanded by the added feature of controlled self-disassembly. This nanocomposite in essence puts itself together and takes itself apart in a very dynamic fashion that is self-propagating and self-propelled due to the built-in GDP/GTP reactions that provide the driving force and energy for the process. MTs undergo a unit-by-unit self-assembly process that spans a wide range of structural dimensions from atoms to amino acid sequences to tubulin monomers to tubulin heterodimers to MTs. The tubulin code allows for the adaptational fine tuning of the overall MT architecture to accommodate a variety of MAP interactions (Bodakuntla et al. 2019).

2.8 What Are the Benefits of Being a Tube?

As its name suggests, tubulin forms tubes. What is the fundamental reason why the tube morphology occurs and what are some of the unique benefits that result from the tubular shape? Fundamentally, economy of time and conservation of material are reasonable considerations. The rate of formation for constructing a shell is more advantageous from a time and materials perspective in comparison to forming a bulk structure with comparable dimensions. The femur provides an example of this. The femur is hollow to optimize mass to strength ratio properties. Knossow et al. (2020) provide a nice description of X-ray crystallography and cryoTEM data that describe how the curvature of MTs is achieved and how MAPs interact with MTs and influence the structure. Tubulin has a curved conformation when in solution but becomes straight within the MT core. A deeper benefit for MTs to form tubes relates to aspects of transport phenomena. One of the many benefits of adopting a tube morphology involves having additional dimensions for storage and transport. MTs are multidimensional, hollow, and allow multiple kinesin and dynein MAPs to transport their macromolecules and organelle-based cargo simultaneously and circumferentially along the outer periphery in different directions on the same track. The MT transportation network (MTN) consists of the tubulin-based nanocomposite MT tracks and the various MAPs that play crucial roles in facilitating transport operations. Transport of proteins, macromolecules, and organelles occurs along the outside of MT via coordinated movements of dynein and kinesin motor proteins. mRNAs that are transcribed from DNA are properly modified and exit the nucleus through nuclear pores via either passive diffusive transport or active movement along MT tracks via dynein, kinesin or myosin transport molecules (Das et al. 2021).

It is interesting to ponder the question, "What types of transport occur within the lumen of MTs?" Water exists within the lumen space along with electrolytes found within cells. The channel can constrain the water within the lumen to organize in quasi-crystalline patterns which accentuate the anomalous behavior of water in confined spaces as reported by Sahu et al. (2013) for single brain microtubules and Knight et al. (2019) for geological based confinement effects. It has been reported that water can exist as a solid at T above the normal boiling point of water and even up to 151 °C within the narrow space in C nanotubes (Agrawal et al. 2017). There are questions related to the pressure that exists within MTs and it would be interesting to model the pressure within a MT-based on how pressure changes with diameter for tube structures. The MT lumen provides a unique zone of quantum confinement that contributes to the quantum characteristics of MTs. There are a lot of additional interesting questions related to unique forms of matter that can exist within MTs such as oxygen transport via nanobubbles within MTs. MAPs can exist in the lumen of MTs. Santos et al. (2023) used cryogenic electron tomography analysis of Drosophila S2 cell protrusions to reveal that a modified form of nested, helical cofilin bound actin (called cofilactin) filaments can form inside the lumen of MTs under certain conditions.

Probably the most uniquely fascinating role for hollow MTs relates to resonance phenomena and quantum effects which they exhibit. Resonance phenomena offer a unique framework for exploring and explaining some very unique aspects of MT function and provide a direct link between classical and quantum physics. Quantum resonance effects have been identified in various biological phenomena such as photosynthesis, sense of smell, bird brains and navigation, and a variety of other interesting effects. Microwaves are a direct consequence of resonance phenomena and have revolutionized various aspects of food and materials processing since the fateful day when the chocolate bar melted. MT length can be varied to match critically significant distance for coupling.

2.9 MT Nucleation and Fractal Branching

Many aspects of the formation of MTs can be modeled using nucleation phenomena. The field of nucleation phenomena is an important topic in thermodynamics of phase transitions and includes aspects of classical nucleation theory (Becker and Doring 1935; Karthika et al. 2016) with homogeneous and heterogeneous nucleation considerations. More recent considerations include contributions from aggregative growth models and self-assembly processes (Bogush and Zukoski 1991). MTs can display aspects of homogeneous nucleation via γ-TuRC and heterogeneous nucleation via branching from existing MTs. Spontaneous formation of MTs can happen in a process that is akin to homogeneous nucleation. However, this process is less likely to happen due to the large energy requirements. The more likely event is that MTs form via heterogeneous nucleation events that involve the formation of γ-TuRC near MT organizing centers which acts as a seed to facilitate MT growth. The bipolar array of MTs that constitutes the mitotic spindle orchestrates the accurate segregation of chromosomes during cell division (Alfaro-Aco and Petry 2017). Spindles contain MT that are nucleated from other MTs (Petry et al. 2013). MT branching shows a low angle of incidence for branching MT units and unique fractal characteristics (Thawani et al. 2019). This is one of two heterogeneous-type nucleation events that contribute to MT formation. The other method involves branching where MAPs such as TPX2 and augmin play a role in facilitating the branching process (Petry et al. 2013; Alfaro-Aco and Petry 2017; Alfaro-Aco et al. 2017). CKAP4 is another protein that is involved in MT branching and can be linked with cancer metastasis (Cai et al. 2023).

2.10 MTs as Inorganic Quasicrystals

The 13-fold translational symmetry of MTs allows them to be classified among a unique class of materials known as quasiperiodic materials or quasicrystals. Quasicrystals were discovered in 1982 by Shechtman based on his observation and analysis of diffraction patterns for Al–Mn alloys (86% Al) that displayed five-fold "forbidden" symmetry (Shechtman et al. 1984). These new crystals defied conventional ideas regarding allowable crystal symmetries. After initial rejection, his icosahedral-based structural model was accepted and he was recognized for this discovery with a Nobel Prize in 2011. Inorganic quasicrystals have received a lot of attention recently due to their unique structures that are partly derived from their extreme synthesis conditions. Quasicrystals typically form under extreme conditions at meteor impact sites or nuclear bomb detonation sites where high impact temperatures and pressures are achieved (Castelvecchi 2021). They are constructed from the hierarchical assembly of unique structural elements such as icosahedral shapes to produce aperiodic structures with uniquely tailored symmetry and beauty. These nanoscale assemblies are not true crystals because they lack certain elements of translational symmetry that are required by crystals. In essence, quasicrystals cannot fill three-dimensional space without leaving gaps in the pattern and can be thought of as three dimensional analogues of Penrose Tiles (Penrose 1974, 1979). Quasicrystals display high levels of elegantly nested symmetry and fractal inspired beauty. The first quasicrystals were metallic in composition. One very fascinating aspect of quasicrystals is that MTs are an important example of organic quasicrystals due to the 13-fold symmetry that they exhibit.

These interstitial spaces provide zones for some very unique and fascinating chemistry to occur. The nanoscale interlayer spaces in materials such as clays and layered double hydroxides provide unique reaction spaces where remarkable chemistry can occur (Wilson et al. 1999). Studies of the behavior of water in confined spaces can provide insight to help guide modeling efforts. Johnston et al. (2010) used molecular dynamics simulations to show that water molecules can undergo a phase transformation to become quasicrystals when confined between closely spaced parallel plates. Additional molecular dynamics studies highlight numerous strange quantum inspired effects can arise when water is confined within spaces in cells and in quasi-crystalline cytoskeletal elements such as MTs. Can water confined in the lumen space of quasicrystals assume quasi-crystalline structure, thus recreating a double quasi-crystalline nanocomposite where both the outer and inner phase are quasicrystals? At the minimum, the water may exhibit enhanced diffusion behavior and solid-like properties and thus enhanced transport properties in relation to wave propagation and resonance phenomena may be enhanced.

3 Properties of MTs

MT properties encompass a wide range of physico-chemical properties including resonance phenomena, dielectric and diamagnetic characteristics, piezoelectric, electrical conductivity and transport phenomena. The unique properties exhibited by MTs such as mechanical properties, sensing, signal conduction, information processing, and electrical transport properties result in very fascinating potential applications including memristors, nanowires, and quantum computers.

3.1 *Modeling of Unique Behaviors Exhibited by MTs*

The unique properties of MTs allow them to be modeled as a wide variety of materials systems. MTs have been shown to generate electrical oscillations (Cantero et al. 2018), exhibit transistor-like properties (Priel et al. 2006), exhibit memristive properties (Cantero et al. 2019), and work is being conducted to develop computational capabilities within thin films of bovine brain MTs (Vissol-Gaudin et al. 2021). Measurement of the electrical properties of MTs under physiological conditions is no trivial matter. Kalra et al. (2020) used electrochemical impedance spectroscopy to measure the resistance and capacitance of MT solutions at physiological conditions. The capacitance and resistance of MT network at physiological tubulin concentrations were 1.27×10^{-5} F and 9.74×10^{4} Ω. This supports the idea that MTs act as charge storage devices using the mechanism of counterionic condensation across a broad frequency spectrum. This indicates that the cell cytoskeleton is electrically tunable with polymerization-state-dependent dielectric properties of tubulin.

3.2 *MTs as Memristors*

The resistance of MTs depends upon the applied voltage and its memory—the history of applied voltage or injected current. Memristors are defined as two-terminal passive circuit elements that provide a functional relationship between electric charge and magnetic flux. MTs have a resistance that has been calculated to be between 1 Ω and 10 kΩ for a 10 μm MT. The relationship between current and voltage follows a pinched hysteresis loop. When voltage is applied to the MT and then removed, the MT will retain the resistance at its last value. Some MTs have demonstrated that the direction of the current flow along the MT determines whether its resistance will increase or decrease with higher voltage. An analogy for this is that when a fluid flows through a pipe of varying diameters, the resistance will increase if the flow is from large diameter to small diameter, but will decrease if the flow is from small diameter to large diameter. Further research is required in this area Tuszynski et al. (2020).

3.3 *Mechanotransduction*

MT transmit mechanical signals within cells. Putnam et al. (2001) reported that the relative concentration of tubulin and MTs changes in response to applied tensile and compressive forces and fibronectin concentration in the absence of applied forces. Muscle cells on an extracellular matrix (ECM) substrate were used in the study. Forces were applied to the muscle cell ECM substrate to generate both 10% tensile and compressive strain levels. The 10% compressive strain resulted in a $40 \pm 6\%$ decrease in MT mass while 10% tensile strain resulted in a $34 \pm 10\%$ increase in MT mass compared to static controls. The density of the ECM ligand fibronectin was found to increase the amount of polymeric tubulin in the cell from 59 ± 11 to $81 \pm 13\%$ as the fibronectin density was increased from 50 to 1000 ng/cm^2 in the absence of an applied force. Crosstalk occurs between MT and the extracellular matrix via integrins which form a bridge that links the interior of the cell with the extracellular environment (LaFlamme et al. 2019).

The role that MTs play in the mechanotransduction of mechanical stimuli in striated cardiac muscles has been studied. When cultured neonatal rat cardiac myocytes muscle cells were subjected to passive stretching, there was an increase in β tubulin mRNA without an increase in beta tubulin gene transcription (Watson et al. 1996). MTs provide shape stability to myocytes by resisting compression and longitudinal shear stress, as well as influencing viscoelasticity. Pressure overload can also increase the density of MTs. These adaptations can lead to contractile dysfunction which can be reversed by MT disruption. Loads can also induce changes in the electrical activity that are dependent upon MTs. The exact nature and significance of how MTs impact the response of cardiac myocytes to mechanical stimulation are yet to be fully determined (White 2011).

3.4 *Piezoelectricity*

Piezoelectricity is a very useful property of certain materials that allows the interconversion of mechanical and electrical signals. Classic ceramic materials like barium titanite and lead magnesium niobate possess crystals structures which are isotropic under no strain conditions, but an externally applied stress will shift the symmetry of the unit cell, and the displacement of a central atom results in a polar arrangement that develops a potential difference. The ability to convert mechanical signals into electrical signals is useful for remote micro positioning systems for space telescopes and devices in computers for energy storage as well as robotics. Hydroxyapatite is a more bio-related piezoelectric material. Piezoelectricity in bone was initially discovered by Fukada and Yashuda (1957), and bone adapts to mechanical stress by growing stronger. It is interesting that organic materials and even biological materials can exhibit piezoelectric properties (Rajabi et al. 2015). Collagen displays piezoelectric properties so bone tissue can exhibit piezoelectric properties from both the inorganic hydroxyapatite phase, as well as the organic collagen phase. It may come as no surprise that MT have been theoretically shown to possess piezoelectric properties via computer modeling (Venkateshwarlu et al. (2025). However, experimental validation has not yet been provided due to experimental difficulty in proving this through measurements.

3.5 Electrical Properties

The unique charge distribution and innate electron carrier behavior of tubulin monomer and dimer units impart a unique ability to MTs to generate electromagnetic fields (Pokorný et al. 2021). MTs exhibit unique electrical properties. Gutierrez et al. (2023) used the loose patch clamp technique to measure the electrical properties of single MTs and found that the electrical properties change when MT stabilizing molecules such as paclitaxel were present. It makes sense that electric field interactions with MTs can be useful in treating diseases such as cancer. Electric fields have been the subject of much study in the search for effective therapies to treat cancer. Tumor-Treating Electric Fields (TTEFs) is an acronym that is used to describe low intensity (1–2 V) and intermediate frequency range (100–300 kHz) electric fields that have shown some evidence for inhibiting cancer cell proliferation and replication (Kirson et al. 2004). The primary target is believed to be MTs and specific mechanisms have been identified including mitotic spindle disruption, improper chromosome segregation and the resulting mitotic catastrophe (Urman and Itzhaki (2015); Giladi et al. 2015; Tuszynski et al. 2016) and electromagnetic modulation of the cell cycle (Shi et al 2025).

3.6 MTs as One-Dimensional Crystals

Sanchez-Castro et al. (2021) studied MTs with the approach that they can be modeled as one-dimensional crystals for electrical transmission. The models are based on mathematical crystal theory with one-dimensional translational symmetry. MTs have electrical properties (see above) based on their outer surface being predominantly negatively charged, attracting positive ions while repelling the negative ions of the cytosol.

3.7 MTs as Resonance Cavities and Resonators

MT exhibit resonance phenomena over many orders of magnitude and function as resonance cavities and resonators and when resonance frequencies are matched in biological systems, unique phenomena occur. MT length can be varied to match critically significant distance for coupling. Each of the tubulin heterodimers, consisting of α and β subunits, is an electric dipole with a negative surface charge. The helical structure, electric dipoles, and water in the MT cavity contribute to the generation of an electric field. The tubulin heterodimers with helical and axial periodic organization containing electric dipoles enable the transfer of the electromagnetic field with a phase shift of one or more oscillation periods. Electromagnetic oscillations in the MT cavity connect the tubulin heterodimers and distribute energy among the heterodimers (Pokorný et al. 2021). Jelínik and Pokorný (2001) compared MTs to circular waveguides and cylindrical resonators. They noted that the cutoff and resonant frequencies of the transverse magnetic and transverse modes of the MT cavities suggest the possibility of interaction of electromagnetic cavity modes with inner electrons in atoms. They noted that the resonant frequencies may be in the infrared region. Pokorný et al. (2021) reported that the broad frequency range electromagnetic field is the only known mechanism to provide the organization, communication, information transfer, and control mechanisms that biological systems require in a fast way at all length scales. The electromagnetic oscillation system can enable control over various chemical reactions, information processing, and associated phenomena.

Resonance phenomena and electric field effects can also be manipulated to disrupt MT-based processes by hindering key aspects of MT involvement in cell replication, the cell cycle and facilitation and promotion of apoptosis. These phenomena can be linked with the idea that resonance phenomena and quantum effects are being used to develop models to expand our understanding of how our senses (smell, touch, hearing, taste, and sight) work. On a larger scale, these phenomena may be linked with aspects of brain function, memory, and consciousness.

3.8 Making Sense Out of What Makes Our Senses Work

How does our sense of smell work? There is some controversy regarding the exact nature of how we smell and how our other senses are able to detect, process, and interpret information from our surroundings. A lock-and-key mechanism is commonly attributed to how we perceive smell. This is akin to the antibody–antigen receptors exhibited by our immune system. However, there is a growing body of evidence that supports an alternative prospect for how we perceive smell. This theory is based on ideas proposed by Dyson (1938) and championed by Turin (1996) who is a world class perfumer and scholar in the area of quantum olfaction. In the book, The Emperor of Scent, highlights of the history of our expanding understanding of how scent is detected and Turin's challenging journey in pursuing funding for his revolutionary ideas which were initially rejected until his determination started to change perceptions (Burr 2002). In the theory of quantum olfaction, our sense of smell is based on vibrational frequencies that are generated by scent molecules or odorants. Our olfactory neurons have hundreds of receptors which previously were thought to bind with odorant molecules based on shape. The newer quantum theory of scent offers the hypothesis that the olfactory neurons are able to sense the vibrational frequencies of odorant molecules and our brains interpret the information as a specific smell. The quantum aspects involve tunneling of electrons. What is the component of the olfactory neurons that can respond to and sense vibrations? Quantum olfaction and smell provide another unique role for MTs. It is important to be able to test the validity of any theory and develop accurate and informative models to advance our understanding. Tirandaz et al. (2017) developed a computational model to test aspects of the quantum olfaction theory. Based on the idea that quantum vibrations may be detected by MTs in olfactory neurons, are there other phenomena exhibited by MTs in neurons that may involve resonance effects? There is even an expansion of this theory to include electron tunneling quantum effects and resonance phenomena in how we process light to see and how we perceive touch (Folger 2018). Not to leave out the fundamental relationship between resonance and sound, there is also a potential role for MT-based resonance effects in hearing. Bieniussa et al. (2023) described the unique role of MTs within the sensory cells that process auditory signals into neuronal action potentials in the organ of Corti which is located in the cochlea. MTs are integrated within cilia (Jenkins et al. 2009), and this highlights their role in various sensory functions such as smell, taste, and hearing. Do you remember learning the alphabet with the ABC song? Music and resonance effects in MT is a viable area of research that in time will yield very promising results to help us understand how music impacts learning (Hameroff 2015).

4 MT Function

MT exhibit a host of unique functions that provide cells with the ability to carry out specialized functions. The next section focuses on unique MT functions and special features within a select catalog of cells. MT function in specific cells and how uniquely tailored features in MTs contribute to behavioral differences in cells including bone cells, RBCs, adipocytes, muscle cells, and cancer cells will be described.

4.1 The Cell Cytoskeleton: Bone Analogues Within Cells

The MTs in cells are structural elements within the cytoskeleton that are analogous to a nanoscale skeleton. Bone tissue in the skeletal system provides structural support for the whole body while the cytoskeleton is the support network of the cell. Bone tissue and MTs share a number of unique characteristics as shown in Table 1. MTs share similarities with bone tissue at the whole tissue level as well as the individual organic collagen, inorganic calcium phosphate phases that occur within bone, and the extracellular matrix component of bone and water (Pasteris et al. 2014). Bone mineral phases and MTs are formed via nucleation, growth, and dissolution processes. The hydroxyapatite (HAp) mineral phase in bone undergoes nucleation and crystal growth processes. Bone and MTs have a hollow region that runs along its axial length. Long bones such as the femur have the intermedullary cavity and MTs have a similar "intermicrotubular" cavity sometimes referred to as the lumen. Bone and MTs exhibit extensive remodeling capabilities which are active response mechanisms to specific environmental cues. Bone and MTs have a major structural protein component that makes up the majority of its composition. Collagen is the main structural protein in bone while tubulin is the main structural protein in MTs. There are a large number of collagen isoforms and there are a large number of tubulin isoforms. There are 28 different structural adaptations for collagen which have been identified in the body while around seven (7) tubulin types with additional isoforms have been discovered and documented. There are a host of other proteins that play important roles in other aspects of fine tuning the structure and function of bone and MTs. Bone has ECM proteins that play key developmental roles in orchestrating HAp nucleation and crystal growth and other important components of bone healing and remodeling. MTs have MAPs that function in a similar manner. Collagen and MTs can mineralize and influence nucleation phenomena. MTs transport matrix vesicles which are integral for key aspects of biomineralization (Bottini et al. 2018; Iwayama et al. 2022). MTs may also play role in the transport of HAp that forms within matrix vesicles. Calcium plays a vitally important role in a majority of biological processes. It is no surprise that calcium plays an important role in bone tissue by combining with phosphate ion to form the HAp reinforcing mineral phase. Calcium ion also plays key roles in MT functions such as influencing the depolymerization of MTs (O'Brien et al. 1997) and regulating how kinesin molecules transport mitochondria (Wang and Schwarz 2009).

One of the more unique aspects of the role of calcium in both bone and MTs involves the inter-relationship and unique implication of a classic model component of bone mineral called Posner's Clusters. Posner clusters have a unique historical place in the development of models for how the mineral phase forms in mammalian hard tissue (Betts and Posner 1974; Mancardi et al. 2017). Posner clusters have the chemical formula $Ca_9(PO_4)_6$ and are on the order of 1 nm in diameter. They have been implicated in various models for mineral formation in bone as well as calcium and phosphate cycling in mitochondria. Posner clusters play an important role in how the mineral phase(s) in bone form(s) via the initial nucleation of amorphous calcium phosphate (ACP) which subsequently crystallizes into hydroxyapatite or other calcium phosphate phases. MTs and Posner clusters also have potential roles in higher order thinking and consciousness. Fisher (2015) and Swift et al. (2018) highlight an additional role for Posner clusters in providing an accommodating environment to enhance the spin coherence time for the six (6) PO_4^{3-} molecules housed within its structure. These phosphate spins have implications for developing a platform for liquid-state nuclear magnetic resonance-based quantum computation, in vivo medical imaging applications with a view for intracellular enzyme sensing (Luo et al. 2021), and a proposed role as "neural qubits" as a component in a hypothetical model to understand the mechanism for quantum processing in the brain.

Table 1 Bone and MT similarities in structural features

Whole bone tissue level
(1) Hollow axial region (2) Extensive remodeling in response to environmental cues (resorption pits, osteoclast activity, stress-induced remodeling, etc.)
Organic matrix phase level
(1) Large protein component (MT—$\alpha\beta$ tubulin, bone—collagen) (2) Intracellular synthesis of protein to help regulate structure and guide formation (ECM vs. MT-associated proteins (MAPs))
Biomineral reinforcing phase level (hydroxyapatite) comparison with tubulin dimer unit
(1) Nucleation-directed growth processes (2) Evidence for homogeneous nucleation and heterogeneous nucleation (3) Self-assembly directed growth processes (4) Fundamental building blocks (atomic elemental level (calcium and phosphate) vs. C, H, O (other elements)), molecular level (Posner cluster vs. polypeptide chain and tubulin monomer/dimer unit) (5) Aggregative growth of base units to yield hierarchical structures (Posner cluster vs. tubulin dimer) (6) Critical importance of Ca^{2+} mediated bioprocess (Ca role in mineral phase formation, Ca role in depolymerization of MT) (7) Exhibition of quantum effects (8) Postulated roles in neural processes (potential role of Posner clusters in aspects of neuron activity and consciousness) (proposed by Fisher (2015) and Swift et al. (2018))

4.2 *MTs and Adipose Cells*

MTs help control the size, distribution, and organization of lipid droplets in adipocytes. Cell organize lipid droplets in adipocytes to influence energy storage and metabolism. MTs are a major component of the cytoskeleton, providing structural support and enabling cell shape changes during adipocyte development. They are also involved in the remodeling of the cytoskeleton, which is crucial for the transition from preadipocytes to mature adipocytes. It is generally known that white adipose cells store fat for energy while brown adipose cells and tissue are more active in heat generation, thermal regulation, and metabolism. MTs may play a role in transporting mitochondria for more efficient energy burning to generate heat in brown adipose cells while MTs may play a role in transporting lipid droplets in white adipose cells. More research is necessary to provide more specific insight regarding how the role of MTs changes in function for White versus Brown adipose cells and tissue. MTs help with adipocyte differentiation during adipogenesis by influencing gene expression of proteins that are needed for these processes to occur. Adipose tissue is composed of white and brown adipose cells and has been elevated to organ status as the adipose organ. The adipose organ is composed of brown adipose tissue, white adipose tissue, and beige adipose tissue which is a mixture of both brown and white adipose cells. The adipose organ is classified as part of the endocrine system with obesity and type 2 diabetes as its main chronic pathological diseases (Cinti and Cinti 2022).

4.3 Adipose Tissue and Insulin Resistance

Insulin resistance is a serious consequence of the imbalance in the relative amounts of white, brown, and beige fat and improper ratio that occurs with obesity. Analogies are powerful tools and one potential analogy for understanding insulin resistance can be borrowed from a famous children's story called The Boy Who Cried Wolf. Many versions of the story have been told over history but the general scope of the story revolves around a young boy who fabricates a false situation where he yells that a wolf is nearby. When the townspeople respond and see that the boy was lying, they disregard his calls when a real wolf appears. Adipocyte heterogeneity is required to mediate the multiple pathways that control systemic glucose tolerance. White adipocytes specialize in sequestering triglycerides away from the liver, muscle, and other tissues to limit toxicity. In contrast, brown/beige adipocytes are very active in directly taking up glucose in response to β adrenergic signaling and insulin and enhancing energy expenditure. Nonetheless, white, beige, and brown adipocytes all share the common feature of secreting factors and possibly exosomes that act on distant tissues to control glucose homeostasis. Obesity exerts deleterious effects on each of these adipocyte functions to cause insulin resistance. Czech (2020) provided an analysis of the mechanisms that cause insulin resistance. A diverse mixture of white, brown, and beige adipose tissue is needed for proper metabolism of glucose through proper insulin signal conduction. This is because the different adipose tissues play different roles in the body where white adipose tissue plays a role in limiting toxicity in the liver and muscles by removing triglycerides. Brown and beige adipose tissue actively respond to insulin signals with direct uptake of glucose to enhance burning energy. However, the common feature among white, brown, and beige adipose tissue is that the respective cells secrete factors and exosomes that help control glucose homeostasis (Czech 2020).

4.4 MT Function in Red Blood Cells (RBCs)

MTs play a role in all cells within the blood and bone marrow including both hematopoeietic stem cells and mesenchymal stem cells with all their progenitor cells, RBCs, and associated cells representing the immune system (white blood cells, B cells, T cells, and others…). MTs provide structural support for healthy rbcs by forming the peripheral ring of MTs called the marginal band that enhances the mechanical properties of RBCs in nonmammalian species, mammalian erythroblasts, and platelets (Dmitrieff et al. 2017). MTs also play an important role regarding the transportation network that carries blood throughout the body to conduct its important function of transporting oxygen to cells and removing wastes products and carbon dioxide. MTs from the endothelial cells that line the inner surface of blood vessels play an important role in maintaining the proper mechanical properties for proper blood flow. Blood vessels, arteries, and veins need to be elastic and flexible with healthy lining of endothelial cells.

Sickle cell anemia is an example of a pathological challenge which can potentially be treated using a MT-derived therapy. Sickle cell disease was one of the first diseases to be understood at the molecular level and is caused by a less than 0.1% error in the amino acid sequence of hemoglobin. Sickle Cell disease has a well-documented history (Smith 1999). Sickle cell was first identified as a disease in 1910 after analysis of the blood of a 20-year-old college student whose rbcs appeared thin and in the shape of a sickle (Herrick 1910). Sickle cell has the distinction of being the first disease to be understood on a molecular basis due to the groundbreaking work of Pauling et al. (1949). A sickle cell crisis occurs when the amount of oxygen decreases below a critical threshold and the abnormal hemoglobin forms fibers which force the rbc morphology to change into the thin crescent shape. This morphology negatively impacts flow characteristics of the deformed rbcs. The pathophysiological reason for this is based on a mutation of the hemoglobin gene where valine is switched for glutamic acid at position 6 (Renaudier 2014).

MTs play a very important role in various aspects of sickle cell disease where the departure from normal MT function in rbcs facilitates the characteristic morphological development when a crisis occurs due to lack of oxygen. MT play a role in sickle cell disease onset and progression and may be a source for the development of treatments. MT defects cause inefficient organization during growth of hemoglobin in sickle cell. In their very high resolution study of the assembly dynamics of sickle cell hemoglobin, Castle et al. (2019) discovered that the abnormal hemoglobin molecules formed fibers that were about 20 nm in diameter in a surprisingly inefficient manner. The self-assembly process efficiency was about 4%. This opens up the door for the development of more effective targeted therapies that can be delivered at lower threshold doses.

4.5 Role of MTs in Cancer Metastasis

4.5.1 What Is Cancer Metastasis?

Metastasis is one of the "Hallmarks of Cancer" (Hanahan and Weinberg 2000, 2011; Hanahan 2022) and is responsible for most cancer-related deaths (Morales et al. 2021). In fact, each of the traditional Hallmarks of Cancer (Hanahan and Weinberg 2000), the revised and more recent recently revised (Hanahan 2022) and the Hallal Marks of Cancer (Alsheri and Wilson 2024) related to food and cancer prevention has a strong inter-relationship with MTs. Metastasis occurs when cancer cells invade the tissue surrounding the tumor stroma and migrate to other organs (D'Andrea et al. 2021). Cancer metastasis is a multistep process that involves five main steps: (i) tumor cell invasion and local infiltration into adjacent tissue, (ii) transendothelial migration of cancer cells into vessels (intravasation), (iii) survival in the circulatory system, (iv) extravasation (exit from blood vessels), and (v) colonization (subsequent proliferation in competent tissue and organs). Cancer cell mechanobiology studies focus on how the mechanical properties and chemical composition of the extracellular matrix (ECM) influence the metastasis of cancer cells. Cancer migration is crucial for several physiological processes, including tissue morphogenesis, immune cell trafficking, wound repair, and metastasis. Cancer mechanobiology studies provide evidence to help explain how forces (such as pressure, tension, and fluid flow) and mechanical properties (including stiffness and elasticity) affect cellular function and tumor progression. This knowledge can be used to develop strategies that impede the dissemination of cancer cells from the initial tumor site, thereby preventing the formation of metastases in other tissues or organs. A brief review of mechanobiology, cancer metastasis, and cancer cell biology is provided to offer background information.

4.5.2 Mechanobiology in Cancer Metastasis

Recent advances in engineering and the physical sciences have revealed critical roles of the mechanical and structural properties of cells and tissues in guiding malignancy and metastasis (Malandrino et al. 2018). Tissue architecture and the mechanical characteristics of tissues and cells play a significant role in cancer progression. The dynamic remodeling of the stromal collagen network is a hallmark of tumor progression. Cancer cells exert various forces against their surrounding environment, creating a complex system for analysis (Kraning-Rush et al. 2012). What are the molecular mechanisms that allow cancer cells to sense solid stress? This elusive question was addressed in a unique way by treating cancer as a thermodynamically driven process that included aspects of liquid phase separation (Sun et al. 2024).

MDA-MB-231 is an invasive human breast cancer cell line widely used for in vitro studies of breast cancer metastasis. This cell line generally exhibits poor metastatic tumorigenic potential (Holliday and Speirs 2011). However, it serves as the foundation for developing metastatic models for in vitro studies following the induction of genetic changes identified by Massague's group (Kang et al. 2003). Breast cancer cells are influenced by collagen matrix alignment and can adjust their migration through contact guidance (Riching et al. 1989; Carey et al. 2016; Ray et al. 2017). Breast and prostate cancers, along with many other cancer types, are mechanically sensitive (Rao et al. 2014; Verbruggen et al. 2021). The connection between cancer response to mechanical loading in the stroma and disease outcome remains somewhat unclear. In vitro cancer cell tissue constructs with in situ force loading can help clarify the role of mechanical forces in modifying the functional behavior of cancer cells.

Taxol, a chemotherapeutic agent, plays a significant role in the mechanobiology of cancer metastasis. Taxol was originally isolated from the stem bark of the western yew, *Taxus brevifolia*, and has also been found in the leaves, stem and roots of a variety of other Taxus species (Patel 1998). The drug is a complex ester taxane derivative containing a rare oxetan ring, and is the first compound of this type to have anti-leukemic and tumor inhibitory properties. Manfredi (1982) found that taxol had the ability to inhibit the replication of HeLa cells by acting as a mitotic spindle "poison." Prior to taxol, colchicines as well as vinblastine were the main drugs of choice for cancer therapy. Taxol is a potent anti-neoplastic drug that binds to the N-terminal region of β-tubulin and promotes the formation of very stable MTs that arrest the cell cycle at the G_2/M phase and prevent normal cell division. This arrest causes rapidly dividing carcinogenic cells to bypass the remaining phases in mitotic cell division and undergo apoptosis (Merkher et al. 2017; Lim et al. 2022). Another potential mechanism for how taxol facilitates the treatment of human cancer cells involves initiation of mitotic slippage and the subsequent arrest of the cell cycle in G1 and accompanying apoptosis (Wilson et al. 1985; Arnal and Wade 1995; Mukhtar et al. 2014). Prolonged exposure of cells to Taxol induces apoptotic cell death via DNA fragmentation (Torres 1998).

Taxol's impact on MT mechanics is profound, as it enhances the stability of lateral interactions between tubulin molecules, thereby altering the mechanical properties of MTs and affecting cellular mechanics (Cannariato et al. 2024). This stabilization is crucial in reducing the mechanobiological invasiveness of metastatic cells, as evidenced by their reduced ability to indent synthetic gels, a proxy for invasive potential (Merkher and Weihs 2017). Taxol can decrease the expression of metastasis associated proteins like VEGF and MMP-9 thereby reducing metastatic spread in models of salivary adenoid cystic carcinoma (Quintero-Fabián et al. 2019). In clinical settings, Taxol is effective in reducing circulating tumor cells, which are precursors to metastasis, as reflected in its significant ability to lower the incidence of bone metastases in experimental models (Stearns 1995). However, resistance to Taxol remains a challenge, often mediated by mechanisms such as the overproduction of P-glycoprotein, which functions as a drug efflux pump, maintaining sub-cytotoxic drug levels within resistant cells (Horwitz et al. 1993). Additionally, Taxol can induce pro-survival phenotypes in cancer cells through stress response pathways, complicating its efficacy in specific contexts (Anderson et al. 1995). Despite these challenges, Taxol remains a cornerstone in the treatment of various cancers, including breast cancer, where it is used both as a monotherapy and in combination with other agents to enhance therapeutic outcomes (Jivani and Shinde 2024). Overall, Taxol's role in mechanobiology is multifaceted, involving direct effects on MT dynamics and indirect impact on cellular signaling pathways that collectively influence cancer metastasis and treatment resistance.

The exploration of cancer therapeutics derived from periwinkle and other natural sources has highlighted the significant roles of JNK, Caspase 9, BRCA-1, and the apoptosome in apoptosis, a critical process for eradicating cancer cells (Goswami et al. 2024). MTs play a significant multifaceted role in apoptosis via reorganization to form the apoptotic MT network (Ávila et al. 2015). JNK, a key player in the MAPK pathway, is involved in stress-induced apoptosis and is activated by various stimuli, including phytochemicals, which can modulate apoptosis in cancer cells (Chen and Tan 1999; Kumar et al. 2024). Caspase 9, part of the intrinsic mitochondrial pathway, is crucial for apoptosis, and its activation is a primary target in cancer therapies, with numerous compounds being investigated for their ability to induce caspase-mediated apoptosis (Debatin 2004; Allani et al. 2024). BRCA-1, a tumor suppressor gene, is involved in DNA repair and apoptosis, with its cleavage by caspases facilitating chemotherapy-induced apoptosis. This cleavage is crucial for the pro-apoptotic function of BRCA-1, which is impaired by certain mutations, affecting the response to chemotherapeutic agents (Quinn et al. 2003; Dizin et al. 2008).

There are a number of additional Specific agents from foods can partner with MTs to help deliver a knockout punch to cancer cells. Sulforaphanes are found in cruciferous vegetables like broccoli, kale, etc. Broccoli sprouts have a unusually high concentration of sulforaphanes. Zhou et al. (2018) found that sulforaphanes can inhibit the growth of a number of cancers, but the relatively short half-life of 2 h limits its use. The metabolites of sulforaphane (sulforaphane-cysteine (SFN-Cys) and sulforaphane-N-acetyl-cysteine (SFN-NAC)) exhibit longer half-lives and exhibited the ability to treat human prostate cancer. The mechanism of action involved triggering the dynamic imbalance of MTs leading to cell apoptosis. Gupta et al. (2006) showed how the antioxidant curcumin inhibits MT assembly through tubulin binding.

Mitochondria play a multifaceted role in apoptosis, not only as energy providers but also as regulators of apoptotic pathways. They are targeted in cancer therapies to induce apoptosis through mitochondrial outer membrane permeabilization, leading to the release of cytochrome C and activation of caspases (Son et al. 2017; Wang et al. 2017). MTs also contribute to apoptosis by forming an apoptotic MT network, which is crucial for inducing apoptosis in response to MT-damaging agents (MDAs). These agents can trigger apoptosis through p53-independent pathways, making them effective even in p53-mutant cancers (Jun et al. 2016). The integration of these pathways and components underscores the complexity and potential of targeting apoptotic mechanisms in cancer therapy, offering promising avenues for overcoming drug resistance and improving therapeutic outcomes (Debatin 2004; Hamilton et al. 2021).

MT acetylation is a post-translational modification of α-tubulin, primarily at lysine 40, which is crucial for stabilizing MTs and supporting cellular processes such as intracellular transport, cell motility, and division (Gupta et al. 2006; Xie et al. 2024). This modification is facilitated by α-tubulin acetyltransferase 1 (αTAT1) and is linked to forming stable MT structures, often involved in cancer cell migration and metastasis (Kwon et al. 2020). In cancer, especially aggressive types such as triple-negative breast cancer (TNBC) and hepatocellular carcinoma (HCC), higher levels of MT acetylation are associated with increased metastatic potential as they promote micro-tentacle formation and support cell adhesion and invasive movement (Yang et al. 2024; Zhong et al. 2021).

Blocking MT acetylation can interfere with these processes, thus reducing cancer metastasis. Overall, blocking MT acetylation appears to be a promising way to stop cancer spread by destabilizing MT and disrupting the cellular mechanisms that enable metastasis (Ruggiero and Lalli 2021; Mangaonkar et al. 2024). MT-targeting drugs that inhibit acetylation can inhibit cancer metastasis. Histone deacetylase strengthens the MT cytoskeleton through acetylation. Histone deacetylase inhibitors possess antimetastatic properties (Mangaonkar et al. 2024). For example, MT acetylation inhibitors like GM-90257 and GM-90631 have been shown to trigger cell death and halt mitosis in TNBC by activating the JNK/AP-1 signaling pathway, leading to apoptosis and decreased tumor growth (Ahn et al. 2023). Similarly, targeting CAMSAP2-driven non-centrosomal MT acetylation in HCC has been found to hinder cell migration and invasion, suggesting that disrupting this modification could be a strategy to prevent metastasis (Li et al. 2020). Moreover, reducing MT acetylation through CDK9 inhibition has demonstrated anti-leukemic effects by destabilizing MTs, highlighting the potential of targeting acetylation pathways across various cancers (Xiao et al. 2023). Furthermore, the absence of tektin4, a MAP, promotes TNBC metastasis through HDAC6-mediated tubulin deacetylation, implying that HDAC6 inhibitors could be a therapeutic option for tektin4-deficient TNBC (Ge et al. 2021). In comparison, other post-translational modifications (PTMs) of tubulin, such as detyrosination, also influence cancer aggressiveness; however, acetylation specifically promotes focal adhesion dynamics and cell movement (Bance et al. 2018, 2019). The potential for using MT-based phenomena in cancer detection and therapeutics was highlighted in a study by Boggs et al. (2015). The study focused on how the acetylation of lysine 40 in α-tubulin promoted the generation of micro-tentacle-like cell protrusions, tumor cell reattachment, and chemotaxis. These characteristic features provide selective advantages for metastatic potential and were particularly enriched in basal-like breast cancers. This provides an interesting opportunity for α-tubulin acetylation to serve as both a diagnostic and therapeutic target for metastatic breast cancer. Emerging therapeutic approaches include using HDAC6 inhibitors, which boost the anti-tumor effects of drugs like eribulin by increasing tubulin acetylation, offering a potential treatment for TNBC (Oba et al. 2021). Additionally, the regulation of MT acetylation by noncoding RNAs, such as long non coding RNAs (lncRNAs) and miRNAs, underscores the complexity of PTM control in cancer development (Kar et al. 2024). Overall, targeting MT acetylation looks promising for cancer treatment, especially in tumors where acetylation is linked to metastasis and drug resistance (Wattanathamsan et al. 2021; Wattanathamsan and Pongrakhananon 2022).

4.6 *Strategic Approaches in MTA Development*

The development of MT-targeting agents (MTAs) has seen significant advancements over the past several decades. Initially, these agents were mainly recognized for their ability to interfere with MT dynamics, disrupting mitosis and inducing cancer cell death. However, as challenges like toxicity, limited selectivity, and the emergence of drug resistance became evident, researchers redirected their focus toward innovative strategies designed to enhance therapeutic efficacy and safety. Key strategies include: the judicious use of stabilizing and destabilizing agents, precision-targeted approaches, and combination therapies.

4.7 Stabilizing Versus Destabilizing Agents

MTAs can be broadly classified based on their effects on MT dynamics into stabilizing and destabilizing agents. Stabilizing agents, such as Taxol (paclitaxel) and epothilones, work by promoting the assembly and stabilization of MTs, thereby preventing their disassembly. This stabilization disrupts the normal dynamic behavior of MTs during cell division, leading to mitotic arrest and subsequent apoptosis. These agents are particularly effective against rapidly dividing cancer cells, making them a cornerstone of chemotherapy regimens for various malignancies (Pasquier and Kavallaris 2008; Wordeman and Vicente 2021). In contrast, destabilizing agents, including Vinca alkaloids like vinblastine and vincristine, inhibit MT polymerization. They bind to tubulin and prevent the assembly of MTs, resulting in mitotic arrest through a different mechanism compared to stabilizing agents. These agents are often used in combination with other chemotherapeutic drugs to enhance treatment efficacy and overcome resistance (Kumar et al. 2017; Zhang et al. 2023). These two classes of agents exploit opposing effects on MT dynamics to interfere with cancer cell proliferation and are vital components of many anticancer treatment strategies.

4.8 Precision-Targeted Approaches

Recent advances in cancer treatments highlight the importance of precision-targeted strategies to improve the selectivity and effectiveness of MT-targeting agents (MTAs). One such strategy involves the development of Antibody-Drug Conjugates (ADCs), which combine the high specificity of monoclonal antibodies with the potent cell-killing effects of MTAs. By attaching a MT-disrupting agent to an antibody that recognizes tumor-specific antigens, ADCs enable targeted delivery of the cytotoxic payload directly to cancer cells, thereby sparing normal tissues and reducing systemic toxicity. For example, trastuzumab-DM1 (ado-trastuzumab emtansine) targets specifically HER2-positive breast cancer cells, delivering the Vinca alkaloid derivative DM1 directly to the tumor, which enhances treatment effectiveness while minimizing adverse effects (Seligmann and Twelves 2013; Collyer et al. 2022). Another innovative strategy involves nanoparticle-based drug delivery systems. Nanoparticles can encapsulate or conjugate MTAs, significantly improving their solubility, stability, and bioavailability. These nanocarriers facilitate targeted delivery by exploiting the enhanced permeability and retention (EPR) effect, allowing higher concentrations of the drug to accumulate within tumor tissues while limiting exposure to healthy tissues. This approach not only enhances therapeutic efficacy but also reduces systemic toxicity, making it a promising avenue for improving the clinical utility of MTAs (Banerjee et al. 2016). These precision-targeted strategies exemplify the shift toward more personalized and effective cancer therapies, leveraging molecular recognition and nanotechnology to optimize drug delivery and improve patient outcomes.

4.9 Combination Therapies

In the changing landscape of cancer treatment, combination therapy has become a key strategy to improve therapeutic results, especially when using MTAs. The reason for this approach is to take advantage of the synergistic effects of drugs with different mechanisms of action, thereby increasing tumor cell death, preventing or slowing the development of resistance, and lowering the chance of relapse. MTAs, such as Taxol (paclitaxel), are especially effective when combined with other chemotherapeutic drugs, targeted therapies, or immunotherapies. For example, in treating breast cancer, Taxol is often used alongside anthracyclines like doxorubicin and alkylating agents such as cyclophosphamide. This combination takes advantage of their complementary mechanisms: while Taxol stabilizes MTs and disrupts cell division, doxorubicin intercalates into DNA and inhibits topoisomerase II, causing DNA damage; cyclophosphamide, on the other hand, alkylates DNA, creating crosslinks that interfere with DNA replication and transcription. Together, these drugs provide a more complete attack on tumor cells, leading to higher response rates, better progression-free survival, and increased overall survival compared to monotherapy (Pasquier and Kavallaris 2008; Wordeman and Vicente 2021). Furthermore, combination regimens can address the heterogeneity within tumors, targeting different subpopulations of cancer cells and circumventing mechanisms that often lead to drug resistance. For example, combining MTAs with agents that inhibit survival pathways or promote apoptosis can sensitize resistant tumor cells to MT disruption. Clinical trials continue to explore various combinations, including MTAs with targeted inhibitors of growth factor receptors or immune checkpoint inhibitors, to develop more effective, less toxic, and durable treatment strategies (Guo et al. 2022; Shi et al. 2024). Overall, the integration of MTAs into combination therapy protocols exemplifies a rational and strategic approach to maximize anticancer efficacy, extend patient survival, and improve quality of life. As understanding of tumor biology deepens, these combination strategies are expected to become even more refined and personalized, paving the way for precision oncology.

4.10 Clinical Applications of MTAs

MTAs are among the most widely utilized chemotherapeutic drugs in oncology, owing to their ability to interfere with cell division and induce apoptosis in rapidly proliferating tumor cells. Their application spans a broad range of malignancies, including solid tumors and hematological cancers. Taxol (Paclitaxel) remains a cornerstone in the treatment of various cancers. It is approved for the treatment of ovarian, breast, and non-small-cell lung cancers, where it effectively induces mitotic arrest by stabilizing MTs. Its efficacy has made it a standard component of many combination regimens, improving survival outcomes in these cancers (Pasquier and Kavallaris 2008; Wordeman and Vicente 2021). Additionally, paclitaxel is used in the management of advanced gastric cancer, cervical cancer, and certain head and neck cancers, often in combination with other chemotherapeutic agents or targeted therapies. Vinca alkaloids, such as vinblastine, vincristine, and vinorelbine, have been integral in the treatment of hematologic malignancies, including lymphomas, leukemias, and multiple myeloma. They are also employed in solid tumors such as testicular cancer, small-cell lung cancer, and breast cancer. Their unique mechanism of inhibiting MT polymerization makes them effective in disrupting tumor cell division, and they are often used in combination with other chemotherapeutics to enhance efficacy (Kumar et al. 2017; Zhang et al. 2023). Epothilones are a newer class of MTAs with a mechanism similar to taxanes but with improved activity in taxane-resistant cancers. They have shown promise in clinical trials for metastatic breast cancer, non-small-cell lung cancer, and prostate cancer, especially in cases where tumors have developed resistance to earlier-generation MTAs (Pasquier and Kavallaris 2008; Wordeman and Vicente 2021). Beyond these, other notable applications include Eribulin, a synthetic analog of halichondrin B, which is approved for metastatic breast cancer and liposarcoma. Eribulin inhibits MT growth and promotes apoptosis (Takahashi et al. 2024). The epothilone analog Ixabepilone is used in metastatic or locally advanced breast cancer, particularly in cases resistant to other MTAs (Pivot et al. 2008). Overall, MTAs are versatile agents with a broad spectrum of clinical applications, and ongoing research continues to expand their therapeutic potential, including the development of new formulations, targeted delivery systems, and combination regimens designed to overcome resistance and improve patient outcomes.

4.11 Challenges and Limitations of MTAs

Despite their widespread clinical success, MT-targeting agents (MTAs) face several challenges that limit their effectiveness and tolerability. One of the main issues is drug resistance, which often develops in cancer cells after long-term exposure to MTAs. Resistance mechanisms include the overexpression of drug efflux pumps, such as P-glycoprotein, which actively pumps drugs out of cancer cells, and mutations in tubulin genes that alter drug binding sites, thereby reducing the effectiveness (Pasquier and Kavallaris 2008; Perez 2009) of drugs. These changes can cause treatment failure and disease progression. Another important limitation is toxicity, as MTAs are linked to various adverse side effects. Patients often face hematological toxicities like neutropenia, neurotoxicities such as peripheral neuropathy, and systemic symptoms including fatigue. These toxicities can significantly affect quality of life and frequently require dose reductions or stopping treatment (Seligmann and Twelves 2013; Wordeman and Vicente 2021). Managing these side effects remains a crucial part of clinical care and ongoing research. Limited specificity is also a significant concern. Many MTAs target MTs indiscriminately, affecting not only cancer cells but also normal proliferating tissues, leading to collateral damage. This lack of selectivity contributes to off-target effects and limits the therapeutic window. The development of more targeted delivery systems and tumor-specific agents aims to overcome this limitation. However, it remains a significant hurdle in the clinical application of MTAs (Banerjee et al. 2016; Collyer et al. 2022). Overall, addressing these challenges, namely, resistance, toxicity, and limited specificity, is crucial for enhancing the efficacy and safety profile of MTAs and expanding their role in cancer therapy.

4.12 Future Directions in MTA Development for Cancer Therapies

The field of MTAs is on the verge of major changes as researchers aim to address long-standing issues like resistance, toxicity, and limited tumor specificity. Several innovative approaches are emerging to enhance the therapeutic potential of MTAs and expand their role in personalized cancer therapy.

(A) **Discovery of Novel Binding Sites and Mechanisms**

A promising area of research involves identifying previously unknown binding sites for tubulin. Beyond the classical taxane, Vinca, and colchicine sites, recent studies utilizing advanced structural biology techniques such as cryo-electron microscopy have revealed additional pockets on tubulin that new agents could target. Developing drugs that bind these alternative sites could result in MTAs with unique mechanisms of action, potentially overcoming resistance associated with classical agents. These novel agents may also offer improved selectivity and reduced toxicity by targeting specific MT conformations or post-translational modifications prevalent in cancer cells (Wang et al. 2023).

(B) **Precision Delivery and Nanotechnology**

Enhancing drug delivery remains a primary goal, with nanotechnology taking a leading role. Researchers are creating nanoparticles, liposomes, and polymer carriers that can encapsulate MTAs to protect them from degradation and allow controlled release. These carriers can be functionalized with ligands or antibodies to target tumor-specific antigens, thereby increasing drug accumulation in cancerous tissues while minimizing effects on healthy cells. Adding stimuli-responsive materials, such as pH-sensitive or enzyme-degradable nanoparticles, further improves delivery by releasing drugs specifically within the tumor environment. These targeted systems can significantly reduce systemic toxicity and enhance treatment effectiveness (Banerjee et al. 2016; Collyer et al. 2022).

(C) **Overcoming Drug Resistance**

Resistance to MTAs remains a significant challenge in clinical oncology. Future research will focus on developing agents that can circumvent standard resistance mechanisms, such as the overexpression of efflux pumps, like P-glycoprotein, or mutations in tubulin genes. For instance, efforts are underway to create epothilones and next-generation taxanes with altered binding affinities that remain effective against resistant tumor cells. Additionally, combination therapies are being explored, pairing MTAs with inhibitors of resistance pathways such as P-glycoprotein inhibitors or modulators of MT-associated proteins to restore drug sensitivity and prolong responses (Wordeman and Vicente 2021).

(D) **Targeting MT Dynamics Beyond Cell Division**

Emerging evidence suggests that MTs play roles beyond mitosis, including regulation of cell migration, intracellular trafficking, and signaling pathways. Future MTA development may focus on agents that selectively modulate non-mitotic MT functions, thereby disrupting tumor invasion and metastasis without affecting normal cell division. Such specificity could improve therapeutic windows and reduce side effects (Ferrara et al. 2016).

(E) **Personalized and Biomarker-Driven Approaches**

The integration of genomics and proteomics into oncology has opened avenues for personalized medicine. Identifying biomarkers predictive of response to specific MTAs could enable clinicians to tailor treatments to individual patients, maximizing efficacy and minimizing adverse effects. For example, tubulin isotype expression profiles or post-translational modifications could serve as indicators for selecting the most effective MT inhibitors (Dinić et al. 2024).

(F) **Combining MTAs with Immunotherapy**

Recent advances in immuno-oncology suggest synergistic potential when combining MTAs with immune checkpoint inhibitors or other immunomodulatory agents. MTAs can modulate the tumor microenvironment and enhance immune recognition, thereby improving responses to immunotherapy. Future studies are expected to optimize such combinations, potentially leading to durable, long-lasting remissions (Serpico et al. 2020).Table 2 provides a number of examples of post translational MT modifications and their specific roles in cancer metastasis.

4.13 Diabetes and MTs

Glucose is a very important molecule and forms the basis for providing the energy that our bodies need to function. This is why there are so many checks and balances and mechanistic pathways which are necessary to ensure proper utilization of this valuable resource. Our brains use most of the glucose that our bodies take in. The importance of glucose has led to some uniquely unfortunate side consequences that adversely impact various aspects of our metabolism. Since glucose is necessary, our bodies have developed a reward system for the consumption of foods that contain glucose or fructose such as fruits or foods that can be broken down during digestion to produce glucose. Sugar is addictive and the pervasive role of sugar in the food industry has resulted in an epidemic proportions of health conditions that are caused,

Table 2 Comparison of microtubule post-translational modifications (PTMs)

PTM	Description	Enzymes involved	Functional impact	Role in cancer metastasis	References
Acetylation (Lys40 of α-tubulin)	Addition of an acetyl group to lysine residue 40 of α-tubulin	αTAT1 (acetyltransferase); HDAC6, SIRT2 (deacetylases)	Stabilizes microtubules, promotes motor protein binding, involved in transport	Promotes cell migration and invasion by stabilizing microtubules, facilitating metastatic spread	Carmona et al. (2023)
Detyrosination	Removal of the C-terminal tyrosine on α-tubulin	Tubulin carboxypeptidases (TCPs)	Enhances microtubule stability, affects motor protein interactions	Elevated detyrosination correlates with increased cell motility and metastatic potential	Nieuwenhuis and Brummelkamp (2019)
Tyrosination	Re-adding tyrosine to detyrosinated α-tubulin	Tubulin tyrosine ligase (TTL)	Marks dynamic microtubules, regulates interactions with microtubule-associated proteins (MAPs)	Increased tyrosination is linked to higher microtubule turnover, promoting invasion and metastasis	Wattanathamsan and Pongrakhananon (2023)
Polyglutamylation	Addition of glutamate chains to tubulin	TTLL (tubulin tyrosine ligase-like) enzymes	Regulates interactions with MAPs and motor proteins, affects microtubule stability	Enhances invasive capacities by promoting microtubule dynamics involved in migration	Das et al. (2014)
Polyglycylation	Addition of glycine chains to tubulin	TTLL enzymes	Influences microtubule stability and interaction with MAPs	Less studied in metastasis but linked to microtubule regulation in invasive cells	Wattanathamsan and Pongrakhananon (2023)
Phosphorylation	Addition of phosphate groups to tubulin or associated proteins	Various kinases (e.g., CDKs, MAP kinases)	Modulates microtubule dynamics, organization, and interactions	Phosphorylation of tubulin or associated proteins can promote cell motility and invasion	Ramkumar et al. (2018)

(continued)

Table 2 (continued)

PTM	Description	Enzymes involved	Functional impact	Role in cancer metastasis	References
Ubiquitination	Addition of ubiquitin to tubulin	E3 ubiquitin ligases	May target tubulin for degradation or alter its interactions	Aberrant ubiquitination may lead to microtubule destabilization, facilitating metastasis	Han et al. (2022)
Novel acylations (e.g., succinylation, crotonylation)	Addition of acyl groups like succinyl or crotonyl groups to lysines	p300/CBP (a versatile acyltransferase) and SIRT family members (deacylases)	Modifies charge and interaction properties; influences stability and dynamics	Emerging evidence suggests they regulate microtubule functions related to cell migration and invasion; potential therapeutic targets for metastasis	Shi et al. (2024)

influenced, and exacerbated by overconsumption of sugar. Books such as sugar, salt, and fat highlight the lengths that food can be used as a weapon of mass destruction when sugar content is manipulated to utilize the addiction appeal of sugar to drive sales. Lustig et al. (2012) discuss the toxic truth about sugar and suggest the idea that the USA should follow the lead of other countries and put warning labels and more healthy limits and guidelines for sugar consumption to help more people steer clear of the dangers of overconsumption of sugar and what it does to our bodies. As a simple introduction, excess sugar in our blood that is not metabolized and used for cell energy production can react with proteins and fat molecules in the body and produce advanced glycation end products or "AGEs" for short. As the acronym suggests, AGEs cause premature aging and cause extensive damage to tissues in the body such as the heart, fine blood vessels, skin, etc. It suppresses our immune system, changes gut microbiome dynamic, impacts cognitive function, and contributes to metabolic syndrome and the number-one disease that is associated with improper glucose utilization, Diabetes. Type I diabetes is sometimes referred to as Juvenile diabetes and can be genetic and/or autoimmune type where the body attacks islet cells where insulin is produced. Type II Diabetes may be linked with insulin resistance and is caused by the body's inability to keep glucose within safe limits. In terms of reference, a fasting blood glucose level of less that 100 mg/dL is considered normal, 100–125 mg/dL is considered prediabetic or having metabolic syndrome, and above 125 mg/dL is considered diabetic. There are a host of simple in home care devices that can measure bgl relatively easily. However, the measurement is just a snapshot in time and the single measurement does not indicate where the values are going. The hemoglobin A1C test is a much more valuable measurement because it takes an average snapshot of your bgl over a three month period based on the amount of glucose that binds to hemoglobin molecules in your circulatory system. The three month window is based on the typical lifetime of a rbc. The development of continuous bgl monitors has been a gamechanger in monitoring bgls effectively by talking multiple measurements for weeks at a time.

The discovery of insulin in 1921 was a phenomenal development and brought a bright ray of hope to the many people worldwide who suffered from this disease which was essentially a death sentence. A very nice description of the history of diabetes, the discovery of insulin by Banting and Best, and the unique controversy which surrounded the awarding of the Nobel Prize for the discovery of insulin only two years after its discovery is presented by Ryden and Lindsten (2021).

There is a common misconception regarding how glucose is taken up by cells. The misconception entails an oversimplification of how glucose enters the cell where insulin binds to glucose and escorts the glucose molecule into the cell. Insulin does not directly bond to glucose molecules. Insulin binds to glucose cell surface receptors and triggers a signal cascade that results in GLUT 4 being transported to the cell surface via the pathway provided by MTs (Batty and Langlais 2021). MTs and glucose play key roles in signaling the cycling of insulin in the cell. Zhu et al. (2015) found that the dynamic balance between MT stability and instability plays an important role in glucose homeostasis and proper insulin secretion, and high levels of glucose tip the dynamic balance toward instability and MT disassembly. This plays a role in glucose stimulated insulin secretion (GSIS). Glucose stimulates pancreatic β cells to nucleate Golgi-derived MTs (GDMTs) through the secretion-regulating cAMP/EPAC2 pathway. Glucose-dependent GDMTs are important for long-term β-cell functionality, replenishment of the insulin granule pool, and to establish and maintain proper insulin secretion levels by delivery of insulin granules to the cell membrane (Trogden et al. 2019). Ho et al. (2020) described how glucose regulates MT disassembly and insulin secretion dose using tau phosphorylation.

Glucagon like peptide 1 (GLP I) is a hormone that regulates blood glucose levels and satiety by slowing down the absorption of food from the stomach during digestion. Research on GLP I began in 1970s as a targeted therapy for duodenal ulcer disease. There is a fascinating link between *H. pylori*, amyloid plaques, duodenal ulcers, and the discovery of GLP1 and its contribution to weight loss and to diabetes treatment drugs based on GLP I. This exogenous peptide was harvested from pigs and administered to flow through the pig pancreas. The fascinating result was that the pig pancreas was stimulated to produce more insulin with a corresponding decrease in glucagon production. This was a double whammy for type II diabetes and presented a dual targeted strategy for blood glucose control. This discovery has been developed into a popular drug named semaglutide which is marketed as Wegovy for weight loss and Ozempic for Type II Diabetes (Nauck et al. 1993; Reynolds 2023).

4.14 Hydration Effects on MT Function and Dynamics

How do MTs serve as hydration sensors to detect levels of hydration in our bodies and facilitate an appropriate response? Aquaporins were discovered in 1992 and play a key role in cellular water transport (Brown 2017). Aquaporins and MTs share a very unique and important relationship. Aquaporins are water channels that direct the transport of water into and out of cells via responses to changes in osmolality. This is a critically important role for aquaporins due to the role of hydration in cell, tissue, and organ health. MTs play an important role of transporting aquaporins to key locations within the cell (Sidhaye et al. 2012).

We have a precedence based on studies with plants to support this idea. Drought conditions signal the biosynthesis of abscisic acid (ABA) in corn plant (*Zea mays*) cells. ABA signals the plant to close stomata and uptake more water through the root system to counteract dehydration stress. Lü et al. (2007) studied the effect of osmotic stress and MT stabilization and destabilization under conditions of root system dehydration. In mammalian species, there is an intricate series of checks and balances to help ensure that cells stay properly hydrated. Hydration is critically important for proper cell function and this cannot be emphasized enough. It can be argued that dehydration is either a direct or indirect factor in many diseases that we face today. Watts and Boyle (2010) studied how dehydration impacted food intake. They reported that anorexia occurred when test animal subjects ingested hypertonic saline and this critical adaptive behavioral response helped conserve fluids during extended periods of cellular dehydration. Anorexia induced multiple inhibitory processes to suppress feeding, and restoration of water intake restored normal feeding behavior.

Vasopressin is a key protein that contributes to how our bodies sense water levels and hydration state for proper allocation of water. Bankir et al. (2017) studied the role of vasopressin in thirst regulation. Vasopressin is often called AVP (arginine-vasopressin) or antidiuretic hormone (ADH). Vasopressin plays a major role in the regulation of water and sodium homeostasis by its antidiuretic action on the kidney which is mediated by special receptors. AVP secretion is triggered by a rise in plasma osmolality, a decline in blood volume or stress. AVP is thought to play a role in blood pressure regulation, potentially through interacting with vascular smooth muscle cells. In addition, AVP may play a role in metabolic pathways such as gluconeogenesis. Bichet (2019) provided a detailed description of the anatomy and physiology of thirst, taste for water, and AVP release. The description is based on anticipatory signals for thirst and a vasopressin release mechanism that is coordinated by homeostatic neurons and circumventricular organs that monitor the composition of blood. Acid-sensing taste receptor cells (TRCs) express otopetrin 1 on type III presynaptic TRCs on the tongue. These TRCs were previously thought to function solely as sour taste sensors, but new evidence indicates that they also mediate taste responses to water. Median Preoptic Nucleus (MnPO) neuron activity is proportional to the intensity of aversive state caused by dehydration. Median Preoptic Nucleus (MnPO) neurons serve as a central detector that discriminates fluid ingestion from solid ingestion and promote acute thirst satiation via the subfornical organ and other downstream targets.

4.15 *MTs, Gut Microbiome, Vitamins, Inflammation, and Cardiac Health*

MTs play an important role in the gut microbiome Immune-based on all the known roles that they play for proper cell function based on cell movement, transport of vital macromolecules and organelles such as proteins, vesicles, and mitochondria, and key aspects of cell division related to kinetochore and mitotic spindle and position of chromosomes. The gut microbiome plays a role in vitamin synthesis. MT play an essential role in the immune system. MT also play a role in vitamin synthesis/transport. Kamimura et al. (1995) determined that MTs play a key role in the intracellular transport of Vitamin D3 and MT integrity plays a role in normal synthesis of this important vitamin. Vitamin D plays many important functions in health in helping our bodies use vitamin C, regulate calcium and phosphorus absorption in the intestines, bone health, cell growth and differentiation, immune system function, and cancer regulation (Kato 2000; Heaney 2008; Aranow 2011; Jeon and Shin 2018). Vitamins also play a role in moderating MT function. B12 helps stabilize MT (Wu et al. 2019), Vitamin K3 destabilizes MTs (Acharya et al. 2009) in the gut and the adaptive and innate immune system (Ilan-Ber and Ilan 2019). The cytoskeleton plays a major role to facilitate a number of immune cell effector functions. MT filaments help direct migratory cells to their final destination and mediate specific cell–cell interactions involving T cells and antigen-presenting cells (Kopf and Kiermaier 2021). MTs play a key role in both initiation and resolution of immune response, and its roles in various aspects of cellular function relation to inflammation can be categorized as the inflammasome (Parthasarathy et al. 2014).

4.16 MT and Digestion

A study by Prisco et al. (2025) demonstrated a fascinating link between the gut microbiome, MTs, and cardiac health. Supplementation of the gut microbiome with *Lactobacillus* was found to restore intestinal health, dampen systemic inflammation, and reduce GP130 ligands and associated right ventricular cardiomyocyte MT remodeling. This provides support for the idea that a novel microbiome-inflammation-MT axis exists which can be cultivated for improving right ventricular dysfunction and improving overall heart health. This also supports the idea of how healthy diet not only impacts gut microbiome health but it plays key roles in overall body system health and we are getting to the point where we can selectively target specific tissues and organs in the body to overcome chronic disease conditions. There is much to discuss about the multifunctional role of MTs in food and health, and this will be the subject of future work.

4.17 MTs and Neurodegenerative Conditions and Disease

MTs play important roles in the progression of neurodegenerative conditions and cognitive decline and depression. MT dysfunction is implicated in many aspects of neurodegenerative diseases. Tau is a MAP which undergoes glycation and has been postulated to play a role in forming the amyloid plaques that are a key indicator of Alzheimer's. MT can also undergo glycation. This is rooted in many pathological conditions beyond Alzheimer's such as diabetes and vascular disease. The lysine residue on tubulin preferentially undergoes glycation (Ledesma et al. 1995). A very important discovery by Bar et al. (2025) revealed that the brain stores excess glucose akin to muscle tissue and the liver. The major drawback to glucose storage in the brain relates to its tendency to accumulate in tau plaques and contribute too neurodegenerative conditions.

5 MT and Quantum Biology Effects: Quantum Link with Consciousness

We have taken time to build a foundation to establish the critically important intracellular roles that MTs play within cells. These roles involve both passive and active control aspects for sensing, signaling, storing, maintaining, and transporting key elements within the cell from the moment of conception throughout each stage of life and development. The importance and interconnectedness of these roles are magnified when we consider the influential role that MTs play in our brain and neurons and nervous system. MTs may provide a link between physical processes and the quantum realm of consciousness and learning. Current ideas consider MTs as having a potential role in quantum consciousness, and associated theories are gaining traction due to philosophical, theoretical, and experimental findings. These ideas can be used to pose an additional question: If MT dysfunction leads to metabolic, neurodegenerative and other disease states, what happens when MT are functioning at peak capacity in relation to learning, memory and consciousness?

5.1 MTs and Orchestrated Objective Reduction (Orch OR) Model for Consciousness

The Orchestrated Objective Reduction (Orch OR) model for consciousness was initially proposed in the mid 1990s by mathematical physicist Sir Roger Penrose and anesthesiologist Stuart Hameroff. Orch OR model for consciousness is a key theory that set the stage for contemplations related to links between neuronal MTs and the origin of consciousness. The theory was initially ridiculed because it was so far from established thoughts for how thinking and learning and consciousness were achieved in our brains. The basic premise for the model involves three key aspects related to quantum phenomena: quantum superposition, ordered reduction, and orchestration. Quantum superposition involves the idea that the tubulin building blocks for MTs can exist in multiple states simultaneously. Ordered reduction involves the concept that consciousness arises from a spontaneous collapse of quantum superposition states caused by interactions with gravity. The concept of orchestration involves the timing of these quantum intercorrelated events and the model suggests that biological processes within the MTs and MAPs in brains influence the timing and outcome of ordered reduction events to "orchestrate" these quantum processes and give rise to consciousness (Hameroff and Penrose 1996, 2014; Hameroff 2001, 2022). After the lukewarm at best reception, the model has been gaining traction since the experimental basis for quantum effects in nature has been reported for photosynthesis and other important biological processes. Marais et al. (2018) provide a timely review of quantum biology and future projections of this fascinating collaboration between biology/molecular biology and classical and quantum physics.

One of the strongest possible connections between MTs and consciousness involves the question of how anesthetic agents work in bringing about a state of unconsciousness. While the exact mechanism behind general anesthesia remains an open question in neuroscience, MTs are proposed as the site where the agents act to bring about the unconscious state. MT-targeting agents such as neurotransmitters dopamine, endorphins, and gamma aminobutyric acid (GABA) are postulated to interact with MTs and promote MT disassembly. As an interesting side note, GABA is also produced by beta islet cells and plays a role in glucagon action (Rorsman et al. 1989). Zadeh-Haghighi and Simon (2022) developed a model that shows how the interrelationships between magnetic fields and radical pairs can provide insight into how xenon works as an anesthetic agent. In the model, MT density changes are the result of magnetic field modulated spin dynamics of naturally occurring radical pairs in MTs. This model provides some support to make a connection between MT-based and radical pair-based quantum theories of consciousness. An additional connection between MTs and the active mechanism for unconsciousness was reported by Khan et al. (2024) in their study of how the MT-binding agent epothilone delayed the onset of unconsciousness in rats by up to 69 s as measured by latency to loss of righting reflex (LORR) in rats injected with 4% isofluorane.

5.2 *MT: From Quantum Computation to Quasars and Beyond*

The pervasive role of MTs in the life and function of the cell can be extended far beyond the boundaries of the outer cell membrane. This chapter touched on some of the exciting properties that MTs exhibit and how they can be used in (1) developing models to further understand the role of MTs in biological functions, (2) targeting pathological processes that can contribute to finding cures for many diseases that affect our bodies, metabolism, and mind, and (3) help enhance our understanding of how our brains work and how learning, memory, and consciousness are interrelated. One of the more recent possibilities for expanding the reach of MT influence involves the area of quantum computation and exploration in AI interfaces. Much progress continues to be made as studies continue to fine tune our understanding of the quantum nature of MTs. Priel et al. (2010) described a physical model that highlighted neural cytoskeleton elements actin and MTs as major players in molecular-level processing of information required for learning and memory storage. This idea is based on the highly charged surfaces of actin filaments and MTs that enable them to conduct electric signals and modulated waves. The MT Actin cytoskeletal network information processing model may underlie certain types of learning and memory. Shirmovsky (2024) described the possibility of quantum teleportation occurring in MTs and his group has contributed quite a bit to the field of Quantum Biology.

There is no telling where our journey to understand the intricate interrelationships that exist among the quantum phenomena that drive atomic and molecular interactions and the biological processes that orchestrate the structure, property and function relationships that support cell, tissue, and organ function will take us. These interactions display fractal aspects that extend beyond the boundaries of Earth to the farthest reaches of our universe. Recent research has established an amazing link between galaxy filaments and neural filaments. Vazza and Feletti (2020) presented compelling arguments that the neuronal network in our brain shares unique patterns in common with structures within the cosmic web of our universe that interconnect galaxies. The largest scale model that could ever be conceived for modeling a biological system is the universe as expressed through the cosmic web. MTs are intimately involved in this model due to their important roles in neurons, axons, and brain structure. The exploration of these and other MT-based mysteries will continue to inspire great thought and questions as we search for clues to uncover the nature of life and consciousness and further define our place in the universe.

6 Summary and Future Directions/Possibilities/ Inspirations

This chapter provides a small glimpse into the immense potential of MTs and the unique capabilities that they present for advanced medicine and materials development. This is directly related to the wide variety of functional adaptations that MTs can adopt based on strategically tailored interactions with appropriate proteins or other macromolecules. The robust nature of these interactions between tubulin heterodimers and MAPs gives rise to the wonderful assortment of biological activities that occur within the cell. MTs play a role in orchestrating events preceding conception throughout the developmental stages in the new life. MTs represent the ultimate composite and can be used as a foundation for a host of powerful and insightful models that span life, maintain health, and even probe the nature of learning and our consciousness.

There are a number of MT-based models that can be developed into physical models for enhanced learning opportunities. Simple elements such as straws, springs and magnets can be used to construct unique models for young scholars to further explore biological structures that are encountered within the cell. For example, a model to explore and visualize the role of MTs in cell division can be designed using straws to highlight the centriole. The centriole is a supramolecular quasicrystal with multiple layers of 3- and 9-fold symmetry. True to life conceptual models that capture the essence of the nanoscale components of the cell can be developed to spark discovery and inspiration. We must continue to foster this inspiration within our young scholars that propel us toward a better understanding of the interrelationships among our bodies, brains, and the environment. This can serve as a catalyst to help us move forward to build better models to enhance health on a global scale and explore phenomena ranging from the quantum world of the quark to interstellar quasars and the vast reaches of the universe. In addition, the intrinsic beauty and symmetry of crystals, quasicrystals and supramolecular assemblies, the macro scale intercellular basis of life and health, and uncovering keys to understanding the driving force for the vast role of MT in life can be explored at a deeper level through appropriate models.

Amazing things lie on the horizon as we continue to learn about the interconnected role of MTs in all aspects of life and learning. Formulating key questions will be an important driver of this process as our understanding of MTs increases and our ability to wisely integrate them into medical treatments and technological resources. Some of the big questions that can start the conversation include the following:

- What are the past discoveries, present capabilities and inspirations, and future possibilities that are encapsulated within MTs?
- To what extent has the discovery of MTs and subsequent advances in our understanding of their structure, properties, and function revolutionized medicine and what are the future possibilities and implications of these discoveries?
- How can MT pathologies and dysfunction be corrected to reverse disease processes and reestablish health?
- What is the exact link between MTs and higher order learning processes and the specific role of MT in learning and consciousness?

These are just a few of the many questions that we can ask to help drive our investigations of this remarkable biomaterial nanocomposite that holds the key to life, health, and learning.

Acknowledgements The authors would like to dedicate this chapter to Dr. Tiffany Omokanwaye, one of our dear colleagues who passed away way before her time. May her light and legacy continue to bring forth fruit as we move closer to finding a pervasive and total cure for all forms of cancer and continue to explore the mysteries of MTs.

References

B.R. Acharya, D. Choudhury, A. Das, G. Chakrabarti, Vitamin K3 disrupts the microtubule networks by binding to tubulin: a novel mechanism of its antiproliferative activity. Biochemistry **48**(29), 6963–6974 (2009). https://doi.org/10.1021/bi900152k. (PMID: 19527023)

K.V. Agrawal, S. Shimizu, L.W. Drahushuk, D. Kilcoyne, M.S. Strano, Observation of extreme phase transition temperatures of water confined inside isolated carbon nanotubes. Nat. Nanotechnol. **12**, 267–273 (2017). https://doi.org/10.1038/nnano.2016.254

S. Ahn, A. Kwon, Y. Oh, S. Rhee, W.K. Song, Microtubule acetylation-specific inhibitors induce cell death and mitotic arrest via JNK/AP-1 activation in triple-negative breast cancer cells. Mol. Cells **46**(6), 387–398 (2023)

R. Alfaro-Aco, S. Petry, How TPX2 helps microtubules branch out. Cell Cycle **16**(17), 1560–1561 (2017)

R. Alfaro-Aco, A. Thawani, S. Petry, Structural analysis of the role of TPX2 in branching microtubule nucleation. J. Cell Biol. **216**(4), 983–997 (2017). https://doi.org/10.1083/jcb.201607060

M. Allani, Akhilesh, V. Tiwari, Caspase-driven cancer therapies: navigating the bridge between lab discoveries and clinical applications. Cell Biochem. Funct. **42**(2), e3944 (2024)
A.M. Alshehri, O.C. Wilson Jr, Biomimetic hydrogel strategies for cancer therapy. Gels. **10**(7), 437 (2024)
C.D. Anderson, J. Wang, G.N. Kumar, J.M. McMillan, U.K. Walle, T. Walle, Dexamethasone induction of taxol metabolism in the rat. Drug Metab. Dispos. **23**(11), 1286–1290 (1995)
C. Aranow, Vitamin D and the immune system. J. Investig. Med. **59**(6), 881–886 (2011)
I. Arnal, R.H. Wade, How does taxol stabilize microtubules? Curr. Biol. **5**, 900–908 (1995)
M. Ávila, A. Fernández-Vega, J. Garrido-Maraver, I. de Lavera, M. de la Mata, M. Cordero, E. Gómez, A. Pavón, M. Álvarez Códoba, D. Cotán, J. Sánchez-Alcázar, Emerging roles of apoptotic microtubules during the execution phase of apoptosis. Cytoskeleton **72**(9), 435–446 (2015). https://doi.org/10.1002/cm.21254
B. Bance, S. Seetharaman, C. Leduc, B. Boëda, S. Etienne-Manneville, Microtubule acetylation but not detyrosination promotes focal adhesion dynamics and cell migration. BioRxiv 425421 (2018)
B. Bance, S. Seetharaman, C. Leduc, B. Boëda, S. Etienne-Manneville, Microtubule acetylation but not detyrosination promotes focal adhesion dynamics and astrocyte migration. J. Cell Sci. **132**(7), jcs225805 (2019)
S. Banerjee, D.J. Hwang, W. Li, D.D. Miller, Current advances of tubulin inhibitors in nanoparticle drug delivery and vascular disruption/angiogenesis. Molecules **21**(11), 1468 (2016)
L. Bankir, D.G. Bichet, N.G. Morgenthaler, Vasopressin: physiology, assessment and osmosensation. J. Intern. Med. **282**(4), 284–297 (2017). https://doi.org/10.1111/joim.12645. (Epub 26 July 2017. PMID: 28649750)
S. Bar, K.A. Wilson, T.A.U. Hilsabeck, S. Alderfer, E.B. Dammer, J.B. Burton, S. Shah, A. Holtz, E.M. Carrera, J.N. Beck, J.H. Chen, G. Kauwe, F. Seifar, A. Shantaraman, T.E. Tracy, N.T. Seyfried, B. Schilling, L.M. Ellerby, P. Kapahi, Neuronal glycogen breakdown mitigates tauopathy via pentose-phosphate-pathway-mediated oxidative stress reduction. Nat. Metab. **7**(7), 1375–1391 (2025)
S.R. Batty, P.R. Langlais, Microtubules in insulin action: what's on the tube? Trends Endocrinol Metab **32**(10), 776–789 (2021)
R. Becker, W. Doring, Kinetische behandlung der keimbildung in ubers attigten dampfen. Ann. Phys. **416**(8), 719–752 (1935)
F. Betts, A.S. Posner, An X-ray radial distribution study of amorphous calcium phosphate, Mater. Res. Bull. **9**(3), 353–360 (1974)
D.G. Bichet, Regulation of thirst and vasopressin release. Annu. Rev. Physiol. **81**, 359–373 (2019). https://doi.org/10.1146/annurev-physiol-020518-114556. (PMID: 30742785)
L. Bieniussa, I. Jain, M.B. Grau, L. Juergens, R. Hagen, C. Janke, K. Rak, Microtubule and auditory function—an underestimated connection. Semin. Cell Dev. Biol. **137**, 74–86 (2023)
S. Bodakuntla, A.S. Jijumom, G.-B. Villablanca, C. Janke, Microtubule-associated proteins: structuring the cytoskeleton. Trends Cell Biol. **29**(10), 804–819 (2019)
A.E. Boggs, M.I. Vitolo, R.A. Whipple, M.S. Charpentier, O.G. Goloubeva, O.B. Ioffe, K.C. Tuttle, J. Slovic, Y. Lu, G.B. Mills, S.S. Martin, α-Tubulin acetylation elevated in metastatic and basal-like breast cancer cells promotes microtentacle formation, adhesion, and invasive migration. Cancer Res. **75**(1), 203–215 (2015)
G.H. Bogush, C.F. Zukoski, Uniform silica particle precipitation: an aggregative growth model. J. Colloid Interface Sci. **142**(1), 19–34 (1991)
G.G. Borisy, E.W. Taylor, The mechanism of action of colchicine. Binding of colchincine-3H to cellular protein. J. Cell Biol. **34**(2), 525–533 (1967a)
G.G. Borisy, E.W. Taylor, The mechanism of action of colchicine. Colchicine binding to sea urchin eggs and the mitotic apparatus. J. Cell Biol. **34**(2), 535–548 (1967b)
M. Bottini, S. Mebarek, K.L. Anderson, A. Strzelecka-Kiliszek, L. Bozycki, A.M.S. Simão, et al., Matrix vesicles from chondrocytes and osteoblasts: Their biogenesis, properties, functions and biomimetic models. Biochim. Biophys. Acta. Gen. Subjects. **1862**(3), 532–546 (2018).

D. Brown, The discovery of water channels (aquaporins). Ann. Nutr. Metab. **70**(Suppl 1), 37–42 (2017)
C Burr, *The Emperor of Scent: A Story of Perfume, Obsession, and the Last Mystery of the Senses* (Random House, 2002)
M. Cai, W. Wu, S. Deng, Q. Yang, H. Wu, H. Wang, J. Zhang, Q. Feng, J. Shao, Y. Zeng, J. Li, Expression of cytoskeleton-associated protein 4 is associated with poor prognosis and metastasis in nasopharyngeal carcinoma. Exp. Biol. Med. (Maywood) **248**(12), 1085–1094 (2023)
A. Calaprice (ed.), *The Ultimate Quotable Einstein*, vol. 475 (Princeton University Press, Princeton, New Jersey, 2010), pp 384–385
M. Cannariato, E.A. Zizzi, J.A. Tuszynski, M.A. Deriu, Multiscale computational analysis of the effect of taxol on microtubule mechanics. ACS Biomater. Sci. Eng. **10**(9), 5666–5674 (2024)
M.R. Cantero, C. Villa Etchegoyen, P.L. Perez et al., Bundles of brain microtubules generate electrical oscillations. Sci. Rep. **8**, 11899 (2018). https://doi.org/10.1038/s41598-018-30453-2
M.R. Cantero, P.L. Perez, N. Scarinci, H.F. Cantiello, Two-dimensional brain microtubule structures behave as memristive devices. Sci. Rep. **9**, 12398 (2019)
S.P. Carey, Z.E. Goldblatt, K.E. Martin, B. Romero, R.M. Williams, C.A. Reinhart-King, Local extracellular matrix alignment directs cellular protrusion dynamics and migration through Rac1 and FAK. Integr. Biol. (Camb.) **8**(8), 821–835 (2016)
B. Carmona, H.S. Marinho, C.L. Matos, S. Nolasco, H. Soares, Tubulin post-translational modifications: the elusive roles of acetylation. Biology **12**(4), 561 (2023)
D. Castelvecchi, First nuclear detonation created 'impossible' quasicrystals. Nature **593**(7860), 487 (2021)
B.T. Castle, D.J. Odde, D.K. Wood, Rapid and inefficient kinetics of sickle hemoglobin fiber growth. Sci. Adv. **5**(3), eaau1086 (2019)
Y.R. Chen, T.H. Tan, Mammalian c-Jun N-terminal kinase pathway and STE20-related kinases. Gene Ther. Mol. Biol. **4**, 83–98 (1999)
R. Chowdhury, T. Mimoso, A.A. Chouaib, N. Mougios, D. Krah, F. Opazo, S. Koster, S.O. Rizzoli, A.H. Shaib, Microtubules as a versatile reference standard for expansion microscopy. Commun. Biol. **8**, 499 (2025)
F. Cinti, S. Cinti, The endocrine adipose organ: a system playing a central role in COVID-19. Cells **11**(13), 2109 (2022)
S.E. Collyer, G.D. Stack, J.J. Walsh, Selective delivery of clinically approved tubulin binding agents through covalent conjugation to an active targeting moiety. Curr. Med. Chem. **29**(31), 5179–5211 (2022)
T.J. Craddock, M. St George, H. Freedman, K.H. Barakat, S. Damaraju, S. Hameroff, J.A. Tuszynski, Computational predictions of volatile anesthetic interactions with the microtubule cytoskeleton: implications for side effects of general anesthesia. PLoS ONE **7**(6), e37251 (2012)
M.P. Czech, Mechanisms of insulin resistance related to white, beige, and brown adipocytes. Mol. Metab. **34**, 27–42 (2020)
M.R. D'Andrea, V. Cereda, L. Coppola, G. Giordano, A. Remo, E. De Santis, Propensity for early metastatic spread in breast cancer: role of tumor vascularization features and tumor immune infiltrate. Cancers **13**(23), 5917 (2021)
V. Das, A. Kanakkanthara, A. Chan, J.H. Miller, Potential role of tubulin tyrosine ligase-like enzymes in tumorigenesis and cancer cell resistance. Cancer Lett. **350**(1), 1–4 (2014)
S. Das, M. Vera, V. Gandin, R.H. Singer, E. Tutucci, Intracellular mRNA transport and localized translation. Nat. Rev. Mol. Cell Biol. **22**, 483–504 (2021)
K.M. Debatin, Apoptosis pathways in cancer and cancer therapy. Cancer Immunol. Immunother. **53**, 153–159 (2004)
J. Dinić, S.J. Stojanov, M. Dragoj, M. Grozdanić, A. Podolski-Renić, M. Pešić, Cancer patient-derived cell-based models: applications and challenges in functional precision medicine. Life **14**(9), 1142 (2024)
E. Dizin, H. Ray, F. Suau, T. Voeltzel, V.N. Dalla, Caspase-dependent BRCA1 cleavage facilitates chemotherapy-induced apoptosis. Apoptosis **13**, 237–246 (2008)

S. Dmitrieff, A. Alsina, A. Mathur, F.J. Nedelec, Balance of microtubule stiffness and cortical tension determines the size of blood cells with marginal band across species. PNAS **114**(17), 4418–4423 (2017)

M. Dogterom, G.H. Koenderink, Actin-microtubule crosstalk in cell biology. Nat. Rev. Mol. Cell Biol. **20**(1), 38-54 (2019)

G. Dyson, The scientific basis of odour. Chem. Ind. **57**, 647–651 (1938)

D.W. Fawcett, W.A. Anderson, D.M. Phillips, Morphogenetic factors influencing the shape of the sperm head. Dev. Biol. **26**(2), 220–251 (1971)

R. Ferrara, S. Pilotto, U. Peretti, M. Caccese, S. Kinspergher, L. Carbognin, N. Karachaliou, R. Rosell, G. Tortora, E. Bria, Tubulin inhibitors in non-small cell lung cancer: looking back and forward. Expert Opin. Pharmacother. **17**(8), 1113–1129 (2016)

L.T. Ferreira, A.C. Figueiredo, B. Orr, D. Lopes, H. Maiato, Dissecting the role of the tubulin code in mitosis. Methods Cell Biol. **144**, 33–74 (2018). https://doi.org/10.1016/bs.mcb.2018.03.040. (PMID: 29804676; PMCID: PMC6402544)

M.P.A. Fisher, Quantum cognition: The possibility of processing with nuclear spins in the brain. Ann. Phys. 362, 593–602 (2015)

T. Folger, How quantum mechanics lets us see, smell, and touch. Discover Magazine, 2018

E. Fukada, I. Yashuda, On the piezoelectric effect of bone. J. Phys. Soc. Japan **12**(10), 1158–1162 (1957)

L.P. Ge, X. Jin, Y.S. Yang, X.Y. Liu, Z.M. Shao, G.H. Di, Y.Z. Jiang, Tektin4 loss promotes triple-negative breast cancer metastasis through HDAC6-mediated tubulin deacetylation and increases sensitivity to HDAC6 inhibitor. Oncogene **40**(12), 2323–2334 (2021)

M. Giladi, R.S. Schneiderman, T. Voloshin, Y. Porat, M. Munster, R. Blat, S. Sherbo, Z. Bomzon, N. Urman, A. Ithaki, S. Cahal, A. Shteingauz, A. Chaudhry, E.D. Kirson, U. Weinberg, Y. Palti, Mitotic spindle disruption by alternating electric fields leads to improper chromosome segregation and mitotic catastrophe in cancer cells. Sci Rep. **5**:18046. 26658786 (2015)

H.V. Goodson, E.M. Jonasson, Microtubules and microtubule-associated proteins. Cold Spring Harb. Perspect. Biol. **10**(6), a022608 (2018)

S. Goswami, S. Adhikary, S. Bhattacharya, R. Agarwal, A. Ganguly, S. Nanda, P. Rajak, The alarming link between environmental microplastics and health hazards with special emphasis on cancer. Life Sci. **355**, 122937 (2024)

L.M. Griffith, T.D. Pollard, Evidence for actin filament-microtubule interaction mediated by microtubule-associated proteins. J. Cell Biol. **78**(3), 958-65. (1978)

Y. Guo, Z. Wang, X. Shi, M. Shen, Engineered cancer cell membranes: an emerging agent for efficient cancer theranostics. Exploration (Beijing) **2**(1), 20210171 (2022)

W. Guo, T.A. Ale, S. Sun, J.E. Sanchez, L. Li, A comprehensive study on the electrostatic properties of tubulin-tubulin complexes in microtubules. Cells **12**(2), 238 (2023). https://doi.org/10.3390/cells12020238. (PMID: 36672172; PMCID: PMC9857020)

K.K. Gupta, S.S. Bharne, K. Rathinasamy, N.R. Naik, D. Panda, Dietary antioxidant curcumin inhibits microtubule assembly through tubulin binding. FEBS J. **273**(23), 5320–5332 (2006)

B.C. Gutierrez, H.F. Cantiello, M. Cantero, The electrical properties of isolated microtubules. Sci. Rep. **13**, 10165 (2023)

S. Hameroff, Consciousness, the brain, and spacetime geometry. Ann. n. y. Acad. Sci. **929**, 74–104 (2001)

S. Hameroff, Is your brain really a computer or is it a quantum orchestra? Interalia Magazine (2015). https://www.interaliamag.org/articles/stuart-hameroff-is-your-brain-really-a-computer-or-is-it-a-quantum-orchestra-tuned-to-the-universe/

S. Hameroff, Consciousness, cognition and the neuronal cytoskeleton—a new paradigm needed in neuroscience. Front. Mol. Neurosci. **15**, 869935 (2022). https://doi.org/10.3389/fnmol.2022.869935

S. Hameroff, R. Penrose, Consciousness in the universe—a review of the Orch OR Theory. Phys. Life Rev. **11**(1), 39–78 (2014)

C. Hamilton, J.P. Fox, D.B. Longley, C.A. Higgins, Therapeutics targeting the core apoptotic machinery. Cancers **13**(11), 2618 (2021)

S. Hameroff and R. Penrose, Orchestrated reduction of quantum coherence in brain microtubules: A model for consciousness, Math. Comput. Simul. 40(3–4), 453–480 (1996)

S. Han, R. Wang, Y. Zhang, X. Li, Y. Gan, F. Gao, P. Rong, W. Wang, W. Li, The role of ubiquitination and deubiquitination in tumor invasion and metastasis. Int. J. Biol. Sci. **18**(6), 2292 (2022)

D. Hanahan, Hallmarks of cancer: new dimensions. Cancer Discov. **12**(1), 31–46 (2022)

D. Hanahan, R.A. Weinberg, The hallmarks of cancer. Cell **100**(1), 57–70 (2000)

D. Hanahan, R.A. Weinberg, Hallmarks of cancer: the next generation. Cell **144**(5), 646–674 (2011)

R.P. Heaney, Vitamin D in health and disease. Clin. J. Am. Soc. Nephrol. **3**, 1535–1541 (2008)

J.B. Herrick, Peculiar elongated and sickle-shaped red blood corpuscles in a case of severe anemia. Arch. Intern. Med. **6**, 517–521 (1910)

K.H. Ho, X. Yang, A.B. Osipovich, O. Cabrera, M.L. Hayashi, M.A. Magnuson, G. Gu, I. Kaverina, Glucose regulates microtubule disassembly and the dose of insulin secretion via Tau phosphorylation. Diabetes **69**(9), 1936–1947 (2020)

T. Hohmann, F. Dehghani, The cytoskeleton—a complex interacting meshwork. Cells **8**(4), 362 (2019)

D.L. Holliday, V. Speirs, Choosing the right cell line for breast cancer research. Breast Cancer Res. **13**(4), 215 (2011)

S.B. Horwitz, D. Cohen, S. Rao, I. Ringel, H.J. Shen, C.P. Yang, Taxol: mechanisms of action and resistance. J. Natl. Cancer Inst. Monogr. **15**, 55–61 (1993)

https://www.cytoskeleton.com/the-structure-of-microtubules-a-brief-history

https://www.discovermagazine.com/the-sciences/how-quantum-mechanics-lets-us-see-smell-and-touch

T. Ilan-Ber, Y. Ilan, The role of microtubules in the immune system and as potential targets for gut-based immunotherapy. Mol. Immunol. **111**, 73–82 (2019)

T. Iwayama, T. Okada, T. Ueda, K. Tomita, S. Matsumoto, M. Takedachi, S. Wakisaka, T. Noda, T. Ogura, T. Okano, P. Fratzl, T. Ogura, S. Murakami, Osteoblastic lysosome plays a central role in mineralization. Sci Adv. **5**(7): eaax0672 (2019)

T. Iwayama, P. Bhongsatiern, M. Takedachi, and S. Murakami, Matrix vesicle–mediated mineralization and potential applications. J. Dental Res. **101**(13), 1554–1562 (2022)

W.R. Jeffery, C.R. Tomlinson, R.D. Brodeur, Localization of actin messenger RNA during early ascidian development. Dev. Biol. **99**, 408–417 (1983)

F. Jelínek, P. Jiří, Microtubules in biological cells as circular waveguides and resonators. Electro- and Magnetobiology. **20**, 75–80 (2001)

P.M. Jenkins, D.P. McEwen, J.R. Martens, Olfactory cilia: linking sensory cilia function and human disease. Chem. Senses **34**(5), 451–464 (2009)

S.M. Jeon, E.A. Shin, Exploring vitamin D metabolism and function in cancer. Exp. Mol. Med. **50**, 1–14 (2018)

A. Jivani, R.K. Shinde, A comprehensive review of taxane treatment in breast cancer: clinical perspectives and toxicity profiles. Cureus **16**(4), e59266 (2024)

J.C. Johnston, N. Kastelowitz, V. Molinero, Liquid to quasicrystal transition in bilayer water. J. Chem. Phys. **133**, 154516 (2010)

D.H. Jun, B.J. Kim, J.H. Park, J.G. Kim, K.C. Chi, J.M. Park, M.K. Kim, H. Kang, Preoperative body mass index may determine the prognosis of advanced gastric cancer. Nutr. Cancer **68**(8), 1295–1300 (2016)

A.P. Kalra, S.D. Patel, A.F. Bhuiyan, J. Preto, K.G. Scheuer, U. Mohammed, J.D. Lewis, V. Rezania, K. Shankar, J.A. Tuszynski, Investigation of the electrical properties of microtubule ensembles under cell-like conditions. Nanomaterials **10**(2), 265 (2020)

S. Kamimura, M. Gallieni, M. Zhong, W. Beron, E. Slatopolsky, A. Dusso, Microtubules mediate cellular 25-hydroxyvitamin D3 trafficking and the genomic response to 1,25-dihydroxyvitamin D3 in normal human monocytes. J. Biol. Chem. **270**(38), 22160–22166 (1995)

Y. Kang, P.M. Siegel, W. Shu, M. Drobnjak, S.M. Kakonen, C. Cordon-Cardo, T.A. Guise, J. Massague, A multigenic program mediating breast cancer metastasis to bone. Cancer Cell **3**(6), 537–549 (2003)

S. Kar, R. Mukherjee, S. Guha, D. Talukdar, G. Das, N. Murmu, Modulating the acetylation of α-tubulin by LncRNAs and microRNAs helps in the progression of cancer. Cell Biochem. Funct. **42**(2), e3953 (2024)

S. Karthika, Radhakrishnan, P. Kalaichelvi, A review of classical and nonclassical nucleation theories. Cryst. Growth Des. **16**(11), 6663–6681 (2016)

S. Kato, The function of vitamin D receptor in vitamin D action. J. Biochem. **127**(5), 717–722 (2000)

M.T. Kelliher, H.A.J. Saunders, J. Wildonger, Microtubule control of functional architecture in neurons. Curr. Opin. Neurobiol. **57**, 39–45 (2019)

M.B. Kelz, G.A. Mashour, The biology of general anesthesia from paramecium to primate. Curr. Biol. **29**, R1199–R1210 (2019)

S. Khan, Y. Huang, D. Timucin, S. Bailey, S. Lee, J. Lopes, E. Gaunce, J. Mosberger, M. Zhan, B. Abdelrahman, X. Zeng, M. Wiest, Microtubule-stabilizer epothilone B delays anesthetic-induced unconsciousness in rats. eNeuro **11**(8), ENEURO.0291-24.2024 (2024)

E.D. Kirson, Z. Gurvich, R. Schneiderman, E. Dekel, A. Itzhaki, Y. Wasserman, R. Schatzberger, Y. Palti, Disruption of cancer cell replication by alternating electric fields. Cancer Res. **64**, 3288–3295 (2004)

A.W. Knight, N.G. Kalugin, E. Coker, A.G. Ilgen, Water properties under nano-scale confinement. Sci. Rep. **9**, 8246 (2019)

M. Knossow, V. Campanacci, L.A. Khodja, B. Gigant, The mechanism of tubulin assembly into microtubules: insights from structural studies. iScience **23**(9), 101511 (2020)

A. Kopf, E. Kiermaier, Dynamic microtubule arrays in leukocytes and their role in cell migration and immune synapse formation. Front. Cell Dev. Biol. **9**, 635511 (2021). https://doi.org/10.3389/fcell.2021.635511

C.M. Kraning-Rush, J.P. Califano, C.A. Reinhart-King, Cellular traction stresses increase with increasing metastatic potential. PLoS ONE **7**(2), e32572 (2012)

S. Kumar, D. Sharma, R. Kumar, Role of macromolecular crowding on stability and iron release kinetics of serum transferrin. J. Phys. Chem. B **121**(37), 8669–8683 (2017)

M. Kumar, S. Kaur, S. Kaur, C-Jun N-terminal kinase (JNK), p38, and caspases: promising therapeutic targets for the regulation of apoptosis in cancer cells by phytochemicals. Curr. Cancer Ther. Rev. **20**(2), 200–211 (2024)

Y.J. Kwon, E.B. Seo, S.H. Kwon, S.H. Lee, S.K. Kim, S.K. Park, K. Kim, S. Park, J.W. Park, Extracellular acidosis promotes metastatic potency via decrease of the BMAL1 circadian clock gene in breast cancer. Cells **9**(4), 989 (2020)

S.E. LaFlamme, S. Mathew-Steiner, N. Singh, D. Colello-Borges, B. Nieves, Integrin and microtubule crosstalk in the regulation of cellular processes. Cell. Mol. Life Sci. **75**(22), 4177–4185 (2019)

J.B. Lawrence, R.H. Singer, Intracellular localization of messenger RNAs for cytoskeletal proteins. Cell **45**, 407–415 (1986)

M.C. Ledbetter, K.R. Porter, A “microtubule” in plant cell fine structure. J. Cell Biol. **19**(1), 239–250 (1963)

M.D. Ledesma, P. Bonay, J. Avila, τ Protein from Alzheimer’s disease patients is glycated at its tubulin-binding domain. J. Neurochem. **65**, 1658–1664 (1995)

D. Li, X. Ding, M. Xie, Z. Huang, P. Han, D. Tian, L. Xia, CAMSAP2-mediated noncentrosomal microtubule acetylation drives hepatocellular carcinoma metastasis. Theranostics **10**(8), 3749 (2020)

P.T. Lim, B.H. Goh, W.L. Lee, Taxol: mechanisms of action against cancer, an update with current research, chap. 3, in *Paclitaxel*, ed. by M.K. Swamy, T. Pullaiah, Z.S. Chen (Academic Press, 2022), pp. 47–71

B. Lü, Z. Gong, J. Wang, J. Zhang, J. Liang, Microtubule dynamics in relation to osmotic stress-induced ABA accumulation in *Zea mays* roots. J. Exp. Bot. **58**(10), 2565–2572 (2007)

J. Luo, Q. Hu, M. Gou, X. Liu, Y. Qin, J. Zhu, C. Cai, T. Tian, Z. Tu, Y. Du, H. Deng, Expression of Microtubule-Associated Proteins in Relation to Prognosis and Efficacy of Immunotherapy in Non-Small Cell Lung Cancer. Front. Oncol. **11**, 680402 (2021)

R.H. Lustig, L.A. Schmidt, C.D. Brindis, Public health: The toxic truth about sugar. Nature. **482**(7383), 27–29 (2012)

A. Malandrino, R.D. Kamm, E. Moeendarbary, In vitro modeling of mechanics in cancer metastasis. ACS Biomater. Sci. Eng. **4**(2), 294–301 (2018)

T.T. Maliekal, D. Dharmapal, S. Sengupta, Tubulin isotypes: emerging roles in defining cancer stem cell niche. Front. Immunol. **13**, 876278 (2022)

S. Mangaonkar, S. Nath, B.P. Chatterji, Microtubule dynamics in cancer metastasis: harnessing the underappreciated potential for therapeutic interventions. Pharmacol. Ther. **263**, 108726 (2024). ISSN 0163-7258

G. Mancardi , C.E. Hernandez Tamargo , D. Di Tommaso, N.H. de Leeuw, Detection of Posner's clusters during calcium phosphate nucleation: A molecular dynamics study. J. Mater. Chem. B. **5**(35), 7274–7284 (2017)

J.J. Manfredi, J. Parness, S.B. Horwitz, Taxol binds to cellular microtubules. J. Cell Biol. **94**(3), 688–696 (1982)

A. Marais, B. Adams, A.K. Ringsmuth, M. Ferretti, J.M. Gruber et al., The future of quantum biology. J. r. Soc. Interface. **15**, 20180640 (2018)

Y. Merkher, D. Weihs, Proximity of metastatic cells enhances their mechanobiological invasiveness. Ann. Biomed. Eng. **45**(6), 1399–1406 (2017)

Y. Merkher, M.B. Alvarez-Elizondo, D. Weihs, Taxol reduces synergistic, mechanobiological invasiveness of metastatic cells. Converg. Sci. Phys. Oncol. **3**(4), 044002 (2017)

H. Mohri, Amino acid composition of "tubulin" constituting microtubules of sperm flagella. Nature **27**, 1053–1054 (1968)

X. Morales, I. Cortes-Dominguez, C. Ortiz-de-Solorzano, Modeling the mechanobiology of cancer cell migration using 3D biomimetic hydrogels. Gels **7**(1), 17 (2021)

A. Moukachar, K. Harvey, E. Roke, K. Sloan, P. Cameron et al., Development and evaluation of a low-cost LEGO 3D bioprinter: from building-blocks to building blocks of life. Adv. Mater. Technol. **8**(6), 2100868 (2023)

E. Mukhtar, V.M. Adhami, H. Mukhtar, Targeting microtubules by natural agents for cancer therapy. Mol. Cancer Ther. **13**(2), 275–284 (2014)

M.A. Nauck, N. Kleine, C. Orskov, J.J. Holst, B. Willms, W. Creutzfeldt, Normalization of fasting hyperglycaemia by exogenous glucagon-like peptide 1 (7–36 amide) in type 2 (non-insulin-dependent) diabetic patients. Diabetologia **36**(8), 741–744 (1993)

J. Nieuwenhuis, T.R. Brummelkamp, The tubulin detyrosination cycle: function and enzymes. Trends Cell Biol. **29**(1), 80–92 (2019)

E.T. O'Brien, E.D. Salmon, H.P. Erickson, How calcium causes microtubule depolymerization. Cell Motil. Cytoskeleton **36**(2), 125–135 (1997)

L. O'Donnell, M.K. O'Bryan, Microtubules and spermatogenesis. Semin. Cell Dev. Biol. **30**, 45–54 (2014)

T. Oba, M. Ono, H. Matoba, T. Uehara, Y. Hasegawa, K.I. Ito, HDAC6 inhibition enhances the anti-tumor effect of eribulin through tubulin acetylation in triple-negative breast cancer cells. Breast Cancer Res. Treat. **186**, 37–51 (2021)

P.T. Parthasarathy, Y. Cho, R. Lockey, N. Kolliputi, An old molecule with a new role: microtubules in inflammasome regulation. Cell Biochem. Biophys. **70**(1), 697–698 (2014)

E. Pasquier, M. Kavallaris, Microtubules: a dynamic target in cancer therapy. IUBMB Life **60**(3), 165–170 (2008)

J.D. Pasteris, C.H. Yoder, B. Wopenka, Molecular water in nominally unhydrated carbonated hydroxylapatite: the key to a better understanding of bone mineral. Am. Miner. **99**(1), 16–27 (2014)

R. Patel, Tour de paclitaxel: biocatalysis for semisynthesis. Ann. Rev. Microbiol. **52**, 361–395 (1998)
L. Pauling, R.B. Corey, A proposed structure for the nucleic acids. Proc. Natl. Acad. Sci. u.s.a. **39**(2), 84–97 (1953a)
L. Pauling, R.B. Corey, Structure of the nucleic acids. Nature **171**(4347), 346 (1953b)
L. Pauling, H.A. Itano, S.J. Singer, I.C. Wells, Sickle cell anemia: a molecular disease. Science **110**, 543–548 (1949)
R. Penrose, The role of aesthetics in pure and applied mathematical research. Bull. Inst. Math. Appl. **10**(7/8), 266–271 (1974)
R. Penrose, Pentaplexity a class of non-periodic tilings of the plane. Math. Intell. **2**(1), 32–37 (1979)
E.A. Perez, Microtubule inhibitors: differentiating tubulin-inhibiting agents based on mechanisms of action, clinical activity, and resistance. Mol. Cancer Ther. **8**(8), 2086–2095 (2009)
S. Petry, A.C. Groen, K. Ishihara, T.J. Mitchison, R.D. Vale, Branching microtubule nucleation in Xenopus egg extracts mediated by augmin and TPX2. Cell **152**, 768–777 (2013)
M.L. Pimm, J.L. Henty-Ridilla, New twists in actin-microtubule interactions. Mol. Biol. Cell, *32*(3), 211–217 (2021)
X. Pivot, C. Villanueva, L. Chaigneau, T. Nguyen, M. Demarchi, T. Maurina, U. Stein, C. Borg, Ixabepilone, a novel epothilone analog in the treatment of breast cancer. Expert Opin. Investig. Drugs **17**(4), 593–599 (2008)
J. Pokorný, J. Pokorný, J. Vrba, Generation of electromagnetic field by microtubules. Int. J. Mol. Sci. **22**(15), 8215 (2021)
A. Priel, A.J. Ramos, J.A. Tuszynski, H.F. Cantiello, A biopolymer transistor: electrical amplification by microtubules. Biophys. J. **90**, 4639–4643 (2006)
A. Priel, J.A. Tuszynski, N.J. Woolf, Neural cytoskeleton capabilities for learning and memory. J. Biol. Phys. **36**(1), 3–21 (2010)
S.Z. Prisco, M. Blake, F. Kazmirczak, R. Moon, B.P. Kremer, L.M. Hartweck, M. Kim, N. Vogel, J.B. Mendelson, D. Moutsoglou, T. Thenappan, K.W. Prins, *Lactobacillus* restructures the micro/mycobiome to combat inflammation-mediated right ventricular dysfunction in pulmonary arterial hypertension. Circ. Heart Fail. **16**, e012524 (2025)
A.J. Putnam, K. Schultz, D.J. Mooney, Control of microtubule assembly by extracellular matrix and externally applied strain. Am. J. Physiol. Cell Physiol. **280**(3), C556–C564 (2001)
J.E. Quinn, R.D. Kennedy, P.B. Mullan, P.M. Gilmore, M. Carty, P.G. Johnston, D.P. Harkin, BRCA1 functions as a differential modulator of chemotherapy-induced apoptosis. Can. Res. **63**(19), 6221–6228 (2003)
S. Quintero-Fabián, R. Arreola, E. Becerril-Villanueva, J.C. Torres-Romero, V. Arana-Argáez, J. Lara-Riegos, M.A. Ramírez-Camacho, M.E. Alvarez-Sánchez, Role of matrix metalloproteinases in angiogenesis and cancer. Front. Oncol. **9**, 1370 (2019)
A.H. Rajabi, M. Jaffe, T.L. Arinzeh, Piezoelectric materials for tissue regeneration: a review. Acta Biomater. **24**, 12–23 (2015). https://doi.org/10.1016/j.actbio.2015.07.010. (Epub 7 July 2015. PMID: 26162587)
A. Ramkumar, B.Y. Jong, K.M. Ori-McKenney, ReMAPping the microtubule landscape: how phosphorylation dictates the activities of microtubule-associated proteins. Dev. Dyn. **247**(1), 138–155 (2018)
S. Rao, U. Tata, V. Lin, J.C. Chiao, The migration of cancer cells in gradually varying chemical gradients and mechanical constraints. Micromachines **5**(1), 13–26 (2014)
A. Ray, Z.M. Slama, R.K. Morford, S.A. Madden, P.P. Provenzano, Enhanced directional migration of cancer stem cells in 3D aligned collagen matrices. Biophys. J. **112**(5), 1023–1036 (2017)
P. Renaudier, Physiopathologie de la drépanocytose [Sickle cell pathophysiology]. Transfus. Clin. Biol. **21**(4–5), 178–181 (2014)
M. Reynolds, What the scientists who pioneered weight-loss drugs want you to know. Wired, 2023. https://www.wired.com/story/obesity-drugs-researcher-interview-ozempic-wegovy/

K.M. Riching, B.L. Cox, M.R. Salick, C. Pehlke, A.S. Riching, S.M. Ponik, B.R. Bass, P. Rorsman, P.O. Berggren, K. Bokvist, H. Ericson, H. Möhler, C.G. Ostenson, P.A. Smith, Glucose-inhibition of glucagon secretion involves activation of GABAA-receptor chloride channels. Nature **341**(6239), 233–236 (1989)

P. Rorsman, P.O. Berggren, K. Bokvist, H. Ericson, H. Mohler, C.G. Ostenson, and P.A. Smith, Glucose-inhibition of glucagon secretion involves activation of GABAA-receptor chloride channels. Nature. **341**, 233–236 (1989)

C. Ruggiero, E. Lalli, Targeting the cytoskeleton against metastatic dissemination. Cancer Metastasis Rev. **40**(1), 89–140 (2021)

L. Rydén, J. Lindsten, The history of the Nobel prize for the discovery of insulin. Diabetes Res. Clin. Pract. **175**, 108819 (2021)

S. Sahu, S. Ghosh, B. Ghosh et al., Atomic water channel controlling remarkable properties of a single brain microtubule: correlating single protein to its supramolecular assembly. Biosens. Bioelectron. **47**, 141–148 (2013). https://doi.org/10.1016/j.bios.2013.02.050

N. Sanchez-Castro, M.A. Palomino-Ovando, P. Singh, S. Sahu, M. Toledo-Solano, J. Faubert, J.E. Lugo, A. Bandyopadhyay, K. Ray, Microtubules as one-dimensional crystals: is crystal-like structure the key to the information processing of living systems? Crystals **11**(3), 318 (2021)

C.V. Santos, S.L. Rogers, A.P. Carter, CryoET shows cofilactin filaments inside the microtubule lumen. EMBO Rep. **24**, e57264 (2023)

E. Schrödinger, *What Is Life? The Physical Aspect of the Living Cell* (Cambridge University Press, Cambridge, 1944). http://www.whatislife.ie/downloads/What-is-Life.pdf

J. Seligmann, C. Twelves, Tubulin: an example of targeted chemotherapy. Future Med. Chem. **5**(3), 339–352 (2013)

A.F. Serpico, R. Visconti, D. Grieco, Exploiting immune-dependent effects of microtubule-targeting agents to improve efficacy and tolerability of cancer treatment. Cell Death Dis. **11**(5), 361 (2020)

D. Shechtman, I. Blech, D. Gratias, J.W. Cahn, Metallic phase with long-range orientational order and no translational symmetry. Phys. Rev. Lett. **53**(20), 1951–1953 (1984)

M.L. Shelanski, E.W. Taylor, Isolation of a protein subunit from microtubules. J. Cell Biol. **34**(2), 549–554 (1967)

J. Shen, J.H. Zhang, H. Xiao et al., Mitochondria are transported along microtubules in membrane nanotubes to rescue distressed cardiomyocytes from apoptosis. Cell Death Dis. **9**, 81 (2018)

H. Shi, W. Cui, Y. Qin, L. Chen, T. Yu, J. Lv, A glimpse into novel acylations and their emerging role in regulating cancer metastasis. Cell. Mol. Life Sci. **81**(1), 76 (2024)

K. Shi, X. Peng, T. Xu, Z. Lin, M. Sun, Y. Li, Q. Xian, T. Xiao, S. Chen, Y. Xie et al., Electromagnetic modulation of the cell cycle and its applications in cancer therapy. Int. J. Mol. Sci. **26**(9), 4445 (2025)

S.V. Shirmovsky, On the possibility of implementing a quantum entanglement distribution in a biosystem: microtubules. Biosystems **245**, 105230 (2024)

V.K. Sidhaye, E. Chau, V. Srivastava, S. Sirimalle, C. Balabhadrapatruni, N.R. Aggarwal, F.R. D'Alessio, D.N. Robinson, L.S. King, A novel role for aquaporin-5 in enhancing microtubule organization and stability. PLoS ONE **7**(6), e38717 (2012)

D.B. Slautterback, Cytoplasmic microtubules: I. Hydra. J. Cell Biol. **18**(2), 367–388 (1963)

T. Smith, First molecular explanation of disease. Nat. Struct. Mol. Biol. **6**, 307 (1999)

C.Y. Son, A. Yethiraj, Q. Cui, Cavity hydration dynamics in cytochrome c oxidase and functional implications. PNAS **114**(42), E8830–E8836 (2017)

M.E. Stearns, Taxol reduces circulating tumor cells to prevent bone metastases in SCID mice. Invas. Metastasis **15**(5–6), 232–241 (1995)

X. Sun, Y. Zhou, S. Sun et al., Cancer cells sense solid stress to enhance metastasis by CKAP4 phase separation-mediated microtubule branching. Cell Discov. **10**, 114 (2024)

M.W. Swift, C.G. Van De Walle, M.P.A. Fisher, Posner molecules: from atomic structure to nuclear spins. Phys. Chem. Chem. Phys. **20**(18), 12373–12380 (2018)

M. Takahashi, Y. Kikawa, K. Kashiwabara, N. Taira, T. Iwatani, K. Shimozuma, S. Ohtani, T. Yoshinami, J. Watanabe, M. Kashiwaba, K.I. Watanabe, M. Kitada, K. Sakaguchi, Y. Tanabe,

T. Aihara, H. Mukai, Eribulin versus S-1 as first or second-line chemotherapy to assess health-related quality of life and overall survival in HER2-negative metastatic breast cancer (RESQ study): a non-inferiority, randomised, controlled, open-label, phase 3 trial. eClinicalMedicine **74**, 102715 (2024)

A. Thawani, H.A. Stone, S. Petry, Spatiotemporal organization of branched microtubule networks. eLife **8**, e43890 (2019)

A. Tirandaz, F. Taher Ghahramani, V. Salari, Validity examination of the dissipative quantum model of olfaction. Sci. Rep. **7**, 4432 (2017)

K. Torres, Mechanism of taxol-induced cell death are concentration dependent. Can. Res. **58**, 3620–3626 (1998)

M. Toya, M. Takeichi, Organization of non-centrosomal microtubules in epithelial cells. Cell Struct. Funct. **41**(2), 127–135 (2016)

M. Toya, S. Kobayashi, M. Kawasaki, G. Shioi, M. Kaneko, T. Ishiuchi, K. Misaki, W. Meng, M. Takeichi, CAMSAP3 orients the apical-to-basal polarity of microtubule arrays in epithelial cells. Proc. Natl. Acad. Sci. u.s.a. **113**(2), 332–337 (2016)

K.P. Trogden, X. Zhu, J.S. Lee, C.V.E. Wright, G. Gu, I. Kaverina, Regulation of glucose dependent Golgi-derived microtubules by cAMP/EPAC2 promotes secretory vesicle biogenesis in β cells. Curr. Biol. **29**(14), 2339-2350.e5 (2019)

L. Turin, A spectroscopic mechanism for primary olfactory reception. Chem. Senses **21**, 773–791 (1996)

J.A. Tuszynski, D. Friesen, H. Freedman, et al., Microtubules as sub-cellular memristors. Sci. Rep. **10**, 2108 (2020).

J. Tuszynski, C. Wenger, D. Friesen, J. Preto, An overview of sub-cellular mechanisms involved in the action of TTFields. Int. J. Environ. Res. Public Health **13**, 1128 (2016)

N. Urman, A. Itzhaki, Mitotic spindle disruption by alternating electric fields leads to improper chromosome segregation and mitotic catastrophe in cancer cells. Sci. Rep. **5**, 18046 (2015)

F. Vazza, A. Feletti, The quantitative comparison between the neuronal network and the cosmic web. Front. Phys. **8**, 525731 (2020). https://doi.org/10.3389/fphy.2020.525731

A. Venkateshwarlu, S.S. Akshayveer, R. Melnik, Piezoelectricity and flexoelectricity in biological cells: the role of cell structure and organelles. Biomech. Model. Mechanobiol. **24**(1), 47–76 (2025)

S.W. Verbruggen, C.L. Thompson, M.P. Duffy, S. Lunetto, J. Nolan, O.M.T. Pearce, C.R. Jacobs, M.M. Knight, Mechanical stimulation modulates osteocyte regulation of cancer cell phenotype. Cancers (Basel) **13**(12) (2021)

K.J. Verhey, J. Gaertig, The tubulin code. Cell Cycle **6**(17), 2152–2160 (2007). https://doi.org/10.4161/cc.6.17.4633

E. Vissol-Gaudin, C. Pearson, C. Groves, D.A. Zeze, H.F. Cantiello, M.D.R. Cantero, M.C. Petty, Electrical behaviour and evolutionary computation in thin films of bovine brain microtubules. Sci. Rep. **11**, 10776 (2021)

X. Wang, T.L. Schwarz, The mechanism of Ca^{2+}-dependent regulation of kinesin-mediated mitochondrial motility. Cell **136**(1), 163–174 (2009)

Y. Wang, W. Gao, X. Shi, J. Ding, W. Liu, H. He, K. Wang, F. Shao, Chemotherapy drugs induce pyroptosis through caspase-3 cleavage of a gasdermin. Nature **547**(7661), 99–103 (2017)

H. Wang, L. Yang, M. Liu, J. Luo, Protein post-translational modifications in the regulation of cancer hallmarks. Cancer Gene Ther. **30**(4), 529–547 (2023)

B. Watson, *The Man Who Changed How Boys and Toys Were Made* (Penguin Group, USA, 2002), 244 pp. ISBN-13978-0142003534

J. Watson, F. Crick, Molecular structure of nucleic acids: a structure for deoxyribose nucleic acid. Nature **171**, 737–738 (1953)

P.A. Watson, R. Hannan, L.L. Carl, K.E. Giger, Contractile activity and passive stretch regulate tubulin mRNA and protein content in cardiac myocytes. Am. J. Physiol. Cell Physiol. **271**(2 Pt 1), C684–C689 (1996)

O. Wattanathamsan, V. Pongrakhananon, Emerging role of microtubule-associated proteins on cancer metastasis. Front. Pharmacol. **13**, 935493 (2022)

O. Wattanathamsan, V. Pongrakhananon, Post-translational modifications of tubulin: their role in cancers and the regulation of signaling molecules. Cancer Gene Ther. **30**(4), 521–528 (2023)

O. Wattanathamsan, R. Thararattanobon, R. Rodsiri, P. Chanvorachote, C. Vinayanuwattikun, V. Pongrakhananon, Tubulin acetylation enhances lung cancer resistance to paclitaxel-induced cell death through Mcl-1 stabilization. Cell Death Discov. **7**(1), 67 (2021)

A.G. Watts, C.N. Boyle, The functional architecture of dehydration-anorexia. Physiol. Behav. **100**(5), 472–477 (2010)

R.C. Weisenberg, G.G. Borisy, E.W. Taylor, The colchicine-binding protein of mammalian brain and its relation to microtubules. Biochemistry **7**(12), 4466–4479 (1968)

E. White, Mechanical modulation of cardiac microtubules. Pflugers Arch. **462**(1), 177–184 (2011)

L. Wilson, H.P. Miller, K.W. Farrell, K.B. Snyder, W.C. Thompson, D.L. Purich, Taxol stabilization of microtubules in vitro: dynamics of tubulin addition and loss at opposite microtubule ends. Biochemistry **24**, 5254–5262 (1985)

O.C. Wilson Jr., T. Olorunyolemi, A. Jaworski et al., Surface and interfacial properties of polymer-intercalated layered double hydroxide nanocomposites. Appl. Clay Sci. **15**, 265–279 (1999)

L. Wordeman, J.J. Vicente, Microtubule targeting agents in disease: classic drugs, novel roles. Cancers **13**(22), 5650 (2021)

F. Wu, K. Xu, L. Liu, K. Zhang, L. Xia, M. Zhang, C. Teng, H. Tong, Y. He, Y. Xue, H. Zhang, D. Chen, A. Hu, Vitamin B_{12} enhances nerve repair and improves functional recovery after traumatic brain injury by inhibiting ER stress-induced neuron injury. Front. Pharmacol. **10**, 406 (2019)

L. Xiao, Y. Liu, H. Chen, L. Shen, Targeting CDK9 with selective inhibitors or degraders in tumor therapy: an overview of recent developments. Cancer Biol. Ther. **24**(1), 2219470 (2023)

X. Xie, B. Zhang, D. Li, J. Gao, J. Li, C. Liu, Y. Dan, P. Xu, L. Yan, X. Huang, Suppression of microtubule acetylation mediates the anti-leukemic effect of CDK9 inhibition. Cancer Cell Int. **24**(1), 1–13 (2024)

C. Yang, H. Liu, X. Feng, H. Shi, Y. Jiang, J. Li, J. Tan, Research hotspots and frontiers of neoadjuvant therapy in triple-negative breast cancer: a bibliometric analysis of publications between 2002 and 2023. Int. J. Surg. **110**(8), 4976–4992 (2024)

H. Zadeh-Haghighi, C. Simon, Radical pairs may play a role in microtubule reorganization. Sci. Rep. **12**, 6109 (2022)

C. Zhang, M. Zhao, G. Wang, Y. Li, Recent progress on microtubule degradation agents. J. Med. Chem. **66**(19), 13354–13368 (2023)

F.J. Zhong, Y.M. Li, C. Xu, B. Sun, J.L. Wang, L.Y. Yang, EB2 promotes hepatocellular carcinoma proliferation and metastasis via MAPK/ERK pathway by modulating microtubule dynamics. Clin. Sci. **135**(7), 847–864 (2021)

Y. Zhou, G. Yang, H. Tian, Y. Hu, S. Wu, Y. Geng, K. Lin, W. Wu, Sulforaphane metabolites cause apoptosis via microtubule disruption in cancer. Endocr. Relat. Cancer **25**(3), 255–268 (2018)

X. Zhu, R. Hu, M. Brissova, R.W. Stein, A.C. Powers, G. Gu, I. Kaverina, Microtubules negatively regulate insulin secretion in pancreatic β cells. Dev. Cell **34**, 656–668 (2015)

Microfluidic Synthesis of Nanoparticles for Biological Applications

Yiqiang Fan, Kexin Gao, Xueqin Chen, and Siyuan Ding

Abstract Nanoparticles have currently been widely used in biological and medical fields, including drug delivery, biosensing, tissue engineering, and vaccines. The conventional fabrication/synthesis methods of nanoparticles usually involve a complex synthesis approach with sophisticated instruments, the synthesized nanoparticles have a wide size distribution with uncontrolled surface structures. Emerging microfluidics technology has been used in biological and medical fields for almost three decades in the areas of point-of-care tests, drug screening, and biosynthesis. The use of the microfluidics technique for the synthesis of nanoparticles has the advantage of precise control of the synthesis process, low contamination, and controllable size with a narrow size distribution, short reaction time, and cost-effectiveness. This study reviewed the most up-to-date approaches to the synthesis of nanoparticles for various biological applications, and an outlook is also provided for the future trend on nanoparticle synthesis and applications in biological and medical fields.

Keywords Microfluidics · Nanoparticle synthesis · Nano-bio material · Microreactor · Micromixer

1 Introduction

Microfluidics is defined as the technique of manipulating fluidic in the micro- or nanoscale. Early microfluidics is sourced from the fluid control mechanism of the MEMS (microelectromechanical) devices (Henning 1998) otherwise known as bio-MEMS (Wang and Soper 2006). The scaling of the microfluidics is in the range of several millimeters to several micrometers, corresponding to a volume of 10^{-9}–10^{-18} L. The advantages of microfluidics on the synthesis of the nanoparticles (NPs) are mainly sourced from the precise manipulation/control of the fluid in low volume and the scaling effect (e.g., increased surface-to-volume ratio) which enables the

Y. Fan (✉) · K. Gao · X. Chen · S. Ding
School of Intelligent Science and Engineering, Nanjing University of Science & Technology, Nanjing, China
e-mail: yiqiang.fan50@gmail.com

R. Narayan (ed.), *Nanostructured Biomaterials and Their Applications*,
https://doi.org/10.1007/978-3-032-16316-5_5

homogeneous mixing (Shepherd et al. 2021a), efficient heat (Wang et al. 2015), mass transfer (van Stee et al. 2022), and low reagent consumption (Theberge et al. 2012).

Microfluidics has been widely used in various fields and proved to be very useful in the sensing or synthesis of substances on a small scale (Abedini-Nassab et al. 2021; Cheng et al. 2021). Some of the most typical examples include microfluidics for point-of-care test in medical fields; precise synthesis of lipid nanoparticles (LNP) for drug delivery (Maeki et al. 2022); organ/tissue on a chip for drug screening (Leung et al. 2022); single-cell/single DNA detection and analysis (Jiang et al. 2023; Ruan et al. 2021); environmental monitoring (Saez et al. 2021).

Nanoparticles are usually defined as particles with size or diameter in the ranges between 1 and 100 nm (Kreuter 2007), however, in the research and application scenarios, this range can further expand to between 1 and 1000 nm. As with microfluidics, the scaling effect of nanoparticles significantly influences the physical, chemical, and biological properties of the nanoparticles (Windolf et al. 2021; Sun et al. 2023a; Joseph et al. 2023), including the significantly increased surface-to-volume ratio, increased stability, increased reactivity, and quantum effects. The nanoparticles, either synthesized by top-down (Fu et al. 2018) or bottom-up (de Oliveira et al. 2020) approaches, can be classified into metal nanoparticles (Falcaro et al. 2016), metal oxide nanoparticles (Sengul and Asmatulu 2020), polymeric nanoparticles (Behl et al. 2020), and lipid-based nanoparticles (Eygeris et al. 2022), carbon-based nanoparticles (Holmannova et al. 2022), ceramic nanoparticles (Wang et al. 2022), and quantum dots (Li et al. 2020). Almost all these types of nanoparticles have been used in various applications in medical or biological fields.

Nanoparticles are widely used in medicine and biological fields, including but not limited to drug delivery (Chandrakala et al. 2022), diagnostics (Yu et al. 2021), cancer treatment (Gavas et al. 2021), vaccines (Nguyen and Tolia 2021), tissue engineering (Godoy-Gallardo et al. 2021), and biosensing (Karnwal et al. 2024). Take drug delivery as an example, nanoparticles can serve as either a nano drug or as drug carrier (for other small molecular drugs) in the drug delivery process, due to their small size, nanoparticles can penetrate through various barriers (Utreja et al. 2020) to reach most of the body parts, and the unload/release of the drug can also be precisely controlled to deliver genes (Mirza and Karim 2021), protein (Hong et al. 2020), and other kinds of reagents (Li et al. 2021).

The conventional synthesis methods for nanoparticles can be classified as bottom-up (Branda et al. 2021) or top-down (Patil et al. 2021) approaches (as shown in Fig. 1). As the name implies, top-down approaches break the large substance into smaller (nano) pieces, usually with a mechanical grinding method (Ali et al. 2014). The mechanical grinding is easily scalable for the industrial fabrication of nanoparticles, but usually with very poor size distribution and lack of control on the formation of nanoparticles (Fu et al. 2018). The bottom-up approach uses the chemical/physical growth of the nanoparticles from clusters formed by atom precursors. Compared with the top-down approach, the bottom-up approach is usually low-cost, rapid, and suitable for small-scale production in the laboratory. However, in the growth/self-assembly process of nanoparticles in the bottom-up approach, the size distribution

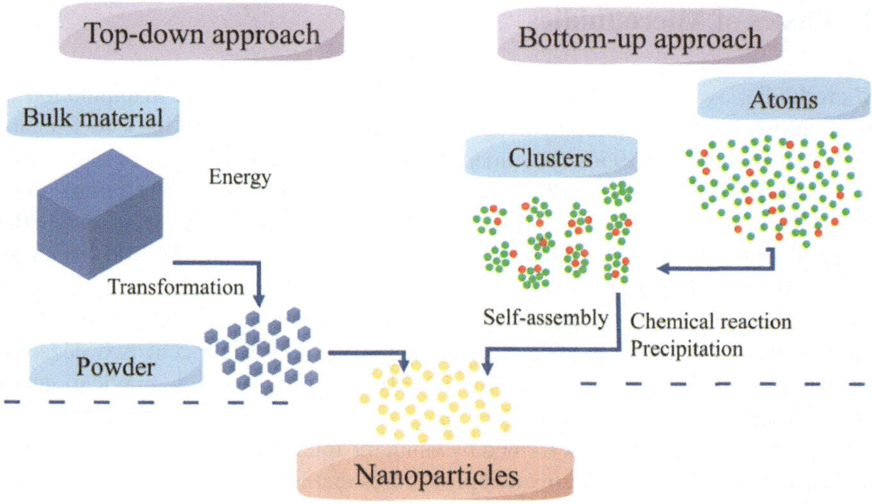

Fig. 1 Illustration of the top-down and bottom-up approaches for the synthesis of nanoparticles

is highly influenced by the parameter in the mixing process and other factors (Rane et al. 2018), in addition, the agglomerate is also a common defect in the bottom-up process (Yeap 2018).

The current synthesis method for nanoparticles with a microfluidic approach is usually a bottom-up approach and can be divided into two categories, single-phase and multiple-phase synthesis (Khizar et al. 2022). Synthesis of nanoparticles with microfluidics has been widely explored in the recent decade. Almost all kinds of nanoparticles as mentioned above have been successfully synthesized with microfluidic approaches, compared with the conventional synthesis methods of nanoparticles, microfluidics is proven to be one of the most promising methods for the precise synthesis of nanoparticles with countless advantages (Gimondi et al. 2023; Nette et al. 2020).

This study will first review the basics of microfluidics techniques for nanoparticle synthesis, including the materials and commonly used fabrication approaches for microfluidics devices. The mixing phenomenon in microfluidic devices for the synthesis of nanoparticles will also be briefly introduced. Then, various synthesis methods (with an emphasis on single and multiple-phase mixing) based on microfluidic techniques for nanoparticles will be introduced. Next, microfluidics synthesis for different types of nanoparticles will be discussed and compared. The applications of microfluidics-synthesized nanoparticles are presented. Finally, the outlook of the future research directions of microfluidic-based nanoparticle synthesis is provided.

2 Basics of Microfluidics

Microfluidics is usually defined as the fluid flow (behavior) and manipulation at the microscale. The development of microfluidics can be traced back to Richard Feynman's talk in the 1950s (Feynman 2018), with the development of microelectronics and MEMS, in the 1980s, early fluid channels (Phillips 1987), pumps (Van Lintel et al. 1988), and valves (Esashi et al. 1989) in microscale were invented with the microfabrication technologies inherited from microelectronics and MEMS (Henning 1998). At the end of the 1980s, the concept of "microfluidics" started to appear at conferences and gradually separated from microelectronics and MEMS and formed a relatively independent field (Gravesen et al. 1993). In the recent two decades, microfluidics technology is developing rapidly driven by the wide applications of microfluidics technology in biological and medical fields (Whitesides 2006). The concept of "Lab-on-a-chip" is formed by using the integrated microfluidic system to replace the complicated experimental procedures that are conducted in a biological, chemical, or medical laboratory (Stone et al. 2004). Thus, with the integrated Lab-on-a-chip microfluidic system, the point-of-care test can be conducted for portable or low-resource settings areas (Chin et al. 2012). Figure 2 shows the publications sourced from the "web of science" platform with the keyword "microfluidics," the count of publications is steadily increasing and increased around 4 times from 2013 to 2023.

The advantages of microfluidics are mainly sourced from the scaling effect (Squires and Quake 2005). Compared with the conventional sensing or synthesis approaches, microfluidics usually has a lower reagent consumption, better sensitivity, single-cell/DNA manipulation capability, automation, and low carbon footprint (Liu and Jiang 2017; Ongaro et al. 2022). In the area of nanoparticle synthesis, compared

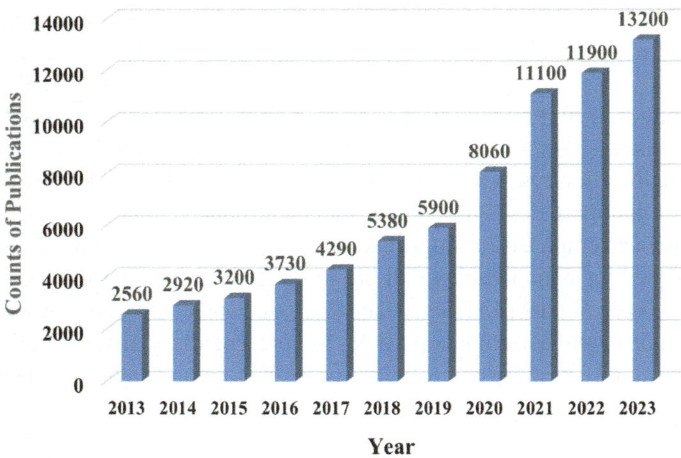

Fig. 2 Counts of publications with the keyword "microfluidics" in the last ten years from the "Web of Science" platform

with the conventional top-down or bottom-up approaches, microfluidic technology has advantages including precise control of the reaction conditions, enhanced mixing efficiency, consistency of the produced nanoparticles, flexibility, and enhanced safety with hazardous chemicals.

2.1 *Materials in Microfluidics*

With the fabrication techniques inherited from microelectronics and microfluidics, early microfluidic devices were usually fabricated with inorganic materials, i.e., silicon and glass (Gravesen et al. 1993). Microstructures (microchannels) were etched on the surface of the silicon or glass wafers with the standard photolithography method and physical/chemical etching methods (as shown in Fig. 3a and b). Then, another layer of silicon/glass wafers was bonded to enclose the microchannel (Raley et al. 1995). Silicon and glass wafers can be processed with a very high precision, even the channels in the nanoscale can be fabricated with the photolithography approaches (Wu et al. 2001). On the other hand, glass capillaries have also been widely used as the droplet generator in microfluidics (Herranz-Blanco et al. 2017).

To be applied in microfluidics, silicon material is opaque in the visible range, which increases the difficulties in the observation of the flow inside the channel. Glass material, due to the amorphous structure, is transparent in the visible range, the quartz material can even be used for Raman spectra (Dochow et al. 2013). Compared with silicon material, the fabrication and bonding approach of glass material is more flexible (Jia et al. 2004). Glass-based microfluidics have also been widely used in high-pressure or continuous chemical reactions (Tiggelaar et al. 2007). It must be mentioned that silicon and glass materials usually need to be processed in the cleanroom with sophisticated fabrication instruments, which has become a barrier for researchers without access to the cleanroom (Qi et al. 2018).

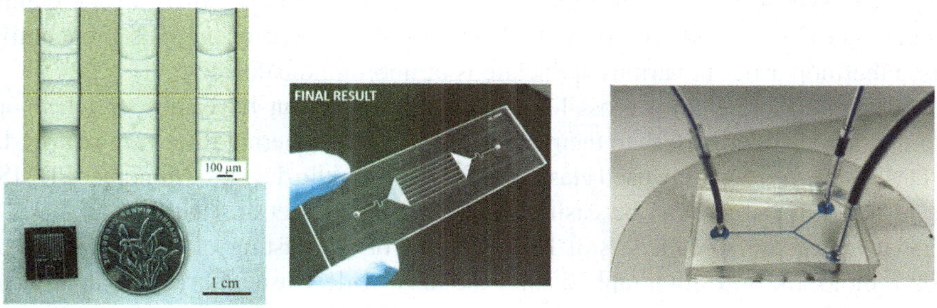

(a) (b) (c)

Fig. 3 Silicon/glass and polymer-based microfluidic devices. (**a**): Silicon-based microfluidic devices (Wang et al. 2024); (**b**): Glass-based microfluidic devices (Wlodarczyk et al. 2019); (**c**) Polydimethylsiloxane (PDMS) microfluidic devices (Al-Ali et al. 2023)

With the fast development of polymer materials in the 1980s and the invention of soft lithography in 1998 (Duffy et al. 1998), polymer material has now become the major player in microfluidic devices. Up to now, polymer materials have been widely used in biological, chemical, medical, environmental, and energy applications of microfluidic devices (Tsao 2016) (an example of polymer-based microfluidics is shown in Fig. 3c). Compared with silicon/glass materials, polymer materials have the following advantages: firstly, polymer materials are much more easier to process (in liquid form before crosslinking, or soften when heated), sometimes can even be processed with conventional lab equipment without cleanroom access (Fan 2018); secondly, the wide selection of polymer materials provides various physical and chemical properties fit for different application requirement, for microfluidics devices, the surface wettability and chemical resistance is critical; thirdly, compared with glass or silicon material, polymer materials are usually much cheaper; fourthly, the fabrication methods for polymer-based microfluidics have been developed for more than 20 years, with various characteristics of low-cost, rapid, massive production, etc. (more information on fabrication techniques on polymer microfluidic devices will be provided in the next session). Finally, compared with silicon/glass materials, the biocompatibility of polymer material is superior. Figure 4 is a bubble chart showing the counts of publications with the keyword "microfluidics" and the corresponding polymer materials. The size of the bubble is proportional to the counts of publications indexed in the "web of science" platform. As shown in Fig. 4, due to the widely adopted soft-lithography method used in microfluidics, the PDMS is the most widely used polymer material, while PS (polystyrene) and PMMA (Polymethyl methacrylate) are the second most popular materials in microfluidics according to the publication in the past ten years.

Polymer materials can be classified in different ways. In this study, based on the application of polymer materials in microfluidics, we classified the polymer materials in microfluidic into two groups: elastomers and thermoplastics. Images of polymer-based microfluidic devices (fabricated with various polymer materials, sourced from the author's lab, all with external dimensions of 25 mm by 75 mm) are shown in Fig. 5: PDMS is the most frequently used elastomers, while PMMA, cyclic olefin copolymer (COC), and polyoxymethylene (POM) are some of the most frequently used thermoplastics in various applications of microfluidic devices.

Elastomers are lightly cross-linked polymers that can be easily stretched or compressed and will return to their original shape once external forces are removed. PDMS is the most widely used elastomer for microfluidic devices. Monomer PDMS is in liquid form and can be easily shaped. Whitesides et al. (Duffy et al. 1998) first invented the so-called "soft lithography" for the casting of PDMS with the SU-8 mold, the soft lithography is still the most widely used fabrication approach by researchers in biological and medical fields. PDMS has the advantages of being low-cost, biocompatible, transparent in the visible range, and gas-permeable. The physical/chemical properties of PDMS can also be easily modified based on the application requirements (Zhou et al. 2010). Some of the drawbacks of PDMS include

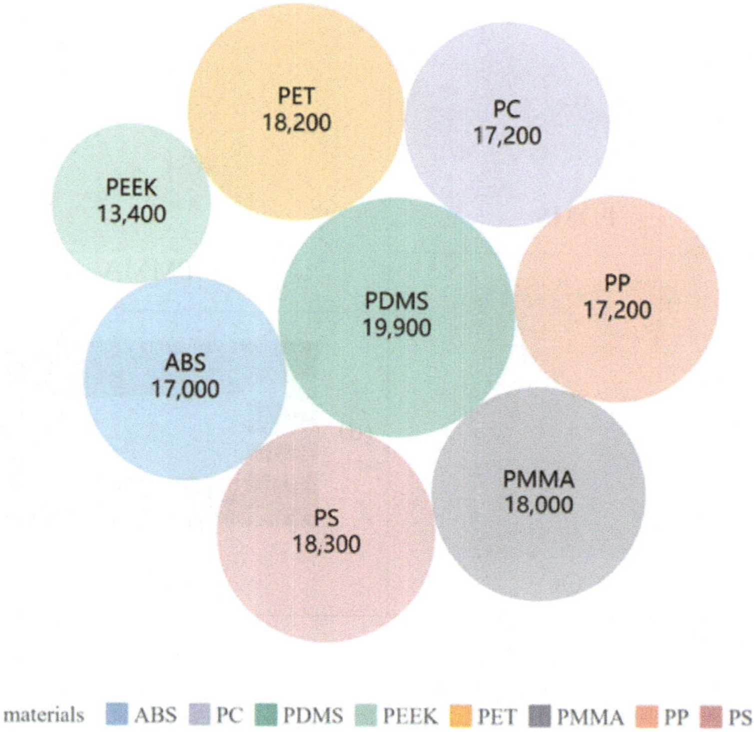

Fig. 4 Bubble chart of various polymer materials: acrylonitrile butadiene styrene (ABS), polycarbonate (PC), PDMS, polyether ether ketone (PEEK), polyethylene terephthalate (PET), PMMA, polypropylene (PP), and PS used in microfluidic devices, size of the bubble representing the counts of publications with the keywords of "microfluidics" and the corresponding materials from the "Web of Science" platform in the past 10 years

swelling under solvent, hydrophobicity, and not suitable for high-pressure applications. Table 1 compares some of the physical properties of the most widely used polymer materials in microfluidics.

Unlike elastomers, thermoplastics soften when heated and solidified when cooled. Thermoplastics can be easily reshaped with a temperature higher than the glass transition temperature (Ma et al. 2020). Thermoplastics can be classified as amorphous plastics and semicrystalline plastics. Some of the most frequently used amorphous plastics include polymethyl methacrylate (PMMA) (Fan et al. 2018), polystyrene (PS) (Tran et al. 2014), polycarbonate (PC), and acrylonitrile butadiene styrene (ABS) (Chen et al. 2021). The most frequently used semicrystalline plastics include polypropylene (PP) (Sun et al. 2019), polyether ether ketone (PEEK) (Song et al. 2004), and polyethylene terephthalate (PET). Compared with PDMS-based microfluidic devices, thermoplastics are more rigid, gas-impermeable, and more resistant to organic solvents. Most importantly, the process speed of thermoplastics is rapid with

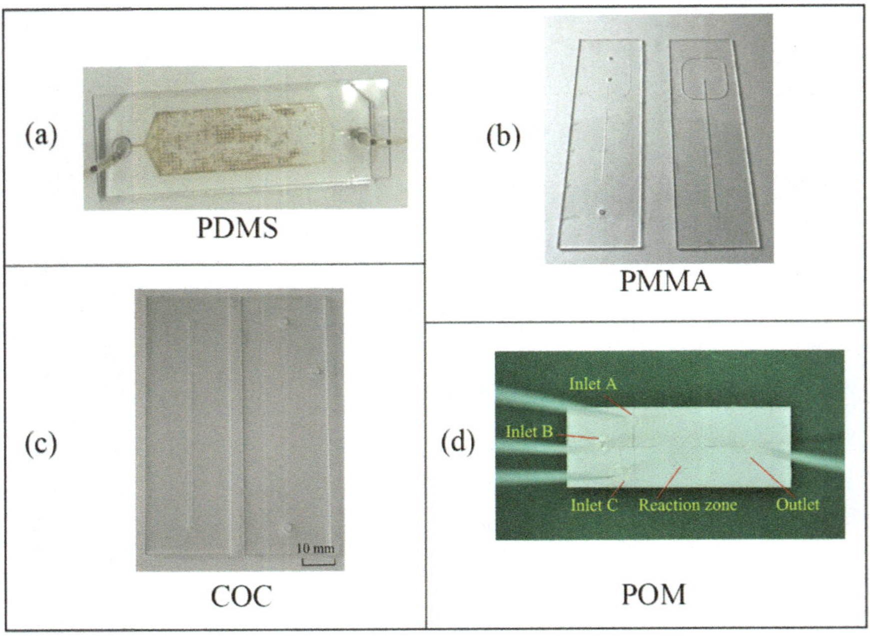

Fig. 5 Polymer-based microfluidic devices (all sourced from the author's lab). (**a**) PDMS-based microfluidic device; (**b**) PMMA-based microfluidics device; (**c**) COC-based microfluidic device; (**d**) POM-based microfluidic device

relatively lower cost. For instance, when using injection molding, thermoplastic-based microfluidic devices can be formed within a minute with negligible material cost in bulk fabrication (Lee et al. 2018).

Besides elastomers and thermoplastics, hydrogel (Yao and Fan 2021) and paper (Sun et al. 2023b) are also temporarily used for microfluidic devices. Since hydrogel- and paper-based microfluidics are currently not used for nanoparticle synthesis, we won't go into much detail on hydrogels and paper material. Another type of organic material we need to mention is photocurable resins (Au et al. 2016), which are usually used in 3D-printed microfluidic devices.

2.2 Fabrication Methods of Microfluidics for Nanoparticle Synthesis

2.2.1 Silicon and Glass Bulk Micromachining

Silicon and glass materials were frequently used in the early stage of microfluidic devices and occasionally used for the synthesis of nanoparticles (Jiang et al. 2015). Bulk micromachining refers to the fabrication of microstructures on the

Table 1 Comparison of the properties of typical polymers used in microfluidics

Polymer	Acronym	T_g (°C)	T_m (°C)	Water absorption (%)	Solvent resistance	Optical transmissivity	
						Visible	UV[a]
Cyclic olefin (co)polymer	COC/COP	70–155	190–320	0.01	Excellent	Excellent	Excellent
Polymethylmethacrylate	PMMA	100–122	250–260	0.3–0.6	Good	Excellent	Good
Polycarbonate	PC	145–148	260–270	0.12–0.34	Good	Excellent	Poor
Polystyrene	PS	92–100	240–260	0.02–0.15	Poor	Excellent	Poor
Polypropylene	PP	− 20	160	0.10	Good	Good	Fair
Polyetheretherketone	PEEK	147–158	340–350	0.1–0.5	Excellent	Poor	Poor
Polyethylene terephthalate	PET	69–78	248–260	0.1–0.3	Excellent	Good	Good
Polyethylene	PE	− 30	120–130	0.01	Excellent	Fair	Fair
Polydimethylsiloxane	PDMS	− 125	− 84~− 41	0.01	Poor	Excellent	Fair

T_g glass transition temperature; T_m melting temperature,
[a]high UV transmissivity often requires the selection of special polymer grades, e.g., without stabilizers or other additives

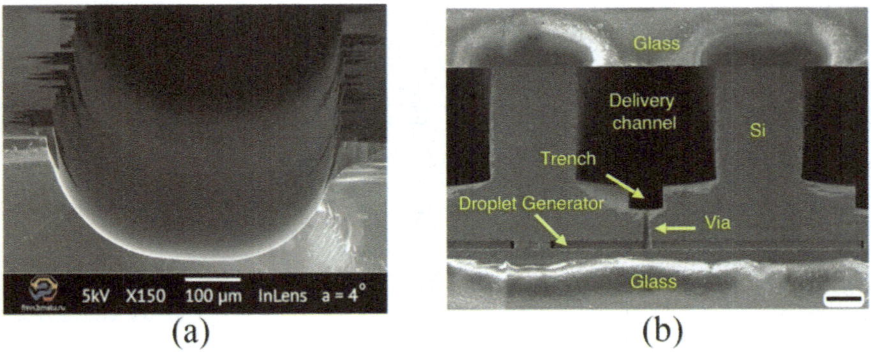

Fig. 6 Microchannels fabricated on glass and silicon wafers. (**a**): Microchannels fabricated on a glass substrate with wet etching (Konstantinova et al. 2023). (**b**): Microchannels fabricated on a silicon wafer (Yadavali et al. 2019)

surface of silicon/glass wafers by chemical/physical etching approaches (Gardeniers et al. 2003). Silicon has a crystalline structure that enables both the isotropic and anisotropic etching, amorphous material like glass is usually processed with the isotropic etching. The commonly used etchants used for anisotropic etching of silicon include KOH (Sato et al. 1998) and NaOH (Brockmeier et al. 2012), in addition, the high aspect ratio patterns can also be fabricated with a DRIE (deep reactive-ion etching) (Horstmann et al. 2024) process on silicon wafers. Glass wafer is usually isotopically etched with hydrofluoric acid (HF) (Shubhava et al. 2022). The patterned silicon and glass wafers can be bonded in the following manners: glass-glass (Funano et al. 2021), silicon-glass (Zhelev et al. 2018), and silicon-silicon. Microchannels fabricated on the surface of glass and silicon wafers are shown in Fig. 6.

2.2.2 Microfabrication Method for Polymer-Based Microfluidics

Compared with silicon/glass-based microfluidics, polymers are the most frequently used materials in nanoparticle synthesis with advantages in flexibility, low-cost, and a wide selection of material properties. In this study, various fabrication methods for polymer-based microfluidics used in nanoparticle synthesis will be briefly introduced.

The first and most used fabrication method in the laboratory is the replica molding of PDMS. The fabrication procedure is shown in Fig. 7. A thick layer of photoresist (typical SU-8) is spin-coated on the surface of the silicon wafer (Fig. 7a), and the thickness is defined by the viscosity of the SU-8 and the spin speed; Then the UV patterning is conducted either with the low-cost film or with the soda-line glass mask (Fig. 7b); The patterned SU-8 served as the mold for the replica molding of PDMS (Fig. 7c); The casting of PDMS is conducted by pouring the mixed PDMS base and curing agent with a weight ratio of 10:1 on the patterned SU-8 (Fig. 7d); The

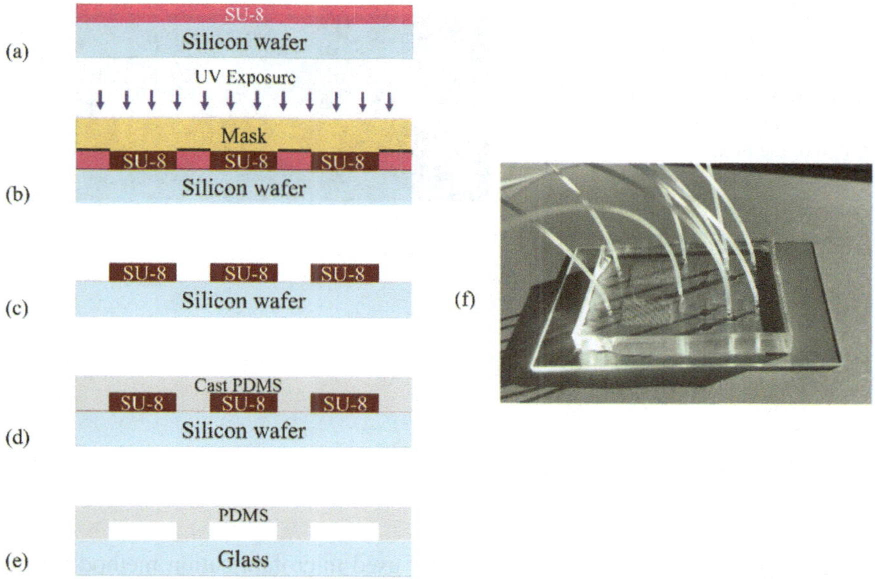

Fig. 7 Fabrication procedure for PDMS-based microfluidics (soft lithography). (**a**) Spin-coating of photoresist (typically SU-8); (**b**) patterning of photoresist using UV with a mask; (**c**) patterned SU-8 structure; (**d**) casting and curing process of the PDMS; (**e**) bonding of the patterned PDMS to a glass slide to enclose the microchannel; (**f**) fabricated PDMS-based microfluidic devices (droplet generator, from author's lab)

final step is bonding, the surfaces of the PDMS and glass are treated with typically with oxygen plasma and then bonded. The fabrication procedure of PDMS can be conducted with or without the cleanroom, which facilitates the adoption of this procedure in conventional chemical or biological laboratories.

PDMS-based microfluidic devices have been widely used for the synthesis of nanoparticles. Hassan et al. used PDMS-based microfluidics operating at laminar flow for the synthesis of iron oxide nanoparticles (Abou Hassan et al. 2008). Lim et al. fabricated a parallel PDMS-based flow-focusing microfluidic device for the synthesis of PLGA-PEG nanoparticles with controllable properties and production rates (Lim et al. 2014a).

Injection molding has also been widely used for commercial microfluidics cartridges for the synthesis of nanoparticles (Lee et al. 2018). In the injection molding process of microfluidics chips, the thermoplastics (e.g., PMMA, COC), were heated until molten, and then injected under high pressure into a metal mold to form the shape of the microfluidic devices. Once the material cools and solidifies, the mold is opened, and the finished part is ejected to finish the patterning. Figure 8 shows the injection molded polymer microfluidic device for the synthesis of LNP (lipid nanoparticle synthesis) (Ripoll et al. 2022).

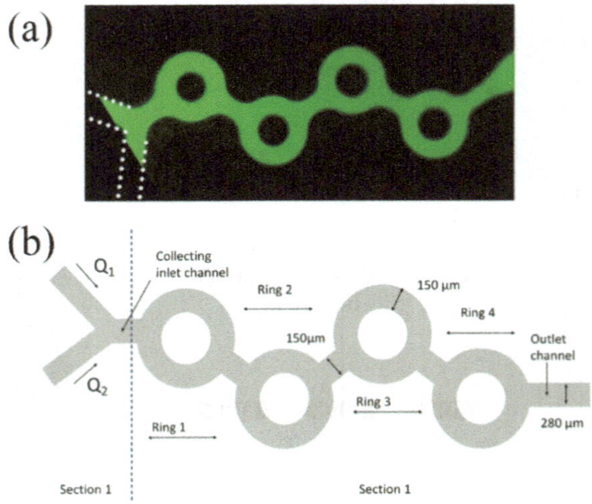

Fig. 8 Injection molded microfluidic cartridge for LNP synthesis (Ripoll et al. 2022). (**a**): Fluid flow inside the microchannel; (**b**): Design of the mixer

Laser ablation is another very frequently used microfabrication method for the rapid prototyping of polymer-based microfluidics used for the synthesis of nanoparticles (Kulkarni et al. 2021). Usually, the CO_2 laser with a wavelength of 10.6 μm is used for the direct ablation on the surface of the thermoplastic materials. Laser with shorter wavelengths may also be used for the fabrication of polymer-based microfluidics (Gao et al. 2019). Laser ablation is purely a thermal process, the laser beam is focused on the surface of the thermoplastics, causing the meltdown and evaporation of the material within a short period, resulting in a Gaussian-like profile of the microchannels (as shown in Fig. 9a), the laser ablated polystyrene-based microfluidic devices is shown in Fig. 9b (Li et al. 2012). The depth and width of the microchannels can be controlled with the adjustment of the laser scanning speed and laser power (Cai et al. 2017). The precision of the laser ablated microchannels mainly depends on the driving mechanism of the laser ablation machine and the stability of the laser source.

Besides laser ablation, direct machining has also been frequently used for the fabrication of microfluidic devices (Behroodi et al. 2020). Direct machining uses computer numerical control (CNC) mill with milling cutters of different sizes for the fabrication of microchannels and other structures on the surface of polymer materials. Compared with injection molding or PDMS casting, direct machining is rapid, low-cost, and with fabrication precision usually higher than CO_2 laser ablation. The machined thermoplastic material can also be used as the mold for the replica molding of PDMS. An example of the direct machined mold for the replica molding of a PDMS-based microfluidic device for the chitosan nanoparticle synthesis is shown in Fig. 9c (Cetin et al. 2013).

In the past few years, with the fast development of 3D-printing technology, more and more 3D-printed microfluidics devices were developed for the synthesis of nanoparticles. Some of the most frequently used 3D-printing techniques for nanoparticle synthesis include stereolithography (SLA) (Shapovalov et al. 2023; Kara et al.

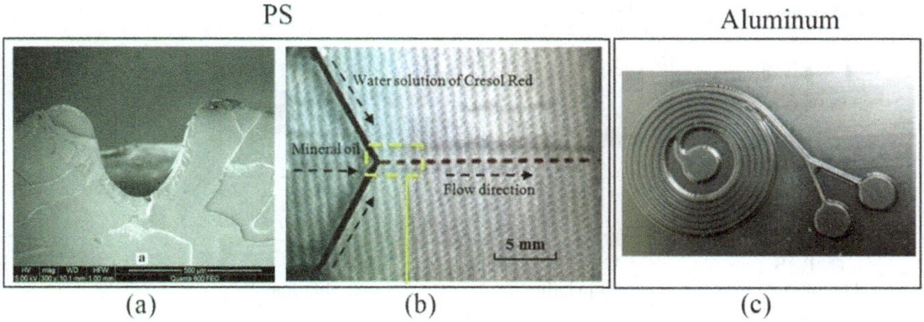

Fig. 9 Laser ablated and machined microfluidic devices for nanoparticle synthesis. (**a**) Cross-section profile of the laser ablated microchannel on PS substrate (Li et al. 2012); (**b**) Laser ablated microfluidic device fabricated on PS (Li et al. 2012); (**c**) CNC direct milled aluminum mold for PDMS casting {Yousuff, 2017 #259}

2021) and fused deposition modeling (FDM) (Bressan et al. 2019; Bressan et al. 2020). Compared with the conventional fabrication approaches for polymer-based microfluidics, the 3D-printing methods are rapid and relatively low-cost. The major drawback of the 3D-printed microfluidic devices used for nanoparticle synthesis is biocompatibility (Bhattacharjee et al. 2016), which limited selection of materials and opacity.

With the wide selection of materials and the fabrication approaches (as illustrated in Fig. 10) for polymer-based microfluidics, there are several aspects to consider when choosing the polymers and fabrication methods. Firstly, the required quantities of the chips, for small baths of nanoparticles with single or several microfluidic devices, PDMS casting, direct milling or 3D printing is usually recommended for the flexibility of chip fabrication and channel precision; Secondly, if the nanoparticles need to be produced in bulk or for commercial use, the injection molded microfluidic chips has the best fabrication repeatability to ensure the quality of the synthesis of the produced nanoparticles; Thirdly, if the high precision micro or even nanofluidic device is needed, the photolithography approach is the best option for glass/silicon-based devices; Finally, some synthesis procedure needs some environmental control of surface physical/chemical properties, which also need to be taken into consideration. Figure 10 compared various fabrication techniques (hot embossing, PDMS casting, injection molding, photolithography, 3D printing, and laser ablation methods.) for microfluidics from aspect of fabrication/material cost (C.), precision of the corresponding fabrication method (P.) and the processing (fabrication) speed (S.). Generally, PDMS casting is suitable for research or small batch fabrication while injection molding is suitable for product development. Glass/silicon-based microfluidic device process with photolithography method has the most precise microstructure, but with highest fabrication cost. The selection of fabrication approaches for microfluidic devices used for nanoparticles needs to take the following aspects into consideration: bulk material for microfluidics devices, material and fabrication cost,

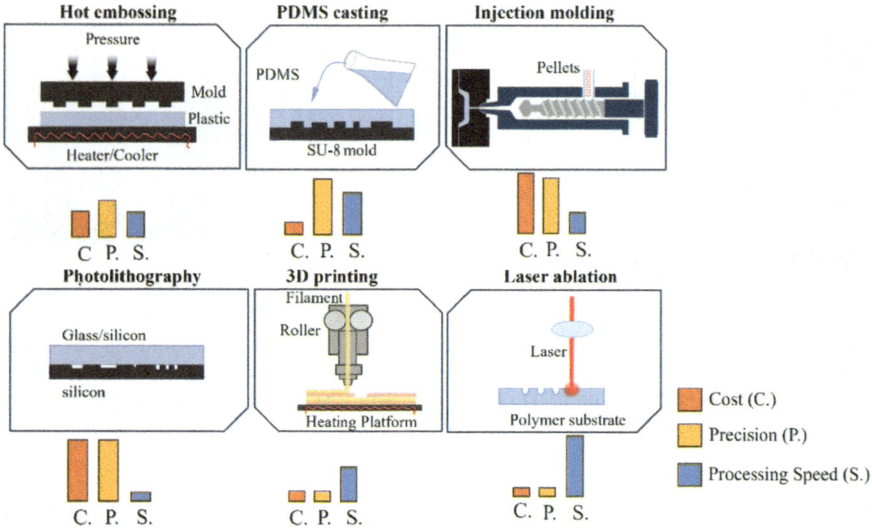

Fig. 10 Comparison of the various fabrication methods of microfluidics for nanoparticle synthesis, including hot embossing, PDMS casting, injection molding, photolithography, 3D printing and laser ablation. These fabrication methods are compared from the aspect of fabrication and material cost, fabrication precision and fabrication speed

precision of the microfabrication, quantity of the devices, and the special chemical/physical requirements of the devices in specific nanoparticle synthesis.

3 Synthesis of Nanoparticles with Microfluidics Approach

Using microfluidic approaches for synthesizing nanoparticles has advantages including but not limited to: controlled synthesis on nanoparticle size and distribution, automated operation, cost effective and low power consumption. In this section, we will first briefly introduce the conventional synthesis methods of nanoparticles, then we will introduce various microfluidics approaches for the synthesis of nanoparticles which are classified into single-phase and multiple phases synthesis approach. Finally, we will discuss the types of nanoparticles that can be synthesized with microfluidics approaches and how to scale up the production of nanoparticles with the microfluidics approaches.

3.1 Conventional Synthesis Methods of Nanoparticles

As shown in Fig. 1 in the previous section, the conventional synthesis methods of nanoparticles can be divided into the bottom-up and top-down approaches. Current microfluidics method for the synthesis of nanoparticles all based on the bottom-up approach. On the other hand, based on the specific synthesis approach, nanoparticle synthesis can also be classified into the physical (Meischein et al. 2021), chemical (Gan et al. 2020), or even biological (Rónavári et al. 2021) approach.

The bottom-up method refers to the synthesis (accumulation) of nanoparticles from even smaller substances (e.g., molecules, clusters). Based on the accumulation process of the building blocks, the bottom-up process can be classified into hydrothermal (Mohan et al. 2020), sol-gel (Arya et al. 2021), chemical vapor deposition (Yang et al. 2022), and biological synthesis (Srivastava et al. 2021). It must be mentioned that the nucleation and growth of nanoparticles is a complicated process, the homogeneous nucleation and the control of nucleation rate is critical to achieve the required size and distribution of the nanoparticles.

The top-down method refers to the crackdown of the substances on the nanoscale. The size-reduction process is usually a physical approach, different from the nucleation process in the bottom-up approach. The top-down method uses ball milling (Tsuzuki 2021), lithography (Chiang et al. 2021), laser ablation (Balachandran et al. 2022), sputtering (Orozco-Montes et al. 2021), and thermal treatment (Abdel-Aziz et al. 2020) to break the bulk material into nanoparticles. Compared with the bottom-up approach, the top-down method is more efficient for large-scale production with low-cost, but with lower uniformity in size distribution. Table 2 compares different conventional nanoparticle production methods with top-down and bottom-up approaches.

Figure 11 illustrates some of the conventional approaches for nanoparticle synthesis. Figure 11a used a "green" approach for the chemical synthesis of metal nanoparticles (Ying et al. 2022), Fig. 11b used sol-gel method for the synthesis of spinel ferrite and transition metals-substituted spinel ferrite nanoparticles (Salih and Mahmood 2023), Fig. 11c shows the laser ablation approaches for the top-down synthesis of metal nanoparticles (Liang et al. 2021).

Compared with the conventional synthesis approaches for nanoparticles which usually involve a complicated multi-step process, microfluidic approaches have the advantages on precise control of the synthesizing process, the pressure, flow rate, reagent concentration, and environmental conditions (e.g., pH, temperature) can be controlled and adjusted to ensure the uniformity of nanoparticles with desired size. In addition, the large surface-to-volume ratio also shortened the reaction time and enhanced the mixing process. In the following sections, we will introduce the microfluidic-based nanoparticle synthesis with the single and multiple phases in the precipitation process.

Table 2 Conventional methods for the fabrication of nanoparticles

Methodology	Synthesis method	Types of nanoparticles	Synthesis process	Refs.
Top-down	Ball milling	ZnO nanoparticles	Ball milling with ethyl alcohol as lubrication aid	Wirunchit et al. (2021)
Top-down	Soft-lithographic	Gold nanoparticles	Scalable nanoparticle chemical lift-off lithography	Chiang et al. (2021)
Top-down	Laser ablation	Au:ZnO (core:Shell) nanoparticles	Ablated in a glass vial 1064 nm pulses generated by a 1 Hz Nd:YAG laser with a pulse duration of 9 ns	Rashid et al. (2021)
Top-down	Plasma sputtering	Platinum nanoparticles	Synthesized in glycerol as a liquid substrate via a magnetron sputtering	Orozco-Montes et al. (2021)
Top-down	Thermal decomposition	Fe_2O_3 nanoparticles	Three different metal cation precursors used in decomposition	Benhammada et al. (2020)
Bottom-up	Chemical vapor deposition	Metal carbides	Buckling and release of MXene carpet to expose fresh surface for reaction	Wang et al. (2023a)
Bottom-up	Hydrothermal	Cobalt ferrite nanoparticles	Hydrothermal process with ammonium hydroxide as surfactant agent	Refat et al. (2022)
Bottom-up	Precipitation	Magnetic iron oxide nanoparticles	Mixing the ferrous/ ferric chloride precursor with the NaOH base solution	Besenhard et al. (2020)
Bottom-up	Sol-gel	ZnO and CuO nanoparticles	Sol–gel process using zinc nitrate and copper (II) nitrate as precursor	Patel et al. (2022)
Bottom-up	Biological	Silver nanoparticles	Synthesized at a 1:3 ratio of leaf extract to $AgNO_3$ solution	Nagime et al. (2024)

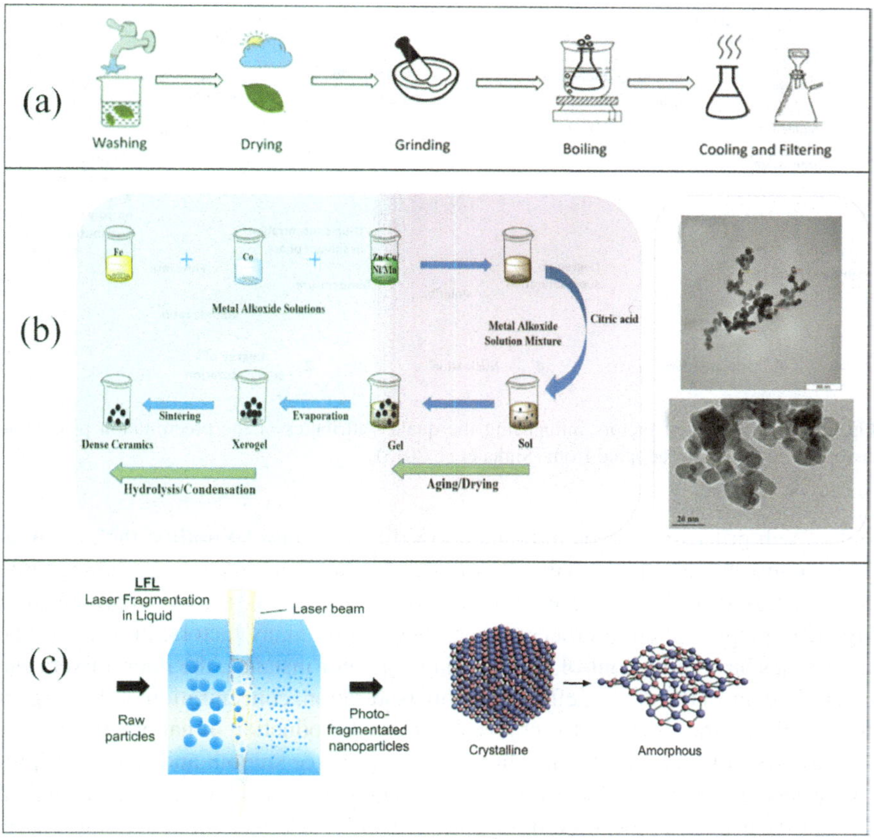

Fig. 11 Conventional synthesis methods for nanoparticles. (**a**): Green synthesis of metal nanoparticles (Ying et al. 2022); (**b**): Synthesis of spinel ferrite and transition metals-substituted spinel ferrite nanoparticles with sol-gel method (Salih and Mahmood 2023); (**c**): Laser fragmentation for the amorphization of metal oxide nanoparticles (Liang et al. 2021)

3.2 Single-Phase Synthesis of Nanoparticles with Microfluidic Approach

Microfluidics approaches for the synthesis of nanoparticles typically use the bottom-up approaches. Streams (usually all in aqueous phase) flow in parallel in the microfluidic channel without turbulent mixing, the diffusion across the stream introduces the nanoprecipitation process, the nanoparticles are formed after nucleation and growth. Take the synthesis of LNP nanoparticles as an example, the reaction reagent (e.g., drug payload, lipid) is dissolved in a solvent (e.g., alcohol), and then mixed with the antisolvent in the microfluidics mixer with various mixer structures inside the microchannels, the LNP nanoparticles are then precipitated after the nucleation

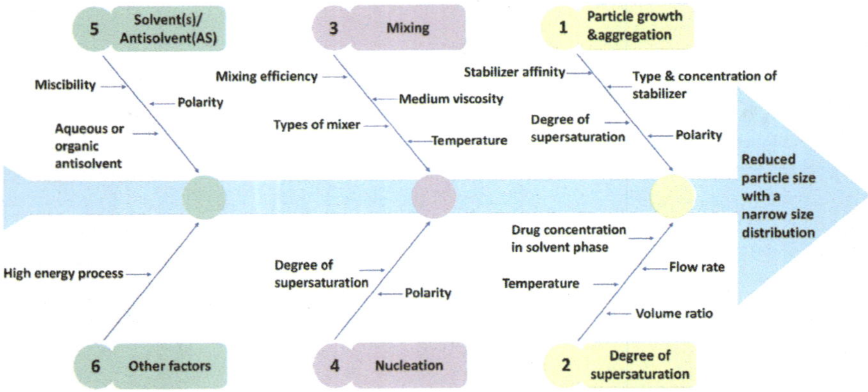

Fig. 12 Interdependent factors influencing the quality attributes of the precipitation process in nanoparticle synthesis, adopted from (Sinha et al. 2013)

and growth process, it needs to be mentioned that besides solubility, the precipitation can also be introduced with other environmental parameters, e.g., temperature and pH. Based on the diagram summarized by Sinha et al. (2013) (reproduced in Fig. 12), the precipitation process was influenced by many factors, in microfluidic approaches have more control over these factors. For instance, the micromixers can precisely control the mixing efficiency, supersaturation, concentration of the reagent and stabilizer, and flow rate to achieve the desired production of nanoparticles.

Based on different mixing mechanisms to introduce smooth and rapid nanoprecipitation in the microfluidic devices to form nanoparticles in biological and medical fields, we can classify the microfluidic devices into single-phase and multiple-phase, and we will introduce these two types of microfluidic devices in this and next section.

The single-phase device is the most frequently used approach for nanoparticle synthesis with the microfluidic technique (based on bottom-up approach). Based on the current publications on nanoparticle synthesis with microfluidic approach, three types of nanoparticles, polymer-based, lipid-based, and inorganic nanoparticles can all be synthesized with the single-phase microfluidic devices.

The illustration of the single-phase mixer (for LNP synthesis) is shown in Fig. 13a. The mixing (finally induced nanoprecipitation) occurs at the interface between the fluid streams. These streams, usually 2–3 streams, are all aqueous based, thus, this system setup belongs to the "single-phase" microfluidic device. Due to the small scale of the microchannels, the fluid streams have very low Reynolds number (Battat et al. 2022) (decided based on size of the channel, fluid viscosity, and flow rate), these streams will flow in parallel without turbulence (Lee et al. 2016), thus, the only mixing mechanism is the diffusion. The diffusion speed only depends on the diffusion coefficient of the molecules, and usually takes a long channel for the homogeneous mixing of the fluid streams. The numerical simulation for the fluid mixing with different Reynolds numbers (controlled by various flow rates is shown in Fig. 13b (Wang et al. 2012).

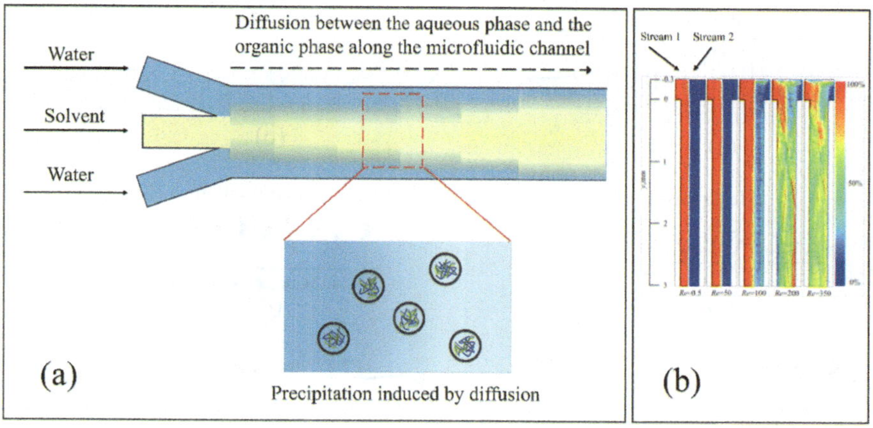

Fig. 13 Illustration of the single-phase mixer. (**a**): Illustration for working principle of diffusion mixer for LNP synthesis; (**b**): Numerical simulation conducted with COMSOL Multiphysics software for mixing of two aqueous streams (Wang et al. 2012)

Due to the slow diffusion mixing rate in the microfluidic devices, conventional single-phase microfluidic devices have a long and straight channel for mixing, which lowers the efficiency of the nanoparticle synthesis. To overcome this issue, researchers used three approaches to enhance the mixing: use hydrodynamic focusing to reduce the diffusion length of the mixing (as shown in Fig. 15a); the second approach is passive mixing with either a complex geometry to twist the flow (Ansari et al. 2018; Lee et al. 2023) (herringbone mixer, as shown in Fig. 14d) or specially designed microstructures inside the microchannel split and recombine the stream (Zhang et al. 2019a; Chen et al. 2019) (e.g., Tesla mixer, as shown in Fig. 14b); the third approach is the active mixing, external pressure (Zhang et al. 2019b), magnetic (Broeren et al. 2023) (as shown in Fig. 14g), acoustic field (Giraldo et al. 2021) (as shown in Fig. 14e), electric field (Wang et al. 2023b), vibration (as shown in Fig. 14f) or even thermal field (Tan 2019) was used to enhance the mixing of the flow.

Figure 15 shows some of the typical single-phase microfluidic devices for nanoparticle synthesis, Fig. 15a shows a PMMA-based hydrodynamic flow-focusing device for alginate-chitosan nanoparticle synthesis (Zamani et al. 2023), Fig. 15b shows a three-player PMMA-based microfluidic for liposomes synthesis (Aranguren et al. 2020), Fig. 15c shows a microfluidic flow-focusing device with rolled up channel ("origami") configuration to enhance the mixing process (Aranguren et al. 2020), Fig. 15d shows a 3D-printed high-throughput lipid nanoparticle synthesis device with four herringbone microchannel to enhance the mixing (Bokare et al. 2019).

Single-phase mixer for nanoparticle synthesis is the most commonly used approach and has proven to be effective and highly controllable in the nanoparticle synthesis process. Passive or active mixing mechanisms can be used to enhance the mixing in the microchannel. Table 3 listed some of the typical approaches for nanoparticle synthesis with single-phase microfluidic mixers. As shown in Table 3, single-phase mixers have been widely used in the synthesis of polymer nanoparticles

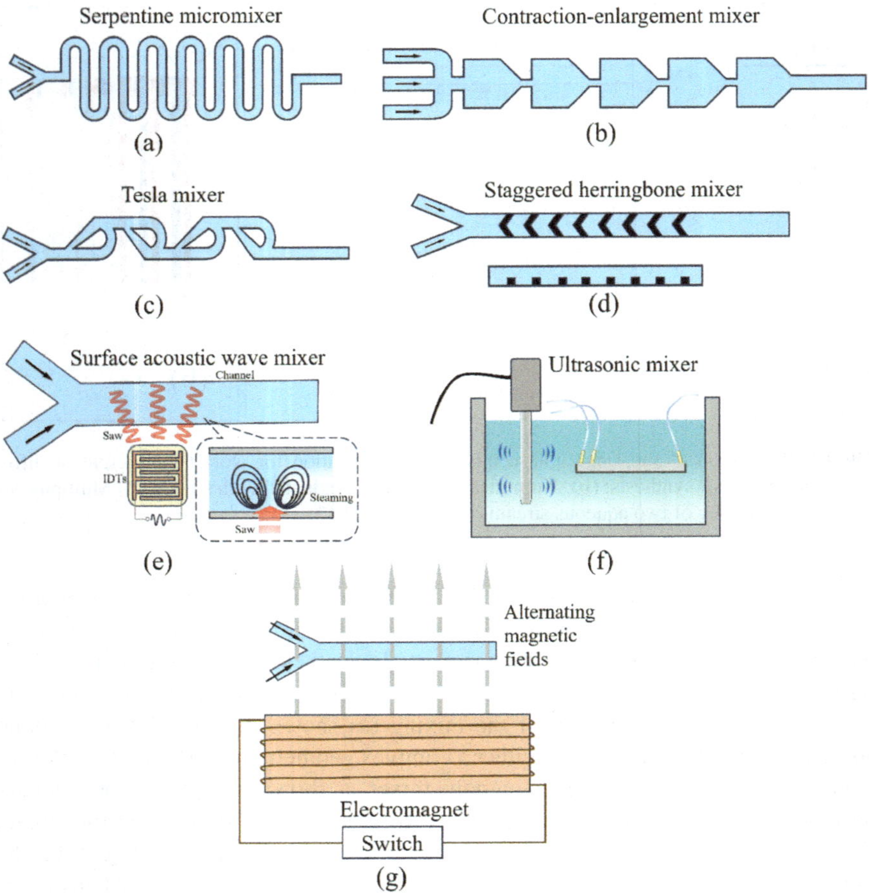

Fig. 14 Illustration of the passive and active mixer (**a**): Serpentine mixer, with elongated microchannel to achieve mixing; (**b**): Contraction-enlargement mixer to enhance the passive mixing; (**c**): Tesla mixer; (**d**): Staggered herringbone mixer, with herringbone structure to cause the chaotic mixing; (**e**): Active mixer, use surface acoustic wave to enhance the mixing at the targeted point; (**f**): Ultrasonic mixer, with external ultrasonic head to induce the active mixing; (**g**): Y-shape microfluidic mixer with alternating magnetic field to enhance the mixing (fluid inside the microchannel is either magnetic fluid or contains magnetic bead)

(usually PLGA-related) and liposomes. On the other hand, PDMS is the most used bulk material of the sing-phase mixer due to easy processing.

Single-phase mixer for nanoparticle synthesis is mainly trapped by the mixing efficiency, thus, various methods have been invented to enhance the mixing efficiency, the passive approach uses the physical structure of the microchannel to enhance the mixing, and the active approach uses the external electrical, thermal, or acoustic field to enhance the mixing (illustrated in Fig. 14). In the microfluidics field, droplet microfluidic which involves the formation of droplets under two phases (typically

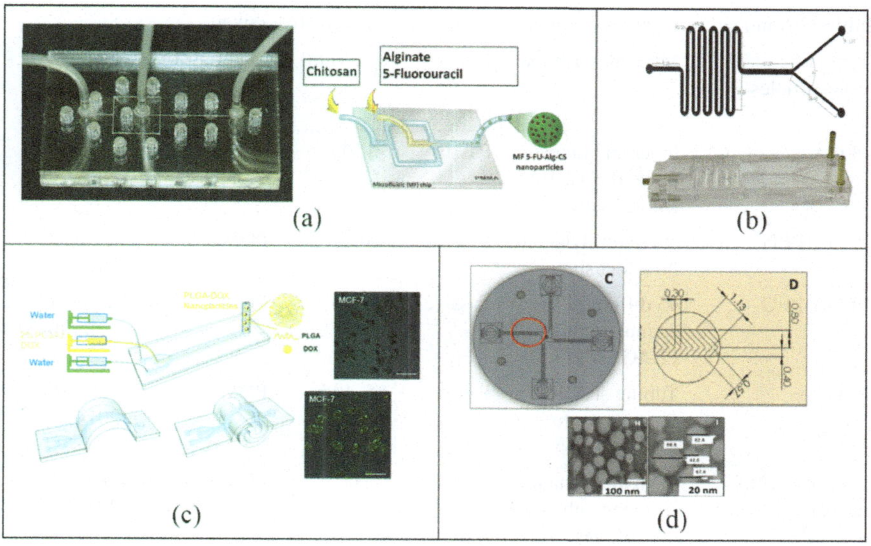

Fig. 15 Various single-phase mixers used for nanoparticle synthesis for biological applications. (**a**) PMMA-based microfluidic device for alginate-chitosan nanoparticle (Zamani et al. 2023); (**b**) three-layer PMMA-based low-cost microfluidic device for liposomes synthesis (Aranguren et al. 2020); (**c**) origami microfluidic chip for synthesizing monodisperse DOX-loaded PLGA nanoparticles (Sun et al. 2013); (**d**) herringbone-patterned 3D-printed devices for lipid nanoparticle synthesis (Bokare et al. 2019)

oil and water-based), has been widely used for the encapsulation of cells (Jiang et al. 2023) and DNA (Hepokoski et al. 2022) for detection or forming micro-scale particles (Baah and Floyd-Smith 2014). Inspired by the droplet microfluidics technique, researchers started to use multi-phase microfluidic devices for the synthesis of nanoparticles for enhanced mixing and process control, which will be introduced in the next section.

3.3 *Multiple-Phase Synthesis of Nanoparticles with Microfluidic Approach*

Multiple-phase microfluidic devices for the synthesis of nanoparticles refer to microfluidic devices with two or more immiscible phases (e.g., aqueous phase, oil phase, and gas) to form droplets (segmented flow) inside the microchannel. The nanoparticles are usually synthesis in the droplets, the physical restriction of the channel wall and the interfacial tension significantly enhanced the mixing inside the droplet to synthesis the nanoparticle with precise control on the size and generation frequency of the droplet (as illustrated in Fig. 16).

Table 3 Nanoparticle synthesized with single-phase passive/active mixer

Types of nanoparticles	Mixer description	Passive/ active mixing	Size (nm)	Materials of the chip	Refs.
PLGA	Inner and outer fluids form a 3D coaxial flow	Passive	~150	Glass capillaries	Liu et al. (2015)
PLGA-PEG	3D hydrodynamic flow focusing	Passive	13–150	PDMS	Lim et al. (2014b)
PLGA-PEG	45 different formulations of PLAGA-PEG	Passive	25–30	PDMS	Valencia et al. (2013)
PLGA	Tubing sustain pressure up to 4.5 MPa	Passive	55–135	PDMS	Wang et al. (2014)
Polymer–DNA nanocomplexes	3D hydrodynamic focusing enhanced by external acoustic	Active	263	PDMS	Lu et al. (2014)
Liposomes	Ultrasound significantly reduced the size of the liposomes	Active	60–190	Glass	Huang et al. (2010)
Lipid nanoparticles	Achieved 50% target gene silencing in hepatocytes in mice	Passive	70	PDMS	Belliveau et al. (2012)
Lipid-PLGA hybrid nanoparticle	Core-shell lipid-PLGA nanoparticle with tunable size	Passive	60–90	PDMS	Feng et al. (2015)
PLGA–DOX nanoparticles	A microfluidic origami chip to synthesize nanoparticle	Passive	100–234	PDMS	Sun et al. (2013)
Lipid nanoparticle	Herringbone structures induce chaotic advection	Passive	20–80	PDMS	Zhigaltsev et al. (2012)
Alginate-chitosan nanoparticle	Alg-CS polyelectrolyte complexes synthesized with flow-focusing method	Passive	~115	PMMA	Zamani et al. (2023)

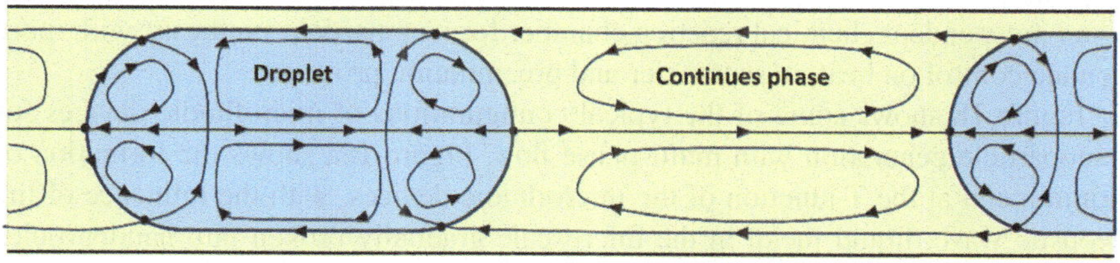

Fig. 16 Flow recirculation in the droplet and continues phase, adopted from (Hodges et al. 2004)

With the development of droplet generators, various configurations of the microfluidic devices have been used for the generation of the droplet in nanoparticle synthesis, as shown in Fig. 17, the droplet can be generated in the cross-flow (T-junction) droplet generator (as shown in Fig. 17a–e), co-flow droplet generator (shown in Fig. 17f and g) or flow-focusing (shown in Fig. 17h) droplet generator. The size and generation speed of the droplet depends on many factors including viscosity of the continue and disperse phase, flow rate of each phase, channel structure, and wettability of the channel surface (Zhu and Wang 2017).

There are several combinations of the continues and disperse (segment) phase for the synthesis of nanoparticles, as listed in Table 4. Two most frequently used combinations are: aqueous phase as disperse phase and oil as continues phase; gas as disperse phase and liquid as continues phase (form slug inside the channel). Gas as a disperse phase is more commonly used due to the easier operation in the experimental process, gas can be pumped inside the microfluidic device either with a syringe pump or pressure pump. For multiple-phase droplet generators, each droplet acts

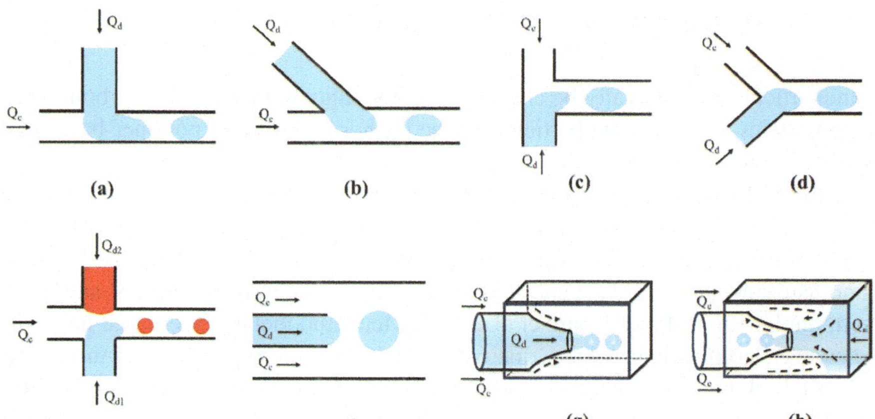

Fig. 17 Illustration of the two or multiple-phase microfluidic devices for nanoparticle synthesis. (**a–d**) Illustration of two-phase T-junction type droplet generation microfluidic device; (**e**) three phases T-junction type droplet generator; (**f, g**) two-phase co-flow droplet generator; (**h**) three-phase flow-focusing droplet generator

as an independent chemical reaction chamber for nanoparticle synthesis, with more actuate control on heat/mass transfer and precipitation process.

Figure 18 shows some of the typical configurations of microfluidic devices for nanoparticle generation with multi-phase flow. Figure 18a shows the formation of liquid metal at the T-junction of the microfluidic devices, with the influence of the acoustic wave, liquid metal in the microscale gradually broken into nanoparticles when propagating long the microchannel (Tang et al. 2018). Figure 18b shows a PDMS-based droplet generator for the synthesis of magnetic nanoparticles (Zou et al. 2022). Figure 18c shows the co-flow droplet generator for the generation of chitosan (CS) or graphene quantum dots (GQD) nanoparticles (Mohebichamkhorami et al. 2023). Figure 18d shows a glass capillary-based flow-focusing microfluidic device for the synthesis of gold nanoparticles (Bandulasena et al. 2019).

Table 4 lists the typical multi-phase microfluidic devices for the synthesis of nanoparticles. Since most of the current study is still at the initial stage in the laboratory, most of the multi-phase microfluidic devices were made with the soft-lithography approach. Different from single-phase microfluidic devices, multiple-phase devices were mainly used for the synthesis of metal, metal oxide, or magnetic nanoparticles.

Multi-phase microfluidic approaches for nanoparticle synthesis are effective methods for the synthesis of inorganic nanoparticles, the precise control of the nano-precipitation process can be conducted inside the droplet: particle size, generation speed, and composition of droplet can be manipulated with the microfluidic devices.

3.4 Types of Nanoparticle Synthesis with Microfluidics for Biological and Medical Applications

Nanoparticles can generally be classified into organic, inorganic, and carbon-based nanoparticles. Organic nanoparticles can be further divided into polymer-based and lipid-based nanoparticles.

Table 5 lists some of the most used types of nanoparticles in biological and medical fields. For the carbon-based nanoparticle, carbon dots can be used in analytical sensor and bioimaging devices (Wang and Qiu 2016); Graphene and graphene oxide-based nanomaterials can be used in gene delivery, cancer treatment, drug delivery, and bone/teeth implantation (Priyadarsini et al. 2018). Metal and metal oxide-based nanoparticles, e.g., gold, cobalt, silver, zinc oxide, and iron oxide, can be used in various fields in biological and medical fields, including, drug delivery, biosensing, antimicrobial, wound healing, and biotoxicity (Nikolova and Chavali 2020; Yadavalli and Shukla 2017). Polymer (e.g., PLA, PLGA, PCL) nanoparticles have been used for drug delivery (Jiaying et al. 2023), tissue regeneration (Martins et al. 2018), and immunotherapy (Li et al. 2024). Chitosan nanoparticle was reported for applications in nanomedicine for drug delivery (Khalaf et al. 2023). Solid liposome nanoparticle is usually used as the carrier for drug delivery (Xu et al. 2022; Hou et al. 2021).

Table 4 Nanoparticle synthesized with multi-phase microfluidic mixer

Types of nanoparticles	Description	Segment/continues phase	Size (nm)	Materials of the chip	Refs.
Silica	Fluorescent silicon alkoxide precursor solution used for synthesis	Alkoxide/fluorine oil	50–350	PDMS	Wacker et al. (2012)
Silver nanoparticles	Synthesized by the reduction of metal salt solutions	$AgNO_3$ solution and $NaBH_4$/mineral oil	~5	PDMS	Xu et al. (2016a)
Gold nanoparticles	Branched gold NPs synthesized in a microfluidics	Metal salt/HFE-7500	~80	PDMS	Abalde-Cela et al. (2018)
Gold and silver nanoparticles	Gold and silver nanoparticles synthesized simultaneously	Ionic liquid/halocarbon	~4	PDMS	Sebastian Cabeza et al. (2012)
Gold nanoparticles	Mixing-reaction conditions precisely tuned	Air, silicone oil toluene/ionic liquid	3–5	Silicon	Sebastian Cabeza et al. (2012)
Silver nanoparticles	FDM-based 3D-printed microfluidic system	$AgNO_3$ solution and $NaBH_4$/mineral oil	7–8	PLA	Bressan et al. (2019)
Silver nanoparticle–chitosan composite	Synthesized with a low-cost laser ablated device	Chitosan, $AgNO_3$/oil	~300 μm	PMMA	Yang et al. (2016)
Liquid metal	Stealthy liquid metal nanoparticles formed with acoustic wave	Liquid metal/bPEG solution	250–400	PDMS	Tang et al. (2018)
Fe_3O_4nanoparticle	Controlled synthesis of magnetic nanoparticles in droplet	Ferric salts/oil	20–30	PDMS	Zou et al. (2022)
Quantum dots	Chitosan or graphene quantum dots are synthesized as drug carriers	Quantum dots/ tripolyphosphate	10–20	PDMS	Mohebichamkhorami et al. (2023)

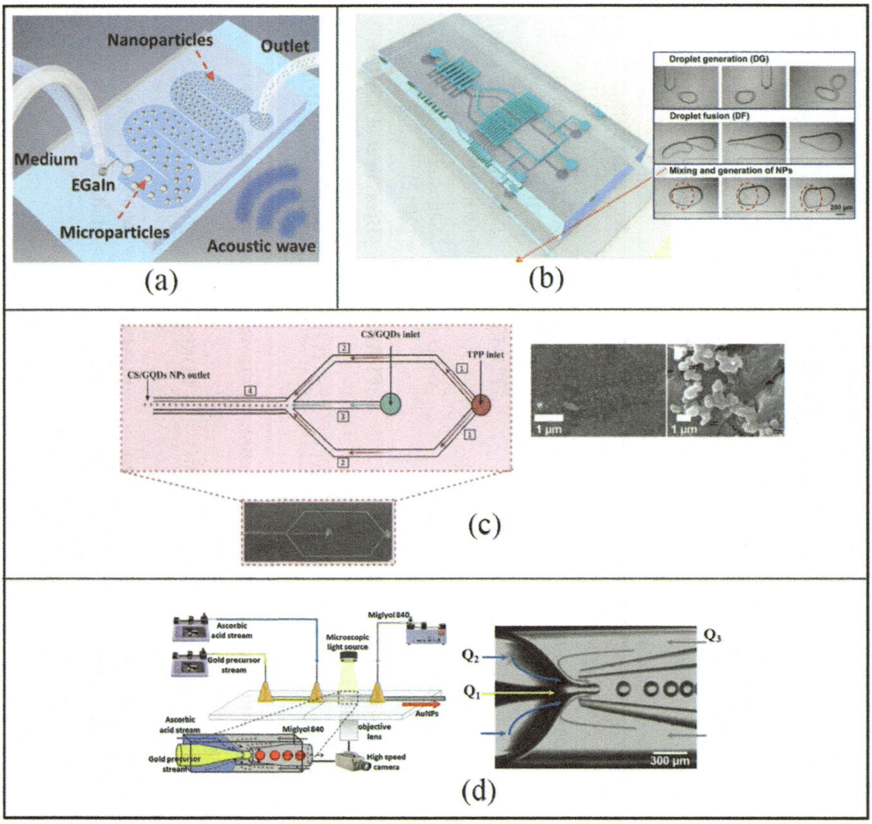

Fig. 18 Multiple-phase microfluidics for the synthesis of nanoparticles. (**a**): Liquid metal micro-droplets are formed at the T-junction with the presence of acoustic waves (Tang et al. 2018); (**b**): PDMS-based microfluidics for magnetic nanoparticle synthesis (Zou et al. 2022); (**c**): Two inlets for CS or GQD and tripolyphosphate solution and one outlet for CS/GQD nanoparticles (Mohebichamkhorami et al. 2023); (**d**): Glass capillaries-based microfluidics devices for gold nanoparticles synthesis (Bandulasena et al. 2019)

3.5 Scaling up the Synthesis of Nanoparticles

Microfluidics has many advantages in the synthesis of nanoparticles, as discussed in the previous sections. However, several drawbacks may hinder the further development of microfluidics' application in nanoparticle synthesis. Clogging may happen due to the small dimension of the microchannels to jam the channel. The biggest challenge, also brought by the scaling effect of the microchannel, is that the throughput (production rate) is very low, compared with the conventional synthesis methods. The current nanoparticle synthesis approach with microfluidic is unsuitable for industrial production. In recent decades, various approaches have been invented for scaling

Table 5 Types of nanoparticle synthesis with microfluidic devices

Classification	Nanoparticles	Application direction in biological and medical fields	Type of mixing	Refs.
Carbon-based	Carbon fiber	Good biocompatibility, porous scaffolds support cell adhesion or use as electrodes	Passive, flow focusing	Hu et al. (2019)
Carbon-based	Carbon dots	Used for targeted drug delivery, or carrier for gene therapy	Passive, precipitation	Shao et al. (2019)
Carbon-based	Graphene oxide exfoliation	Used for drug delivery and controlled release, and molecular detection	Passive, droplet mixing	Qiu et al. (2020)
Inorganic-metal	Gold	Used for bioimaging, biosensors and drug delivery	Passive, flow focusing	Lazarus et al. (2010)
Inorganic-metal	Silver	Used in antibacterial, antifungal and cancer therapy	Passive, droplet mixing	Xu et al. (2016b)
Inorganic-metal	Zinc oxide	Used in biosensors, antimicrobial and drug delivery.	Passive, single-phase mixing with obstacle	Popa et al. (2023)
Inorganic-metal	Iron oxide	Enhancing magnetic resonance imaging, also used in tissue emerging	Passive, droplet mixing	James et al. (2020)
Inorganic-metal	Cobalt	Antimicrobial, antioxidant, antifungal, and enzyme inhibition	Passive, single-phase mixing	Yang et al. (2020)
Organic-polymer	PLGA	Used for drug encapsulation, delivery and cancer therapy	Passive	Varani et al. (2021)
Organic-polymer	PLA	Immunoregulation, packaging	Passive, single-phase, flow focusing	Heshmatnezhad and Nazar (2020)

(continued)

Table 5 (continued)

Classification	Nanoparticles	Application direction in biological and medical fields	Type of mixing	Refs.
Organic-polymer	PCL	Cancer therapy, wound treatment, antibacterial study	Passive, single-phase, flow focusing	Heshmatnezhad et al. (2021)
Organic-polymer	Chitosan	Drug deliver, anticancer drugs	Active	Chai et al. (2021)
Organic-polymer	Alginate	Delivery of drugs and chemotherapies, tissue reparation and regeneration	Passive, droplet mixing	Singh et al. (2020)
Organic-lipid-based	Therapeutic liposomes	Deliver drugs for cancer, infections, or chronic diseases	Passive, droplet mixing	Gkionis et al. (2021)
Organic-lipid-based	Diagnostic liposomes	Imaging agents for applications in MRI, CT, or fluorescence imaging	Passive, single phase	Lv et al. (2021)
Organic-lipid-based	Vaccine liposomes	Deliver antigens and enhance immune responses	Passive, single phase	Xiu et al. (2024)
Organic-lipid-based	Cosmetic liposomes	Delivering active ingredients like vitamins or moisturizers	Passive, single phase	Bochicchio et al. (2020)

up the throughput of microfluidic devices, which may also be used in nanoparticle synthesis.

To increase the throughput of microfluidic devices for nanoparticle synthesis, the most practical approach is increasing the quantity of mixers in one microfluidic device. Several dozen or even hundreds of mixers can be arranged on one microfluidic device and work in parallel for the synthesis of nanoparticles. As shown in Fig. 19a, three-layer PDMS-based microfluidic devices were designed and fabricated for the parallel generation of MPEG-PLGA nanoparticles with a single-flow flow-focusing approach (Kang et al. 2013). Dozens of flow-focusing mixers work in parallel to significantly increase the throughput of the nanoparticle synthesis. A similar configuration can also be found in Fig. 19b, multi-layer PDMS microfluidic devices were used for the synthesis of PLGA-PEG nanoparticles (Lim et al. 2014a). Ladder-like microfluidic devices were also fabricated as shown in Fig. 19c for the synthesis of LNPs, herringbone structures were embedded in the microchannels to enhance the mixing (Shepherd et al. 2021b).

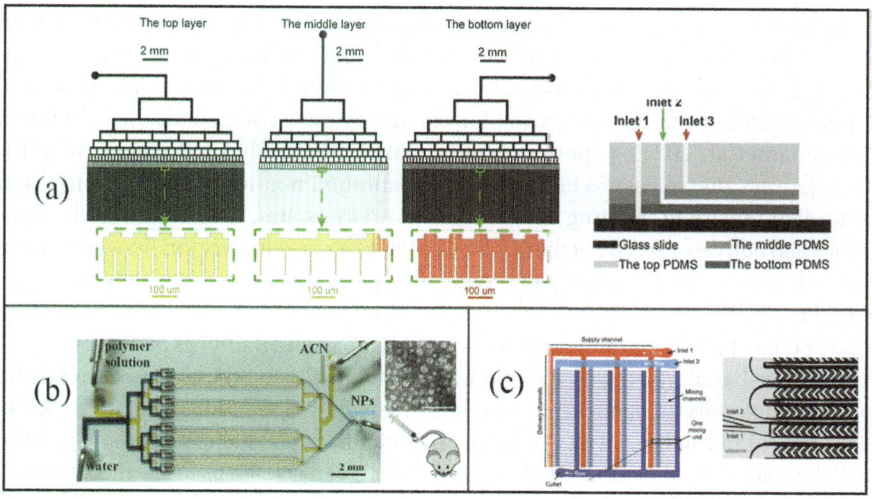

Fig. 19 Parallel microfluidic devices used to enhance the throughput of the microfluidic devices. (**a**) Three-layer PDMS-based microfluidic device with parallel flow-focusing microchannels for MPEG–PLGA nanoparticles synthesis (Kang et al. 2013). (**b**) 3D flow-focusing device for PLGA-PEG nanoparticles synthesis (Lim et al. 2014a); (**c**) Parallelized microfluidic device with herringbone micromixers for LNP synthesis (Shepherd et al. 2021b)

However, in scaling up the production rate of nanoparticles with a microfluidics approach, parallel seems to have the following limitations: Firstly, the quantity of the integrated mixers has limitations, unlike the transistors in the IC industry, the dimension of the microchannel significantly influences the working patterns of the microfluidic devices, more mixers makes the microfluidic devices bigger and impractical for operation; Secondly, flow control in parallel microchannels, both in synthesis of nanoparticles and other applications, is always challenging, to ensure the homogeneous liquid supply to large quantity of microchannels is not yet fully realized by researchers. Thus, the future changes of the scaling up the throughput of the microfluidics method for nanoparticle synthesis is to find a robust and preferable, low-cost microfluidic configuration and fluid control algorithm, the possible solution may include but not limited to a parallel microchannel approach and using AI to assist the flow control.

4 Application of Nanoparticles in Biological and Medical Fields

This section will briefly introduce the application of nanoparticles synthesized with microfluidics approaches in the biological and medical fields.

Lipid-based nanoparticles. Lipid-based nanoparticles can be synthesized with various microfluidic devices, usually with the single-phase approach (Shan et al. 2023). Lipid nanoparticles can be divided into solid nanoparticles and liposomes. Liposomes are sphere vesicles with bilayers, liposomes exist naturally, e.g., in blood (Glassman et al. 2021). Liposomes are the most frequently used nanoparticle for drug delivery due to easy synthesis, biocompatibility, non-toxic, drug stability, and controlled release in the drug delivery process. Drugs are capsuled inside the liposomes and delivery directly at the targeted point, as a non-viral vector, liposomes have been widely used in the delivery of protein into the cytoplasm of cells. Polymer (typically PEG) was used for the modification of the liposomes to elongate the circulating time and has been used in the treatment of breast cancer (Badivi et al. 2024).

Polymer-based nanoparticles. Some of the most commonly used synthetic polymer materials for nanoparticle synthesis including PLGA, PLA, and PCL (Mulla et al. 1967; Łukasiewicz et al. 2021), and natural materials, such as chitosan, gelatin, and alginate (Aibani et al. 2021; Feng et al. 2020) can also be used for the synthesis of nanoparticles. Most of the current microfluidics approaches for the synthesis of polymer nanoparticles use a PDMS-based microfluidic approach with a single-phase approach. Polymer nanoparticles have been successfully used in cancer treatment (Karlsson et al. 2018), with the advantages of drug safety, increased drug permeability in tissue/cell, and controlled release, various clinical trials have been conducted worldwide (Namiot et al. 2023; Zheng et al. 2021).

Inorganic nanoparticles, including metal and metal oxide nanoparticles and carbon-based nanoparticles. Metal nanoparticles, e.g., gold nanoparticles, have intrinsic antibacterial (Aguilar-Garay et al. 2024) and antifungal (Nikhil et al. 2024) properties and can be used to enter tissue and attach immune cells, which is useful in immunotherapy (Hammami et al. 2021). Polymer and gold can also be combined to form gold metallic nanoparticles (AuNPs) and used in cancer imaging and cancer therapy (e.g., chemo-radio therapy, thermo-chemo-therapy) (Wu et al. 2024). Silver nanoparticles also have antimicrobial properties, and were used for enhancing the activity of drugs (Hashem et al. 2024), and used in wearable biosensors (Naysmith et al. 2024). Metal oxide nanoparticles can be used in dentistry wound healing (Farazin et al. 2023) and regenerative medicine (Shineh et al. 2024). Since the cancer cell is more sensitive to heat damage, iron oxide magnetic nanoparticles can target the cancer cell without damaging the regular cells (Hedayatnasab et al. 2023). Zinc oxide nanoparticles are also a good candidate for drug delivery applications with biodegradable properties (Jiang et al. 2018).

5 Conclusion

With the precise control of the synthesis process, the microfluidics technique has been widely used in the synthesis of nanoparticles. Microfluidics usually uses a bottom-up approach, with either single-phase or multiple phases for the precipitation process. Due to the scaling effect, the mixing inside the microfluidics is usually laminar flow, and the mixing needs to be enhanced either passively or actively. Various glass/polymer materials and fabrication methods have been used for the fabrication of microfluidics devices for nanoparticle synthesis. Synthesized nanoparticles have been used in various fields including drug delivery, imaging, immunotherapy, and cancer treatment.

Further development of nanoparticle synthesis with the microfluidic approach is mainly restricted to the production efficiency of the microfluidics approach. Due to the small scale of the microfluidic devices, it seems the only practical way is parallelization: hundreds or even thousands of microfluidic devices working in parallel to promote the yield of nanoparticle production. However, the precise control of the microfluidic devices working in parallel is very challenging, AI may help with the feedback control of the nanoparticle synthesis processes.

Some other future development areas on nanoparticle synthesis with a microfluidics approach include: functional nanoparticles for targeted drug delivery, green synthesis of nanoparticle with microfluidics method, personalized medicine/vaccine, and advanced quality control of synthesis process.

Acknowledgement This study was supported by the 2025 Autonomous Research Program of Nanjin University of Science and Technology (30925010534).

References

S. Abalde-Cela, P. Taladriz-Blanco, M.G. de Oliveira, C. Abell, Droplet microfluidics for the highly controlled synthesis of branched gold nanoparticles. Sci. Rep. **8**(1), 2440 (2018). https://doi.org/10.1038/s41598-018-20754-x

M.H. Abdel-Aziz, M.S. Zoromba, M. Bassyouni, M. Zwawi, A.A. Alshehri, A.F. Al-Hossainy, Synthesis and characterization of Co-Al mixed oxide nanoparticles via thermal decomposition route of layered double hydroxide, (in English). J. Mol. Struct. **1206**, 127679 (2020). https://doi.org/10.1016/j.molstruc.2020.127679

R. Abedini-Nassab, M. Pouryosef Miandoab, M. Sasmaz, Microfluidic synthesis, control, and sensing of magnetic nanoparticles: a review. Micromachines (Basel) **12**(7), 768 (2021). https://doi.org/10.3390/mi12070768

A. Abou Hassan, O. Sandre, V. Cabuil, P. Tabeling, Synthesis of iron oxide nanoparticles in a microfluidic device: preliminary results in a coaxial flow millichannel. Chem. Commun. (Camb.) **15**, 1783–1785 (2008). https://doi.org/10.1039/b719550h

R. Aguilar-Garay et al., A comprehensive review of silver and gold nanoparticles as effective antibacterial agents, (in English). Pharmaceuticals **17**(9), 1134 (2024). https://doi.org/10.3390/ph17091134

N. Aibani, R. Rai, P. Patel, G. Cuddihy, E.K. Wasan, Chitosan nanoparticles at the biological Interface: implications for drug delivery, (in English). Pharmaceutics **13**(10), 1686 (2021). https://doi.org/10.3390/pharmaceutics13101686

A. Al-Ali, W. Waheed, F. Dawaymeh, N. Alamoodi, A. Alazzam, A surface treatment method for improving the attachment of PDMS: acoustofluidics as a case study. Sci. Rep. **13**(1), 18141 (2023)

M.E. Ali, M. Ullah, A. Maamor, S.B. Abd Hamid, Surfactant assisted ball milling: a simple top down approach for the synthesis of controlled structure nanoparticle, (in English). Nanosci.,

Nanotechnol. Nanoeng. **832**, 356–361 (2014). https://doi.org/10.4028/www.scientific.net/AMR.832.356

M.A. Ansari, K.Y. Kim, S.M. Kim, Numerical and experimental study on mixing performances of simple and vortex micro T-mixers. Micromachines (Basel) **9**(5), 204 (2018). https://doi.org/10.3390/mi9050204

A. Aranguren, C.E. Torres, C. Munoz-Camargo, J.F. Osma, J.C. Cruz, Synthesis of nanoscale liposomes via low-cost microfluidic systems. Micromachines (Basel) **11**(12), 1050 (2020). https://doi.org/10.3390/mi11121050

S. Arya et al., Review-influence of processing parameters to control morphology and optical properties of sol-gel synthesized ZnO nanoparticles, (in English). ECS J. Solid State Sci. Technol. **10**(2), 023002 (2021). https://doi.org/10.1149/2162-8777/abe095

A.K. Au, W. Huynh, L.F. Horowitz, A. Folch, 3D-printed microfluidics. Angew. Chem. Int. Ed. **55**(12), 3862–3881 (2016)

D. Baah, T. Floyd-Smith, Microfluidics for particle synthesis from photocrosslinkable materials, (in English). Microfluid. Nanofluid. **17**(3), 431–455 (2014). https://doi.org/10.1007/s10404-014-1333-y

S. Badivi et al., Targeted delivery of bee venom to A549 lung cancer cells by PEGylate liposomal formulation: an apoptotic investigation. Sci. Rep. **14**(1), 17302 (2024). https://doi.org/10.1038/s41598-024-68156-6

A. Balachandran, S.P. Sreenilayam, K. Madanan, S. Thomas, D. Brabazon, Nanoparticle production via laser ablation synthesis in solution method and printed electronic application-a brief review. Results Eng. **16**, 100646 (2022)

M.V. Bandulasena, G.T. Vladisavljevic, B. Benyahia, Droplet-based microfluidic method for robust preparation of gold nanoparticles in axisymmetric flow focusing device, (in English). Chem. Eng. Sci. **195**, 657–664 (2019). https://doi.org/10.1016/j.ces.2018.10.010

S. Battat, D.A. Weitz, G.M. Whitesides, Nonlinear phenomena in microfluidics. Chem. Rev. **122**(7), 6921–6937 (2022). https://doi.org/10.1021/acs.chemrev.1c00985

A. Behl, V.S. Parmar, S. Malhotra, A.K. Chhillar, Biodegradable diblock copolymeric PEG-PCL nanoparticles: synthesis, characterization and applications as anticancer drug delivery agents, (in English). Polymer **207**, 122901 (2020). https://doi.org/10.1016/j.polymer.2020.122901

E. Behroodi, H. Latifi, Z. Bagheri, E. Ermis, S. Roshani, M. Salehi Moghaddam, A combined 3D printing/CNC micro-milling method to fabricate a large-scale microfluidic device with the small size 3D architectures: an application for tumor spheroid production. Sci. Rep. **10**(1), 22171 (2020). https://doi.org/10.1038/s41598-020-79015-5

N.M. Belliveau et al., Microfluidic synthesis of highly potent limit-size lipid nanoparticles for in vivo delivery of siRNA. Mol. Ther. Nucleic. Acids **1**(8), e37 (2012). https://doi.org/10.1038/mtna.2012.28

A. Benhammada, D. Trache, M. Kesraoui, A.F. Tarchoun, S. Chelouche, A. Mezroua, Synthesis and characterization of α-Fe2O3 nanoparticles from different precursors and their catalytic effect on the thermal decomposition of nitrocellulose. Thermochim. Acta **686**, 178570 (2020)

M.O. Besenhard et al., Co-precipitation synthesis of stable iron oxide nanoparticles with NaOH: new insights and continuous production via flow chemistry, (in English). Chem. Eng. J. **399**, 125740 (2020). https://doi.org/10.1016/j.cej.2020.125740

N. Bhattacharjee, A. Urrios, S. Kang, A. Folch, The upcoming 3D-printing revolution in microfluidics. Lab Chip **16**(10), 1720–1742 (2016). https://doi.org/10.1039/c6lc00163g

S. Bochicchio, A. Dalmoro, V. De Simone, P. Bertoncin, G. Lamberti, and A. A. Barba,Simil-microfluidic nanotechnology in manufacturing of liposomes as hydrophobic antioxidants skin release systems. Cosmetics 7(2), 22 (2020). [Online]. Available: https://www.mdpi.com/2079-9284/7/2/22

A. Bokare et al., Herringbone-patterned 3D-printed devices as alternatives to microfluidics for reproducible production of lipid polymer hybrid nanoparticles. ACS Omega **4**(3), 4650–4657 (2019). https://doi.org/10.1021/acsomega.9b00128

F. Branda et al., Structure and bottom-up formation mechanism of multisheet silica-based nanoparticles formed in an epoxy matrix through an *In Situ* process, (in English). Langmuir **37**(29), 8886–8893 (2021). https://doi.org/10.1021/acs.langmuir.1c01363

L.P. Bressan et al., 3D-printed microfluidic device for the synthesis of silver and gold nanoparticles, (in English). Microchem. J. **146**, 1083–1089 (2019). https://doi.org/10.1016/j.microc.2019.02.043

L.P. Bressan, T.M. Lima, G.D. da Silveira, J.A. da Silva, Low-cost and simple FDM-based 3D-printed microfluidic device for the synthesis of metallic core–shell nanoparticles. SN Appl. Sci. **2**(5), 984 (2020)

A. Brockmeier, F.J.S. Rodriguez, M. Harrison, U. Hilleringmann, Surface tension and its role for vertical wet etching of silicon, (in English). J. Micromech. Microeng. **22**(12), 125012 (2012). https://doi.org/10.1088/0960-1317/22/12/125012

S. Broeren, I.F. Pereira, T. Wang, J. den Toonder, Y. Wang, On-demand microfluidic mixing by actuating integrated magnetic microwalls. Lab Chip **23**(6), 1524–1530 (2023). https://doi.org/10.1039/d2lc01168a

J.C. Cai et al., Rapid prototyping of cyclic olefin copolymer based microfluidic system with CO laser ablation, (in English). Microsyst. Technol. Micro Nanosyst. -Inf. Storage Process. Syst. **23**(10), 5063–5069 (2017). https://doi.org/10.1007/s00542-017-3282-3

B. Cetin, M.D. Asik, S. Taze, Design and fabrication of a microfluidic device for synthesis of chitosan nanoparticles. J. Nanotechnol. Eng. **4**(3), 031004 (2013)

Y. Chai, Y. Wang, B. Li, W. Qi, R. Su, Z. He, Microfluidic synthesis of lignin/chitosan nanoparticles for the pH-responsive delivery of anticancer drugs. Langmuir **37**(23), 7219–7226 (2021). https://doi.org/10.1021/acs.langmuir.1c00778

V. Chandrakala, V. Aruna, G. Angajala, Review on metal nanoparticles as nanocarriers: current challenges and perspectives in drug delivery systems. Emerg. Mater. **5**(6), 1593–1615 (2022)

P.C. Chen, C.C. Chou, C.H. Chiang, Systematically studying dissolution process of 3D printed acrylonitrile butadiene styrene (ABS) mold for creation of complex and fully transparent polydimethylsiloxane (PDMS) fluidic devices, (in English). Biochip J. **15**(2), 144–151 (2021). https://doi.org/10.1007/s13206-021-00009-0

X.Y. Chen, S. Zhang, Z.L. Wu, Y. Zheng, A novel Koch fractal micromixer with rounding corners structure, (in English). Microsyst. Technol. Micro Nanosyst. -Inf. Storage Process. Syst. **25**(7), 2751–2758 (2019). https://doi.org/10.1007/s00542-019-04296-4

Y. Cheng, S.D. Ling, Y.H. Geng, Y.D. Wang, J.H. Xu, Microfluidic synthesis of quantum dots and their applications in bio-sensing and bio-imaging (in English). Nanoscale Adv. **3**(8), 2180–2195 (2021). https://doi.org/10.1039/d0na00933d

N. Chiang et al., Large-scale soft-lithographic patterning of plasmonic nanoparticles. ACS Mater. Lett. **3**(3), 282–289 (2021). https://doi.org/10.1021/acsmaterialslett.0c00535

C.D. Chin, V. Linder, S.K. Sia, Commercialization of microfluidic point-of-care diagnostic devices. Lab Chip **12**(12), 2118–2134 (2012). https://doi.org/10.1039/c2lc21204h

P.F. de Oliveira, R.M. Torresi, F. Emmerling, P.H. Camargo, Challenges and opportunities in the bottom-up mechanochemical synthesis of noble metal nanoparticles. J. Mater. Chem. A **8**(32), 16114–16141 (2020)

S. Dochow et al., Quartz microfluidic chip for tumour cell identification by Raman spectroscopy in combination with optical traps. Anal. Bioanal. Chem. **405**(8), 2743–2746 (2013). https://doi.org/10.1007/s00216-013-6726-3

D.C. Duffy, J.C. McDonald, O.J. Schueller, G.M. Whitesides, Rapid prototyping of microfluidic systems in poly (dimethylsiloxane). Anal. Chem. **70**(23), 4974–4984 (1998). https://doi.org/10.1021/ac980656z

M. Esashi, S. Shoji, A. Nakano, Normally closed microvalve and mircopump fabricated on a silicon wafer. Sensors Actuators **20**(1–2), 163–169 (1989)

Y. Eygeris, M. Gupta, J. Kim, G. Sahay, Chemistry of lipid nanoparticles for RNA delivery. Acc. Chem. Res. **55**(1), 2–12 (2022). https://doi.org/10.1021/acs.accounts.1c00544

P. Falcaro et al., Application of metal and metal oxide nanoparticles@MOFs (in English). Coord. Chem. Rev. **307**, 237–254 (2016). https://doi.org/10.1016/j.ccr.2015.08.002

Y. Fan, Low-cost microfluidics: materials and methods. Micro Nano Lett. **13**(10), 1367–1372 (2018)

Y.Q. Fan, K.X. Gao, J. Chen, W.G. Li, Y.J. Zhang, Low-cost PMMA-based microfluidics for the visualization of enhanced oil recovery, (in English). Oil Gas Sci. Technol.-Rev. d'Ifp Energies Nouvelles **73**, 26 (2018). https://doi.org/10.2516/ogst/2018026

A. Farazin, M. Mohammadimehr, H. Naeimi, Flexible self-healing nanocomposite based gelatin/tannic acid/acrylic acid reinforced with zinc oxide nanoparticles and hollow silver nanoparticles based on porous silica for rapid wound healing. Int. J. Biol. Macromol. **241**, 124572 (2023). https://doi.org/10.1016/j.ijbiomac.2023.124572

Q. Feng et al., Microfluidic based high throughput synthesis of lipid-polymer hybrid nanoparticles with tunable diameters. Biomicrofluidics **9**(5), 052604 (2015). https://doi.org/10.1063/1.4922957

X. Feng et al., Properties of Pickering emulsion stabilized by food-grade gelatin nanoparticles: influence of the nanoparticles concentration. Colloids Surf. B Biointerfaces **196**, 111294 (2020). https://doi.org/10.1016/j.colsurfb.2020.111294

R. Feynman, There's plenty of room at the bottom, in *Feynman and Computation*, (CRC Press, 2018), pp. 63–76

X. Fu, J. Cai, X. Zhang, W.D. Li, H. Ge, Y. Hu, Top-down fabrication of shape-controlled, monodisperse nanoparticles for biomedical applications. Adv. Drug Deliv. Rev. **132**, 169–187 (2018). https://doi.org/10.1016/j.addr.2018.07.006

S.-i. Funano, N. Ota, Y. Tanaka, A simple and reversible glass–glass bonding method to construct a microfluidic device and its application for cell recovery. Lab Chip **21**(11), 2244–2254 (2021)

Y.X. Gan, A.H. Jayatissa, Z. Yu, X. Chen, M.H. Li, Hydrothermal synthesis of nanomaterials, (in English). J. Nanomater. (2020). https://doi.org/10.1155/2020/8917013

K. Gao, J. Liu, Y. Fan, Y. Zhang, Ultra-low-cost fabrication of polymer-based microfluidic devices with diode laser ablation. Biomed. Microdevices **21**(4), 83 (2019). https://doi.org/10.1007/s10544-019-0433-6

J.G. Gardeniers, R. Oosterbroek, A. van den Berg, Silicon and glass micromachining for µTAS, in *Lab on a Chip*, (Elsevier, 2003), pp. 37–64

S. Gavas, S. Quazi, T.M. Karpinski, Nanoparticles for cancer therapy: current progress and challenges. Nanoscale Res. Lett. **16**(1), 173 (2021). https://doi.org/10.1186/s11671-021-03628-6

S. Gimondi, H. Ferreira, R.L. Reis, N.M. Neves, Microfluidic devices: a tool for nanoparticle synthesis and performance evaluation. ACS Nano **17**(15), 14205–14228 (2023). https://doi.org/10.1021/acsnano.3c01117

K.A. Giraldo, J.S. Bermudez, C.E. Torres, L.H. Reyes, J.F. Osma, J.C. Cruz, Microfluidics for multiphase mixing and liposomal encapsulation of nanobioconjugates: passive vs acoustic systems. Fluids **6**(9), 309 (2021)

L. Gkionis, H. Aojula, L.K. Harris, A. Tirella, Microfluidic-assisted fabrication of phosphatidylcholine-based liposomes for controlled drug delivery of chemotherapeutics. Int. J. Pharm. **604**, 120711 (2021). https://doi.org/10.1016/j.ijpharm.2021.120711

P.M. Glassman et al., Red blood cells: The metamorphosis of a neglected carrier into the natural mothership for artificial nanocarriers, (in English). Adv. Drug Deliv. Rev. **178**, 113992 (2021). https://doi.org/10.1016/j.addr.2021.113992

M. Godoy-Gallardo et al., Antibacterial approaches in tissue engineering using metal ions and nanoparticles: from mechanisms to applications. Bioact. Mater. **6**(12), 4470–4490 (2021). https://doi.org/10.1016/j.bioactmat.2021.04.033

P. Gravesen, J. Branebjerg, O.S. Jensen, Microfluidics-a review. J. Micromech. Microeng. **3**(4), 168 (1993)

I. Hammami, N.M. Alabdallah, A. Al Jomaa, M. Kamoun, Gold nanoparticles: synthesis properties and applications, (in English). J. King Saud Univ. Sci. **33**(7), 101560 (2021). https://doi.org/10.1016/j.jksus.2021.101560

M. Hashem, R.A. Sobh, M. Abd El-Ghaffar, pH-responsive bionanocomposite pectin grafted with dimethylaminoethyl methacrylate and acrylic acid copolymer along with silver nanoparticles for breast cancer drug delivery. Polym. Eng. Sci. (2024)

Z. Hedayatnasab, A.R. Saadatabadi, H. Shirgahi, M. Mozafari, Heat induction of iron oxide nanoparticles with rational artificial neural network design-based particle swarm optimization for magnetic cancer hyperthermia. Mater. Res. Bull. **157**, 112035 (2023)

A.K. Henning, Microfluidic mems, in *1998 IEEE Aerospace Conference Proceedings (Cat. No. 98TH8339)*, vol. 1, (IEEE, 1998), pp. 471–486

M.L. Hepokoski et al., Absolute quantification of plasma mitochondrial DNA by droplet digital PCR marks COVID-19 severity over time during intensive care unit admissions. Am. J. Physiol. Lung Cell. Mol. Physiol. **323**(1), L84–L92 (2022). https://doi.org/10.1152/ajplung.00128.2022

B. Herranz-Blanco, E. Ginestar, H. Zhang, J. Hirvonen, H.A. Santos, Microfluidics platform for glass capillaries and its application in droplet and nanoparticle fabrication. Int. J. Pharm. **516**(1–2), 100–105 (2017). https://doi.org/10.1016/j.ijpharm.2016.11.024

F. Heshmatnezhad, A.R.S. Nazar, On-chip controlled synthesis of polycaprolactone nanoparticles using continuous-flow microfluidic devices, (in English). J. Flow Chem. **10**(3), 533–543 (2020). https://doi.org/10.1007/s41981-020-00092-8

F. Heshmatnezhad, A.R.S. Nazar, H. Aghaei, J. Varshosaz, Production of doxorubicin-loaded PCL nanoparticles through a flow-focusing microfluidic device: encapsulation efficacy and drug release, (in English). Soft Matter **17**(47), 10675–10682 (2021). https://doi.org/10.1039/d1sm01070k

S.R. Hodges, O.E. Jensen, J.M. Rallison, The motion of a viscous drop through a cylindrical tube, (in English). J. Fluid Mech. **501**, 279–301 (2004). https://doi.org/10.1017/S0022112003007213

D. Holmannova, P. Borsky, T. Svadlakova, L. Borska, Z. Fiala, Carbon nanoparticles and their biomedical applications, (in English). Appl. Sci.-Basel **12**(15), 7865 (2022). https://doi.org/10.3390/app12157865

S. Hong, D.W. Choi, H.N. Kim, C.G. Park, W. Lee, H.H. Park, Protein-based nanoparticles as drug delivery systems, (in English). Pharmaceutics **12**(7), 604 (2020). https://doi.org/10.3390/pharmaceutics12070604

B. Horstmann et al., Cryogenic DRIE processes for high-precision silicon etching in MEMS applications, (in English). J. Micromech. Microeng. **34**(7) (2024). https://doi.org/10.1088/1361-6439/ad5563

X. Hou, T. Zaks, R. Langer, Y. Dong, Lipid nanoparticles for mRNA delivery. Nat Rev Mater **6**(12), 1078–1094 (2021). https://doi.org/10.1038/s41578-021-00358-0

X.L. Hu et al., Structure-tunable graphene oxide fibers via microfluidic spinning route for multifunctional textiles, (in English). Carbon **152**, 106–113 (2019). https://doi.org/10.1016/j.carbon.2019.06.010

X. Huang et al., Ultrasound-enhanced microfluidic synthesis of liposomes. Anticancer Res. 30(2), 463–466 (2010). [Online]. Available: https://www.ncbi.nlm.nih.gov/pubmed/20332455

M. James, R.A. Revia, Z. Stephen, M. Zhang, Microfluidic synthesis of iron oxide nanoparticles. Nanomaterials (Basel) **10**(11), 2113 (2020). https://doi.org/10.3390/nano10112113

Z.J. Jia, Q. Fang, Z.L. Fang, Bonding of glass microfluidic chips at room temperatures, (in English). Anal. Chem. **76**(18), 5597–5602 (2004). https://doi.org/10.1021/ac0494477

B. Jiang et al., Design and packaging of a highly integrated microreactor system for high-temperature on-board hydrogen production, (in English). Chem. Eng. J. **275**, 206–219 (2015). https://doi.org/10.1016/j.cej.2015.03.133

J. Jiang, J. Pi, J. Cai, The advancing of zinc oxide nanoparticles for biomedical applications. Bioinorg. Chem. Appl. **2018**(1), 1062562 (2018). https://doi.org/10.1155/2018/1062562

Z.Q. Jiang, H.R. Shi, X.Y. Tang, J.L. Qin, Recent advances in droplet microfluidics for single-cell analysis, (in English). Trac-Trends Anal. Chem. **159**, 116932 (2023). https://doi.org/10.1016/j.trac.2023.116932

Y. Jiaying et al., Arenobufagin-loaded PEG-PLA nanoparticles for reducing toxicity and enhancing cancer therapy. Drug Deliv. **30**(1), 2177362 (2023). https://doi.org/10.1080/10717544.2023.2177362

T.M. Joseph et al., Nanoparticles: taking a unique position in medicine. Nanomaterials (Basel) **13**(3), 574 (2023). https://doi.org/10.3390/nano13030574

X.J. Kang et al., Mass production of highly monodisperse polymeric nanoparticles by parallel flow focusing system, (in English). Microfluid. Nanofluid. **15**(3), 337–345 (2013). https://doi.org/10.1007/s10404-013-1152-6

A. Kara et al., Engineering 3D printed microfluidic chips for the fabrication of nanomedicines. Pharmaceutics **13**(12), 2134 (2021). https://doi.org/10.3390/pharmaceutics13122134

J. Karlsson, H.J. Vaughan, J.J. Green, Biodegradable polymeric nanoparticles for therapeutic cancer treatments. Annu. Rev. Chem. Biomol. Eng. **9**(1), 105–127 (2018). https://doi.org/10.1146/annurev-chembioeng-060817-084055

A. Karnwal et al., Gold nanoparticles in nanobiotechnology: from synthesis to biosensing applications. ACS Omega **9**(28), 29966–29982 (2024). https://doi.org/10.1021/acsomega.3c10352

E.M. Khalaf et al., Recent progressions in biomedical and pharmaceutical applications of chitosan nanoparticles: A comprehensive review. Int. J. Biol. Macromol. **231**, 123354 (2023). https://doi.org/10.1016/j.ijbiomac.2023.123354

S. Khizar, N. Zine, A. Errachid, N. Jaffrezic-Renault, A. Elaissari, Microfluidic-based nanoparticle synthesis and their potential applications. Electrophoresis **43**(7–8), 819–838 (2022)

T. Konstantinova et al., Deep multilevel wet etching of fused silica glass microstructures in BOE solution. Sci. Rep. **13**(1), 5228 (2023)

J. Kreuter, Nanoparticles—a historical perspective. Int. J. Pharm. **331**(1), 1–10 (2007)

M.B. Kulkarni, J. Us, K. Amreen, S. Goel, Portable thermal management platform for synthesis of ZnO nanoparticle in a microfluidic device: validated for electrochemical sensing and glucose fuel cell applications, (in English). IEEE Trans. Electron Devices **68**(8), 4070–4076 (2021). https://doi.org/10.1109/Ted.2021.3091954

L.L. Lazarus, A.S. Yang, S. Chu, R.L. Brutchey, N. Malmstadt, Flow-focused synthesis of monodisperse gold nanoparticles using ionic liquids on a microfluidic platform. Lab Chip **10**(24), 3377–3379 (2010). https://doi.org/10.1039/c0lc00297f

B. Lee et al., Characterization of passive microfluidic mixer with a three-dimensional zig-zag channel for cryo-EM sampling, (in English). Chem. Eng. Sci. **281**, 119161 (2023). https://doi.org/10.1016/j.ces.2023.119161

C.Y. Lee, W.T. Wang, C.C. Liu, L.M. Fu, Passive mixers in microfluidic systems: a review, (in English). Chem. Eng. J. **288**, 146–160 (2016). https://doi.org/10.1016/j.cej.2015.10.122

U.N. Lee et al., Fundamentals of rapid injection molding for microfluidic cell-based assays. Lab Chip **18**(3), 496–504 (2018). https://doi.org/10.1039/c7lc01052d

C.M. Leung et al., A guide to the organ-on-a-chip. Nat. Rev. Methods Prim. **2**(1), 33 (2022)

F. Li et al., Oral immunization with *lactobacillus casei* expressing the porcine circovirus type 2 cap and LTB induces mucosal and systemic antibody responses in mice. Viruses **13**(7), 1302 (2021). https://doi.org/10.3390/v13071302

G.X. Li, Q. Li, R. Cheng, S. Chen, Synthesis of quantum dots based on microfluidic technology, (in English). Curr. Opin. Chem. Eng. **29**, 34–41 (2020). https://doi.org/10.1016/j.coche.2020.02.005

H.W. Li, Y.Q. Fan, R. Kodzius, I.G. Foulds, Fabrication of polystyrene microfluidic devices using a pulsed CO laser system, (in English). Microsyst. Technol. Micro Nanosyst. -Inf. Storage Process. Syst. **18**(3), 373–379 (2012). https://doi.org/10.1007/s00542-011-1410-z

Y. Li et al., Facile synthesis of rapamycin-loaded PEG-b-PLA nanoparticles and their application in immunotherapy. J. Polym. Sci. **62**(10), 2215–2230 (2024)

S.X. Liang, L.C. Zhang, S. Reichenberger, S. Barcikowski, Design and perspective of amorphous metal nanoparticles from laser synthesis and processing. Phys. Chem. Chem. Phys. **23**(19), 11121–11154 (2021). https://doi.org/10.1039/d1cp00701g

J.M. Lim et al., Parallel microfluidic synthesis of size-tunable polymeric nanoparticles using 3D flow focusing towards in vivo study. Nanomedicine **10**(2), 401–409 (2014a). https://doi.org/10.1016/j.nano.2013.08.003

J.-M. Lim et al., Parallel microfluidic synthesis of size-tunable polymeric nanoparticles using 3D flow focusing towards in vivo study. Nanomed. Nanotechnol. Biol. Med. **10**(2), 401–409 (2014b)

D. Liu, S. Cito, Y. Zhang, C.F. Wang, T.M. Sikanen, H.A. Santos, A versatile and robust microfluidic platform toward high throughput synthesis of homogeneous nanoparticles with tunable properties. Adv. Mater. **27**(14), 2298–2304 (2015). https://doi.org/10.1002/adma.201405408

Y. Liu, X. Jiang, Why microfluidics? Merits and trends in chemical synthesis. Lab Chip **17**(23), 3960–3978 (2017). https://doi.org/10.1039/c7lc00627f

M. Lu, Y.P. Ho, C.L. Grigsby, A.A. Nawaz, K.W. Leong, T.J. Huang, Three-dimensional hydrodynamic focusing method for polyplex synthesis. ACS Nano **8**(1), 332–339 (2014). https://doi.org/10.1021/nn404193e

S. Łukasiewicz, A. Mikołajczyk, E. Błasiak, E. Fic, M. Dziedzicka-Wasylewska, Polycaprolactone nanoparticles as promising candidates for nanocarriers in novel nanomedicines. Pharmaceutics **13**(2), 191 (2021)

S. Lv et al., One-step microfluidic fabrication of multi-responsive liposomes for targeted delivery of doxorubicin synergism with Photothermal effect. Int. J. Nanomedicine **16**(null), 7759–7772 (2021). https://doi.org/10.2147/IJN.S329621

X. Ma, R. Li, Z. Jin, Y. Fan, X. Zhou, Y. Zhang, Injection molding and characterization of PMMA-based microfluidic devices. Microsyst. Technol. **26**, 1317–1324 (2020)

M. Maeki, S. Uno, A. Niwa, Y. Okada, M. Tokeshi, Microfluidic technologies and devices for lipid nanoparticle-based RNA delivery. J. Control. Release **344**, 80–96 (2022). https://doi.org/10.1016/j.jconrel.2022.02.017

C. Martins, F. Sousa, F. Araujo, B. Sarmento, Functionalizing PLGA and PLGA derivatives for drug delivery and tissue regeneration applications. Adv. Healthc. Mater. **7**(1), 1701035 (2018). https://doi.org/10.1002/adhm.201701035

M. Meischein, X. Wang, A. Ludwig, Unraveling the formation mechanism of nanoparticles sputtered in ionic liquid, (in English). J. Phys. Chem. C **125**(43), 24229–24239 (2021). https://doi.org/10.1021/acs.jpcc.1c07621

Z. Mirza, S. Karim, Nanoparticles-based drug delivery and gene therapy for breast cancer: recent advancements and future challenges, in *Seminars in Cancer Biology*, vol. 69, (Elsevier, 2021), pp. 226–237

S. Mohan, M. Vellakkat, A. Aravind, U. Reka, Hydrothermal synthesis and characterization of zinc oxide nanoparticles of various shapes under different reaction conditions. Nano Express **1**(3), 030028 (2020)

F. Mohebichamkhorami et al., Microfluidic synthesis of ultrasmall chitosan/graphene quantum dots particles for intranasal delivery in Alzheimer's disease treatment. Small **19**(40), e2207626 (2023). https://doi.org/10.1002/smll.202207626

M.Z. Mulla, M.R.T. Rahman, B. Marcos, B. Tiwari, S. Pathania, Poly lactic acid (PLA) nanocomposites: effect of inorganic nanoparticles reinforcement on its performance and food packaging applications. Molecules **26**(7) (1967). https://doi.org/10.3390/molecules26071967

P.V. Nagime et al., Facile synthesis of silver nanoparticles using *Calotropis procera* leaves: unraveling biological and electrochemical potentials. Discov. Nano **19**(1), 139 (2024). https://doi.org/10.1186/s11671-024-04090-w

E.D. Namiot, A.V. Sokolov, V.N. Chubarev, V.V. Tarasov, H.B. Schioth, Nanoparticles in clinical trials: analysis of clinical trials, FDA approvals and use for COVID-19 vaccines. Int. J. Mol. Sci. **24**(1), 787 (2023). https://doi.org/10.3390/ijms24010787

A. Naysmith, N.S. Mian, S. Rana, A. Hewitt, Multifunctional green synthesized silver nanoparticle and polypyrrole-based e-textile for wearable thermoregulation applications, (in English). Green Chem. Lett. Rev. **17**(1), 2419003 (2024). https://doi.org/10.1080/17518253.2024.2419003

J. Nette, P.D. Howes, A.J. deMello, Microfluidic synthesis of luminescent and plasmonic nanoparticles: fast, efficient, and data-rich. Adv. Mater. Technol. **5**(7), 2000060 (2020)

B. Nguyen, N.H. Tolia, Protein-based antigen presentation platforms for nanoparticle vaccines. NPJ Vaccines **6**(1), 70 (2021). https://doi.org/10.1038/s41541-021-00330-7

A. Nikhil et al., Vancomycin-conjugated polyethyleneimine-stabilized gold nanoparticles attenuate germination and show potent antifungal activity against *Aspergillus* spp (in English). Appl. Sci.-Basel **14**(16), 6926 (2024). https://doi.org/10.3390/app14166926

M.P. Nikolova, M.S. Chavali, Metal oxide nanoparticles as biomedical materials, (in English). Biomimetics **5**(2), 27 (2020). https://doi.org/10.3390/biomimetics5020027

A.E. Ongaro et al., Engineering a sustainable future for point-of-care diagnostics and single-use microfluidic devices. Lab Chip **22**(17), 3122–3137 (2022). https://doi.org/10.1039/d2lc00380e

V. Orozco-Montes et al., Synthesis of platinum nanoparticles by plasma sputtering onto glycerol: effect of argon pressure on their physicochemical properties, (in English). J. Phys. Chem. C **125**(5), 3169–3179 (2021). https://doi.org/10.1021/acs.jpcc.0c09746

M. Patel, S. Mishra, R. Verma, D. Shikha, Synthesis of ZnO and CuO nanoparticles via sol gel method and its characterization by using various technique. Discov. Mater. **2**(1), 1 (2022)

N. Patil, R. Bhaskar, V. Vyavhare, R. Dhadge, V. Khaire, Y. Patil, Overview on methods of synthesis of nanoparticles. Int. J. Curr. Pharm. Res. **13**(2), 11–16 (2021)

R.J. Phillips, *Forced-Convection, Liquid-Cooled, Microchannel Heat Sinks* (Massachusetts Institute of Technology, 1987)

M.L. Popa, M.D. Preda, I.A. Neacsu, A.M. Grumezescu, O. Ginghina, Traditional vs. microfluidic synthesis of ZnO nanoparticles. Int. J. Mol. Sci. **24**(3), 1875 (2023). https://doi.org/10.3390/ijms24031875

S. Priyadarsini, S. Mohanty, S. Mukherjee, S. Basu, M. Mishra, Graphene and graphene oxide as nanomaterials for medicine and biology application, (in English). J. Nanostructure Chem. **8**(2), 123–137 (2018). https://doi.org/10.1007/s40097-018-0265-6

Z. Qi et al., Disposable silicon-glass microfluidic devices: precise, robust and cheap. Lab Chip **18**(24), 3872–3880 (2018). https://doi.org/10.1039/c8lc01109e

H. Qiu, X.J. Wu, R. Hong, G. Wu, S. Chen, Microfluidic-oriented synthesis of graphene oxide nanosheets toward high energy density supercapacitors, (in English). Energy Fuel **34**(9), 11519–11526 (2020). https://doi.org/10.1021/acs.energyfuels.0c02143

N.F. Raley, J.C. Davidson, J.W. Balch, Examination of glass-silicon and glass-glass bonding techniques for microfluidic systems, in *Micromachining and Microfabrication Process Technology*, vol. 2639, (SPIE, 1995), pp. 40–45

A.V. Rane, K. Kanny, V. Abitha, S. Thomas, Methods for synthesis of nanoparticles and fabrication of nanocomposites, in *Synthesis of Inorganic Nanomaterials*, (Elsevier, 2018), pp. 121–139

T.M. Rashid, U.M. Nayef, M.S. Jabir, F.A.H. Mutlak, Synthesis and characterization of Au:ZnO (core:shell) nanoparticles via laser ablation, (in English). Optik **244**, 167569 (2021). https://doi.org/10.1016/j.ijleo.2021.167569

N.M. Refat, M.Y. Nassar, S.A. Sadeek, A controllable one-pot hydrothermal synthesis of spherical cobalt ferrite nanoparticles: synthesis, characterization, and optical properties. RSC Adv. **12**(38), 25081–25095 (2022). https://doi.org/10.1039/d2ra03345c

M. Ripoll et al., Optimal self-assembly of lipid nanoparticles (LNP) in a ring micromixer. Sci. Rep. **12**(1), 9483 (2022). https://doi.org/10.1038/s41598-022-13112-5

A. Rónavári et al., Green silver and gold nanoparticles: biological synthesis approaches and potentials for biomedical applications. Molecules **26**(4), 844 (2021)

Q. Ruan et al., Sensitive, rapid, and automated detection of DNA methylation based on digital microfluidics. ACS Appl. Mater. Interfaces **13**(7), 8042–8048 (2021). https://doi.org/10.1021/acsami.0c21995

J. Saez, R. Catalan-Carrio, R.M. Owens, L. Basabe-Desmonts, F. Benito-Lopez, Microfluidics and materials for smart water monitoring: a review. Anal. Chim. Acta **1186**, 338392 (2021). https://doi.org/10.1016/j.aca.2021.338392

S.J. Salih, W.M. Mahmood, Review on magnetic spinel ferrite (MFe(2)O(4)) nanoparticles: from synthesis to application. Heliyon **9**(6), e16601 (2023). https://doi.org/10.1016/j.heliyon.2023.e16601

K. Sato et al., Characterization of orientation-dependent etching properties of single-crystal silicon: effects of KOH concentration. Sensors Actuators A: Phys. **64**(1), 87–93 (1998)

V. Sebastian Cabeza, S. Kuhn, A.A. Kulkarni, K.F. Jensen, Size-controlled flow synthesis of gold nanoparticles using a segmented flow microfluidic platform. Langmuir **28**(17), 7007–7013 (2012)

A.B. Sengul, E. Asmatulu, Toxicity of metal and metal oxide nanoparticles: a review (in English). Environ. Chem. Lett. **18**(5), 1659–1683 (2020). https://doi.org/10.1007/s10311-020-01033-6

H. Shan et al., One-step formation of targeted liposomes in a versatile microfluidic mixing device. Small **19**(7), 2205498 (2023)

M. Shao et al., Continuous synthesis of carbon dots with full spectrum fluorescence and the mechanism of their multiple color emission. Lab Chip **19**(23), 3974–3978 (2019). https://doi.org/10.1039/c9lc00683d

V.V. Shapovalov et al., 3D-printed microfluidic system for the in situ diagnostics and screening of nanoparticles synthesis parameters. Micro Nano Eng. **20**, 100224 (2023). https://doi.org/10.1016/j.mne.2023.100224

S.J. Shepherd, D. Issadore, M.J. Mitchell, Microfluidic formulation of nanoparticles for biomedical applications. Biomaterials **274**, 120826 (2021a). https://doi.org/10.1016/j.biomaterials.2021.120826

S.J. Shepherd et al., Scalable mRNA and siRNA lipid nanoparticle production using a parallelized microfluidic device. Nano Lett. **21**(13), 5671–5680 (2021b). https://doi.org/10.1021/acs.nanolett.1c01353

G. Shineh, M. Mobaraki, E. Afzali, F. Alakija, Z.J. Velisdeh, D.K. Mills, Antimicrobial metal and metal oxide nanoparticles in bone tissue repair. Biomed. Mater. Devices, 1–24 (2024)

A. Shubhava, G.K. Jayarama, S. Kannarpady, S.P. Kale, R. Pinto, Chemical etching of glasses in hydrofluoric acid: a brief review, (in English). Mater. Today-Proc. **55**, 46–51 (2022). https://doi.org/10.1016/j.matpr.2021.12.110

I. Singh, C.S. Lacko, Z. Zhao, C.E. Schmidt, C. Rinaldi, Preparation and evaluation of microfluidic magnetic alginate microparticles for magnetically templated hydrogels. J. Colloid Interface Sci. **561**, 647–658 (2020). https://doi.org/10.1016/j.jcis.2019.11.040

B. Sinha, R.H. Muller, J.P. Moschwitzer, Bottom-up approaches for preparing drug nanocrystals: formulations and factors affecting particle size. Int. J. Pharm. **453**(1), 126–141 (2013). https://doi.org/10.1016/j.ijpharm.2013.01.019

Y. Song, C.S. Kumar, J. Hormes, Fabrication of an SU-8 based microfluidic reactor on a PEEK substrate sealed by a 'flexible semi-solid transfer' (FST) process. J. Micromech. Microeng. **14**(7), 932 (2004)

T.M. Squires, S.R. Quake, Microfluidics: fluid physics at the nanoliter scale, (in English). Rev. Mod. Phys. **77**(3), 977–1026 (2005). https://doi.org/10.1103/RevModPhys.77.977

S. Srivastava et al., Biological Nanofactories: Using living forms for metal nanoparticle synthesis. Mini Rev. Med. Chem. **21**(2), 245–265 (2021). https://doi.org/10.2174/13895575209992011116163012

H.A. Stone, A.D. Stroock, A. Ajdari, Engineering flows in small devices: microfluidics toward a lab-on-a-chip, (in English). Annu. Rev. Fluid Mech. **36**(1), 381–411 (2004). https://doi.org/10.1146/annurev.fluid.36.050802.122124

H. Sun et al., Reliable and reusable whole polypropylene plastic microfluidic devices for a rapid, low-cost antimicrobial susceptibility test. Lab Chip **19**(17), 2915–2924 (2019). https://doi.org/10.1039/c9lc00502a

J. Sun et al., A microfluidic origami chip for synthesis of functionalized polymeric nanoparticles. Nanoscale **5**(12), 5262–5265 (2013). https://doi.org/10.1039/c3nr01289a

K. Sun, Y. Fan, M. Hebda, Y. Zhang, Origami microfluidics: a review of research progress and biomedical applications. Biomed. Mater. Devices **1**(1), 388–401 (2023b)

L. Sun et al., Smart nanoparticles for cancer therapy. Signal Transduct. Target. Ther. **8**(1), 418 (2023a). https://doi.org/10.1038/s41392-023-01642-x

H. Tan, Numerical study of a bubble driven micromixer based on thermal inkjet technology (retracted article), (in English). Phys. Fluids **31**(6), 062006 (2019). https://doi.org/10.1063/1.5098449

S.Y. Tang et al., Microfluidic mass production of stabilized and stealthy liquid metal nanoparticles. Small **14**(21), e1800118 (2018). https://doi.org/10.1002/smll.201800118

A.B. Theberge, E. Mayot, A. El Harrak, F. Kleinschmidt, W.T. Huck, A.D. Griffiths, Microfluidic platform for combinatorial synthesis in picolitre droplets. Lab Chip **12**(7), 1320–1326 (2012). https://doi.org/10.1039/c2lc21019c

R.M. Tiggelaar et al., Fabrication, mechanical testing and application of high-pressure glass microreactor chips, (in English). Chem. Eng. J. **131**(1–3), 163–170 (2007). https://doi.org/10.1016/j.cej.2006.12.036

R. Tran et al., Simplified prototyping of perfusable polystyrene microfluidics. Biomicrofluidics **8**(4), 046501 (2014). https://doi.org/10.1063/1.4892035

C.W. Tsao, Polymer microfluidics: simple, low-cost fabrication process bridging academic lab research to commercialized production. Micromachines (Basel) **7**(12), 225 (2016). https://doi.org/10.3390/mi7120225

T. Tsuzuki, Mechanochemical synthesis of metal oxide nanoparticles. Commun. Chem. **4**(1), 143 (2021). https://doi.org/10.1038/s42004-021-00582-3

P. Utreja, S. Verma, M. Rahman, Use of nanoparticles in medicine. Curr. Biochem. Eng. **6**(1), 7–24 (2020)

P.M. Valencia, E.M. Pridgen, M. Rhee, R. Langer, O.C. Farokhzad, R. Karnik, Microfluidic platform for combinatorial synthesis and optimization of targeted nanoparticles for cancer therapy. ACS Nano **7**(12), 10671–10680 (2013). https://doi.org/10.1021/nn403370e

H. Van Lintel, F. Van de Pol, S. Bouwstra, A piezoelectric micropump based on micromachining of silicon. Sensors Actuators **15**(2), 153–167 (1988)

J. van Stee, P. Adriaenssens, S. Kuhn, K. Binnemans, T. Van Gerven, Liquid-liquid mass transfer in microfluidic reactors: assumptions and realities of non-ideal systems. Chem. Eng. Sci. **248**, 117232 (2022)

M. Varani et al., Synthesis and biodistribution of Tc-Labeled PLGA nanoparticles by microfluidic technique, (in English). Pharmaceutics **13**(11), 1769 (2021). https://doi.org/10.3390/pharmaceutics13111769

J.B. Wacker, I. Lignos, V.K. Parashar, M.A. Gijs, Controlled synthesis of fluorescent silica nanoparticles inside microfluidic droplets. Lab Chip **12**(17), 3111–3116 (2012). https://doi.org/10.1039/c2lc40300e

B. Wang et al., General synthesis of high-entropy alloy and ceramic nanoparticles in nanoseconds. Nat. Synth. **1**(2), 138–146 (2022)

D. Wang et al., Direct synthesis and chemical vapor deposition of 2D carbide and nitride MXenes. Science **379**(6638), 1242–1247 (2023a). https://doi.org/10.1126/science.add9204

G.L. Wang, D.W. Yang, Y. Wang, D. Niu, X.L. Zhao, G.F. Ding, Heat transfer and friction characteristics of the microfluidic heat sink with variously-shaped ribs for chip cooling. Sensors (Basel) **15**(4), 9547–9562 (2015). https://doi.org/10.3390/s150409547

H. Wang et al., Convenient two-step method constructed silicon-based microfluidic chip for fast CYP2C19 SNPs detection. RSC Adv. **14**(36), 26007–26015 (2024). https://doi.org/10.1039/d4ra03913k

J. Wang et al., A microfluidic tubing method and its application for controlled synthesis of polymeric nanoparticles. Lab Chip **14**(10), 1673–1677 (2014). https://doi.org/10.1039/c4lc00080c

J.L. Wang, J.J. Qiu, A review of carbon dots in biological applications, (in English). J. Mater. Sci. **51**(10), 4728–4738 (2016). https://doi.org/10.1007/s10853-016-9797-7

W. Wang, S.A. Soper, *Bio-MEMS: Technologies and Applications* (CRC Press, 2006)

W. Wang, S. Zhao, T. Shao, Y. Jin, Y. Cheng, Visualization of micro-scale mixing in miscible liquids using μ-LIF technique and drug nano-particle preparation in T-shaped micro-channels. Chem. Eng. J. **192**, 252–261 (2012)

X.P. Wang, H.Y. Xu, H.T. Qi, Mixing performance of an expansive mixer on viscoelastic solutions under alternating current electric field, (in English). Phys. Fluids **35**(10) (2023b). https://doi.org/10.1063/5.0172045

G.M. Whitesides, The origins and the future of microfluidics. Nature **442**(7101), 368–373 (2006). https://doi.org/10.1038/nature05058

H. Windolf, R. Chamberlain, J. Quodbach, Predicting drug release from 3D printed oral medicines based on the surface area to volume ratio of tablet geometry. Pharmaceutics **13**(9), 1453 (2021) https://doi.org/10.3390/pharmaceutics13091453

S. Wirunchit, P. Gansa, W. Koetniyom, Synthesis of ZnO nanoparticles by ball-milling process for biological applications, (in English). Mater. Today-Proc. **47**, 3554–3559 (2021). https://doi.org/10.1016/j.matpr.2021.03.559

K.L. Wlodarczyk, D.P. Hand, M.M. Maroto-Valer, Maskless, rapid manufacturing of glass microfluidic devices using a picosecond pulsed laser. Sci. Rep. **9**(1), 20215 (2019). https://doi.org/10.1038/s41598-019-56711-5

M. Wu, Y. Xiao, R. Wu, J. Lei, T. Li, Y. Zheng, Aggregable gold nanoparticles for cancer photothermal therapy. J. Mater. Chem. B **12**(33), 8048–8061 (2024). https://doi.org/10.1039/d4tb00403e

S.Y. Wu, Q. Lin, Y. Yuen, Y.C. Tai, MEMS flow sensors for nano-fluidic applications, (in English). Sensors Actuators Phys. **89**(1–2), 152–158 (2001). https://doi.org/10.1016/S0924-4247(00)00541-0

X. Xiu et al., Novel 3D integrated microfluidic device: design, construction, and application to the preparation of liposomes for vaccine delivery. J. Drug Delivery Sci. Technol. **91**, 105191 (2024). https://doi.org/10.1016/j.jddst.2023.105191

L. Xu, J.H. Peng, M. Yan, D. Zhang, A.Q. Shen, Droplet synthesis of silver nanoparticles by a microfluidic device, (in English). Chem. Eng. Process.-Process Intensif. **102**, 186–193 (2016a). https://doi.org/10.1016/j.cep.2016.01.017

L. Xu, J. Peng, M. Yan, D. Zhang, A.Q. Shen, Droplet synthesis of silver nanoparticles by a microfluidic device. Chem. Eng. Process.: Process Intensif. **102**, 186–193 (2016b)

Y. Xu et al., Lipid-coated CaCO(3) nanoparticles as a versatile pH-responsive drug delivery platform to enable combined chemotherapy of breast cancer. ACS Appl. Bio Mater. **5**(3), 1194–1201 (2022). https://doi.org/10.1021/acsabm.1c01234

S. Yadavali, D. Lee, D. Issadore, Robust microfabrication of highly parallelized three-dimensional microfluidics on silicon. Sci. Rep. **9**(1), 12213 (2019)

T. Yadavalli, D. Shukla, Role of metal and metal oxide nanoparticles as diagnostic and therapeutic tools for highly prevalent viral infections. Nanomedicine **13**(1), 219–230 (2017). https://doi.org/10.1016/j.nano.2016.08.016

C.H. Yang et al., Microfluidic assisted synthesis of silver nanoparticle-chitosan composite microparticles for antibacterial applications. Int. J. Pharm. **510**(2), 493–500 (2016). https://doi.org/10.1016/j.ijpharm.2016.01.010

M. Yang, L.M. Luo, G.W. Chen, Microfluidic synthesis of ultrasmall co nanoparticles over reduced graphene oxide and their catalytic properties, (in English). AICHE J. **66**(6), e16950 (2020). https://doi.org/10.1002/aic.16950

M. Yang et al., One-step chemical vapor deposition fabrication of Ni@NiO@graphite nanoparticles for the oxygen evolution reaction of water splitting. RSC Adv. **12**(17), 10496–10503 (2022). https://doi.org/10.1039/d2ra00947a

Y. Yao, Y. Fan, CO_2 laser fabrication of hydrogel-based open-channel microfluidic devices. Biomed. Microdevices **23**(4), 47 (2021). https://doi.org/10.1007/s10544-021-00584-x

S.P. Yeap, Permanent agglomerates in powdered nanoparticles: formation and future prospects, (in English). Powder Technol. **323**, 51–59 (2018). https://doi.org/10.1016/j.powtec.2017.09.042

S.X. Ying et al., Green synthesis of nanoparticles: current developments and limitations, (in English). Environ. Technol. Innovation **26**, 102336 (2022). https://doi.org/10.1016/j.eti.2022.102336

Z. Yu et al., Nanoparticles: a new approach to upgrade cancer diagnosis and treatment. Nanoscale Res. Lett. **16**(1), 88 (2021). https://doi.org/10.1186/s11671-021-03489-z

M.H. Zamani, A. Khatibi, B. Tavana, P. Zahedi, S. Aghamohammadi, Characterization of drug-loaded alginate-chitosan polyelectrolyte nanoparticles synthesized by microfluidics, (in English). J. Polym. Res. **30**(2), 86 (2023). https://doi.org/10.1007/s10965-023-03468-1

M. Zhang et al., Comparison of micro-mixing in time pulsed Newtonian fluid and viscoelastic fluid, (in English). Micromachines **10**(4), 262 (2019b). https://doi.org/10.3390/mi10040262

S. Zhang, X.Y. Chen, Z.L. Wu, Y. Zheng, Numerical study on stagger Koch fractal baffles micromixer, (in English). Int. J. Heat Mass Transf. **133**, 1065–1073 (2019a). https://doi.org/10.1016/j.ijheatmasstransfer.2019.01.009

N. Zhelev et al., Fabrication of microfluidic cavities using Si-to-glass anodic bonding. Rev. Sci. Instrum. **89**(7), 073902 (2018). https://doi.org/10.1063/1.5031837

X. Zheng et al., An overview of polymeric nanomicelles in clinical trials and on the market, (in English). Chin. Chem. Lett. **32**(1), 243–257 (2021). https://doi.org/10.1016/j.cclet.2020.11.029

I.V. Zhigaltsev et al., Bottom-up design and synthesis of limit size lipid nanoparticle systems with aqueous and triglyceride cores using millisecond microfluidic mixing. Langmuir **28**(7), 3633–3640 (2012). https://doi.org/10.1021/la204833h

J. Zhou, A.V. Ellis, N.H. Voelcker, Recent developments in PDMS surface modification for microfluidic devices. Electrophoresis **31**(1), 2–16 (2010). https://doi.org/10.1002/elps.200900475

P. Zhu, L. Wang, Passive and active droplet generation with microfluidics: a review. Lab Chip **17**(1), 34–75 (2017)

L. Zou et al., Microfluidic synthesis of magnetic nanoparticles in droplet-based microreactors. Mater. Chem. Phys. **276**, 125384 (2022). https://doi.org/10.1016/j.matchemphys.2021.125384

Reactive Organic Functionality Linked to Trimethoxysilane in Designing Nanostructured Material with Exceptional Properties for Technological Applications

Prem C. Pandey

Abstract The presence of organic functional groups behaving as electrophile/nucleophile linked with especially trimethoxysilane allows the formation of useful nanomaterials of unparalleled technological interest as a function of Lewis acid/Lewis base strength of functional trimethoxysilane. Such functional groups like: alkyl amine, epoxycyclohexylethyl, glycidoxy propyl, hydrogen linked especially with trimethoxysilane referred to as functional methoxysilanes allowed the formation and tailoring of nanomaterials properties for variety of applications especially: (1) functional trimethoxysilane-derived biocompatible thin film of organically modified silicate, (2) functional trimethoxysilane-derived metal organic framework in nanostructured network of organically modified silicate, (3) functional trimethoxysilane-mediated synthesis of processable monometallic, bimetallic and trimetallic noble metal nanoparticles, (4) synthetic insertion of metal nanoparticles and their cheaper transition metal analogues within mesoporous matrix, (5) functional trimethoxysilane-derived fluorescent nanoparticles, (6) functional trimethoxysilane-derived self-assembling siloxane–metal nanoparticles polymeric nanofluid, (7) functional trimethoxysilane-derived porous Nanostructured Palladium–Cobalt–Silica as Heterogeneous Catalysts, and (8) functional trimethoxysilane-derived functional Prussian blue nanoparticles. The exceptional property of such silica-derived nanomaterial is reviewed in this chapter.

Keywords Electrochemical biosensors · Noble metal nanoparticles · Organically modified silicate · Sol-gel processing · Trimethoxysilane

P. C. Pandey (✉)
Department of Chemistry, Indian Institute of Technology (BHU), Varanasi, India
e-mail: pcpandey.apc@itbhu.ac.in

R. Narayan (ed.), *Nanostructured Biomaterials and Their Applications*,
https://doi.org/10.1007/978-3-032-16316-5_6

1 Introduction

Metal alkoxides are a class of compounds acting as precursors in sol-gel processes through hydrolysis/condensation/polycondensation/densityfication via controlling at nanoscale mastering of the materials preparation and directed huge attentions of world scientists during last few decades to yield metal oxide nanoparticles that has boosted the introduction of suitable remedy of many unsolved issues. Pioneering researches conducted by Late Ram Charan Mehrotra and his group (Bradley et al. 1978) in India on metal alkoxide which has been unique to extend such innovations for subsequent introduction of variety of commercial products and companies at global scenario especially via converting thermodynamically stable silica (SiO_2) to metallic silica and thereafter into alkoxysilane that has been major breakthrough for mastering them at nanoscale. The acid/base-catalyzed key steps namely hydrolysis, condensation, polycondensation and densityfications controlled the sol-gel processing of metal alkoxide in tailoring nanostructured material. Replacing the metal on such alkoxide by silica resulted the formation of nanostructured silicate with exceptional properties and same is followed in natural material evolution. Earlier findings demonstrated the susceptibility on the relative kinetics of hydrolysis of alkoxide residue in the order of methoxy > ethoxy groups that directed the use of trimethoxy group linked to silica for exploring real-time functional reactivity of organic functional group linked to trimethoxysilane.

The introduction of silica linked to trimethoxy group through sol-gel processing yielded the formation of nanostructures silica network bridging the gap between physics, chemistry, biology, medial and engineering sciences (Schmidt et al. 1984) and is normally catalyzed by either acid or base. Accordingly, the strength of Lewis acid and or Lewis base character of organic functionality of trimethoxy precursors drastically control on precise evolution of silica-derived nanostructured material of controlled morphology via real-time controlling the sol-gel processing through the participation of such reactive organic functionalities linked to trimethoxyoxysilanes (Boonstra and Mulder 1988). The presence of these functionalities not only control the sol-gel processing of trimethoxysilane however enable specific interaction between reactive organic functional groups leading to introduction of specific porous morphology and wettability for meeting in situ requirement of innovative technological applications. Four types of such reactive functionalities: 3-aminopropyltrinethoxyoxysilane, [2-(3,4-Epoxycyclohexyl) ethyl] trimethoxysilane, 3-Glycidoxypropyltrimethoxysilane and trimethoxysilane are primarily reviewed and explored in our group for yielding nanostructured domains in variety of formulation as discussed in following sections.

Reactive Organotrimethoxysilanes-Derived Biocompatible Thin Film of Organically Modified Silicate. Requirement of biocompatible matrix for biomedical application especially the development of electrochemical biosensor technology as shown in Fig. 1 directed us for innovative specific development in material chemistry where the success of operational sensor for practical electrochemical biosensor is the function of close interaction between sensing component and signal transduction element

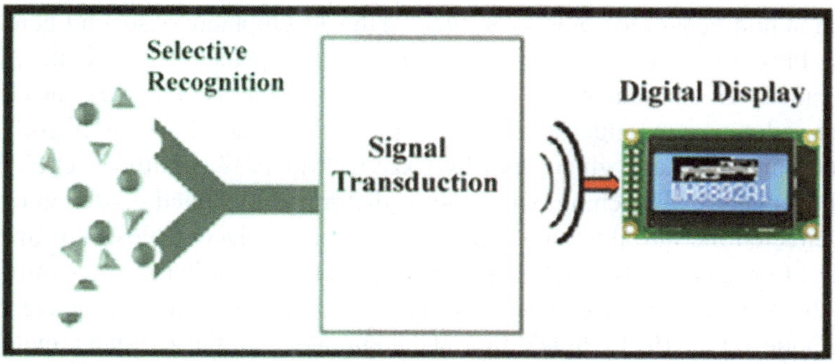

Fig. 1 Schematic diagram showing the main components of a biosensor. "Selective recognition" event allow specific interaction of targeted analyte with biocatalyst resulting change in physical parameter sensing component followed by "signal transduction" into "digital display" as a function of analyte concentration

during biosensing. For example, an electrochemical mode of signal transduction based on current measurement requires the participation of electroactive species that may be either the reaction product or the sensing components itself; this has led to three generation of glucose biosensor when glucose oxidase enzyme is used as biocomponent have been described when electron exchange from glucose and typical glucose oxidase-catalyzed reaction is considered as given below:

Example. Equation 1 Reaction scheme for the first-generation glucose biosensor

$$\beta - \mathrm{D} - \mathrm{glucose} + \mathrm{O_2} \overset{\mathrm{GOD}}{\rightarrow} \mathrm{D} - \mathrm{gluocono} - 1,5 - \mathrm{lactone} + \mathrm{H_2O_2}$$

Example Reaction scheme for the second-generation glucose biosensor.

$$\begin{gathered} \mathrm{glucose} + \mathrm{GOD[FAD]} \rightarrow \mathrm{gluconolactone} + \mathrm{GOD[FADH_2]} \\ \mathrm{GOD[FADH_2]} + \mathrm{Med(ox)} \rightarrow \mathrm{GOD[FAD]} + \mathrm{Med(red)} \\ \mathrm{Med(red)} \rightarrow \mathrm{Med(ox)} + \mathrm{e}^- \end{gathered}$$

Example Reaction scheme for the third-generation glucose biosensor.

$$\begin{gathered} \mathrm{glucose} + \mathrm{GOD[FAD]} \rightarrow \mathrm{gluconolactone} + \mathrm{GOD[FADH_2]} \\ \mathrm{GOD[FADH_2]} \overset{\mathrm{[TCNQ-TTF]}}{\rightarrow} \mathrm{GOD[FAD]} + \mathrm{e}^- \end{gathered}$$

Reaction scheme as shown in Fig. 1 determine the overall response and selectivity of a biosensor design for commercial applications. In first-generation biosensor, the sensor response is the function of either consumption of oxygen involving oxygen electrode or via oxidation of hydrogen peroxide generated as a function glucose oxidase catalyzed reaction. Lack of sufficient oxygen tension at the site of enzymatic reaction in first-generation biosensor directed the development of second-generation glucose biosensor where requirement of oxygen is replaced by synthetic electron transfer mediator and sensor response is dependent on the second order rate constant between redox enzyme/glucose oxidase and redox mediator that subsequently innovated commercial blood glucometer by Exac tech in 1987 (Matthews et al. 1987). Certain problem like leaching out of the mediator and mediated oxidation of interferent directed the introduction of third generation of glucose biosensor involving the role of organic electrocatalyst like TCNQ-TTF and similar other is introduced where the response of the sensor is the function of the efficiency of the electrocatalyst (Pandey et al. 1991). In addition, the components of these organic metals like TCNQ or TTF itself acts as redox mediator justifying their role attributed to second generation of enzyme electrode (Pandey et al. 1991, 1992, 1993, 1994a, b, 1995, 1997, 1998a, b, 1999a; Pandey 1994, 1998; Pandey and Weetall 1994, 1995a; Lima Filho et al. 1996).

Overall, while designing of electrochemical biosensor, also referred to as enzyme electrodes, the key point is the integration of electrode and enzyme requiring biocompatible material forming thin membrane. Out of variety of membrane materials have been tested including conducting polymer (Pandey and Mishra 1988; Pandey 1988) and organic prepolymer (Tran-Minh et al. 1990) and many more have been successfully explored. However, several of them have their own limitations either associated to leaching out of the sensing components from membrane matrix or morphological variation in polymeric domains as a function of time affecting overall response of enzyme electrode and directed us for biocompatible membrane material suitable for encapsulating the same under easily controlled experimental conditions and the role of functional alkoxysilane for biocompatible organically modified silicate suitable for encapsulating bacteriorhodopsin protein has been sought (Pandey et al. 1996). where the use of tetraorthosilicate has been demonstrated via acid controlled hydrolysis of the same associated to slow conversion of tetraorthosilicate into silicate matrix as shown in Fig. 2 with subsequent slow densitification of the silicate matrix making as generated material unsuitable for enzyme electrode design. Although several reviews have been published on (i) Controlled pore formation in organotrialkoxysilane-derived hybrids: from aerogels to hierarchically porous monoliths (Kazuyoshi and Kazuki 2011); (ii) Silica-based nanoparticles: a versatile tool for the development of efficient imaging agents (Claudia et al. 2015), (iii) Mesoporous materials and electrochemistry (Walcarius 2013; Yadong and Dmitri 2013). However all the specific review articles are mostly limited to sol-gel processing of alkoxide and does not expand the finding on the lewis acid an lewis base character of organic functionally participating in chemical interaction and subsequently controlling the sol-gel processing of as made nanomaterials into variety of technological formulations from single concept based on the participation of reactive functionality linked to trialkoxysilnes and first time covered herein.

The subsequent reaction scheme as shown in Fig. 2 allows the formation of Si–O–Si linkages and the conversion rate is to the presence of acids and bases serving as catalysts and the of Si–O–Si linkages tend to undergo densityfication converting into xerogel which is unsuitable for technological design and essentially require to

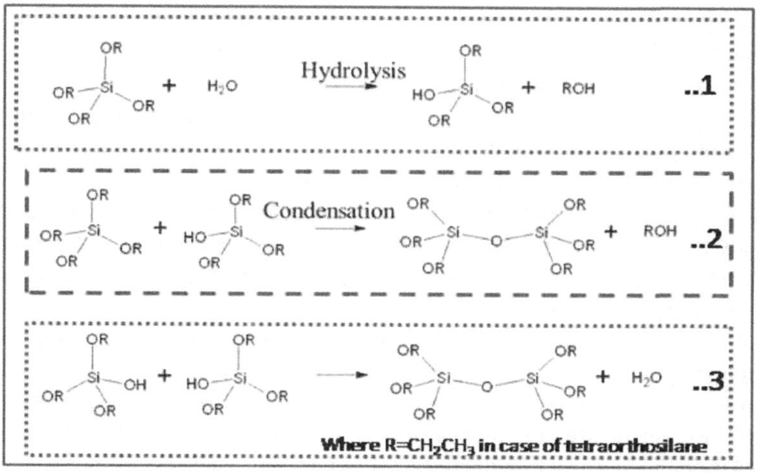

Fig. 2 Sol-gel processing of tetra-alkoxysilane

control the wet ability of the silicate matrix. Further the initial porous morphology of silicate matrix tend to be converted into xerogel accordingly introduction of functional group that may simultaneously allow to incorporate porous morphology through chemical interaction of reactive functional groups together initial porous silicate matrix as such to enable mass transfer dynamics during biochemical interactions. We have first time innovated the role of specific interaction of organic functionality linked to trimethoxyysilane. 3-Aminopropyltrimethoxysilane and-[2-(3,4-Epoxycyclohexyl)ethyl]trimethoxysilane were found to undergo specific interaction based on their Lewis acid and Lewis base character forming polymetric domains of in situ generated morphology as a function targeted sensing component followed by introduction of –Si–O–Si– domains of controlled nanostructured network of organically modified silicate under ambient conditions retaining the biological activity of sensing components (Pandey et al. 1999b, c, d, 2001a) thereby introducing novel approach of integrating the sensing component together physio-chemical transducer potentially needed in chemical sensors/biosensors designs. Such nanostructured network ultimately controlled the diffusion of analytes across the sensing components followed by controlling the stability of immobilized components for practical applications. Apart from the specific role of organically modified silicate in immobilizing the sensing components, options to control the nanostructured network that manipulate both (i) analyte diffusion kinetics and (ii) electron/ion transfer dynamics could also be manipulated (Pandey et al. 1999c, d) by introducing conductive graphite powder and water leachable material within porous network of organically modified silicate (ORMOSIL). The advantages of such organically modified silicate was not only limited to immobilization of sensing components, and simultaneously allowed controlled transport of analyte and electron hopping sites, the nanostructured domain but introduced catalysis during sensing event. Such configuration of modified silicate has innovated the electrochemical oxidation of hydrogen peroxide that was in situ generated as a function oxidase enzyme-catalyzed reaction at relatively lower over-potential (Fig. 3) which normally require high overvoltage on electrochemical oxidation of the same causing major limitations of first-generation glucose sensor (Pandey et al. 1999b, c, d, e, 2001a). The use of 3-Aminopropyltrimethoxysilane and 2-(3,4-Epoxycyclohexyl) ethyltrimethoxysilane in deriving nanostructured thin film is shown in YouTube link (Pandey 2025a). As made thin film of ORMOSIL is biocompatible and display inherent property of bio molecule during opto-electrochemical application. A typical example showing fluorescence microscopy of pyrroloquinoline quinine (PQQ) encapsulated ormisil film is shown in Fig. 4 based on fluorescence activity of PQQ (Joshi et al. 2004). These finding clearly confirmed the variety of applications of biocompatible nanostructed domains of organically modified silicate especially in the areas: (1) organically modified silicate-based nanostructured domain for chemical sensing, (2) encapsulation/immobilization of sensing components within organically modified silicate for opto-electrochemical applications, (3) manipulation in nanostructured network of organically modified silicate film; which has been innovated by our group.

Reactive Organotrimethosilanes-Derived Metal Organic Framework in Nanostructured Network of Organically Modified Silicate Second generation of enzyme electrode as shown in reaction scheme-1 are associated to the participation of redox molecules like ferrocene/derivative of ferrocene/TCNQ/TTF together biological sensing component within immobilized membrane matrix to eliminated the limitations of first-generation enzyme electrode (Pandey et al. 1991, 1992, 1993, 1994a, b, 1995, 1997, 1998a, b, 1999a; Pandey 1994, 1998; Pandey and Weetall 1994, 1995a; Lima Filho et al. 1996). When such configuration was tried in organically modified silicate matrix derived from reactive organic functionalities, being one of potent ceramic nanostructured material, electrochemical behavior was normally associated to sluggish redox electrochemistry (Fig. 5a) of encapsulated redox molecules (Pandey et al. 1999e) The sluggish electrochemistry was normally associated to the availability of poor electron hopping sited within ceramic matrix and directed us for the search of suitable remedy to manipulate

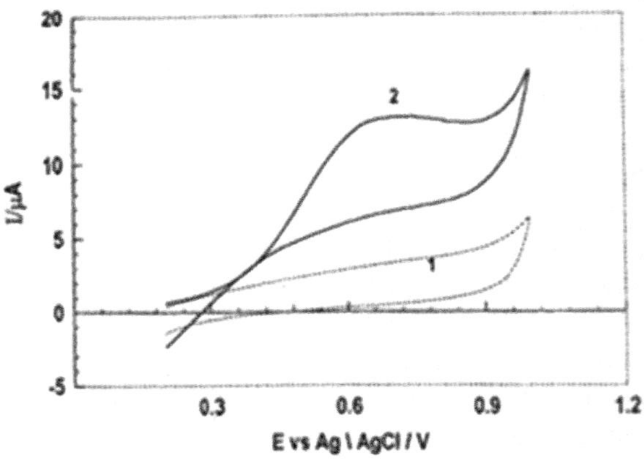

Fig. 3 Cyclic voltammograms of glucose oxidase encapsulated organically modified electrode in absence and the presence of 200 mM glucose in 0.1 M phosphate buffer pH 5.0 at scan rate of 5 mV/s

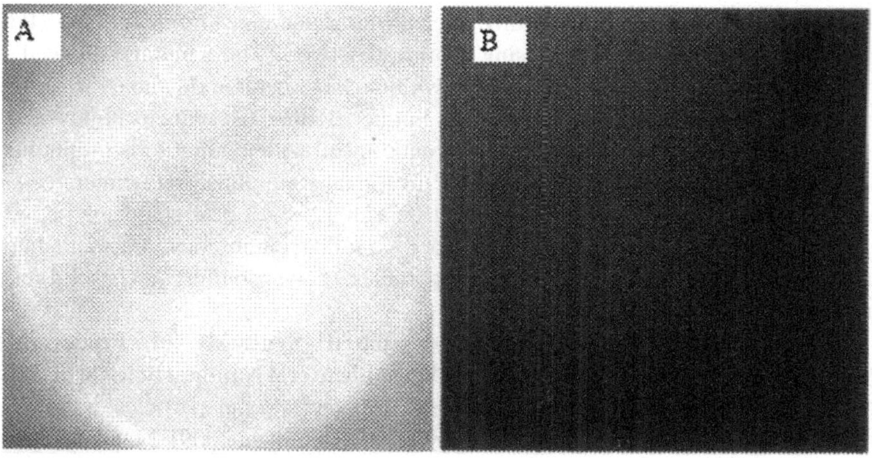

Fig. 4 Image of PQQ-encapsulated ormosil before (**A**) and after fluorescence imaging

the same for efficient electron exchange at a measurable rate (Pandey 2025a). Accordingly we intended to fasten the charge transfer process by incorporating conducting components within nanostructured domain of organically modified silicate using graphite microparticles (Pandey et al. 1999c, d, e). Although such incorporation yielded better electrochemical behavior of ormosil'encapsulated redox moieties however size of such material which was to the order of 1–50 μ further restricted their use to limited applications at a suitable measurable rate. Subsequently, while understanding the role of palladium cations with reactive organic precursors of trimethoxysilane especially 3-glycidoxypropyltrimehoxysilane and [2-(3,4-Epoxycyclohexyl)ethyl]trimethoxysilane, we observed novel finding on the introduction of palladium nanoparticles within ormosil film based on specific interaction of palladium cations and reactive organic groups like glycidoxy- and epoxycyclohexyl leading to the reduction of the same into palladium nanoparticles (Pandey 1999; Pandey et al. 1999e, 2001b, c, d, 2003; Pandey and Upadhyay 2001; Pandey and Singh 2008) and shown in video link (Pandey 2018a, 2025b). These reactive moieties not only allowed the formation of palladium nanoparticles with subsequent introduction of –Pd–C– linkage forming palladium linked ormosil but enable the formation of –Pd–Si– linkage along with –Pd–C– linkage while dealing with reactive trimethoxysilane as one of the components in ormosil formation converting the nanostructured network of silicate into solid solution that displayed excellent redox electrochemistry of ferrocene monocarboxylic acid better than that recorded in homogeneous solution (Fig. 5b) and subsequently allowed the development of commercial blood glucometer with better performance. On the other hand these materials have already proved as an efficient combination displaying excellent redox bioelectrochemistry that made the introduction of commercial blood glucometer for sensing blood glucose level in a drop of blood sample as shown in video link (Pandey 2018b,

2024a). Trimethoxysilane specifically reacted with palladium chloride forming –Pd–Si– bonding during sol-gel processing of ormosil network. These findings allowed to designs a library of electrocatalytic sites within nanostructured domains for variety of applications (Pandey and Singh 2008). Further, Trimethosysilane is highly reactive and allowed the formation of transparent ormosil with number of hydrophobilc trimethoxysilane retaining the reactivity of functional group attached to trimethoxysilane. A typical example of such ormosil made from [2-(3,4-Epoxycyclohexyl)ethyl] trimethoxysilane and trimethoxysilane underogo self assemble converting palladium cation into self assembled palladium nanoparticles on ormosil film even in solid state as shown in Fig. 6 (Pandey et al. 2001b).

Reactive Organotrimethosysilanes-Mediated Synthesis of Processable Monometallic, Bimetallic, and Trimetallic Noble Metal Nanoparticles In ancient times, the most spectacular effect of nanoscale material (nanoparticles, NPs) was seen as color pigment in glass and luster industry (Colomban 2009). Metal nanoparticles (MNPs) have been used to color glasses. Lycurgus cup, kept in British museum is one very famous example of nanoparticles used in coloring glasses. In this case gold nanoparticles (AuNPs) have been used to give ruby red color to the cup. Romans

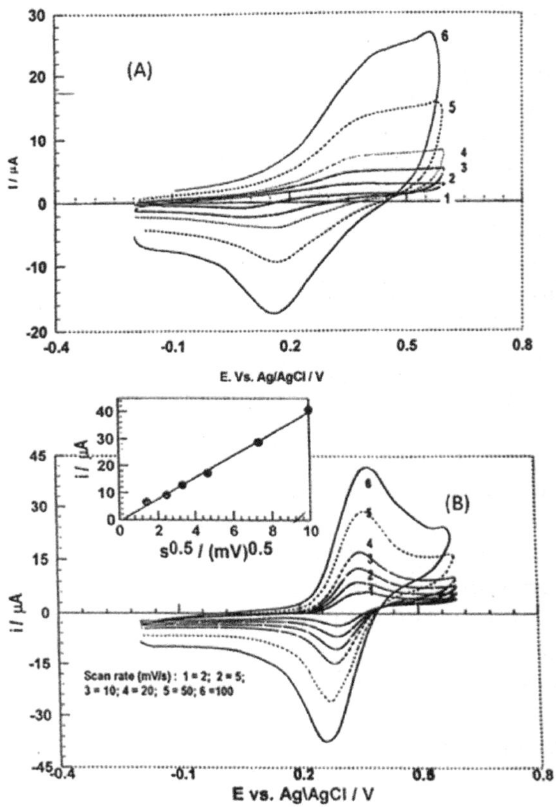

Fig. 5 **a** Cyclic voltammograms of ferrocene monocarboxylic encapsulated organically modified electrode and **b** ferrocene monocarbylic acid ncapsulated palladium linked ormosil with –Pd–Si– linkage in 0.1 M phosphate buffer pH 5.0 at varying scan rate

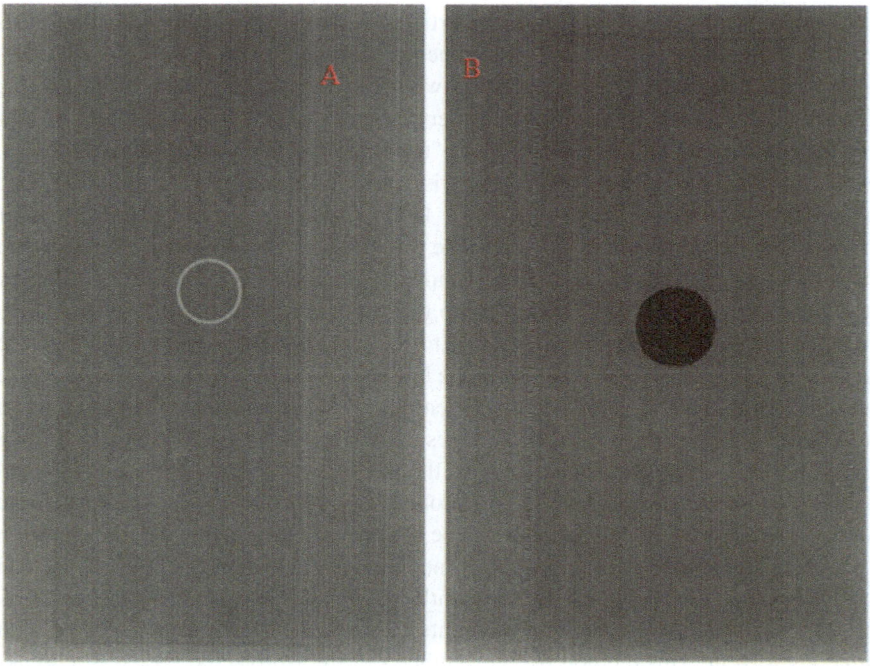

Fig. 6 Photograph of a mixture of trimethoxysilane and 2-(3,4-epoxycyclohexyl) ethyltrimethoxysilane **a** without palladium chloride treatment and **b** with palladium chloride treatment

manufactured this cup in fourth century, it appears green in daylight and red when illuminated from inside (Leonhardt 2007; Freestone et al. 2007). The attention received by MNPs from scientific community can be ascribed to the large surface to volume ratio, intriguing physical and chemical characteristics and surface electronic properties (Daniel and Astruc 2004). The use of metal nanoparticles for applications like molecular recognition, biomedicine, energy transfer, sensors and as catalysts is well established (Otsuka et al. 2013; Saha et al. 2012, Williams et al. 2015) and further open the excitability in innovating artificial enzyme to design selective biosensor. Noble metal nanoparticles have shown the possibility of mimicking peroxidase enzyme activity. AuNPs have received tremendous attention on these lines because of many important features. First, they exhibit unique size dependent physico-chemical and optical properties. Second, these properties can be tuned by controlling the size, shape, and surrounding environment (solvent, ligand etc.). Third, these AuNPs are sub-cellular, non cytotoxic and biocompatible. Fourth, Stable NPs of desired shape can be synthesized easily. One very important property of AuNPs is multifunctionalization that has been exploited for detection of small molecules and biological targets. These finding directed considerable attention of researcher to develop a convenient platform for making nanoparticles most suitable for practical applications in both homogeneous and heterogeneous formulations. Accordingly, considerable efforts have been devoted since last two decades for the synthesis of NPs with a focus on control over its size, shape, dispersibility and functionality. The approaches for the preparation of NPs include both "top-down" and "bottom-up" approaches. After Faraday (Thompson 2007), Turkevisch in 1951 developed a method referred as Turkevisch Method (Turkevich et al. 1951) which remained the most popular method for the synthesis of NPs till date due to the ease of synthesis, cheap and non-toxic nature of stabilizer. In this method sodium citrate is used both as stabilizer and reducer. It initially acts as reducer to noble metal cations producing respective nanoparticles and then as stabilizer due to the electrostatic repulsion between the negatively charged oxygen on citrate. The NPs thus produced are spherical with size around 20 nm Later, another scientist (Frens 1973) extended the work of Turkevisch and successfully synthesized variable sizes of NPs by varying the ratio of satabilizer and gold salt. Further, he also noticed that the size of NPs were inversely proportional to the stabilizer concentration, i.e., to produce larger particles, less sodium citrate should be added while smaller NPs can be obtained by increasing the concentration of citrate. This method utilizes aqueous medium for the synthesis of NPs hence can be used in aqueous phase only. Subsequently, Brust Method was given by Brust et al. (1994) to produce NPs in organic solvents that normally form separate layer with aqueous solvent. This method for the synthesis of thiol-protected NPs was a breakthrough in the field of NPs synthesis. It is a two-phase synthesis strategy in which thiol-metal cations interactions are used to protect gold nanoparticles from agglomeration using thiol ligands. Synthetic protocol involves the transfer of $AuCl_4^-$ from aqueous to toluene media by the use of surfactant tetraoctylammonium bromide and reduced by sodiumborohydride in the presence of octane thiol. A change in color from yellow to deep brown takes place in organic media on addition of sodium borohydride, $NaBH_4$ (Brust et al. 1994). The NPs obtained in this case have a size range 1.5–5 nm. These NPs exhibit higher stability due to superior Au-thiol interaction. The AuNPs can be further dried and redispersed in organic solvent of choice. The AuNPs obtained in this case show dispersibility in organic phase. Simultaneously, Martin method was developed for the production of "naked AuNPs" (Martin et al. 2010). The trick is to stabilize AuNPs, produced by the action of $NaBH_4$ on aqueous $HAuCl_4$ solution, without using stabilizer like citrate or alkanethiols. The NPs produced through this method are monodispersed with diameter ranging from 3.2 to 5.2 nm. Martin method is further modified to give octanethiol stabilized AuNPs. The naked NPs obtained through this method can be coated with dodecanethiol and might be phase-transferred to hexane by shaking with mixture of acetone, water and hexane for 30 min. Apart from these methods a variety of methods have been explored for making gold nanoparticles using variety of capping and reducing agents. AuNPs can be stabilized by using sodium citrate or by exploiting the strong Au-thiol interactions. While mostly thiol ligands have been used for AuNPs functionalization a variety of other ligands have also been used. Amines are also important as stabilizer because they are omnipresent, i.e., present everywhere in biological and environmental system. The first report on the use of amine for AuNPs synthesis was reported (Leff et al. 1996). These workers produced hydrophobic AuNPs by using dodecylamine or oleylamine in place of dodecanethiol of Brust-Schiffrin method. Thus, this method is also regarded as a modified type of Brust–Schiffrin method. The precursor made by the interaction between Au^{3+} and long chain containing primary amine [$AuCl(NH_2R)$] result in AuNPs upon decomposition in air or in tetrahydrofuran (Gomez et al. 2000). Further, phase transfer technique has been used to generate organically soluble monodispersed AuNPs using amines like Laurylamine and octadecylamine (Kumar et al. 2013). Oleyl amine (Aslam et al. 2004), amino acids (Newman and Blanchard 2006; Bhargava et al. 2005) diamines (Selvakannan et al. 2004), tetraoctylammonium (Isaacs et al. 2005), porphyrins (Kotiaho et al. 2010) and hyperbranched polyethylenimine (Duan and Nie 2007) have been used as reducing/capping agents in synthesis of AuNPs, while a direct one-pot synthesis of amine-stabilized AuNPs using 3-(trimethoxysilylpropyl)-diethylenetriamine has been reported (Zhu et al. 2005). The controlled synthesis of NPs by simple heating in ionic liquid has been developed recently, for which quaternary ammonium-based room-temperature ionic liquids was employed as a solvent, a reducing agent, and as a stabilizer (Huang et al. 2002). Piperazine derivatives have also been used as reducing/capping agents during gold nanoparticles synthesis. These outcome certainly direct further insight on synthetic strategy of noble metal nanoparticles, especially on gold nanoparticles for real-time synthesis and applications.

The conventional routes of NPs synthesis described above have been used exhaustively by scientific community for its application in different fields. These methods have been further modified by the addition of several reagents like PVP, PAP etc. to make the NPs conducive for the concerned applications. However, such techniques for NPs synthesis have following limitations: (i) Generally the AuNPs are produced as aqueous suspension. The use of such NPs in organic solvent causes agglomeration. Similarly the NPs having compatibility with organic solvent (Brust–Schiffrin method) are not compatible in aqueous system. (ii) The NPs fabricated through conventional routes are generally produced as dilute solution. The initial concentration of NPs precursor is very low. (iii) The NPs made through conventional routes are not very stable to changes in pH- and Salt- concentration which limits there use for several applications and the NPs have to be modified to serve the purpose. The NPs made through Turkevisch method agglomerate on addition of single drop of salt. The NPs should be able to adapt to different conditions (change of solvent, change of pH and change of salt concentration) without undergoing any change in its size or shape. (iv) Attempt to convert the homogenous suspension of NPs to heterogeneous matrix by adsorbing over some solid support (TiO_2, Al_2O_3 etc.) causes an increase in size of the NPs, i.e., undergo agglomeration. To meet these challenges, sol-gel science and technology, which is most widely accepted methods of creating nanomaterials seems to be more reasonable. Synthesis of sol-gel glasses involving functional trimethosysilane has received widespread attention because of its applications in various directions as discussed above (Pandey et al. 1999b, c, d, 2001a). Accordingly, the use of several functionalized trimethoxysilanes in optimum ratio of hydrophilic character [trimethoxysilane, 3-APTMS] and hydrophobic character 2-(3,4-Epoxycyclohexyl)ethyltrimethoxysilane, 3-glycidoxypropyltrimethoxysilane (3-GPTMS)] have been demonstrated for yielding organically modified thin films for multiple applications. Functional trimethoxysilanes have been used for casting thin films (through sol-gel processing) that can be used for encapsulating enzymes (glucose oxidase), redox material (ferrocene, ferricyanideetc) and noble metal ions (palladium, ruthenium) and for its use as biosensor. The property of the thin film depends on the concentration and composition of the reactive trimethoxysilane and justified by functional reactivity of the moiety linked to trimethoxysilane while fabricating nanostructured thin films of organically modified silicates through the reduction of palladium cations. Some of the functional trimethoxysilane like 3-GPTMS and trimethoxysilane have potential to act as reducing agent for Palladium chloride ($PdCl_2$) that allowed the introduction of Pd within nanostructured network of organically modified silicates (Pandey et al. 1999e, 2001b, c, d, 2003; Pandey 1999, 2018a, b, 2024a, 2025a, b; Joshi et al. 2004; Pandey and Upadhyay 2001; Pandey and Singh 2008). Accordingly, such findings directed to examine the role of reactive functionality linked to trimethoxysilane during the synthesis of noble metal nanoparticles and indeed real-time synthesis of all noble metal nanoparticles together their multimetallic analogues have been made involving the active role 3-APTMS and 3-GPTMS for the first time under ambient conditions (Pandey and Chauhan 2010, 2012, 2013a, b, 2014a, b; Pandey and Pandey 2014a, b, 2016; Pandey et al. 2015a, 2016, 2017; Pandey and Singh 2014, 2015a, b) with further innovation on noble metal nanoparticle synthesis by incorporating microwave exposure of 3-APTMS and 3-GPTMS modulated nanoparticle synthesis with few seconds (Pandey et al. 2015b) as shown in video link (Pandey 2018a, b, c). In order to control the concentrations of reactive trimethoxysilane during nanoparticle synthesis under microwave the mehanolic solution of precursors containing small amount of ethylene glycol may also be followed as shown in You Tube links (Pandey et al. 2021a). These findings described the use of two functional alkoxysilanes as reducing and stabilizing agents overcoming the limitations of conventional routs of noble metal nanoparticles synthesis and their multimetallic. As disclosed earlier, process was further innovated introducing the role of microwave irradiation that allowed rapid conversion of functional alkoxysilanes assisted formation of noble metal nanoparticles and its multimetallic analogues (Pandey et al. 2015b). These findings precisely demonstrated reactive trimethoxysilane assisted controlled and rapid synthesis of noble metal nanoparticles and its multimetallic analogues. Although the use of functional trimethoxysilanes in yielding Ag-NP or other noble metal nanoparticles are most effective however, the Ag-NP formulation that can be converted into: (i) thin film over the surface for biomedical applications like surgical catheter or normal catheter or like, (ii) Ag–NP spray allowing assembling of Ag–NP over any desired substrate just by spraying, (iii) embedding the Ag–NP over the nylon cloth or other cotton cloth are of further potential applications. The properties of organotrialkoxysilane-derived noble metal nanoparticles may further be controlled via replacing 3-glycidoxypropyltrimethoxysilane by small electrophiles as described earlier (Pandey and Pandey 2016) and enable rapid formation of noble metal nanoparticles in the presence of 3-Aminopropyltrimethoxysilane as shown in video link (Pandey 2020a, 2024b, c).

Organotrimethoxysilanes-mediated seeding of bimetallic and trimetallic has been precisely studied under controlled condition. The ratio of Pd–Au during bimetallic metal nanoparticles has drastically affected the nucleation of bimetallic nanoparticles and also on the pattern of bimetallic process. When Palladium salt (80%) and gold salt (20%) are allowed to interact under simultaneous (Fig. 7) and Sequential method (Fig. 8) of bimetallic formation variable nanostructure of the same was observed. Palladium salt (20%) and gold salt (80%) as shown in Fig. 9 under simultaneous and Fig. 10 under simultaneous results remarkable variation in bimetallic arrangements.

The presence of Organotrimethoxysilane during bimetallic nanoparticles formation precisely control arrangement of bimetallic orientation and transition from bimetallic to alloying is noted when the lattice constant of two metals undergoing interaction was very close. A typical example is the case gold and silver as shown in

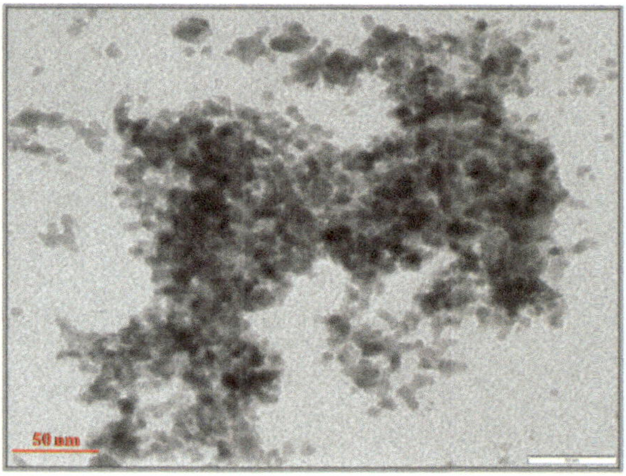

Fig. 7 TEM image of simultaneously made organotrialoxysilane-derived 80% Pd–Au 20%

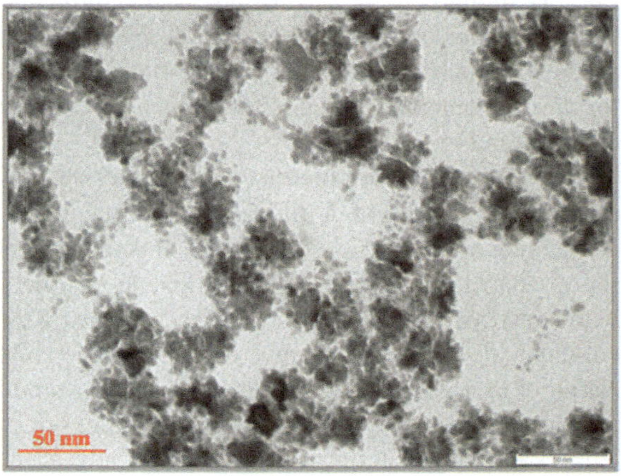

Fig. 8 TEM image of sequentially s made organotrialoxysilane-derived 80% Pd–Au 20%

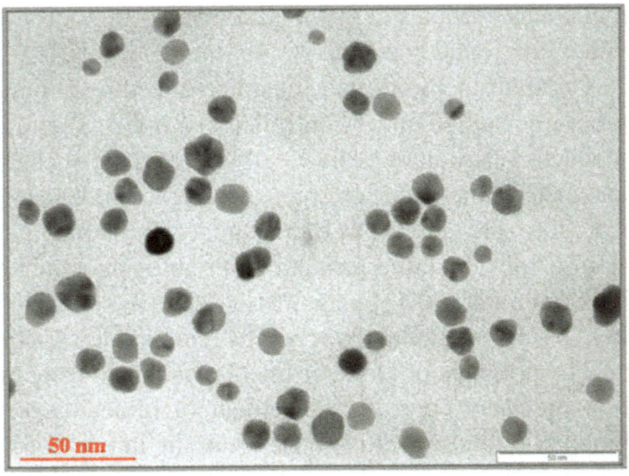

Fig. 9 TEM image of simultaneously made organotrialoxysilane-derived 20%Pd–Au 80%

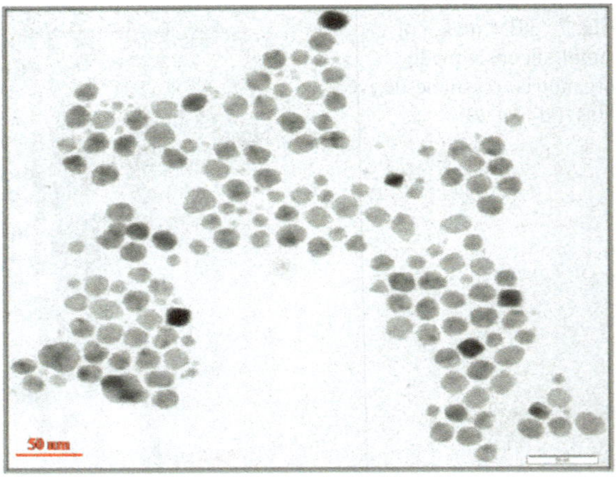

Fig. 10 TEM image of sequentially synthesized 20% Pd–Au 80%

Fig. 11. Similarly reactive trimethoxysilane further control arrangement in trimetallalic orientation as shown in Fig. 12. These bimetallic/trimetallic nanoparticles under specific reaction condition allow the formation if screen printable ink most suitable for making nanoparticles modified screen printed electrode made in our laboratory as shown in Fig. 13.

Reactive Organotrimethoxysilanes-Derived Siloxane—Nanoparticle Self-assembling Nanofluid A siloxane is the functional group found in organosilicon compounds that contain the Si–O–Si linkage commonly used to create materials for variety of applications. These siloxane polymers are used to prepare surfaces with superhydrophobic properties. Accordingly, a direct synthetic route yielding a colloidal siloxane polymer in a volatile organic solvent would enable facile fabrication of thin membranes with controlled permeability. Siloxane polymers may be used as membranes for gas exchange applications (e.g., artificial skin and soft contact lenses) and has been of great attention of advanced research program. Generally,

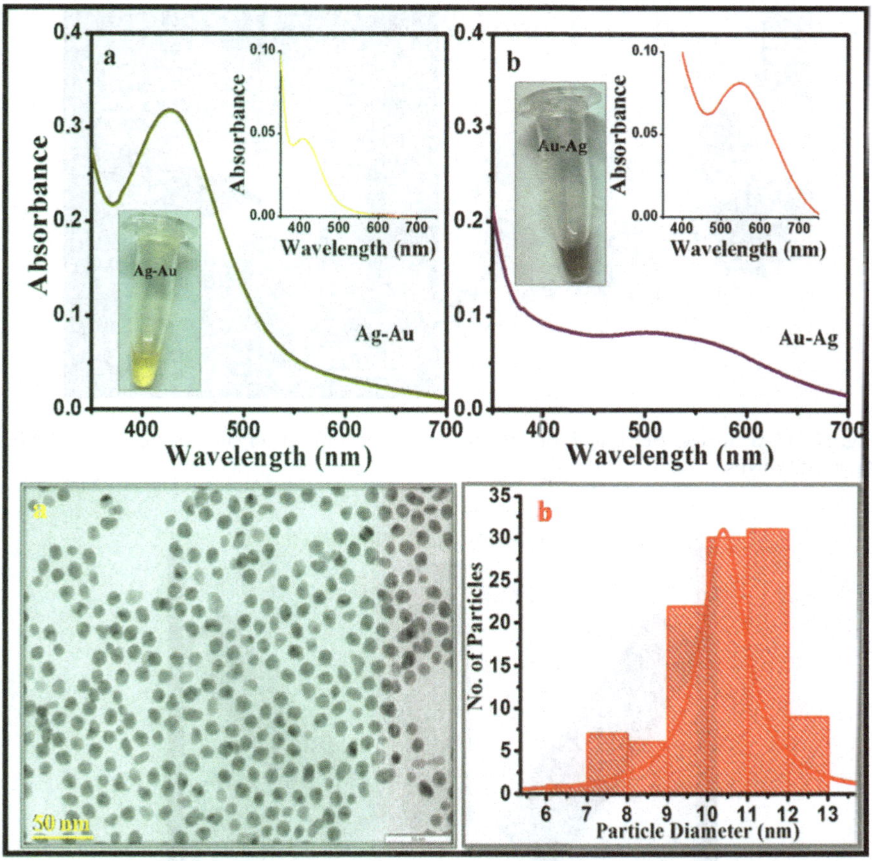

Fig. 11 Top: The UV-Vis spectra of the corresponding organotrialkoxysilane-derived Ag–Au and Au–Ag and the insets shows the UV-Vis spectra of monometallic 80Ag 20%Au and 80%Au20%Ag; bottom: TEM image of Au–Ag, **b** particle size distribution

alkylsilane with active participation of –Si-H linkages has been reported for making siloxane polymer. High reactivity of –Si-H functionality restricted the proper exploration of while making siloxane and directed us to make such polymer using reactive organotrimethoxysilane. Recently, acetone-induced polymerization of 3-APTMS in chloroform has been observed leading to the formation of siloxane. Using 1H, 13C, and 29SiNMR techniques they have proved that acetone reacts with the propylamine of trimethoxysilane to form an imine [(CH3)$_2$C=N(CH$_2$)$_3$Si(OCH$_3$)$_3$], IPTMS or N-isopropylidene-3-aminopropyltrimethoxysilane. The water that is released during the imine formation hydrolyzes the trimethoxysilane inducing thereby the formation of siloxane containing Si–O–Si bridges. Further we have also observed that IPTMS formed from 3-APTMS and acetone showed catalytic activity in reduction of noble metal cations into respective nanoparticles forming AuNPs and siloxane polymer nanofluid (Pandey et al. 2017, 2020a; Pandey and Pandey 2017; Tiwari et al.

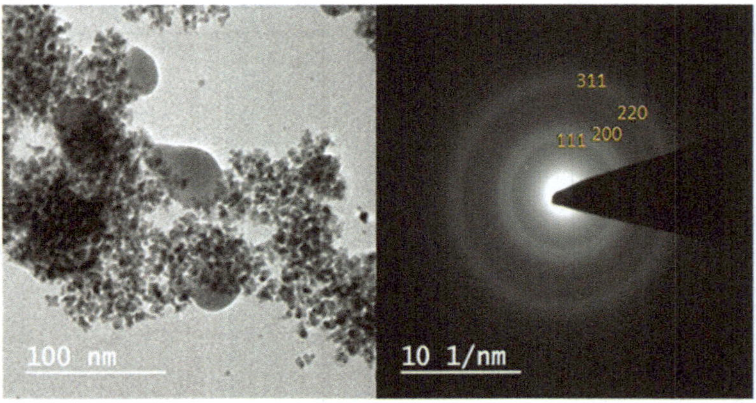

Fig. 12 TEM image (left) and diffraction pattern (right) of organotrialkoxysilane-derived Ag@(AuPd)NPs

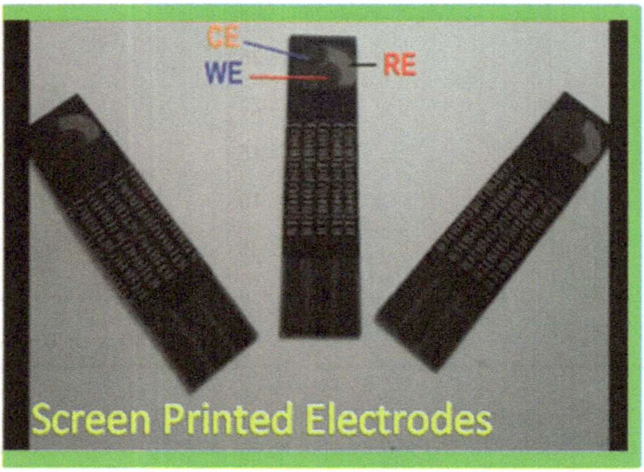

Fig. 13 Organotrialkoxysilane-derived PdNP modified screen printed electrodes

2023). We further demonstrated the controlled polymerization of indole monomers in various organic solvents (Pandey and Prakash 1998a, b; Pandey et al. 2009, 2012, 2024). These findings directed us to understand gold cation-induced polymerization of indole monomer, which forms a Lewis acid–base adduct with gold cations to form a polyindole–gold nanoparticle nanofluid. This type of conversion has been recorded in other volatile solvents such as chloroform, acetonitrile, and dichloromethane (Pandey et al. 2020a). Both siloxane-gold nanoparticles and polyindole–gold nanoparticle nanofluid underwent self-assembly. The nanofluid with Ag–NP can be made which acts as disinfectant against bacterial and viruses (Pandey 2020b) made by mixing:(1) Ag–NP made using 3-APTMS and 3-GPTMS in methanol in appropriate ratio under microwave exposure and if required small amount of ethylene glycol may also be added in methanolic solution of nanoparticle's precursors and (2) conversion of 3-APTMS into siloxane in acetone under ambient conditions. As made nanofluid can further be diluted in acetone or methanol as per requirement and can be used as spray for self-assembling on suitable surface including mask, PPE, surgical catheter and also could be used as bandage for burn infections as demonstrated in you tube link (Pandey 2020c, d). Such material open new horizon on developing extremely stable membrane for biosensor design analogous to that of biological membrane in thickness and also in realizing in molecular recognition of channel forming protein.

Functional Trimethoxysilane-Mediated Synthetic Insertion of Metal Nanoparticles and Their Cheaper Transition Metal Analogues Within Mesoporous Matrix. Porous silica nanoparticles (NPs)/mesoporous silica has been another important materials for variety of application due to their unique properties, such as a large specific surface area and pore volume, controllable particle size and excellent biocompatibility. Mesoporous silica nanoparticles (MSNPs) with a pore size ranging from 2 to 50 nm have been proved as are excellent candidates for drug delivery and biomedical applications. Accordingly, ordered mesoporous silica of M41S family was first reported in the early 1990s, followed by subsequent innovations for variety of applications especially in; (1) a large surface area and pore volume for drug adsorption and loading within the pore channels, (2) options for tuning adjustable pore size to control over drug loading and drug release kinetics, (3) for controlled and targeted drug delivery, (4) in vivo biosafety, biodegradation, biodistribution and excretion, (5) combinations with magnetic and/or luminescent compounds potentially useful for bioimaging, and (6) synthetic incorporation of metal nanoparticles and their multimetallic analogues for variety of excitable applications ranging from assets for carbon free energy devices and options for achieving tuneable catalytic activity and as bioactive materials for bone regeneration. These mesoporous silica are originally derived from tri/tetra-alkoxysilane and proved to be excellent nanomaterial for further innovations with functional trimethoxysilane-derived formulations even before or after achieving controlled mesoporous geometry (Pandey 2017, 2019). Accordingly we attempted to explore the roles of functional trimethoxysilane in both synthetic incorporation of metal nanoparticles and their multimetallic analogues of cheaper transition metals as shown in Fig. 14 most suitable for hydrogen evolution reaction (Pandey 2016, 2018c, 2021; Pandey et al. 2020b, 2021b, c, d; Pandey and Singh 2018).

Reactive Organotrimethoxysilane-Derived Fluorescent Nanoparticles. Generally, gold or silver NPs display weak fluorescence however their use in imaging HeLa cells has been demonstrated (He et al. 2008; Lu and Chen 2012) where variety of parameters such as particle size, decay times, ligands on surfaces, metal atom valence states, and crystallinity imparted the fluorescence spectra of such NPs. Accordingly the role of surface functionalization of gold nanoparticles has been another way to control the fluorescence activity of gold nanoparticles and the role of amine functionalized organotrimethoxysilane have been demonstrated in our group (Pandey et al. 1999b, c, d, e, 2001a, b, c, d; Pandey 1999, 2018a, 2025a; Joshi et al. 2004; Pandey and Upadhyay 2001, 2003; Pandey and Singh 2008). As described in preceeding section,

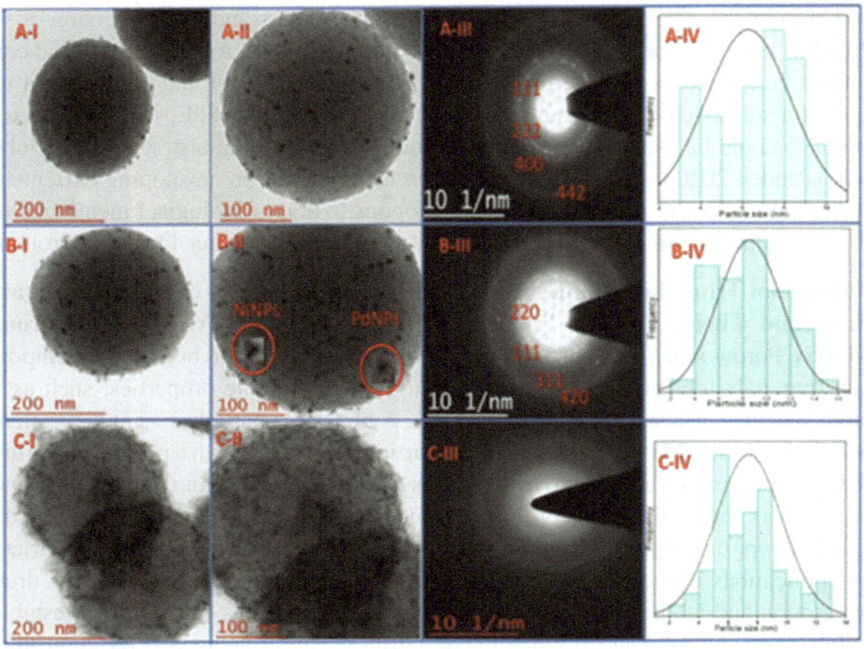

Fig. 14 TEM images, SAED pattern and of PdNPs inserted mesoporous silica nanoparticles (A-i–A-iv), Pd–Ni bimetallic [Pd–Ni (1:1 ratio)](B-i–B-iv) and Pd–Ni bimetallic [Pd–Ni(1:2 ratio)] (C-i–C-iv)

3-GPTMS efficiently allow the reduction of 3-APTMS capped noble metal cations apart from direct reducing ability of 3-GPTMS to palladium cations. The process of nanoparticles and their multimettalic analogue formation has been recorded at room temperature and does not require any additional reagent however the process can be drastically fastened limited within minute under microwave exposure. It has been found that the gold nanoparticles made in absence and under microwave exposure are fluorescent and the fluorescencent activity and the same can further be controlled by controlling 3-APTMS/3-GPTMS ratio (Mitra and Pandey 2022; Mitra et al. 2022). An increase in 3-GPTMS amount caused reduction in size of gold nanoparticles facilitating the fluorescent activity of the same. These finding extended the introduction of sensitive optical sensors for variety of applications since imaging of emission spectroscopy especially fluorescence emission introduce selectivity in analysis. Accordingly, fluorescence spectroscopy played central role in identifying the specific interaction in biomolecules while undergoing the interaction of fluorescence polarization, normally associated to either shift in fluorescence emission as a function of specific electrostatic interaction with the bonding associated to emission spectra (Pandey and Weetall 1995b, c). Fluorescence polarization has further proved as an efficient tool in bioimaging of antigen antibody interaction when tubulin complexed to metal free phorphyrin like metal free tetrakis(4-carboxyphenyl)porphyrin (TCPP) in the presence of antimitotic agents (Morais et al. 2003). Cephalomannine caused the induction of a new fluorescence peak at 651 nm only above 1 μM. These findings justified the role of fluorescence polarization in the presence of specific molecule that undergo interaction with bonding of fluorescent molecules (Morais et al. 2003).

The role of reactive organotrimethoxysilane-derived noble metal nanoparticles has been further examined recently by our group while dealing with fluorescence spectroscopy of well-known fluorophores (e.g., fluorescein, rhodamine, and L-tryptophan) (Pandey et al. 2020c). Reactive organotrimethoxysilane in one way protect the nanogeometry of noble metal nanoparticles and on the other hand may also undergo faster electromeric interaction with known fluorescent probe and act as spacer between fluorescent probe and metal nanoparticles (Pandey et al. 2020c; Tiwar et al. 2025). When the concentrations of spacer is altered that ultimately change the distance between metal nanoparticles and spacer was followed by variation of fluorescence intensity of standard fluorophore either through fluorescence enhancement or quenching and finally tune either to decrease or increase the nanogeometry of noble metal nanoparticles causing significant variation of emission spectra (Pandey et al. 2020c). Another way of exploring the fluorescence spectroscopy associated to metal nanoparticles in analytical diagnostics is the measurement of resonance Rayleigh scattering under the condition when excitation and emission wavelength are allowed to be same i.e. $\Delta\lambda = 0$ (Pandey et al. 2021e). Such finding has been demonstrated in non-enzymatioc sensing of blood glucose and hydrazine-an organic molecule that can precisely explored in hydrogen evolution reaction (Pandey et al. 2021b). Reactive Organotrimethoxysilane one way allowed synthetic incorporation of Pd–Ni bimetallic within mesoporous silica/silica nanoparticles having efficient catalytic activity for decomposition of hydrazine into hydrogen and nitrogen and other hand organotrimethoxysilane-derived gold nanoparticles acted as efficient nanomaterial for probing the decomposition of the hydrazine based on monitoring RRS signal of organotrimethoxysilane derived gold nanoparticles (Pandey et al. 2021b, e). Hydrazine concentration's dependent RRS signal is recorded and were explored in identifying complete decomposion of hydrazine as shown in Fig. 15.

Reactive organotrimethoxysilane-derived gold nanoparticles has been found to display efficient fluorescence emission and the emission intensity is found as a function of 3-APTMS/3-GPTMA ratio that ultimately controlled the size of gold nanoparticles (Mitra et al. 2022). Further the emission spectra of as made gold nanoparticles has also been found as a function of excitation wavelength. At the excitation wavelength of 360 nm the fluorescence emission spectra of organotrimethoxysilane functionalized gold nanoparticles is recorded at 460 nm and has been explored in sensitive dopamine present in cerebrospinal fluid (Mitra et al. 2022). The nature of emission spectra is also found depending on the organotroalkoxysilane-mediated synthetic strategy whether made under microwave exposure or under ambient condition however, both types of gold nanoparticles are fluorescent as shown in Fig. 16. Recent finding demonstrated that organotrimethoxysilanes mediate the syntheses of fluorescent gold nanoparticles and TiO_2-Supported Ag–Ni nanocatalyst for selective decomposition of hydrazine (Mitra et al. 2023). These finding opened a new rout of sensing and catalytic application in dealing with many unresolved scientific issues.

Fig. 15 Synchronous fluorescence spectra at delta $\lambda = 0$, recorded before (ii) and after (iii) hydrous hydrazine decomposition

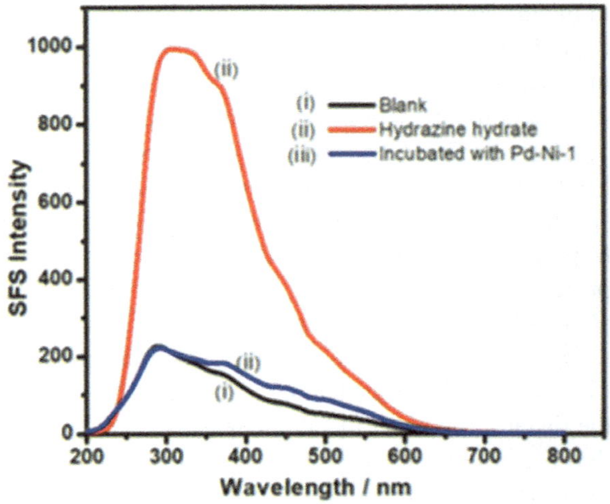

Fig. 16 Fluorescence spectra of AuNP made through control over 3-APTMS and 3-GPTMS ratio under microwave exposure (AuNP-1 and AuNP-2) and the same without microwave exposure (AuNP-AM)

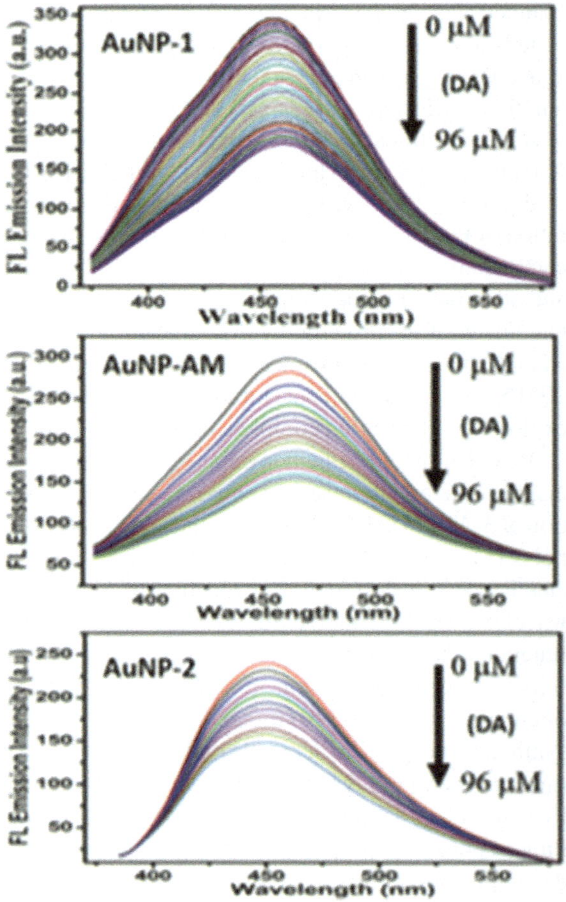

Reactive Organotrimethoxysilane-Derived Functional Prussian Blue Nanoparticles. Metal-hexacyanoferrates (MHCF) have played an important role in variety of scientific applications especially in the field of molecular magnets, as electrode materials in rechargeable battery design, and as electrochromic, ion-exchange, ion-sensing, photomagnetic and electrocatalytic materials. Two metal centers among which when both of them is Fe, when coordinates with CN group, a three dimensional framework of cubic symmetry is formed having octahedral coordination and the compounds are known as Prussian blue (PB). Such materials are made either through a co-precipitation method or by electro-synthesis imparting the precise control of the stoichiometric ratio of two metals in the three dimensional frameworks results into rapid nucleation and the PB obtained under this conditions lack functional nanogeometry and processability for specific application thus many unique properties of PB remain in question for practical designs. Accordingly, a new synthetic route is required for the synthesis of PB nanoparticles using organic moieties as the active reagents that allow: (i) the simultaneous nucleation of PBNP, (ii) solubility of the resulting pigment in targeted reaction medium, and (iii) stabilization of the resulting mixed nanogeometry of PB during practical applications. Reactive Organotrimethoxysilane like 3-aminopropyltrimethoxysilane (Pandey et al. 2013, 2018a, b, 2021f, g; Pandey and Pandey 2013c) and 2-(3,4-Epoxycyclohexyl)ethyltrimethoxysilane in the presence of cyclohexanone allowed controlled synthesis of Prussian blue nanoparticles and their multimetallic analogue for variety of potential applications (Pandey et al. 2018a). As made Prussian blue nanoparticles behave as peroxidase mimetic and the efficiency of enzymatic like activity can be tuned from the nanogeometry of processable Prussian blue nanoparticles.

Reactive Organotrimethoxysilane-Derived Porous Nanostructured Palladium–Cobalt–Silica as Heterogeneous Catalysts for Oxygen Evolution Reaction. The potential for the need of cheaper electrolyzers in water splitting reaction especially derived from nickel/cobalt is very well documented however their use has been restricted due to stability for their exploration in targeted medium that has been one of the main challenging issue of world researchers and variety of approaches are being investigated (Medina et al. 2025). Nanostructured silica has been very well documented as suitable matrix for such stabilization of Nickel/Cobalt nanoparticles. Accordingly we have reported the stabilization of both Ni and Co catalayst within nanostrucrtured silica derived from organotrimethoxysilane. Organotrimethoxysilane-mediated formation of Co@Pdnps were made using Co–NTA nanowires acting as a precursor made through hydrothermal synthesis of cobalt salt and Nitrilotriacetic acid (NTA) (Pandey 2022, 2023a; Pandey and Singh 2023, 2024). Co@Pdnps were synthesized using variable content of organotrimethoxysilane in an N-doped carbon matrix (Co@Pdnps) to control the presence of nanostructured silica after calcinations at 600–700 °C useful in OER (Pandey 2022, 2023a; Pandey and Singh 2023) using cobalt-NTA (nitrilotriacetic acid) that justified that an increase in silica content enhances the catalytic property of electrolyzer. We have

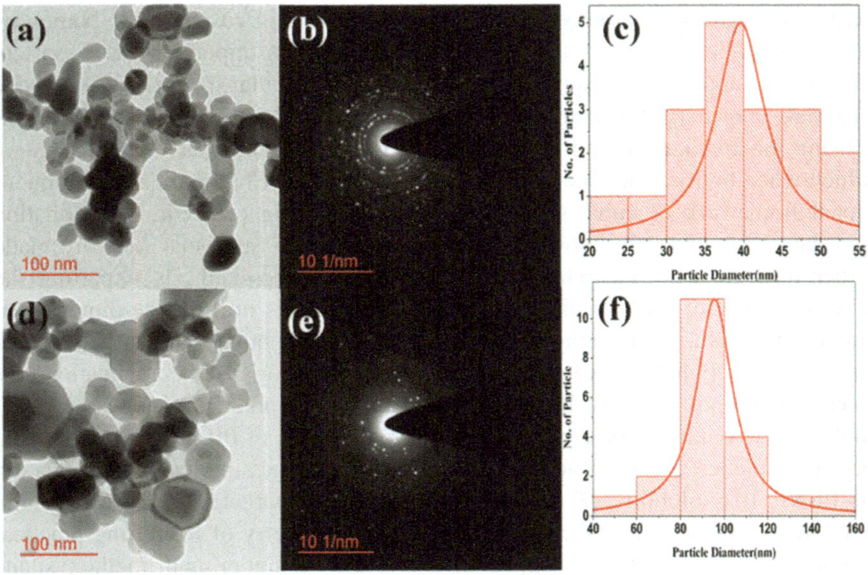

Fig. 17 TEM images, SAED pattern, and particles size distribution of CoPd@NC-1 (**a–c**) and CoPd@NC-2 (**d–f**), respectively

further innovated this finding in making porous Nanostructured Palladium–Cobalt–Silica by controlling the organized reaction between palladium/cobalt/Nickel in the presence of reactive trimethoxysilane and NTA followed by calcinations at 600–700 °C as heterogeneous porous nanocatalysts as shown in Fig. 17 justifying several fold enhancement in catalytic activity during water splitting reaction (Pandey and Singh 2024; Pandey 2023b).

2 Conclusion

Reactive organotrimethoxysilanes having organic functionalities like alkylamine, Epoxycyclohexyl-, glycidoxy- and even trimethoxysilane have been found to create novel nanostructured materials for real applications most suitable for biosensor design as support matrix, electrocatalyst, enzyme mimetics. Our contribution on (1) Reactive organotrimethoxysilanes-derived biocompatible thin film of organically modified silicate, (2) Reactive organotrimethoxysilanes-derived metal organic framework in nanostructured network of organically modified silicate, (3) Reactive organotrimethoxysilanes-mediated synthesis of processable monometallic, bimetallic and trimetallic noble metal nanoparticles, (4) Reactive organotrimethoxysilanes-mediated synthetic insertion of metal nanoparticles and their cheaper transition metal analogues within mesoporous matrix,

(5) Reactive organotrimethoxysilanes-derived fluorescent nanoparticles, (6) Reactive organotrimethoxysilanes-derived functional Prussian blue nanoparticles and (7) Reactive organotrimethoxysilanes-derived Porous Nanostructured Palladium–Cobalt–Silica as Heterogeneous Catalysts are reviewed justifying their potential significance in real practical applications.

Competing Interests The author declare no conflict of interest.

Ethics Approval Not required.

References

M. Aslam, L. Fu, M. Su, K. Vijayamohanan, V.P. Dravid, Novel one-step synthesis of amine-stabilized aqueous colloidal gold nanoparticles. J. Mater. Chem. **14**, 1795–1797 (2004). https://doi.org/10.1021/la060045z

S.K. Bhargava, J.M. Booth, S. Agrawal, P. Coloe, G. Kar, Gold nanoparticle formation during Bromoaurate reduction by amino acids. Langmuir **21**, 5949–5956 (2005)

A.H. Boonstra, C.A.M. Mulder, Effect of hydrolytic polycondensation of tetraethoxysilane on specific surface area of SiO_2 gels. J. Non-Cryst. Solids **105**, 201–206 (1988)

D.C. Bradley, R.C. Mehrotra, D.P. Gaur, *Metal Alkoxides* (Academic Press, New York, 1978), p. 27

M. Brust, M. Walker, D. Bethell, D.J. Schiffrin, R. Whyman, Synthesis of thiol-derivatised gold nanoparticles in a two-phase liquid–liquid system. J. Chem. Soc. Chem. Commun. **7**, 801–802 (1994). https://doi.org/10.1039/C39940000801

C. Claudia, B. Alexandre, G. Alessandra, M. Riccardo, Silica-based nanoparticles: a versatile tool for the development of efficient imaging agents. Chem. Soc. Rev. **44**, 4645–4671 (2015)

P. Colomban, The use of metal nanoparticles to produce yellow, red and iridescent colour, from bronze age to present times in lustre pottery and glass: Solid state chemistry, spectroscopy and nanostructure. J. Nano Res. **8**, 109–132 (2009)

M.-C. Daniel, D. Astruc, Gold nanoparticles: assembly, supramolecular chemistry, quantum-size-related properties, and applications toward biology, catalysis, and nanotechnology. Chem. Rev. **104**, 293–346 (2004)

H. Duan, S. Nie, Etching colloidal gold nanocrystals with hyperbranched and multivalent polymers: a new route to fluorescent and water-soluble atomic clusters. J. Am. Chem. Soc. **129**(9), 2412–2413 (2007). https://doi.org/10.1021/ja067727t

I. Freestone, N. Meeks, M. Sax, C. Higgit, The Lycurgus cup–a Roman nanotechnology. Gold Bull. **40**, 270–277 (2007)

G. Frens, Controlled nucleation for the regulation of the particle size in monodisperse gold suspensions. Nat. Phys. Sci. **241**, 20–22 (1973)

S. Gomez, K. Philippot, V. Collière, B. Chaudret, F. Senocq, P. Lecant, Gold nanoparticles from self-assembled gold(i) amine precursors Chem. Ther. Communities, 1945–1946 (2000). https://doi.org/10.1039/B005327I

H. He, C. Xie, J. Ren, Non bleaching fluorescence of gold nanoparticles and its applications in cancer cell imaging. Anal. Chem. **80**(15), 5951–5957 (2008)

S. Huang, K. Minami, H. Sakaue, T. Shingubara Sm Takahagi, Optical spectroscopic studies of the dispersibility of gold nanoparticle solutions. J. Appl. Phys. **92**, 7491 (2002). https://doi.org/10.1063/1.1518758

S.R. Isaacs, E.C. Cutler, J.-S. Park, T.R. Lee, Y.-S. Shon, Synthesis of Tetraoctylammonium-protected gold nanoparticles with improved stability. Langmuir **21**(13), 5689–5692 (2005)

K.A. Joshi, P.C. Pandey, W. Chen, A. Mulchandani, Ormosil encapsulated Pyrroloquinoline Quinone-modified electrochemical sensor for thiols. Electroanalysis **16**(23), 1938–1943 (2004). https://doi.org/10.1002/elan.200303040

K. Kazuyoshi, N. Kazuki, Controlled pore formation in organotrialkoxysilane-derived hybrids: from aerogels to hierarchically porous monoliths. Chem. Soc. Rev. **40**, 754–770 (2011)

A. Kotiaho, R. Lahtinen, A. Efimov, H. Lehtivuori, N.V. Tkachenko, T. Kanerva, H. Lemmetyinen, Synthesis and time-resolved fluorescence study of porphyrin-functionalized gold nanoparticles. J. Photochem. Photobiol. A Chem. **212**, 129–134 (2010)

A. Kumar, X. Zhang, X.-J. Lian, Gold nanoparticles: Emerging paradigm for targeted drug delivery system. Biotechnol. Adv. **31**, 593–606 (2013). https://doi.org/10.1016/j.biotechadv.2012.10.00

D.V. Leff, L. Brandt, J.R. Heath, Synthesis and characterization of hydrophobic, organically-soluble gold nanocrystals functionalized with primary amines. Langmuir **12**, 4723–4730 (1996)

U. Leonhardt, Invisibility cup. Nature Photon **1**, 207–208 (2007)

J.L. Lima Filho, P.C. Pandey, H.H. Weetall, An amperometric flow injection analysis enzyme sensor for sucrose using a tetracyanoquinodimethane modified graphite paste electrode. Biosens. Bioelectron. **11**, 719–723 (1996). https://doi.org/10.1016/0956-5663(96)85922-7

Y. Lu, W. Chen, Sub-nanometre sized metal clusters: from synthetic challenges to the unique property discoveries. Chem. Soc. Rev. **41**(9), 3594–3623 (2012)

M.N. Martin, J.I. Basham, P. Chando, S.-K. Eah, Charged gold nanoparticles in non-polar solvents: 10-min synthesis and 2D self-assembly. Langmuir **26**(10), 7410–7417 (2010). https://doi.org/10.1021/la100591h

D.R. Matthews, E. Bown, A. Watson, R.R. Holman, J. Steemson, S. Hughes, D. Scott, Pen-sized digital 30-second blood glucose meter. Lancet **329**(8536), 778–779 (1987)

O.E. Medina, A.A. Amell, D. Lopez, A. Santamaría, Comprehensive review of nickel-based catalysts advancements for CO_2 methanation. Renew. Sust. Energ. Rev. **249**, 114926 (2025). https://doi.org/10.1016/j.rser.2024.114926

M.D. Mitra, P.C. Pandey, Functional trialkoxysilane mediated controlled synthesis of fluorescent goldnanoparticles and fluoremetric sensing of dopamine. Opt. Mater. **132**, 112810 (2022)

M.D. Mitra, P.C. Pandey, S. Shukla, Functional trialkoxysilane mediated controlled synthesis of fluorescent gold nanoparticles and fluoremetric sensing of dopamine. Opt. Mater. **132**, 112810 (2022). https://doi.org/10.1016/j.optmat.2022.112810

M.D. Mitra, H. Singh, R. Singh, P.C. Pandey, Organotrialkoxysilanes Mediate the Syntheses of Fluorescent Gold Nanoparticles and TiO_2-Supported Ag−Ni nanocatalysts for selective hydrazine sensing and decomposition. Chem. Select **8**, e202302161 (2023). https://doi.org/10.1002/slct.202302161

S. Morais, P.C. Pandey, W. Chen, A. Mulchandani, A novel bioassay for screening andquantification of Taxanes. Chem. Commun. **10**, 1188–1189 (2003). https://doi.org/10.1039/B302112B

J.D.S. Newman, G.J. Blanchard, Formation of gold nanoparticles using amine reducing agents. J. Mater. Chem. **14**, 1795–1797 (2006). https://doi.org/10.1021/la060045z

I. Otsuka, M. Osaka, Y. Sakai, C. Travelet, J.-L. Putaux, B. Redouane, Self-assembly of Maltoheptaose-block-polystyrene into micellar nanoparticles and encapsulation of gold nanoparticles. Langmuir **29**(49), 5224–15230 (2013)

P.C. Pandey, A new conducting polymer-coated glucose sensor. J. Chem. Soc. Faraday Trans. **1 84**, 2259–2265 (1988)

P.C. Pandey, Tetracyanoquinodimethane-mediated flow injection analysis electrochemical sensor for NADH coupled with dehydrogenase enzymes. Anal. Biochem. **221**(2), 392–396 (1994). https://doi.org/10.1006/abio.1994.1431

P.C. Pandey, Mediated bioelectrochemistry within graphite paste electrode. Trans Indian. Inst. met. **51**, 319–325 (1998)

P.C. Pandey, A process for the preparation of ferrocene encapsulated palladium-linked organically modfied sol-gel glass (Pd-ormosil), Indian Patent 196900, Oct 1999

P.C. Pandey, (2016), A process for making functional alkoxysilane stabilized nickel palladium bimetallic nanocrystallite for catalytic hydrogen evolution there from Indian Patent 357915, Dec 2016

P.C. Pandey, (2017), A process for making self assembled siloxane-polyindole-gold nanoparticles nanocomposite, Indian Paten 343403 filed on 09-12-2017 and granted on 05-08-2020

P.C. Pandey, (2018a), https://youtu.be/kZ-DvLKmOjs. 16 Sep, 2018

P.C. Pandey, (2018b), https://youtu.be/d6369j-SG78. 16 Sep. 2018

P.C. Pandey, (2018c), https://youtu.be/kyzTY14GibY. 22 June 2018

P.C. Pandey, (2018d), https://youtu.be/rVydRLrGOY8. 22 Jun 2018

P.C. Pandey, (2018e), A process for making functional alkoxysilane mediated silica-zeolite supported nickel-palladium bimetallic nanocrystallite for catalytic hydrogen evolution there from Indian Patent 201811021635, June 2018

P.C. Pandey, (2019), A process for microwave assisted functional alkoxysilanes mediated synthesis of monometallic, bimetallic and trimetallic noble metal nanoparticleS, Indian Patent 201911021365, filed on 29/05/2019 and published on 201911021365

P.C. Pandey, (2020a), https://youtu.be/MkSvBJJABcE24. Apr 2020

P.C. Pandey, (2020b), A process on amine-functionalized alkoxysilane derived silver nanoparticles as potentioal antimicrobial and antiviral agengts. Indian Patent 202011014527, filed on 01/04/2020 and published on 08/10/2021

P.C. Pandey, (2020c), https://youtu.be/ViQ9ivQ8msg. 13 Apr 2020

P.C. Pandey, (2020d). https://youtu.be/FeWbw2aH8m8. 16 Jan 2025

P.C. Pandey, (2021), A process for organotrialkoxysilane functionalized palladium-cobalt nanoparticles as potent catalysts for oxygen evolution reaction, Indian Patent 202111060340 Dec 2021

P.C. Pandey, (2021a). https://youtu.be/Zl-QT574j8Q. 17Jul 24, 2021

P.C. Pandey, (2022), A process making porous nanostructured silica with option of tuning carbon, nitrogen, palladium, cobalt/nickel in desired ratio for potential catalytic applications with example in water splitting. Indian Patent 202211058096, Oct 2022

P.C. Pandey, (2023a), A process for making porous nanostructured silicate encapsulated palladium-cobalt-nickel trimetallic nanoparticles for green hydrogen production. Indian Patent 202311002062, Jan 2023

P.C. Pandey, (2023b), https://youtu.be/ViQ9ivQ8msg. 4 Feb 2023

P.C. Pandey, (2024a), https://youtu.be/SsmJn66_Irk. 16 May 2024

P.C. Pandey, (2024b), https://youtu.be/GzWWUq4H8Ds; https://youtu.be/Zl-QT574j8Q. 17 May 2024

P.C. Pandey, (2024c), https://youtu.be/GiZnSmHv4j4. 11 Feb 2020

P.C. Pandey, (2025a), https://youtu.be/yXjwfu1bEQQ. 7 Jan 2025

P.C. Pandey, (2025b), https://youtu.be/aFGt1GbMnSA, 7 Jan 2025

P.C. Pandey, D.S. Chauhan, A process for in-situ generation of noble metal nanoparticles and thereafter core shell of the same. Indian Patent 331496 Oct 2010

P.C. Pandey, D.S. Chauhan, 3-Glycidoxypropyltrimethoxysilane mediated in situ synthesis of noble metal nanoparticles: application to hydrogen peroxide sensing. Analyst **137**, 376–385 (2012)

P.C. Pandey, A.P. Mishra, Conducting polymer-coated enzyme microsensor for urea. Analyst **113**, 329–331 (1988)

P.C. Pandey, A. Pandey, Novel synthesis of Prussian blue nanoparticles and nanocomposite sol: electro-analytical application in hydrogen peroxide sensing. Electrochim. Acta **87**, 1–8 (2013a). https://doi.org/10.1016/j.electacta.2012.08.069

P.C. Pandey, A. Pandey, Cyclohexanone and 3-aminopropyltrimethoxysilane mediated controlled synthesis of mixed nickel-iron hexacyanoferrate nanosol for selective sensing of glutathione and hydrogen peroxide. Analyst **138**, 952–959 (2013b)

P.C. Pandey, A. Pandey, Novel synthesis of super peroxidase mimetic polycrystalline mixed metal hexacyanoferrates nanoparticles dispersion. Analyst **138**, 2295–2301 (2013c)

P.C. Pandey, G. Pandey, Role of organic functionalities linked to alkoxysilane precursors in nanomaterials synthesis and their biomedical applications. MRS Online Proc. Libr. **1719**, 11–20 (2014a). https://doi.org/10.1557/opl.2015.635

P.C. Pandey, G. Pandey, Tunable functionality and nanogeometry in tetrahydrofuran hydroperoxide and 3-aminopropyl-trimethoxysilane mediated synthesis of gold nanoparticles; functional application in glutathione sensing. J. Mater. Chem. B **2**, 3383–3390 (2014b)

P.C. Pandey, G. Pandey, One-pot two-step rapid synthesis of 3-aminopropyltrimethoxysilane mediated highly atalytic Ag@(PdAu) trmetallic nanoparticles. Catal. Sci. Technol. **6**, 3911–3917 (2016)

P.C. Pandey, G. Pandey, A process for making self-assembled siloxane-polyindole-gold nanoparticle nanocomposite. Indian Patent 343403, granted Sept 2017

P.C. Pandey, R. Prakash, Electrochemical synthesis of polyindole-a study for rechargeable battery application. J. Electrochem. Soc. **145**, 999–1003 (1998a)

P.C. Pandey, R. Prakash, Characterization of electropolymerized polyindole-application in the construction of a solid-state ion-selective electrode. J. Electrochem. Soc. **145**, 4103–4107 (1998b)

P.C. Pandey, B. Singh, Library of electrocatalytic sites in nano-structured domains: electrocatalysis of hydrogen peroxide. Biosens. Bioelectron. **24**, 42–848 (2008)

P.C. Pandey, R. Singh, Tetrahydrofuran hydroperoxide and 3- Aminopropyltrimethoxysilanemediated controlled synthesis of Pd, Pd-Au, Au-Pd nanoparticles: role of palladium nanoparticles on the redox electrochemistry of ferrocenemonocarboxylic acid. Electrochim. Acta **138**, 163–173 (2014)

P.C. Pandey, R. Singh, Controlled synthesis of functional silver nanoparticles dispersible in aqueous and non-aqueous medium. J. Nanosci. Nanotechnol. **15**, 5749–5759 (2015a)

P.C. Pandey, R. Singh, Controlled synthesis of Pd, Pd-Au, nanoparticles; effects of organic amine and silanol groups on the morphology and polycrystallinity of nanomaterials. RSC Adv. **5**, 10964–10973 (2015b)

P.C. Pandey, S. Singh, A process for synthetic insertion of palladium and Prussian blue nanoparticles within mesoporous silica nanoparticles, and their application in selective dopamine sensing, Indian Patent 2018201811006295, (Feb 2018)

P.C. Pandey, S. Singh, Synthesis and properties of Organotrialkoxysilane functionalized palladium–cobalt heterogeneous catalysts for oxygen evolution reaction. Russ. J. Electrochem. **59**(8), 604–615 (2023). https://doi.org/10.1134/S1023193523080074

P.C. Pandey, S. Singh, Studies on porous nanostructured palladium–cobalt–silica as heterogeneous catalysts for oxygen evolution reaction. Russ. J. Electrochem. **60**(9), 749–759 (2024)

P.C. Pandey, S. Upadhyay, Bioelectrochemistry of glucose oxidase immobilized on ferrocene encapsulated ormosil modied electrode. Sens. Actuators B Chem B **76**, 193–198 (2001)

P.C. Pandey, H.H. Weetall, Application of photochemical reaction in electrochemical detection of DNA intercalation. Anal. Chem. **66**(8), 1236–1241 (1994)

P.C. Pandey, H.H. Weetall, Peroxidase- and Tetracyanoquinodimethane-modified graphite paste electrode for the measurement of glucose/lactate/glutamate using enzyme-packed bed reactor. Anal. Biochem. **224**(1), 428–433 (1995a). https://doi.org/10.1006/abio.1995.1062

P.C. Pandey, H.H. Weetall, Detection of aromatic hydrocarbon based on DNA intercalation using an evanescent wave biosensor. Anal. Chem. **67**, 787–792 (1995b)

P.C. Pandey, H.H. Weetall, Evanescent wave Fluorobiosensor for the detection of polyaromatic hydrocarbon based on DNA intercalation. Appl. Biochem. Biotechnol. **55**, 87–94 (1995c)

P.C. Pandey, C. Tran-Minh, F. Lantreibecq, Electrochemical studies on tetrathiafulvalene-tetracyanoquinodimethane modified acetylcholine/choline sensor. Appl. Biochem. Biotechnol. **31**, 145–158 (1991). https://doi.org/10.1007/BF02921785

P.C. Pandey, A.M. Kayastha, V. Pandey, Amperometric enzyme sensor for glucose based on graphite paste-modified electrodes. Appl. Biochem. Biotechnol. **33**, 139–144 (1992). https://doi.org/10.1007/BF02950782

P.C. Pandey, V. Pandey, S. Mehta, A new glucose biosensor based on graphite paste modified with tetracyanoquinodimethane. Indian J. Chem. **32A**, 667–672 (1993)

P.C. Pandey, V. Pandey, S. Mehta, An amperometric enzyme electrode for lactate based on graphite paste modified with tetracyanoquinodimethane. Biosens. Bioelectron. **9**, 365–372 (1994a). https://doi.org/10.1016/0956-5663(94)80037-5

P.C. Pandey, S. Glazier, H.H. Weetall, An Amperometric flow-injection analysis biosensor for glucose based on graphite paste modified with Tetracyanoquinodimethane. Anal. Biochem. **214**(1), 233–237 (1994b). https://doi.org/10.1006/abio.1993.1482

P.C. Pandey, R.W. Aston, H.H. Weetall, Tetracyanoquinodimethane mediated glucose sensor based on a self-assembling alkanethiol/phospholipid bilayer. Biosens. Bioelectron. **10**, 669–674 (1995). https://doi.org/10.1016/0956-5663(95)96957-Z

P.C. Pandey, S. Upadhyay, B.C. Upadhyay, H.H. Weetall, P.K. Chem, Reversal in the kinetics of M-state decay of D96N mutant bacteriorhodopsin. Sensors Actuators **B35-36**, 270–276 (1996)

P.C. Pandey, S. Upadhyay, B.C. Upadhyay, Peroxide biosensors and mediated electrochemical regeneration of redox enzymes. Anal. Biochem. **252**(1), 136–142 (1997). https://doi.org/10.1006/abio.1997.2291

P.C. Pandey, S. Singh, B.C. Upadhyay, H.C. Pathak, C.M.D. Pandey, Sensitivity, selectivity and reproducibility of some mediated electrochemical biosensors/sensors. Anal. Lett. **31**, 2327–2348 (1998a). https://doi.org/10.1080/00032719808005310

P.C. Pandey, S. Upadhyay, B.C. Upadhyay, H.C. Pathak, Ethanol biosensors and electrochemical oxidation of NADH. Anal. Biochem. **260**(2), 136–142 (1998b). https://doi.org/10.1006/abio.1998.2679

P.C. Pandey, S. Upadhyay, B. Upadhyay, H.C. Pathak, C.M.D. Pandey, I. Tiwari, Electrochemical oxidation of ascorbic acid at the surface of chemically modified electrode. Bull. Electrochem. **15**, 438–448 (1999a)

P.C. Pandey, S. Upadhyay, H.C. Pathak, A new glucose biosensor based on sandwiched configuration of organically modified sol-gel glass. Electroanalysis **11**, 59–65 (1999b)

P.C. Pandey, S. Upadhyay, H.C. Pathak, A new glucose biosensor based on encapsulated glucose oxidase within organically modified sol-gel glass. Sensors Actuators **B60**, 83–89 (1999c)

P.C. Pandey, S. Upadhyay, I. Tiwari, V.S. Tripathi, Studies on glucose biosensors based on nonmediated and mediated electrochemical oxidation of reduced glucose oxidase encapsulated within organically modified sol-gel glasses. Electroanalysis **11**(17), 1251–1258 (1999d)

P.C. Pandey, S. Upadhyay, H.C. Pathak, A new ferrocene-linked organically modified electrode sol-gel glass and its application in the construction of ion-selective electrode. Electroanalysis **11**, 950–958 (1999e)

P.C. Pandey, S. Upadhyay, I. Tiwari, V.S. Tripathi, Ormosil-based peroxide biosensor—a comparative study on direct electron transport from horseradish peroxidase. Sensors Actuators B **72**, 224–232 (2001a)

P.C. Pandey, S. Upadhyay, I. Tiwari, S. Sharma, A novel ferrocene-encapsulated palladium-linked ormosil-based electrocatalytic biosensor. Role React. Funct. Group, Electroanal. **13**, 1519–1527 (2001b)

P.C. Pandey, S. Upadhyay, I. Tiwari, V.S. Tripathi, A novel ferrocene encapsulated palladium linked ormosil based electrocatalytic dopamine biosensor. Sensors Actuators B Chem **75**, 48–55 (2001c)

P.C. Pandey, S. Upadhyay, I. Tiwari, V.S. Tripathi, An organically modified silicate-based ethanol biosensor. Anal. Biochem. **288**, 39–45 (2001d)

P.C. Pandey, S. Upadhyay, S. Sharma, Functionalized ormosil-based biosensor. Probing a horseradish peroxidase catalyzed reactions. J. Electrochem. Soc. **150**, H85–H92 (2003)

P.C. Pandey, D.S. Chauhan, V. Singh, Poly(indole-6-carboxylic acid) and tetracyanoquinodimethane-modified electrode for selective oxidation of dopamine. Electrochim. Acta **54**, 2256–2260 (2009)

P.C. Pandey, D.S. Chauhan, V. Singh, Effect of processable polyindole and nanostructured domains on selective sensing of dopamine. Mater. Sci. Eng. C **32**, 1–11 (2012)

P.C. Pandey, D.S. Chauhan, A. Pandey, Novel synthesis of Prussian blue nanoparticles and nanocomposite sol: electro-analytical application in hydrogen peroxide sensing. Electrochim. Acta **87**, 1–8 (2013)

P.C. Pandey, A.K. Pandey, G. Pandey, Functionalized alkoxysilane mediated controlled synthesis of noble metal nanoparticles dispersible in aqueous and non-aqueous medium. J. Nanosci. Nanotechnol. **14**, 6606–6613 (2014a)

P.C. Pandey, D. Pandey, G. Pandey, 3-Aminopropyltrimethoxysialne and organic electron donors mediated synthesis of functional gold nanoparticles and their bioanalytical applications. RSC Adv. **4**, 60563–60573 (2014b)

P.C. Pandey, S. Shukla, Y. Pandey, 3-Aminopropyltrimethoxysilane and graphene oxide/reduced graphene oxide-induced generation of gold nanoparticles and their nanocomposites electrocatalytic and kinetic activity. RSC Adv. **56**(2015), 80549–805569 (2015a)

P.C. Pandey, R. Singh, Y. Pandey, Controlled synthesis of functional Ag, AgAu/AuAg nanoparticles and its nanocomposite with Prussian blue for bioanalytical applications. RSC Adv. **5**, 49671–49679 (2015b)

P.C. Pandey, G. Pandey, G. Pandey, J. Haider, Role of organic carbonyl moiety and 3-aminopropyltrimethoxysilane on the synthesis of gold nanoparticles specific to pH and salt tolerance. J. Nanosci. Nanotechnol. **16**, 6155–6163 (2016)

P.C. Pandey, G. Pandey, G. Pandey, A. Walcarius, 3-Aminopropyltrimethoxysilane mediated solvent induced synthesis of gold nanoparticles for biomedical applications. Mater. Sci. Eng. C **79**, 45 (2017)

P.C. Pandey, S. Singh, S.N. Sawant, Functional alkoxysilane mediated controlled synthesis of Prussian blue nanoparticles, enabling silica alginate bead development; nanomaterial for selective electrochemical sensing. Electrochim. Acta **287**, 37–48 (2018a)

P.C. Pandey, S. Singh, A. Walcarius, Palladium-Prussian blue nanoparticles; as homogeneous and heterogeneous electrocatalysts. Electroanal. Chem. **780**, 747–754 (2018b)

P.C. Pandey, N. Katiyal, G. Pandey, R.J. Narayan, Synthesis of self-assembled siloxane–polyindole–gold nanoparticle polymeric nanofluid for biomedical membranes. MRS Commun. **10**, 482–486 (2020a)

P.C. Pandey, S. Shukla, G. Pandey, R.J. Narayan, Organotrialkoxysilane-mediated synthesis of functional noble metal nanoparticles and their bimetallic for electrochemical recognition of L-tryptophan. MRS Adv. **5**, 2429–2444 (2020b). https://doi.org/10.1557/adv.2020.305

P.C. Pandey, S. Shukla, G. Pandey, R.J. Narayan, Organotrialkoxysilane-mediated controlled synthesis of noble metal nanoparticles and their impact on selective fluorescence enhancement and quenching. J. Vac. Sci. Technol. B **38**, 052801 (2020c)

P.C. Pandey, M.D. Mitra, R.J. Narayan, Organo-trialkoxysilane mediated rapid and controlled synthesis metal nanoparticles in both homogeneous and heterogeneous phase and their catalytic applications. MRS Adv. **6**, 43–53 (2021a)

P.C. Pandey, M.D. Mitra, S. Shukla, R.J. Narayan, Organotrialkoxysilane-functionalized mesoporous Pd–Ni nanocatalyst for selective hydrazine decomposition and sensing. MRS Commun. **11**, 78–85 (2021b). https://doi.org/10.1557/s43579-021-00018-y

P.C. Pandey, M.D. Mitra, A.K. Tiwari, S. Singh, Synthetic incorporation of palladium-nickel bimetallic nanoparticles within mesoporoussilica/silica nanoparticles as efficient and cheaper catalyst for both cationic and anionic dyes degradation. J. Environ. Sci. Health A **56**(4), 460–472 (2021c). https://doi.org/10.1080/10934529.2021.1886793

P.C. Pandey, S. Shukla, R.J. Narayan, Organotrialkoxysilane-mediated synthesis of Ni–Pd nanocatalysts at lower concentrations of noble metal: Catalysts for faster hydrogen evolution kinetics. J. Vac. Sci. Technol. B **39**, 032802 (2021d). https://doi.org/10.1116/6.0000881

P.C. Pandey, M.D. Mitra, S. Shukla, R.J. Narayan, Organotrialkoxysilane-functionalized Noble metal monometallic, bimetallic, and Trimetallic nanoparticle mediated non-enzymatic sensing of glucose by resonance Rayleigh scattering. Biosensors **11**, 122 (2021e). https://doi.org/10.3390/bios11040122

P.C. Pandey, S. Shukla, R.J. Narayan, Organotrialkoxysilane-functionalized Prussian blue nanoparticles-mediated fluorescence sensing of arsenic(III). Nano **11**, 1145 (2021f). https://doi.org/10.3390/nano11051145

P.C. Pandey, H.P. Yadav, S. Shukla, R.J. Narayan, Electrochemical sensing and removal of Cesium from water using Prussian blue nanoparticle-modified screen-printed electrodes. Chem **9**, 253 (2021g). https://doi.org/10.3390/chemosensors9090253

P.C. Pandey, A.K. Tiwari, R.J. Narayan, Optimization of solvents, electrolytes, and mediators for polyindole-based electrochemical sensors. Sens. Diagn **3**, 1392–1405 (2024). https://doi.org/10.1039/D4SD00175C

K. Saha, S.S. Agasti, C. Kim, X. Li, V.M. Rotello, Gold nanoparticles in chemical and biological sensing. Chem. Rev. **112**(5), 2739–2779 (2012)

H. Schmidt, H. Scholze, A. Kaiser, Principles of hydrolysis and condensation reaction of alkoxysilanes. J. Non-Cryst. Solids **63**, 1–11 (1984)

P.R. Selvakannan, K.P. Senthil, A.S. More, R.D. Shingte, P.P. Wadgaonkar, M. Sastry, One pot, spontaneous and simultaneous synthesis of gold nanoparticles in aqueous and nonpolar organic solvents using a diamine-containing Oxyethylene linkage. Langmuir **20**, 295–298 (2004)

D. Thompson, Michael faraday's recognition of ruby gold: the birth of modern nanotechnology. Gold Bull. **40**, 267–269 (2007)

A.K. Tiwar, P.C. Pandey, R.J. Narayan, Role of different polymer-stabilized metal nanoparticles in fluorescein reporter–based turn-off-on glutathione detection. MRS Commun. **15**, 227–234 (2025). https://doi.org/10.1557/s43579-025-00696-y

A.K. Tiwari, M.K. Gupta, G. Pandey, P.C. Pandey, Siloxane-silver nanofluid as potential self-assembling disinfectant: a preliminary study on the role of functional alkoxysilanes. Nano **4**, 1 (2023) https://ojs.wiserpub.com/index.php/NAT/article/view/1576/1455

C. Tran-Minh, P.C. Pandey, S. Kumaran, Studies on acetylcholine sensor and its analytical application based on the inhibition of cholinesterase. Biosensor. Bioelectron. **5**, 461–471 (1990)

J. Turkevich, P.C. Stevenson, J. Hillier, A study of the nucleation and growth processes in the synthesis of colloidal gold. Discuss. Faraday Soc. **11**, 55–75 (1951)

A. Walcarius, Mesoporous materials and electrochemistry. Chem. Soc. Rev. **42**, 4098–4140 (2013)

K. Williams, J. Milner, M.D. Boudreau, K. Gokulan, C.G. Cerniglia, S. Khare, Effects of subchronic exposure of silver nanoparticles on intestinal microbiota and gut-associated immune responses in the ileum of Sprague-Dawley rats. Nanotoxicology **9**, 279–289 (2015)

Y. Yadong, T. Dmitri, The chemistry of functional nanomaterials. Chem. Soc. Rev. **42**, 2484–2487 (2013)

H. Zhu, Z. Pan, E.W. Hagaman, C. Liang, S.H. Overbury, S. Dai, Facile one-pot synthesis of gold nanoparticles stabilized with bifunctional amino/siloxy ligands. J. Colloid Interface Sci. **287**, 360–365 (2005). https://doi.org/10.1016/j.jcis.2005.01.106

Synthesis and Biomedical Applications of Cationic Polymer Coated Noble Metal Nanoparticles

Govind Pandey, Tharuna Chandra Pandey, and Shivangi Pandey

Abstract Polyethyleneimines (PEI) is a cationic polymer and has proven viability for variety of biomedical application especially in (i) facilitating stronger attachments with negatively charge outer surface of the cells and (ii) polymeric transfection agent releasing the polymer-DNA complex into the cytoplasm. The use of PEI as active reagent in controlled synthesis of noble metal nanoparticles enabled the formation of cationic polymer coated nanoparticles that manifest the functional ability of PEI during biomedical applications and is reviewed in this chapter. Some typical applications of PEI-functionalized gold and silver nanoparticles with added emphasis on gene therapy in Pediatrics are documented.

1 Introduction

Nanotechnology is an attracting interface between scientific, engineering, agriculture, and medical fields with variety of applications (Shi et al. 2010). Such innovation has been attributed through the functional tunable nanosized materials for industrial, biomedical, and scientific purposes, which provides a set of techniques that allow the manipulation of structural and functional properties on a microscale. Such functional nanogeometry innovate biomedicinal involvement of nanoparticles (NPs), which are used as the backbone in the vaccine to formulate "nanovaccines," nanomaterial-based antiviral agents. Such nanomaterials are not only limited to MDR disinfectants; which inhibit the multiplication within the host or inactivate them outside the host, but also the application of designed nanorobots to detect and repairs of tissue defects at the cellular level (Leon et al. 2020). Unlike the conventional drug formulations, nanoparticles target a desired part of the body for action with further option in exploring surface-functionalized nanoparticles that explicitly targeting lymphatic organs and

G. Pandey (✉) · T. C. Pandey
Department of Pediatrics, Dr. Ram Manohar Lohia Institute of Medical Science, Lucknow, India
e-mail: gvnd121@gmail.com

S. Pandey
Motilal Nehru Medical College, Prayagraj, India

R. Narayan (ed.), *Nanostructured Biomaterials and Their Applications*,
https://doi.org/10.1007/978-3-032-16316-5_7

immune cells to provoke better immune responses. Nevertheless, localized infections are challenging medical task that can be overcome with nanovaccines with specific cells or organ-targeting molecules. The functionality linked to enhance the solubility of hydrophobic compounds manifest for effective remedy in targeting tissue. These systems are helpful to protect the antigens from degradation and stabilize a large number of therapeutic biological components, such as peptides, proteins, and nucleic acids on the substrate with potentiality in viral infections (Mungrue 2014). Nevertheless, functionality linked to biocompatible nanoparticles especially gold and silver nanoparticles have justified boon to human health and is being reviewed herein using cationic polymer of desired dimension.

The presence of carboxylic acid group and amine functionality in amino acid introduce the susceptibility for Zwitter ion formation which subsequently control variety of vital function in living creature. Amines can behave as Brønsted–Lowry bases by accepting a proton from the acid to form corresponding conjugate acids. Due to a lone pair of non-bonding electrons, aliphatic amines can also act as Lewis bases by forming a covalent bond with an electrophile. Accordingly, the organic amine linked to aliphatic chain allows extra event due to the presence of loan pair of non-bonding electrons that under desired experimental condition allows the reduction of especially noble metal cation like gold and silver cations followed by stabilizing the as generated metal nanoparticles and generate the concept of functional noble metal nanoparticles synthesis that has been innovated by Pandey (2010), Pandey and Chauhan (2012), Pandey et al. (2014), Pandey and Singh (2015) and represent the theme of this chapter. Polyethylenimine (PEI) is an organic molecule containing repeating units of the amine group and two carbon aliphatic CH_2CH_2 spacers displaying polycationic character and under varying molecular weights and are explored for synthesis and applications of functional gold and silver nanoparticles with functionality dependent biomedical applications.

1.1 Polyethylenimine Mediated Synthesis of Gold Nanoparticles

The synthesis of AuNPs utilizing active role of amines as capping and reducing agent has been reported by Pandey (2010), Pandey and Chauhan (2012), Pandey et al. (2014), Pandey and Singh (2015). The findings demonstrated that in the presence of only aliphatic amine containing moiety, the time required for AuNPs formation varied from 2 to 40 h depending on the ratio of amine-/Au^{3+}. Since gold cations are relatively stable hence very slow conversion is noticed, however silver cations are relatively more reactive and may undergo complex formation that inhibit the slow conversion of silver cations into silver nanoparticles. These findings revealed that organic amine containing aliphatic spacer initiate the reduction of stable noble metal cations however, require the presence of and electrophile for real time conversion of noble metal cations into respective nanoparticles. Accordingly, a series of electrophile like aldehyde and ketones have been attempted (Pandey et al. 2016) along with polyethylenimine of specific molecular weight as Lewis base for real time conversion of noble metal cations especially gold into respective nanoparticles (Pandey and Pandey 2014; Pandey and Pandey 2016a, b). *The ratio of amine-/Au^3* has been demonstrated to control the nanogeometry of as made nanoparticles. PEI having three different molecular weight: MW 750,000 Da; MW 60,000 Da; MW 1300 Da was chosen for such investigation in order to evaluate the cytotoxicity of PEI during biomedical applications. It was concluded that PEI of MW 1300 Da does not show any cytotoxicity although PEI of all molecular weight allow the formation of gold nanoparticles (Tiwari et al. 2020).

The typical procedure PEI (50 wt% in H_2O) of specific molecular weight was diluted to 8% in methanol. 10 μl of tetrachloroauric acid (10 mM) was mixed with 10 l of methanolic solution of polyethylenimine followed by the addition of 10 l of formaldehyde. The mixture was homogenized on vertex mixture and allowed to stand at room temperature. The formation of PEI-functionalized AuNPs is triggered within 2 min after the addition of formaldehyde as described earlier (Tiwari et al. 2020).

1.2 *Polyethylenimine Mediated Synthesis of Silver Nanoparticles*

The electronegativity of gold is more than that of silver accordingly the reduction of silver cations is relatively difficult than that of gold cations as observed by Pandey and Singh (2015) while investigating the comparative organic amine mediated conversion of gold and silver cations. In addition silver cations are also susceptible to respective oxide formation and undergo precipitation during prolonged incubation in aqueous solution. Accordingly, the synthesis of silver nanoparticles is not analogous to that of gold nanoparticles under identical conditions and slight advancement in synthetic protocol was adopted. Since the amine functionality of cationic polymer is sensitive under microwave irradiation, it is desirable to control the reduction of the noble metal cation under microwave incubation. Interestingly, we have observed rapid synthesis of PEI-coated silver nanoparticles within less than 1 min under microwave incubation. In order to make the microwave irradiation more amenable for nanoparticle synthesis, use of high boiling solvent like ethylene glycol containing Ethylene glycol di-acetate miscible with water and some reagent like 1-vinyl 2-pyrrolidone that prevent heterogeneity of the reaction medium undergoing microwave irradiation has been attempted (Tiwari et al. 2020).

In the typical process of nanoparticle synthesis, ethylene glycol (120 μL) and a methanolic solution of 1-vinyl 2-pyrrolidone (50 μL of a 250 mM solution) were placed in 2 mL glass vial, followed by the addition of a methanolic solution of $AgNO_3$ (10 μL of a 10 mM solution), PEI (150 μL of a 4 mg/mL solution), and 20 μL cyclohexanone. The reaction mixture was thoroughly mixed on a vortex mixer for 30 s and placed in a microwave oven for 15 s. The cycle was repeated four to six times in the microwave oven, resulting in the appearance of a deep yellow color that indicated the real time formation of PEI-functionalized AgNP. PEI having three different molecular weight: MW 750,000 Da; MW 60,000 Da; MW 1300 Da was chosen for such investigation as reported earlier (Tiwari et al. 2020).

1.3 Characterization of PEI-Functionalized Gold Nanoparticles

The gold cations have shown specific interaction with PEI that is susceptible for rapid conversion into AuNPs in the presence of formaldehyde/acetaldehyde cyclohexanone/acetylacetone/tetrahydrofuran hydroperoxide/t-butyl methyl ketone as reported earlier (Pandey and Pandey 2016a, b). On the addition of PEI in methanolic solution of gold cations, the color of the suspension turned into dark yellow suggesting the specific interaction of gold cations with PEI. When organic reducing i.e., formaldehyde is added into the suspension, the conversion of gold cations into AuNPs is recorded within < 2 min. Figure 1 shows time dependent synthesis of PEI-functionalized AuNPs. Within less than 15 min there is significant change in the absorption maxima at 518 nm, characteristic of AuNPs between 1 and 10 nm. It is found that the concentration of gold cations, while keeping the similar concentrations of formaldehyde and PEI, precisely control the size of AuNPs as shown in Fig. 2 based on UV-vis spectroscopy. The UV-VIS spectra recorded on blue, purple, and red AuNPs are shown in Fig. 2. The results shown in Fig. 2 provide interesting finding on the variation of surface plasmon resonance of AuNPs. Curve-1 (Fig. 2) shows absorption at 518 nm whereas curve-2 and curve-3 of AuNPs made from similar synthetic rout justify remarkable variation in absorption maxima and reflects the advantage of the current process. The size of AuNPs can be precisely controlled from the concentrations of either gold cations or PEI. An increase in the concentration of gold cations at constant PEI results an increase in nanogeometry. A decrease in PEI concentration causes increase in nanogeometry. AuNPs of all SPR could be made from the present process within finite time. The choice of organic reducing agent also controls the nanogeometry and dispersibility in desired medium. The use of formaldehyde results into the AuNPs dispersible in all buffering system whereas the use of tert-butyl methyl ketone may be better useful in both aqueous and non-aqueous medium. In addition to that the organic reducing agent also controls the synthesis of AuNPs while changing the M.W. of PEI between 800 and 25 kD. PEI of higher molecular wt i.e., M.W. ~ 60,000 and higher also enable the synthesis of AuNPs. Figure 3 shows the TEM images of as synthesized AuNPs. The process precisely controls the homogeneous distribution of AuNPs with excellent polycrystalline pattern as confirmed from SAED shown in Fig. 4. The average size of AuNPs is found to be 7 nm under current condition having homogeneous distribution between 6 and 9 nm. The SAED pattern shows face centered lattice with excellent polycrystallinity. It should be noted that even the use of organic polymer results the formation of excellent polycrystalline materials. PEI shows specific interaction with gold cations. In methanolic solution gold ions are reduced in the presence of electron donating group like formaldehyde or similar other reagents. Then conversion of gold ions into AuNPs results electrostatic conformation with PEI. Such process allows to control the charge density on PEI stabilized AuNPs based on suitable choice of organic reducing agents like formaldehyde/acetaldehyde/acetone/acetyl acetone/tert-butyl methyl ketone/cyclohexanone/tetrahydrofuran hydroperoxide.

•

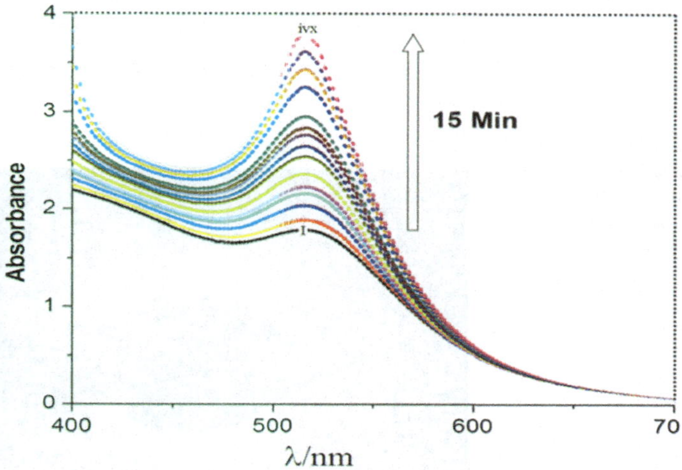

Fig. 1 Time dependent synthesis of AuNPs through active participation of PEI (M.W. 10 kD) and formaldehyde in methanolic solution

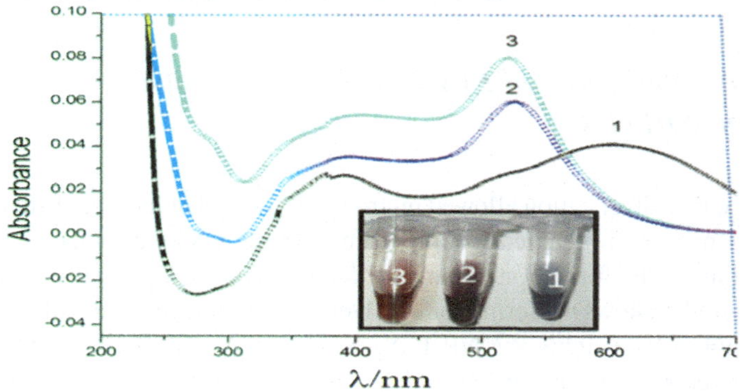

Fig. 2 UV-VIS spectra of PEI stabilized AuNPs made at three different concentrations of chloroauric acid [0.5 mM (1), 0.9 mM (2), 1.5 mM (3)] containing same concentrations of FEI and formaldehyde. The inset shows the respective photographs of AuNPs

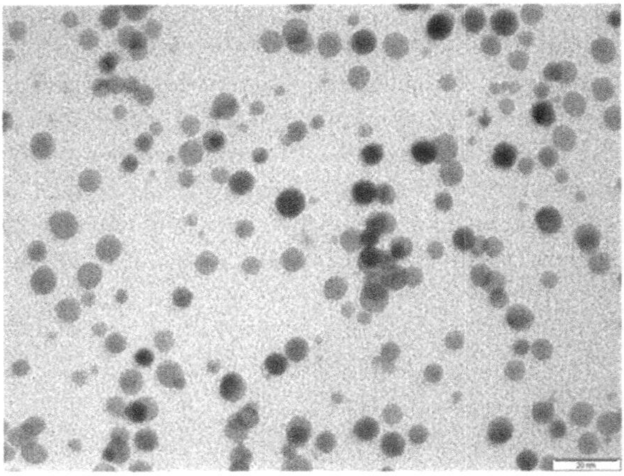

Fig. 3 Time dependent synthesis of AuNPs through active participation of PEI (M.W. 10 kD) and formaldehyde in methanolic solution

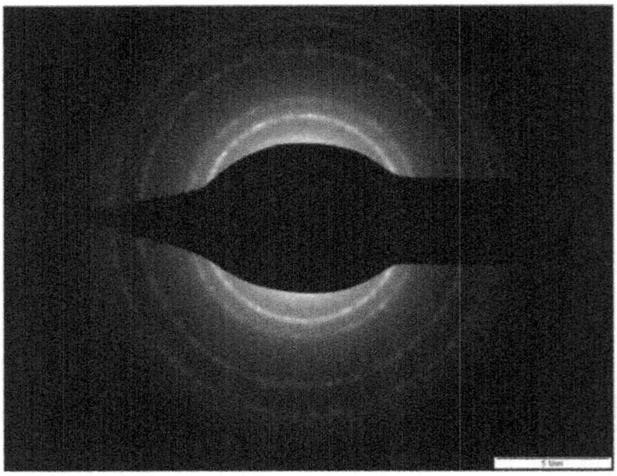

Fig. 4 Selected area electron diffraction pattern of PEI stabilized AuNPs shown in Fig. 3

1.4 Characterization of PEI-Functionalized Silver Nanoparticles

The PEI-capped silver cation allowed microwave-assisted reduction of silver cations in the presence of an organic reducing agent, namely cyclohexanone or formaldehyde, leading to the formation of three different silver nanoparticles (Tiwari et al. 2020). Figure 5A shows the formation of silver nanoparticles coated with PEI of three different molecular weights, Ag-NP-1, Ag-NP-2, and Ag-NP-3. Figure 5A(a) shows the results recorded from Ag-NP-1, Fig. 5A(b) shows the results recorded from Ag-NP-2, and Fig. 5A(c) shows the results recorded from Ag-NP-3. The process allowed for rapid formation of Ag-NPs regardless of molecular weight. The properties of Ag-NP-1, Ag-NP-2, and Ag-NP-3 differed as a function of molecular weight.

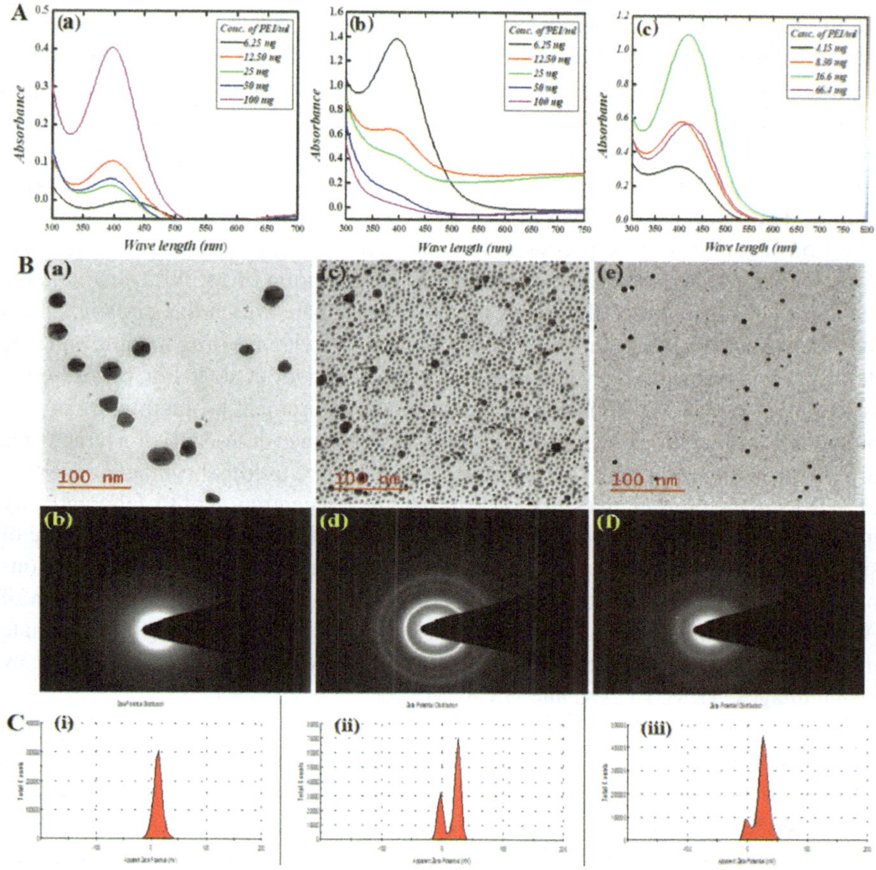

Fig. 5 **A** UV–Vis spectra of **a** Ag-NP-1, **b** Ag-NP-2, and **c** Ag-NP-3. **B** TEM images along with the respective SAED pattern of **a**, **b** Ag-NP-1, **c**, **d** Ag-NP-2 and **e**, **f** Ag-NP-3. **C** Zeta potential of (i) Ag-NP-1, (ii) Ag-NP-2, and (iii) Ag-NP-3

The concentration of PEI also affected the synthesis of Ag-NPs. The Ag-NPs were characterized by TEM (Fig. 5B) and by zeta potential measurements (Fig. 5C).

1.5 *Polyethylenimine Mediated Synthetic Insertion of Gold Nanoparticles into Mesoporous Silica Nanoparticles*

The gold nanoparticles having surface functionalization with suitable agents allow for both selective imaging and photothermal killing of cancer cells by using light with longer wavelengths (Huang et al. 2006). Further Mesoporous silica nanoparticles (MSNP) has been used as safe carrier for drug delivery since mesoporous architecture can easily be explored for selective drug loading (Xia et al. 2009). Further, the use of

AuNPs has been very well demonstrated as biomedicine (Aznar et al. 2016) therefore, synthetic insertion of AuNPs has been desirable in MSNP which can be further explored for specific drug loading. Synthetic approach reported earlier (Pandey and Pandey 2016a, b) may allow PEI mediated synthetic insertion of AuNPs in MSNP of controlled nanogeometry providing novel platform for drug loading along with efficient bio catalytic activity which has been one of the major objective of current finding. The modification of MSNP by PEI is found as an important step for synthetic insertion of AuNPs in mesoporous architecture. Accordingly, we intended to enhance the selective binding of PEI through surface modification of MSNP using suitable reagent like 3-trihydroxysilylpropyl methylphosphonate which has already shown as effective surface modifier for PEI modification for selective drug loading and safe delivery of the same (Pandey and Pandey 2016a, b; Pandey et al. 2017a, b). Although control over size of MSNP is one of an important requirement for facilitating in vivo biomedical applications of AuNPs inserted MSNP however, MSNP of average size of 200 nm with mesoporous architecture of 4–6 nm are used for synthetic insertion of AuNPs in the present investigation. Further, the concentration of PEI dramatically influences the synthetic incorporation of AuNPs within mesoporous architecture of silica nanoparticles accordingly, the results recorded at two different concentrations of PEI involving constant concentrations of formaldehyde in synthetic insertion of AuNPs within unmodified MSNP and 3-trihydroxysilylpropyl methylphosphonate modified MSNP are reported. AuNPs inserted MSNP has been characterized by visual images, TEM, EDAX, and HR SEM.

The typical procedure for synthetic insertion of gold nanoparticles within controlled size of mesoporous silica nanoparticles may be followed by two different approaches as reported earlier (Pandey et al. 2017a, b) namely (1) Surface modification of MSNP by 3-Trihydroxysilylpropyl methyl phosphonate and (2) Polyethylenimine mediated synthetic insertion of AuNPs into mesoporous architecture of MSNP. In Approach-1 50 mg of MSNP was suspended in 1 ml distilled water containing 5% w/v 3-Trihydroxysilylpropyl methyl phosphonate and stirred for 2 h at 40 °C. The modified MSNP was cooled and collected by centrifugation followed by careful washing with water followed by ethanol. The 3-Trihydroxysilylpropyl methyl phosphonate functionalized MSNP was dried at 60 °C overnight. Whereas in approach (2) both unmodified and 3-Trihydroxysilylpropyl methyl phosphonate modified MSNP were used for PEI mediated synthetic insertion of AuNPs. Two stock solutions of PEI in lower aliphatic alcohol i.e., (8 mg/ml and 5 mg/ml) are chosen for modification of MSNP. 200 μl ethanolic solution of PEI (9% w/v) was added into 10 mg of unmodified/modified MSNP with continuous stirring for 1–2 h at 25 °C. The PEI treated MSNP was collected by centrifugation and washed several time to ensure removal of unbound PEI. Into 200 μl ethanolic suspension of PEI treated MSNP, 50 μl formaldehyde solution in ethanol (40% w/v) was added followed by constant stirrings of the reaction system for 2 h at 25 °C. The as made AuNPs within unmodified/modified MSNP was collected by centrifugation followed by washing with lower aliphatic alcohol/ethanol for several time to ensure complete removal of any unbound AuNPs. AuNPs inserted MSNPs were finally dried at 60 °C for overnight.

The as made AuNPs inserted MSNP was evaluated by visual photographs, transmission electron microscopy, energy dispersive X-ray analysis (EDAX) and HR SEM. AuNPs inserted unmodified MSNP made at two concentrations of PEI; (L = 5 mg/ml and H = 8 mg/ml is shown in Fig. 6 whereas AuNPs inserted MSNP functionalized with 3-trihydroxysilylpropyl methyl phosphonate and made at two concentrations of PEI; (L = 5 mg/ml and H = 8 mg/ml) is shown in Fig. 7. These TEM images as shown in Figs. 6 and 7 justify efficient insertion of gold nanoparticles within mesoporous architecture of silica nanoparticles. The size of nanoparticles and its overall distribution represent novelty of the as reported synthetic approach for making nanoparticles in mesoporous architecture.

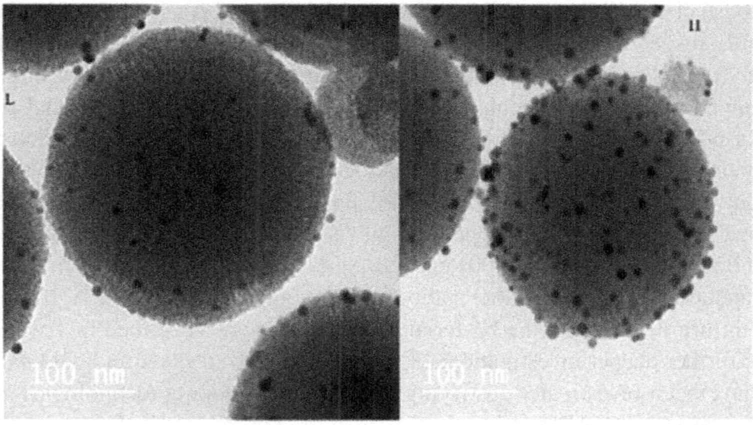

Fig. 6 TEM images AuNPs inserted unmodified MSNP made at two concentrations of PEI (L = 5 mg/ml and H = 8 mg/ml)

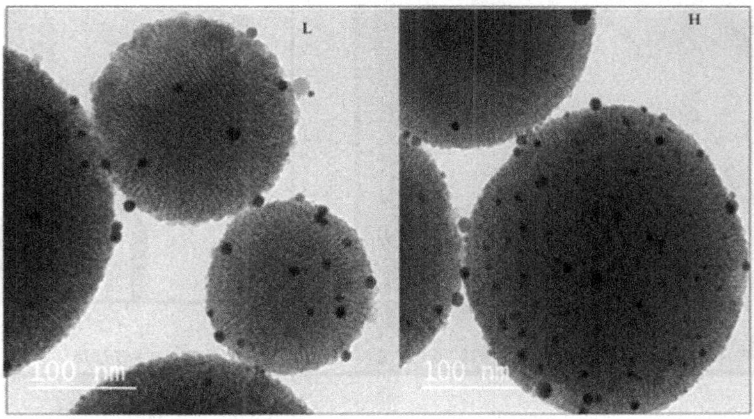

Fig. 7 TEM images AuNPs inserted MSNP functionalized with 3-trihydroxysilylpropyl methyl phosphonate and made at two concentrations of PEI (L = 5 mg/mL and H = 8 mg/mL)

1.6 Bactericidal Activity of PEI-Functionalized AgNPs

PEI-coated silver nanoparticles of three different types were made as a function of the molecular weight of PEI as described earlier (Tiwari et al. 2020). The three Ag-NPs showed bactericidal activity against A. baumannii and other multidrug resistant bacteria; a variation in bactericidal activity was noted on the basis of MW of PEI as shown in (Fig. 8a). The minimum inhibitory concentration (MIC) and minimum bactericidal concentration (MBC) values of each silver nanoparticle (AgNP) were determined by the broth microdilution method in flat bottom sterile microtiter plates. The MBC values for Ag-NP-1, Ag-NP2, and Ag-NP3 against the strain of A. baumannii were 5, 10, and 5 μg/mL, respectively as described in (Tiwari et al. 2020). The MBC values for Ag-NP-1, Ag-NP2, and Ag-NP3 were 10, 20, and 10 μg/mL, respectively and confirmed molecular weight of PEI dependent antibacterial activity as described (Tiwari et al. 2020). Furthermore, it was observed that Ag-NPs capped with high-molecular-weight PEI had more potent bactericidal activity than Ag-NPs capped with low-molecular-weight PEI. The differential bactericidal activity may be attributed to the differences in branching of PEI among the samples; the highly branched PEI (MW 750,000)-capped Ag-NPs (Ag-NP-1) and moderate branched PEI (MW 60,000)-capped Ag-NPs (Ag-NP-4) showed lower MIC values than unbranched PEI (MW 1300)-capped Ag-NPs (Ag-NP-2). As such, it appears that branched PEI interacts more stably with the outer membrane of A. baumannii, which in turn destabilizes the bacterial cell membrane as described in Tiwari et al. (2020). further deeper investigations of PEI-functionalized silver and gold nanoparticles have been investigated justifying novelty in developing technologies against MDR bacteria and COVID-19 pandemic as reported in series of publications (Tiwari et al. 2023).

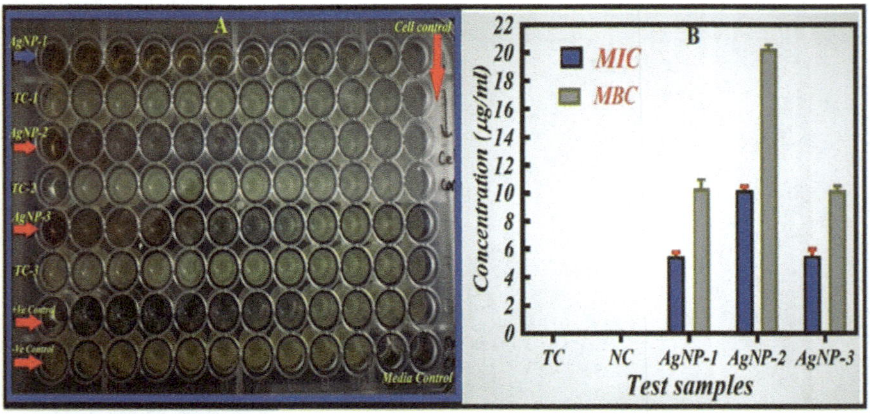

Fig. 8 **a** The antibacterial property assessment plate and **b** MIC and MBC (μg/mL) values of each Ag-NPs against A. baumannii planktonic cells. TC represents test control and NC represents negative control

1.7 Molecular Dynamics of PEI-Functionalized Noble Metal Nanoparticles

The extracellular polymeric substance (EPS) supports intercellular interactions in biofilm communities and protects bacterial cells from a harsh environment. Thus, the EPS matrix contributes to antimicrobial drug tolerance and enhanced antimicrobial resistance compared with planktonic cells. The main matrix components are extracellular DNA (eDNA), structurally complex polysaccharides, and proteins. Extracellular DNA plays an indispensable role in bacterial adhesion within the biofilm, bacterial aggregation within the biofilm, biofilm formation, biofilm structure maturation, maintenance of biofilm integrity, as well as intercellular communication or QS for transfer of genetic information (Srivastava and Bhargava 2016; Kassinger and van Hoek 2020). Therefore, eDNA is potentially a target molecule for eradicating bacterial biofilms. PEI-functionalized gold and silver nanoparticles have a strong affinity toward biofilm extracellular DNA; they show different types of interactions depending on the microenvironment of the biofilm (Kassinger and van Hoek 2020). When a PEI-functionalized nanoparticle penetrates a biological system, it rapidly acquires a corona of biomolecules over its surface in either monolayer or multilayer form (Joo and Aggarwal 2018). As such, cationic interactions involving PEI-functionalized Au nanoparticles and Ag nanoparticles with biofilm components are also affected by this corona (Joo and Aggarwal 2018). Moreover, it has been shown that a change in the concentration of salt leads to changes in the kinetics of interaction of eDNA with PEI-functionalized Au nanoparticles and Ag nanoparticles. As eDNA has a polyanionic nature, electrostatic interactions play a significant role in the case of Au nanoparticles and Ag nanoparticles that are coated by positively charged molecules. Carnerero et al. showed that gold nanoparticles form covalent and non-covalent interactions with a polyanionic DNA backbone. As discussed earlier (Pandey et al. 2017a, 2017b) PEI has justified as an efficient DNA delivery vehicle both in vitro and in vivo. It has been shown that PEI-DNA complexes enter the cells by endocytosis and escape from endosomes participating through proton exchange process. Accordingly PEI-functionalized gold nanoparticles opens paths to development of more efficiency vectors to improve gene therapy treatment and the new generation of DNA vaccines especially in pediatrics.

Gene therapy in pediatrics represents a cutting-edge therapeutic strategy for treating a range of genetic disorders at early age involving the modification or correction of a mutated gene or the introduction of a functional gene into a patient's cells via ex vivo gene therapy and in vivo gene therapy (Gol et al. 2024). Currently, a noteworthy array of gene therapy products has received valid market authorization, with several others in various stages of the approval process. Additionally, a multitude of clinical trials are actively underway, underscoring the dynamic progress within this field. Pediatric genetic disorders in the fields of hematology, oncology, vision and hearing loss, immunodeficiencies, neurological, and metabolic disorders are areas for gene therapy interventions. This chapter initiate the synthetic strategy for making functional biomaterial serving as a guide for pediatric clinicians to get a quick overview of the situation of clinical studies and approved gene therapy products for future generation.

Acknowledgments Thanks to Ex Professor Prem C Pandey of Chemistry Department, IIT BHU for innovating and providing theme of current outcome reviewed in this chapter.

Competing Interests The authors declare no conflict of interest.

Ethics Approval Ethics approval is not needed.

References

E. Aznar, M. Oroval, L. Pascual, J.R. Murguía, R. Martínez-Máñez, F. Sancenón, Gated materials for on-command release of guest molecules. Chem. Rev. **116**(2), 561–718 (2016). https://doi.org/10.1021/acs.chemrev.5b00456

T.M. Gol, F. Zahedipour, P. Trosien, G. Ureña-Bailén, M. Kim, J.S. Antony, M. Mezger, Gene therapy in pediatrics—clinical studies and approved drugs. Life Sci. **348**, 122685 (2024). https://doi.org/10.1016/j.lfs.2024.122685

X. Huang, H. Ivan, M.A. El-Sayed, W. Qian, M.A. El-Sayed, Cancer cell imaging and photothermal therapy in the near-infrared region by using gold nanorods. J. Am. Chem. Soc. **128**(6), 2115–2120 (2006). https://doi.org/10.1021/ja057254a

S.H. Joo, S. Aggarwal, Factors impacting the interactions of engineered nanoparticles with bacterial cells and biofilms: mechanistic insights and state of knowledge. JEM **225**(1), 62–74 (2018). https://doi.org/10.1016/j.jenvman.2018.07.08

S.J. Kassinger, M.L. van Hoek, Biofilm architecture: an emerging synthetic biology target. Synth. Syst. Biotechnol. **5**(1), 1–10 (2020)

L. Leon, E.J. Chung, C. Rinaldi, A brief history of nanotechnology and introduction to nanoparticles for biomedical applications, in *Nanoparticles for Biomedical Applications*, ed. by E.J. Chung, L. Leon, C. Rinaldi (2020), pp. 1–4. https://doi.org/10.1016/b978-0-12-816662-8.00001-1

K. Mungrue, The laboratory diagnosis of dengue virus infection, a review. Adv Lab. Med. Int. **4**, 1–8 (2014)

P.C. Pandey, A process for insitu generation of noble metal nanoparticles and thereafter coreshell of the same. Indian Patent 331496, Oct 2010

P.C. Pandey, D.S. Chauhan, 3-glycidoxypropyltrimethoxysilane mediated in situ synthesis of noble metal nanoparticles: application to hydrogen peroxide sensing. Analyst **137**, 376–345 (2012). https://doi.org/10.1039/C1AN15843K

P.C. Pandey, G. Pandey, A process for the polyethylenimine and organic reducing agent-mediated synthesis of noble metal nanoparticles, and prussian blue nanoparticles therefrom. Indian patent 340262, Dec 2014

P.C. Pandey, G. Pandey, A process for polyethylenimine and organic reducing agent mediated synthetic insertion of gold nanoparticles within mesoporous silica nanoparticles and their biomedical applications. Indian Patent 341050, Dec 2016 (2016a)

P.C. Pandey, G. Pandey, Novel synthesis of gold nanoparticles mediated by polyethylenimine and organic reducing agents for biomedical applications. ASEM **8**, 43–48 (2016b)

P.C. Pandey, R. Singh, Controlled synthesis of functional silver nanoparticles dispersible in aqueous and non-aqueous medium. J. Nanosci. Nanotechnol. **15**, 5749–5759 (2015). https://doi.org/10.1166/jnn.2015.10045

P.C. Pandey, A.K. Pandey, G. Pandey, Functionalized alkoxysilane mediated controlled synthesis of noble metal nanoparticles dispersible in aqueous and non-aqueous medium. J. Nanosci. Nanotechnol. **14**, 6606–6613 (2014). https://doi.org/10.1166/jnn.2014.9378

P.C. Pandey, G. Pandey, J. Haider, G. Pandey, Role of organic carbonyl moiety and 3-aminopropyltrimethoxysilane on the synthesis of gold nanoparticles specific to pH- and salt-tolerance. J. Nanosci. Nanotechnol. **16**, 6155–6163 (2016). https://doi.org/10.1166/jnn.2016.11104

P.C. Pandey, G. Pandey, R.J. Narayan, Controlled synthesis of polyethylenimine coated gold nanoparticles: application in glutathione sensing and nucleotide delivery. J. Biomed. Mater. Res. B Appl. Biomater. **105**, 1191–1199 (2017a). https://doi.org/10.1002/jbm.b.33647

P.C. Pandey, G. Pandey, R.J. Narayan, Polyethylenimine-mediated synthetic insertion of gold nanoparticles into mesoporous silica nanoparticles for drug loading and biocatalysis. Biointerphases **12**, 011005 (2017b). https://doi.org/10.1116/1.4979200

P.C. Pandey, G. Pandey, R.J. Narayan, Polyethylenimine-mediated controlled synthesis of Prussian blue-gold nanohybrids for biomedical applications. J. Biomater. Appl. **36**(1), 26–35 (2021). https://doi.org/10.1177/0885328220975575

J. Shi, A.R. Votruba, O.C. Farokhzad, R. Langer, Nano Lett. **10**, 3223 (2010)

S. Srivastava, A. Bhargava, Biofilms and human health. Biotechnol. Lett. **38**, 1–22 (2016)

A.K. Tiwari, M.K. Gupta, G. Pandey, R.J. Narayan, P.C. Pandey (2020) Molecular weight of polyethylenimine-dependent transfusion and selective antimicrobial activity of functional silver nanoparticle. J. Mater. Res. **35**, 2405–2415. https://doi.org/10.1557/jmr.2020.183

A.K. Tiwari, A. Mishra, G. Pandey, M.K. Gupta, P.C. Pandey, Nanotechnology: a potential weapon to fight against COVID-19. Part. Syst. Charact. **39**, 2100159 (2022). https://doi.org/10.1002/ppsc.202100159

A.K. Tiwari, M.K. Gupta, R.J. Narayan, P.C. Pandey, A whole cell fluorescence quenching-based approach for the investigation of polyethyleneimine functionalized silver nanoparticles interaction with Candida albicans. Front. Microbiol. **14**, 1131122 (2023). https://doi.org/10.3389/fmicb.2023.1131122

T. Xia, M. Kovochich, M. Liong, H. Meng, S. Kabehie, S. George, J.I. Zink, A.E. Nel, Polyethyleneimine coating enhances the cellular uptake of mesoporous silica nanoparticles and allows safe delivery of siRNA and DNA constructs. ACS Nano **3**(10), 3273–3286 (2009)

Synthesis and Nano-Structure Control of Four Morphs of Calcium Carbonate

Akiyoshi Osaka

Abstract The present chapter provides a basic understanding of calcium carbonate (CC) formation and utilization. Topics include synthesis routes, morphology, nanostructure control, interactions with microorganisms, metal ion adsorption or incorporation in the CC lattices, and biomedical applications such as cancer treatments. Some stress is placed on the ionic cluster units entangled with smaller macromolecular chains and phase separation within the precursor solutions.

Keywords Biomedical applications · Biomineralization · Calcium carbonate · Metal ion incorporation · Polymer-induced liquid precursors

1 Introduction

Calcium carbonate (CC) is one of the oldest raw materials, dating back billions of years to the time when microorganisms first emerged. It is employed in diverse industrial fields as blocks, powders, and micro- or nanoparticles. In addition, many types of marine life construct body frames by forming composites. CC is solidified in four morphs: calcite (Calc), aragonite (Arag), vaterite (Vat), and amorphous (ACC) phases. Calc (rhombohedral) is the most thermochemically stable phase among the three crystalline polymorphs, followed by Arag (orthorhombic), while Vat (hexagonal) is the least stable. Konopacka-Łyskawa documented the preparation of Vat spheres in one of their review papers (Konopacka-Łyskawa 2019), providing details of the synthesis before 2019. Figure 1 shows the lattice model and typical morphology of the three morphs (Huang et al. 2022). However, the morphology of CC particles depends on the preparation or manufacturing conditions and the additives or impurity species in the system. Hence, countless studies have been conducted over the past few decades. The present monograph will introduce only a portion of such studies, which are relevant not only to synthesis pathways and conditions, crystallization mechanisms, clusters present in depositing systems, and roles of microorganisms,

A. Osaka (✉)
Faculty of Engineering, Okayama University, Okayama, Japan
e-mail: akiosaka@okayama-u.ac.jp

R. Narayan (ed.), *Nanostructured Biomaterials and Their Applications*,
https://doi.org/10.1007/978-3-032-16316-5_8

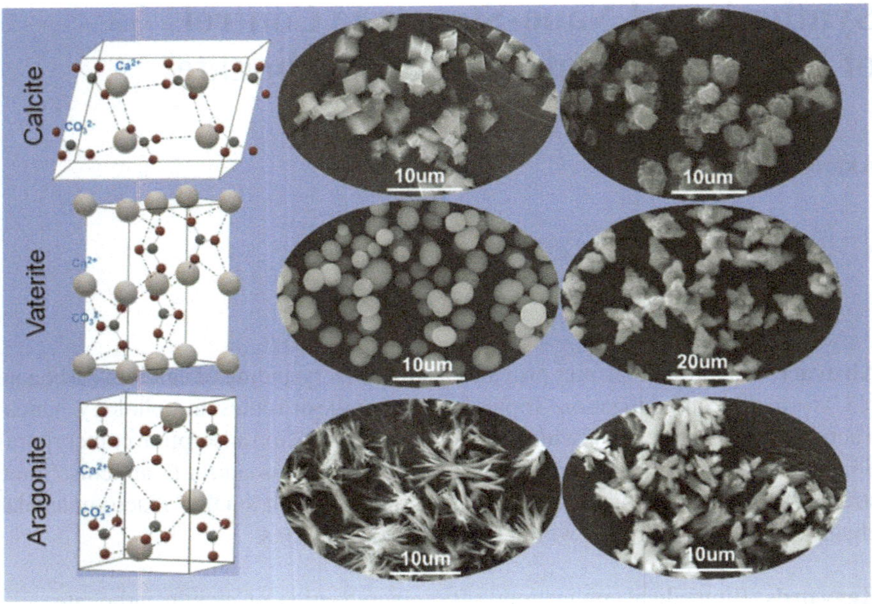

Fig. 1 Three crystalline polymorphs of calcium carbonate (calcite, vaterite, and aragonite) exhibit their typical morphology when precipitated from an aqueous system. Huang et al. (2022) (an open access paper; MDPI)

but also to applications such as CO_2 capture, energy storage, metal restoration and adsorption, medical treatments, and drug delivery systems.

All preparation schemes involve both calcium salts and carbonate sources: $CaCl_2$, $Ca(OH)_2$, CO_2, bicarbonate (HCO_3^-), and carbonate (CO_3^{2-}) ions. It must be emphasized that equilibria are established in aqueous systems among CO_2, HCO_3^-, and CO_3^{2-} under strict correlations to the pH of the system. Here, (aq) is the hydrated state of the species, and H^+(aq) is conventionally preferred, although H_3O^+(aq) is the correct form. All presentations of the activity and state are reproduced as described by Pourbaix [Atlas of electrochemical equilibria in aqueous solutions, 1974: ISBN 9780915567980].

$$CO_2 + H_2O \rightarrow H_2CO_3(aq) \quad \log\,(H_2CO_3)/p(CO_2) = 1.43 \tag{1}$$

$$CO_2 + H_2O \rightarrow HCO_3^-(aq) + H^+(aq) \quad \log\left(HCO_3^-\right)/p(CO_2) = -7.84 + pH \tag{2}$$

$$CO_2 + H_2O \rightarrow CO_3^{2-}(aq) + 2H^+(aq) \quad \log\left(CO_3^{2-}\right)/p(CO_2) = -18.14 + 2pH \tag{3}$$

Equations (4) and (5) represent the equilibrium of dissolved carbonate species.

$$H_2CO_3(aq) \rightarrow HCO_3^-(aq) + H^+(aq) \quad \log\left(HCO_3^-\right)/(H_2CO_3) = -6.38 + pH \tag{4}$$

$$HCO_3^-(aq) \rightarrow CO_3{}^{2-}(aq) + H^+(aq) \quad \log\left(CO_3{}^{2-}\right)/\left(HCO_3^-\right) = -10.34 + pH \tag{5}$$

Thus, the dominant state of carbonate ions depends on the pH of the reaction solution. The CC formation reaction is frequently described as the inverse of the Solvay process:

$$CaCl_2 + Na_2CO_3 \rightarrow CaCO_3 + 2NaCl \tag{6}$$

This Eq. (6) shows only one basic scheme. We can use a variety of combinations of sources, solvents, and additives, as well as different reaction temperatures and periods. In addition, the reaction conditions vary with time as the reaction proceeds; for example, the pH of the solution should decrease as sodium carbonate is consumed. If necessary, we could swing back the pH by adding the carbonate to the system. This makes it difficult to compare the morphologies, sizes, and other properties of CC products from different research groups. (Ogino et al. 1987) stressed the importance of the temperature and time dependence of the ion activity product (IAP). Sawada (1997) developed this concept and discussed the mechanisms of the formation and transformation of CC from one to the other. Ogino visualized the results in Fig. 2, a diagram representing the relative abundance of each morph of CC versus time (Ogino et al. 1987) and temperature (Sawada 1997). The supersaturated system was adjusted to involve 19.3 mM (mM=10^{-3} mol/L) Ca^{2+} and 9.24 mM $CO_3{}^{2-}$ using 6.7 mM $CaCl_2$ and 9.24 mM Na_2CO_3. Figure 1a shows that under the given reaction conditions, ACC first appears, and both Vat and Cal appear in 3 min in pace with the disappearance of ACC. In contrast, Fig. 2b demonstrates that Vat was the dominant phase at 30–40 °C within the earlier reaction stage, and the thermodynamically unstable aragonite phase became dominant at temperatures above 50 °C. Liendo et al. (2020) seemed inspired by the works above in their study on capturing CO_2 from combustion gases. They provided a comprehensive review of the factors that are effective in synthesizing CC (Liendo et al. 2022).

Considering the issues above, this monograph introduces a basic understanding of CC formation and a few applications in the environmental and biomedical fields. The topics include synthesis routes, morphology control, interactions of microorganisms, metal ion adsorption or incorporation in the CC lattices, drug delivery, and cancer therapy. To diminish our environmental load, many research groups have been elaborately engaged in using wastes from industries, construction, or agricultural activities as raw sources of Ca or carbonates. However, little is known about them, partly because the essential reactions are the same as in the CC routes from pure raw chemicals, and partly because the waste compositions are very diverse. Hence, it is difficult to elucidate any common concepts from detailed analyses. Some stress was placed on the ionic cluster units entangled with the smaller molecular chains. In addition, it is intended to attract the interest of readers, especially starters, in the material science and engineering of calcium carbonate. It is also regretful that

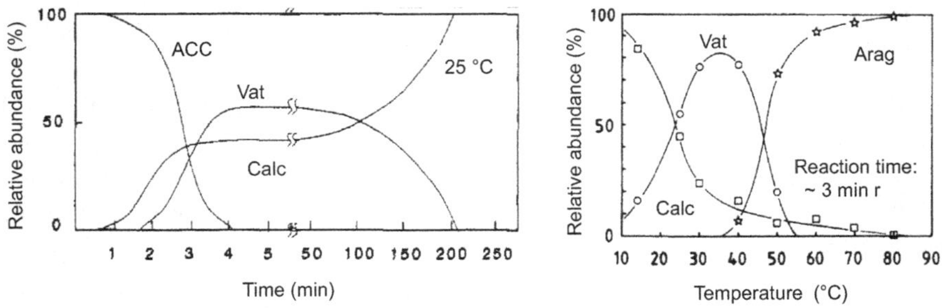

Fig. 2 Polymorphic abundance versus **a** reaction time at 25 °C (Sawada 1997) and **b** temperature for a reaction time of ~3 min (Ogino et al. 1987). ACC: amorphous calcium carbonate, Calc: calcite, Vat: vaterite, Arag: aragonite. (with permission from Elsevier)

only a limited number of publications could be presented, and almost all should be left uncommented here because of space constraints. The present author would like the readers to start with a review "A brief history of biomineralization studies" by Dauphin (2023).

2 Capturing Guest Ions in the Reaction Solutions

2.1 Divalent Metal Ions

Aqueous solutions are typical systems used for CC preparation. In the precipitation of the CC of any of the polymorphs, the system pH must be maintained at alkaline conditions, where the co-existing metal cations are present as hydroxides or carbonates. Table 1 lists the solubility products (Ksp) of some compounds.

Magnesium Ions

Magnesium ions are sometimes added as essential ingredients to control polymorphs and morphology. Ksp is a measure of the solubility of the relevant species. Suppose that Mg and Ca coexist in a certain alkaline carbonate system. Table 1 strongly suggests that the Ca ions formed $CaCO_3$ before the Mg ions precipitated $MgCO_3$. If the system does not contain carbonate ions, Mg^{2+} forms $Mg(OH)_2$, while Ca^{2+} remains free.

Magnesium salts sometimes play a key role in controlling the phase and morphology of CC. For example, Ota et al. (1995) prepared aragonite whiskers due to the carbonation process at 80 °C: blowing CO_2/air (1/20 in volume) into a 2 L aqueous suspension of $Ca(OH)_2$ (0.5 mol) and $MgCl_2$.(0.76 mol). Careful gas injection was performed to maintain the system pH at ~9. Due to the inhibition of Calc nucleation by Mg, the resulting Arag whiskers were several tens of μm long, with aspect ratios of 20 ~ 80. The experimental conditions were in accordance with the aragonite stability zone shown in Fig. 1. They diligently discussed the effects

Table 1 Solubility of carbonates and hydroxides of divalent metals

Compounds	Ksp	Ref.	Compounds	Ksp	Ref.
$MgCO_3$	6.82e-6	a	$Mg(OH)_2$	5.61e-12	a
$CaCO_3$*	3.31e-9 (Calc)	a	$Ca(OH)_2$	5.02e-6	a
	4.61e-9 (Arag)	a			
	1.22e-8 (vat)	a			
$SrCO_3$	5.60e-10	a			
$BaCO_3$	2.59e-9	a			
$Fe(II)CO_3$	3.13e-11	a	$Fe(II)(OH)_2$	4.87e-17	a
$NiCO_3$	1.42e-7	a	$Ni(OH)_2$	5.48e-16	a
$Cu(II)CO_3$	3.55e-12	b	$Cu(OH)_2$	2.20e-20	b
$CdCO_3$	1.0e-12	b	$Cd(OH)_2$	7.2e-15	b
$PbCO_3$	7.40e-14	a	$Pb(OH)_2$	1.43e-20	a

a: CRC Handbook (100th Ed.) p. 4–43, 4–188
b: Wikipedia, USA
*: Calc: calcite, Arag: aragonite, Vat: vaterite

of pH and carbonate ion state on Arag deposition. A mini-review of CC whisker preparation is available (Saulat et al. 2020), while Jing et al. (2018) reviewed the mechanical strength of polypropylene (PP) composited with Cal and Arag whiskers. With reinforcement with CC whiskers, the PP fibrils rationally exhibited improved strength; however, unfortunately, the whisker preparation details were not disclosed.

Mavromatis et al. (2022) studied the incorporation of Mg in Arag that was newly deposited on the surface of added Arag seeds within the systems consisting of (Na_2CO_3 + NaCl), ($CaCl_2$ + $MgCl_2$ + LiCl), and the seed crystallites. Air was bubbled into the solution and held in a 500 mL reaction vessel to control the pH at 8.1 ~ 8.4. In Fig. 3, D_{Mg} (the Mg distribution) is plotted as a function of the supersaturation of the reaction solution Ω_{Arag} with respect to aragonite. The reaction temperatures were 5, 15, and 25 °C. Here, D_{Mg} is defined as

$$D_{Mg} = (Mg/Ca)_{new\ phase}/(Mg/Ca)_{liq} \tag{7}$$

An important aspect is that Ω_{Arag} and D_{Mg} were lower for the higher reaction temperatures. This indicates that the solubility of Arag in the reaction solution was lower at higher temperatures. That is, CC generally becomes less soluble with increasing temperature and is denoted as retrograde solubility. Such behavior is very rarely found and is controversial with ordinary materials, for which the solubility increases with temperature. They also discussed the incompatibility of Mg accommodation in the carbonate lattices. They interpreted the results as showing that the incorporation of Mg in Arag likely occurs at defect sites on the growing mineral surface, as is commonly observed for the ions being incompatible with incorporation into host carbonate lattices. They added that phases with larger degrees of lattice

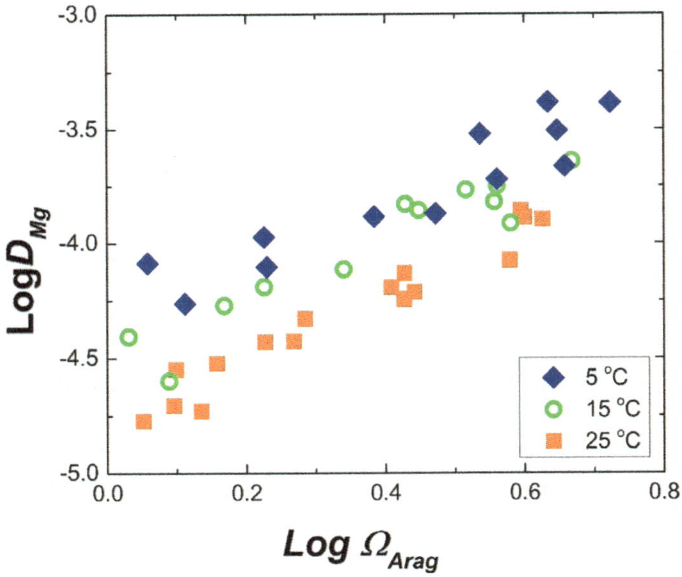

Fig. 3 Magnesium distribution coefficients (D_{Mg}) plotted as a function of the degree of saturation of the reaction solution (Ω_{Arag}) with respect to aragonite. Mavromatis et al. (2022) (with permission from Elsevier)

defects would accommodate such foreign ions. This comment suggests a greater possibility of accommodating foreign ions/species in amorphous CC.

Xiang et al. (2006) reported magnesium substitution in Calc by adding $MgCl_2$ during the slaking stage of $Ca(OH)_2$. Like many others, Ksp was not considered for $M(OH)_2$ (listed above) or for the availability of lattice sites. Therefore, a more detailed analysis is necessary before endorsing the conclusions.

Miscellaneous Metal Ions

By presenting a table of the thermochemical dissociation constants of the species beforehand, Nassrallah-Aboukaïs et al. (1999) discussed the transformation of Vat to Calc when the Vat particles were soaked for up to 17 days in dilute $CuCl_2$ solutions (0.1, 1, and 10 mM). The cupric salt solution is acidic (pH: around 3.6 for a 0.2 M solution (Merck Index, (#2623 cupric chloride 2013))). The Vat particles gradually dissolved, releasing Ca^{2+} and $CO_3{}^{2-}$. These two ions were adsorbed on the Vat surface together with Cu(II), and such adsorption might affect Vat conversion. However, it was concluded that the Vat-to-Calc transformation was influenced by the $CuCO_3 \cdot Cu(OH)_2$ crystallites that formed independently within the systems, but not on the Vat particle surface.

Effects of Seeding on Guest Ion Incorporation

Seeding is an effective tool for incorporating metal ions into the CC lattices in dilute solutions. Feng et al. (2024), for example, discussed the procedure of controlling the calcium ion contents in water (hard water) using Cal particles. They provided brief and comprehensive comments on the nucleation-growth process or seeding in the Introduction part of their paper. Fang et al. (2022) set up an experiment of coprecipitating Cr(III) with Vat, using $CrCl_3$, $CaCl_2$, and Na_2CO_3, and analyzed the resulted CC precipitates in terms of particle and surface morphology as well as atomic environments around relevant species due to EXAFS (X-ray absorption fine structure) and XANES (X-ray absorption near edge structure) for the Cr K-edge region. They suggested that Cr(III) may occupy interstitial voids in the crystals or substitute the Ca^{2+} sites of Vat in the form of $[Cr^{III}(OH)]^{2+}$. In addition, Cr(III) can stimulate Vat precipitation, likely due to the $Cr^{III}(OH)_3$ hydroxide on the Vat surface, suppressing the transformation of Vat to Calc. They also noted that the presence of Cr(III) could distort the Vat lattice structure. Wen et al. (2020) reported a mechanical activation process to recover metal ions from wastewater.

2.2 *Scavenging Metal Ions with Calcium Carbonates*

Ocean water contains various metal ions, which are essential for daily activities. A few groups have used CC polymorphs to extract metal ions from water through coprecipitation. Evans et al. (2020) conducted an extensive experiment on the incorporation of Li, B, Na, Mg, Mn, Sr, Ba, and U into amorphous calcium magnesium carbonates precipitated from seawater under various carbonate chemistries, Mg/Ca ratios, and in the presence of aspartic and glutamic acid. These amino acids, commonly abbreviated as Asp and Glu, are the most prevalent intracrystalline types found in foraminifera and corals. Aspartic acid is discussed later in this monograph regarding the cluster units within the CC precipitating solutions. Some of their conclusions (Evans et al. 2020) are as follows: (1) several aspects of trace element incorporation into ACC mirror those of the seawater-calcite system, (2) ACC outperforms Calc in terms of the element distribution coefficient (D: Metal in solid/metal in seawater), and (3) the D of Mn for ACC precipitated with aspartic acid is lower than that for Calc. It is essential to note that the definition of the term distribution can vary depending on the research group. Readers interested in changing carbonate levels in corals and seawater (referred to as Dissolved Inorganic Carbon (DIC)) may wish to consult (McCulloch et al. 2017). Despite being a minor element in seawater, they focused on the behavior of boron, likely considering the pH buffering capability of $B(OH)_3$ in conjunction with other carbonate species.

Donnelly et al. (2017) used dry ice as a CO_2-supplying and cooling agent to prepare nearly pure Vat. A few years later, for preparing Eu^{3+} and Tb^{3+}-doped Calc with 10 μm in average size, Donnelly et al. (2019) employed dry ice that facilitated the retrograde solubility of CC. Dry ice pellets were added into a solution of CaO/H_2O and lanthanide ions until the solution pH reached 7. According to the X-ray diffraction analysis, the calcite unit cell volume slightly increased by 0.45% at the first Eu doping (0.5%), but it decreased to the level of the undoped Cal with 1.7% doping. Thus, at lower dopant levels, Eu^{3+} ions are likely incorporated into the calcite lattice, while at higher doping levels, they predominantly occupy the surface sites of CC. The same applies to Tb^{3+} ions. Figure 4a and b show the bowtie morphology of the Calc doped with Eu^{3+}. They interpreted the morphology as having a central nucleation point, which grew through acicular structures to form an anisotropic material. (c) shows the Calc powders luminescent in red (Eu) and green (Tb) owing to UV (393 nm) excitation. They stated that these Calc powders could only be derived via the dry ice route, but with other specific reaction conditions unchanged. Alvarez demonstrated (Alvarez et al. 2021) that nickel isotopes can be fractionated due to Ni coprecipitation with Calc. This appears strange because the isotopes of an element have the same electronic structure, leading to equivalent chemical behavior. Lin et al. (2020) prepared Vat granules (~0.4 mm in diameter) from discarded oyster shells to absorb heavy metal ions. They also touched on some studies on removing transition metal ions in periods 5 and 6 with CC conducted in two decades (2000s ~ 2020s).

Herein, additional examples of metal ion elimination are presented. Courtois et al. (2024) prepared spherical hybrid particles of CC (phase not specified) and ε-poly(lysine) for uranium extraction from seawater (UES procedure). (Zhou et al. 2018) reported calcite-based uranium harvesting from seawater due to microparticles of CC combined with polydopamine. Fiorito et al. (2022) prepared Pb absorbents, while Guerrero et al. (2024) reported Cu and Pb adsorption on CC composites with alginate and chitosan.

Seeding uses the surface of seed crystals, expecting epitaxial or topotaxial effects on nucleation and growth (Mavromatis et al. 2022). Jeon et al. (2020) took a piece of Calc single crystal as the substrate for growing a layer of CC. The initial pH was

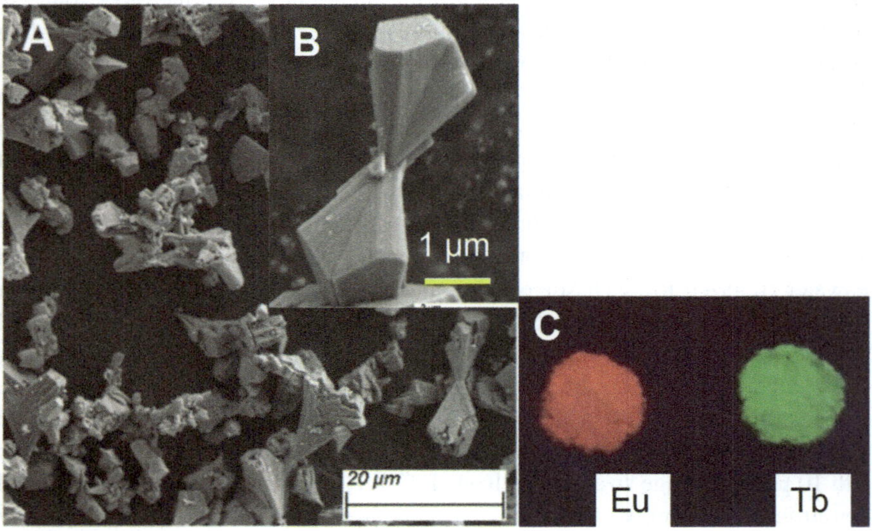

Fig. 4 **a** and **b** bow-tie-like morphology of Calc particles doped with 3.4 mol % Eu^{3+}. **c** Luminescence of Eu^{3+} and Tb^{3+} doped in Calc due to UV (393 nm) excitation. Donnelly et al. (2019) (with permission from Elsevier)

adjusted to 13 with 0.50 M NaOH. A layer of ACC was first deposited, and with the time of exposure, the ACC was transformed to Vat and Calc (~15 min) and finally to Calc after 90 min. Further study indicated that the cleaved plane {104} was stabilized with a layer of ACC particles. In this case, Calc microcrystals (~1 μm) completely coated the surface within 15 min, and they grew to a few μm in size. They further discussed the pathways that led to these layers. With the aid of ultrasound (US) application, Surmeneva et al. (2020a) successfully coated the Ti64 ($Ti_{90}Al_6V_4$) alloy surface with a mixture of Cal and Vat when the alloy surface was oxidized beforehand with 5 M NaOH. The alkali oxidation of the Ti alloy was already conducted by Kim et al. (1996) to ensure the bone compatibility of the alloy surface. It was proposed that for the coating reactions, ultrasound (US) irradiation played a key role because US treatment was expected to drive the surrounding solution deeper into the rough surface. However, Surmeneva et al. found that the alkali-treated surface was already (super)hydrophilic. Therefore, US application might have different effects.

2.3 *Amorphous or Single Crystalline CC*

As discussed later, the existence of amorphous CC (ACC) phases has been accepted over the past few decades. The distorted or highly disordered structure of ACC should be more flexible to accommodate the relevant ionic species. Shuseki et al. (2022) attempted to use the ACC structure for removing Sr^{2+} ions from aqueous systems and found the ACC samples were ~ 70 times as effective as crystalline CC particles. They derived ACC by rapidly adding 0.1 M $CaCl_2$ to 0.1 M Na_2CO_3 + 0.1 M NaOH and carefully analyzed the ACC structure using high-energy X-ray and neutron diffraction. They found that Sr replaced 1% of Ca in the Arag phase transformed from ACC.

In the studies mentioned above, the products were polycrystalline CC. Kezuka et al. (2017) challenged to prepare single-crystalline Calc needles where they first prepared a precursor aqueous suspension 1.5 mass % $Ca(OH)_2$ and 4.3 mass % $MgCl_2$ (the molar ratio Ca/Mg = 1/2.3). A gas mixture of $0.3CO_2$–0.7air (in volume) was blown from the bottom of the vessel into the suspension until the pH reached 6.7. The products were needle-like Arag crystallites that were 3–10 μm thick and 130–280 μm long (the aspect ratio: 10–30). When calcined at 500 °C for 1 h, the calcite XRD peaks fully replaced the aragonite peaks, while the width and length of the needle-like morphology remained unchanged. According to transmission electron micrograph (TEM) observations, the Arag needle had a smoother surface, while the Calc needle showed a rough (zig-zagging) surface, reflecting the rhombohedral lattice of Calc. It is emphasized that the selected area electron diffraction (SAED) spots showed no splitting, confirming that the needle was single crystalline. Kezuka et al. also devoted themselves to the fabrication of Calc nanoparticles under the effects of trace Si impurities (Kezuka et al. 2022), single-crystalline Calc nanorings, or nanorods with a Calc-core and Mg-Ca calcite shell structure (Kezuka et al. 2019). Figure 5a shows nano-sized (~60 nm) hollow single-crystalline Calc cubes, denoted

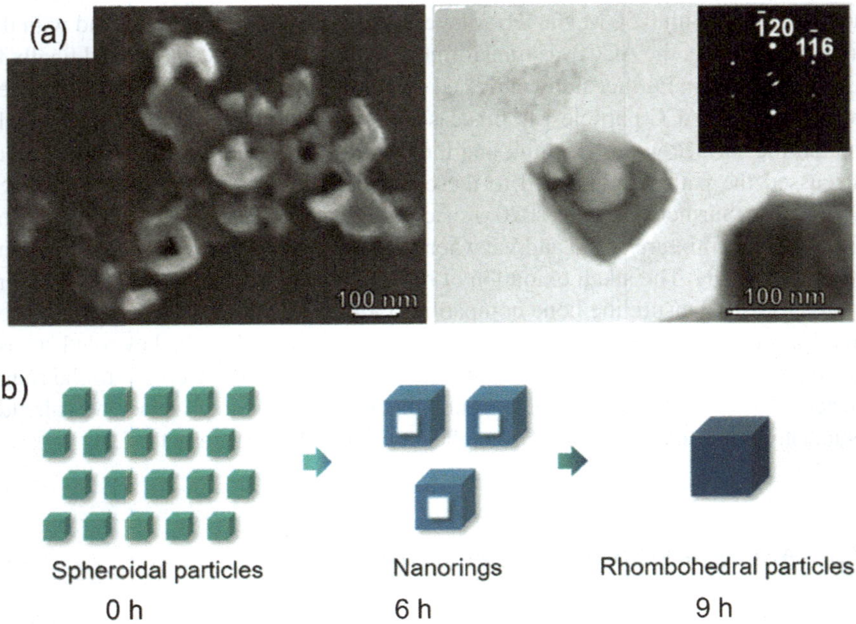

Fig. 5 **a** SEM (left) and TEM (right) images of Cal nano-rings (60 nm). The inserted ASED confirms that the particles are single crystals. **b** Growth model of Cal spheroid NPs to solid NPs (~80 nm) via the nano-rings due to heating Cal slurry at 95 °C. Bar: 100nm. (SAED: selected area electron diffraction). Kezuka et al. (2019) (an open access paper; the Royal Society of Chemistry)

as nanorings, prepared by heating an aqueous slurry of spheroidal ~30 nm-sized Cal nanoparticles up to 95 °C (Kezuka et al. 2018). Aging at 95 °C for 6 h converted these nanorings into solid rhombohedral single-crystalline nanoparticles (NPs; ~80 nm in size). All the facets were {104} planes. Figure 5b schematically shows the process leading to single-crystalline NPs. Takasaki et al. (1994) were interested in the effects of Fe(III) on inhibiting Cal growth from the viewpoint of preventing scale deposition on pipeline walls. Gao et al. (2023) applied FT-IR spectroscopy to track the pathway through which Mg-involved ACC transformed to crystalline forms. They confessed that although they obtained spectral differences clear enough to track the conversion of the Mg-containing ACC, their FIR data did not provide evidence to suggest whether the ACC samples should start as proto-crystalline phases or instead as heterogeneous amorphous phases.

2.4 Anions: Incorporation and Morphology Control

It is common for component ions in crystalline lattices to be replaced by foreign ions to form solid solutions or, in some cases, double salts. With larger carbonate ions, the CC lattice may accommodate anions such as SO_4^{2-}, CrO_4^{2-}, or SeO_4^{2-}. To clarify the effects of sulfate ions (SO_4^{2-}) and the ratio (SO_4^{2-}) /(CO_3^-) on CC precipitation, Mayorga et al. (2019) prepared well-designed aqueous solutions of $5CaCl_2$, $NaHCO_3$, and appropriate amounts of Na_2SO_4 to maintain the ratio (SO_4^{2-})/(CO_3^-) at 0–67.6, with an initial pH of 7.64 ± 0.03. They found that high sulfate ion concentrations in the solution stabilized the precipitated Vat and inhibited Calc formation. On the other hand, Arag was only formed because of a dissolution-precipitation process under a high (SO_4^{2-}) /(CO_3^-) ratio, but it required a long reaction time. Nguyen et al. (2024) prepared some alkyl biphosphonate molecules (BP: $(((HO)_2OP)_2CH$–R), R: an alkyl group) with varied lengths of chain and functional groups of R, and studied their effects on the CC precipitation. The solutions (50 mM $CaCl_2$, 50 mM $NaHCO_3$; pH depended on the composition: 7.5 ~ 9.2) with BP molecules enabled the supersaturated growth of metastable ACC. Their basic concept is that the effects of stabilizing ACC particles depend on the length of the alkyl groups on the BP molecules. The conclusions are summarized in Fig. 6. In the absence of BP in the solution, homogeneous nucleation and growth proceed with repeated dissolution and redeposition, so that ACC is driven to mineralization. The BP molecules reduce the calcium ion activity in the solutions due to the chelation ability of their $-P(=O)(OH)_2$ end group and "slow down" the ACC dissolution, preventing the crystallization of ACC to Calc or Vat. Another precipitation mechanism may work for ACC precursors hybridized with organic oligomers, as will be discussed later in this monograph.

Using a first-principles modeling approach, Feng et al. (2021) analyzed the fluorine sites in the three polymorphs of CC based on their geochemical importance. One possibility is the substitution of one CO_3^{2-} site by 2 F^-, and the other is replacing one of the three oxygen atoms to be present as $[FCO_2]^-$. The carbonate lattice is distorted in both cases, whereas the degree of distortion depends on the polymorphs. Their model calculations concluded that (1) the substitution of a carbonate ion by two fluoride ions is the most favorable incorporation scheme for all polymorphs, and (2) the F concentration in CC increases Calc << Arag ≤ Vat.

In relevance to Molnár et al. (2023) in Sect. 2.5: Silicate minerals consist of a variety of component unit structures derived by the polymerization of orthosilicate (H_4SiO_4): Si-OH + HO-Si → Si-O-Si +H_2O. Minerals composed of sheet-type phyllosilicate units are called smectite. For example, montmorillonite consists of two sheets of tetrahedral silica ($SiO_{4/2}$)* sandwiching a central sheet of octahedral alumina ($AlO_{4/2}(OH)_2$), and is chemically described as $(Na,Ca)_{0.33}(Al,Mg)_2(Si_4O_{10})(OH)_2 \cdot nH_2O$. Kaolinite, with a similar structure but without nH_2O in the lattice, $Al_2Si_2O_5(OH)_4$, is another member of clay minerals. * $O_{4/2}$ is a bridging O shared by two adjacent Si or Al atoms.

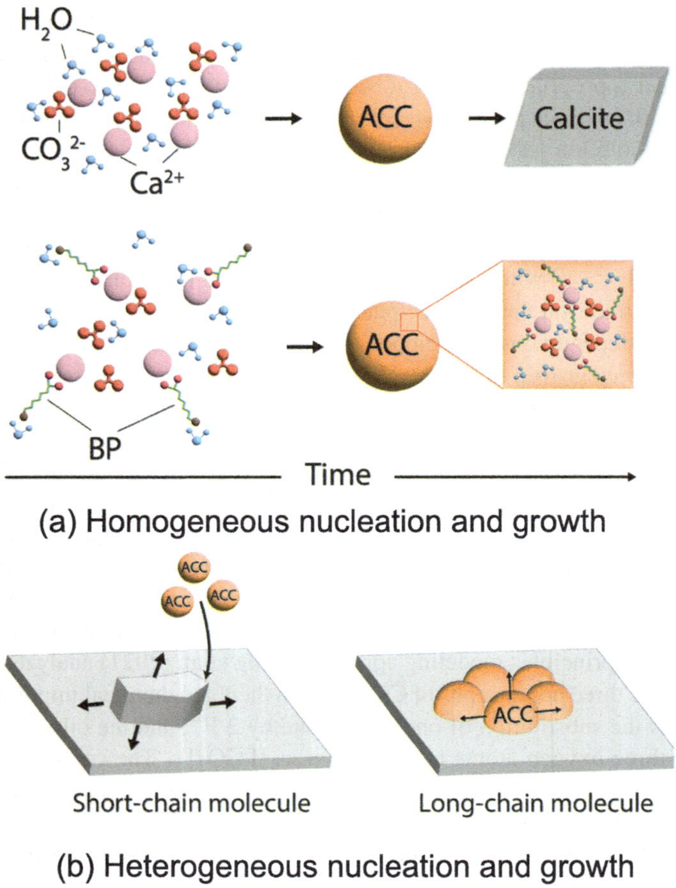

Fig. 6 **a** Homogeneous nucleation procedure: ACC may transform to calcite without BP molecules, whereas BP stabilizes ACC owing to complexation interactions with Ca^{2+} ions within ACC and prevents Cal nucleation. **b** Heterogeneous nucleation on pre-existing CC crystalline planes: regardless of the presence of BP, CC precipitation proceeds with a morphology that depends on the chain length of the BP molecules. Nguyen et al. (2024) (with permission from the American Chemical Society)

2.5 Carbonate Formation in Natural or Artificial Seawater

ACC and its Transformation to Crystalline CC

Our ancestors collected calcium and carbonate ions from the ocean and used them in crystalline (Cal and Arag) and amorphous forms to construct their frames and skeletal parts. Becker et al. (2003) analyzed the ACC structure deposited in the crustacea *Porcellio scaber*. The ACC has a similar EXAFS structure without a strong Ca-Ca correlation around 0.4 nm, indicating a high degree of disorder. Addadi et al. (2003) listed several examples of biogenic ACC in marine organisms and calcifiers. ACC itself is unstable and, in the meantime, is converted into crystalline forms.

Thus, stabilizing effects must be active in calcifiers because some of them require CC for molting. An earlier work (1997) by Beniash et al. (1997) confirmed this transformation using infrared spectroscopy: Cal has no absorption at a specific site, but ACC shows a sharp/strong one. Later, Molnár et al. (2023) attempted to understand the role of ACC in the heterogeneous nucleation of Cal and Vat on silicate minerals touched upon above, or in other words, studied the stability of ACC on their surface. Consequently, they suggested that only smectite strongly enhanced the ACC to Calc transformation, probably because the ACC particles could grow faster and be destabilized, favoring dissolution-recrystallization to Calc. The surfaces of the other two (quartz and kaolinite) slightly stabilized the amorphous state where the ACC particles, as shown by the TEM images in Fig. 7, were present on the edge site of the silicate substrates, forming individual globular particles. This caused a slower transformation than those that remained separated. Sun et al. (2023) prepared rod-shaped Arag and granular Vat from their own Mg-containing synthetic seawater involving Na_2CO_3 and $NaHCO_3$ of varied mixing molar ratios, 1:3 (70 °C; Arag) and 8:1(30 °C; Vat). In addition, they suggested that the presence of Mg^{2+}, K^+, or $SO_4{}^{2-}$ in the solutions favored Arag precipitation, whereas the Mg-free systems favored Vat.

Correlation to Calcium Phosphates

Besides carbonates, many kinds of organisms employ the calcium phosphate family for their hard tissues. The development of artificial hard tissues begins with in vitro experiments before applying them to in vivo experiments. Human plasma is supersaturated with respect to hydroxyapatite, which has the greatest affinity for hard tissue. Thus, when a substrate deposited with CC of any morph is in contact with plasma (pH 7.4), the Ca^{2+} and carbonate ($HCO_3{}^-$ and $CO_3{}^{2-}$) ions in the vicinity of

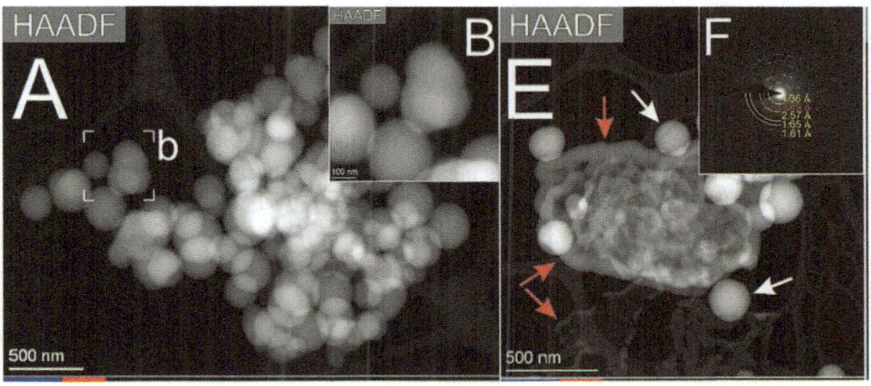

Fig. 7 **a, b** STEM HAADF images of quartz and ACC particles. The ACC particles enveloped preexisting quartz particles. **e** A similar image of kaolinite with ACC (white arrows) formed mainly on the edges of kaolinite particles but also appeared as individual globular particles. Red arrows: merging ACC particles. **f** SAED pattern. Yellow arcs indicate the d-values of kaolinite platelets. The red arc and number mark the diffuse ring with the corresponding d value produced by the ACC particles. Molnár et al. (2023) (with permission from Elsevier)

the CC surface immediately form calcium phosphates, with which the substrate is chemically bonded to the surrounding hard tissue. In a preliminary study, Oral et al. (2020a) demonstrated that Calc, Arag, and Vat particles with varied shapes (rhombohedral, ellipsoidal, and bowknot-like) well proliferated human osteoblast (hOB) cells. Considering the equilibrium of carbonate-related species, Tas (2015) developed artificial seawater with five new recipes and controlled the deposition of any of the three CC forms. Every solution set involved NaCl, $MgCl_2$, Na_2SO_4, $CaCl_2$, KCl, $NaHCO_3$, KBr, H_3BO_3, $SrCl_2$, and NaF (in the order of decreasing contents), while the ionic strength ranges from 0.73 to 0.82, and 0.29 for a set involving only $MgCl_2$, $CaCl_2$, and $NaHCO_3$. No other additives, inorganic or organic, were employed. Figure 8 shows Arag spherules (ooid) depositing from a solution set on the Ultra High Molecular Weight Polyethylene (UHMWPE) surface after soaking for 48 h at 30 °C. This polyethylene surface is chemically inert and inactive to deposit calcium phosphate minerals in the plasma. Kim et al. (2022a) used their own seawater as one of the systems for depositing spherical Vat particles (~10% porous, ~8 μm in diameter). They collected several cases of Vat precipitation in the presence of additives from the literature and summarized them in a table. In their recent review paper, Min et al. (2024a) discussed the behaviors of Ca-based materials, such as CC, tricalcium phosphate (TCP; $Ca_3(PO_4)_2$), and Ca_2SiO_4, on bone regeneration. They provided lists of CC and calcium silicate-based materials to be useful in bone regeneration applications. It is a little regretful, however, that they have not commented on whether chemical bonding could be achieved between their materials and bone tissues [refer to the note in the box below]. Recently, Umemoto (2021) studied the sintering of Calc microparticles into porous Calc granules and bone formation for dental applications. The porous green compacts of Calc were first calcined to eliminate binder at 500 °C for 16 h and then heated at 800 °C for 1 h under flowing CO_2. The sintered bodies have pores larger than 100 μm in diameter. The in vivo test showed better resorption than β-tricalcium phosphate (β-TCP) ceramics and angiogenesis in the pore (generation of new blood vessels). Such high-temperature calcination is conventional in ceramic research and industry. As an alternative, a low-temperature sintering process, denoted as the cold sintering process (CSP), has emerged because it is considered energy-saving or energy-efficient. In CSP, a powder compact containing a small portion of a properly selected aqueous solution is pressed into dense ceramics at temperatures < 300 °C under uniaxial pressures of < 500 MPa. The key steps were dissolution and reprecipitation. According to Seo et al. (2024), "the ceramic particles undergo partial dissolution, forming supersaturated phases, and the phases facilitate the reprecipitation of dissolved components among the particles." For example, Yamaguchi and Hashimoto (2022) applied CSP to densify homemade Vat powder from an ethanol/water solution containing $Ca(OAc)_2$ (AcO: $CH_3C(=O)O$) and $(NH_4)_2CO_3$. The green compacts contained 10 mass % water and were subjected to a uniaxial pressure of 270 MPa. Figure 9 schematically shows the sintering model. From the given sketches (Yamaguchi and Hashimoto 2022), a probable scenario is as follows: (a) The pressure induces further dissolution of the component ions into the water near the contact regions due to stress concentration, and the ions are squeezed into the bulk water region of low pressure. (b) They recrystallized in the newly deposited layer. The residual ions were subsequently crystallized owing to the continued pressurization as well as evaporation of water. Incidentally, Seo et al. produced transparent hydroxyapatite (HAp) ceramics using CSP on HAp compacts with 10 mass % simulated body fluid (SBF), known as the Kokubo solution (Kokubo and Yamaguchi 2019; Kokubo and Takadama 2006; Bohner and Lemaitre 2009).

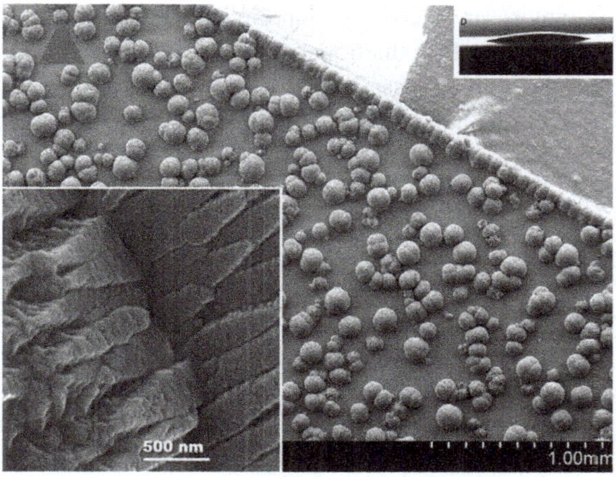

Fig. 8 SEM images of aragonite spherules deposited on UHMWPE (see text) in artificial seawater (48h, 30 °C). Inserts: 0.2~0.3 μm thick layer of mortar-and-brick-type stacking. Insert: Contact angle (water droplet) of superhydrophobic surface of UHMWPE substrate. Tas (2015) (with permission from Elsevier)

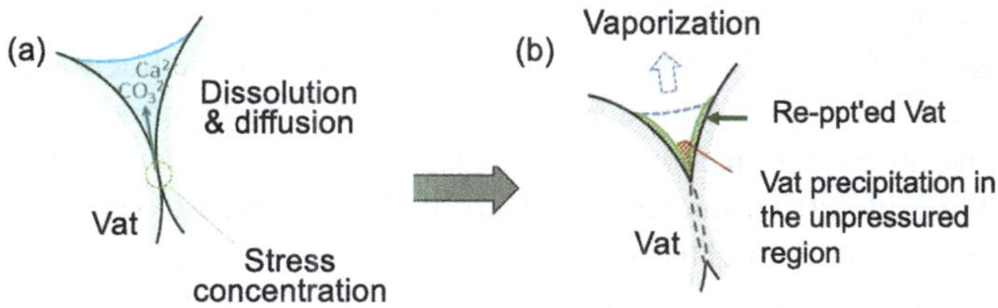

Fig. 9 Steps of cold sintering process (CSP) of Vat. **a** Beginning stage: Dissolution of components near the contact region into the solvent (water) and diffusion to the free surface. **b** Later stages: re-precipitation (re-ppt) on the free surface (green region) and precipitation near the contact region with the released pressure. Modified sketch, Yamaguchi and Hashimoto (2022) (with permission from Elsevier)

Ceramic biomaterials with bone-bonding ability

In 1969, Prof. L. Hench of the University of Florida, USA, opened the era of modern ceramic biomaterials by the invention of Bioglass® (J Am Ceram Soc., 74 (1991)1497). This glass family, with glass coded 45S5 in the center, is the first artificial material group to form chemical bonds directly with bone systems and even soft tissues (e.g., eardrum). This has led to extensive researches to explore another bone-bonding composition and system. Please refer to the book: "An Introduction to Bioceramics," second Ed., edit. by LL Hench, Imperial College Press, 2013, or "Bioceramics from Macro to Nanoscale," edit. by A. Osaka and R. Narayan, Elsevier, 2021.

2.6 *Organic Molecules in the CC Precipitation Solutions*

A few organic molecules are often added to CC precipitating solutions. Functional groups such as -COOH, -OH, -NH_2, and -NH- may have chelating (complexation) interactions with the precipitating components in the solution to modify the activity. However, in the literature, it is rarely suggested how the added molecules interact with the ions to control CC nucleation or crystallization. Yu et al. (2020) used sodium stearate ($C_{17}H_{35}COONa$) and oleate ($C_{17}H_{33}COONa$) to prepare CC particles for filler application. According to Polat (2019), adding sodium laurate ($C_{11}H_{23}COONa$) to solutions of $CaCl_2$ and Na_2CO_3 (pH 8.5, 30 °C) increased the fraction of Vat from 35%Vat-65% Calc to 88% Vat-12% Calc, while the particle morphology changed from cubic to ellipsoidal. In contrast, the average particle size decreased from 32 μm to 14 μm. Tao et al. (2020) studied the effects of Mg and glucose on the precipitating CC phase and morphology. They obtained spindle-like Calc particles with the molar ratio of Mg/Ca <0.5, while at a ratio of ~0.6 rod-like Arag particles appeared and their amount and length increased with the ratio. Moreover, glucose suppressed the effects of Mg on the morphology; the solution with ~1.5 mass % glucose provided all spindle-like particles. Persano et al. (2022) prepared a mixture of ethylene glycol (EG): H_2O (1:5 v/v) and mixed it with equivalent volumes of 0.1 M solutions of $CaCl_2$·and Na_2CO_3. Vat-Calc mixed spherical particles 0.2 ~ 1 μm in size were obtained. Although their SEM images showed a wider size distribution, they achieved a sharper size distribution (monodispersion). The size and Vat fraction depended on the precipitation conditions, including the EG content, precipitation temperature, and reaction time. A set of conditions of 4 °C and salt content of 25 mM for 20 h resulted in the sharpest particle distribution (134 ± 3 nm). The Calc: Vat ratio slightly increased with time, for example, 42:58 (30 min) and 32:68 (180 min). Qi and Zhu (2006) prepared a CC suspension by mixing 0.75 M $Ca(OAc)_2$ (2 mL), 0.75 M Na_2CO_3 (2 mL), EG (10 mL), and SDS (3 mM) prior to heating the suspension with microwave (2.45 GHz, 300 W) up to 100 °C and kept there for 8 min. The final

CC precipitates were spindle-shaped Vat (~5 μm long and ~ 1 μm thick) with no impurities in the XRD chart. In contrast, dagger-like crystallites precipitated due to oil bath heating. With CTAB, instead of SDS, smaller Vat particles (~1 μm) as an assembly of nm-sized grains were precipitated with a trace amount of Calc.

2.7 Polymers (Oligomers and Fibrils) in the CC Precipitation Solutions: Templates

Synthetic Polymers

Linear polymer fibrils or oligomers are found useful for regulating CC particle size, morphology, and polymorphs because most of them have active groups like -OH, $-NH_2$, -NH-, and -COOH, to name a few. The pKa or pKb values of the groups are diverse, and each provides a specific partial or formal charge due to acid–base dissociation in accordance with the solution pH. For example, amino groups hydrolyze water to generate OH^- and $-NH_3^+$ or modify the pH of the system.

$$-NH_2 + H_2O \rightarrow -NH_3^+ + OH^- \tag{8}$$

The resulting partial charges distributed on the fibrillar chains to generate cationic and anionic sites. These sites would regulate or stabilize the arrangement (conformation) of the component species and hence the fibrils are sometimes denoted as template oligomers. This also applies to polysaccharides, amino acid oligomers (peptides), collagen, and their derivatives. They might be within the category of stimulus-responsive polymers (e.g., Issue 1 of Polymer Chemistry, 2017). One of the most impressive examples is chitosan and the other is poly(aspartic acid) (pAsp), alginic acid (alginate), or poly(acrylic acid) (PAA: [-C-C(COOH)-]$_n$). Grant et al. (1973) showed in 1973 that chitosan fibrils embraced cations like Ca^{2+}, forming an "egg box." Figure 10 is a two-dimensional drawing taken from their original paper: each chain has three-fold screw symmetry and is assembled in three dimensions. Polyethylene glycol (PEG) is taken by Siva et al. (2017) to discuss the phase and morphology of CC at the precipitation from a mixture of 0.1 M Na_2CO_3, 0.1 M $CaCl_2$, and 0.01 M PEG incubated at 60 °C (pH control was not given). They expected PEG to behave similarly to PAA, and concluded that PEG promoted Arag and Vat deposition. Liposomes may affect CC precipitation because of their different types of groups. Erceg et al. (2022) reported negatively charged 1, 2-dimyristoyl-sn-glycero-3-phospho-L-serine (DMPS) derived ~2 μm-sized hollow Vat spheres consisting of ~0.2 μm grains. According to Nahi et al. (2023) C_4 and C_7 polyamines and branched or linear polyamines regulate the formation of Arag over Calc or Vat. When they placed $(NH_4)_2CO_3$ powder and 1–50 mM $CaCl_2$ solution in a sealed desiccator, CO_2 and NH_3/NH_4OH due to the decomposition of $(NH_4)_2CO_3$ were gradually supplied to the Ca solution, resulting in CC precipitation. This process is known as a gas-diffusion process (Sect. 4.1). For example, Fig. 11 shows stacked layers of hexagonal aragonite platelets co-aligned along their c-axes, derived from branched polyamines.

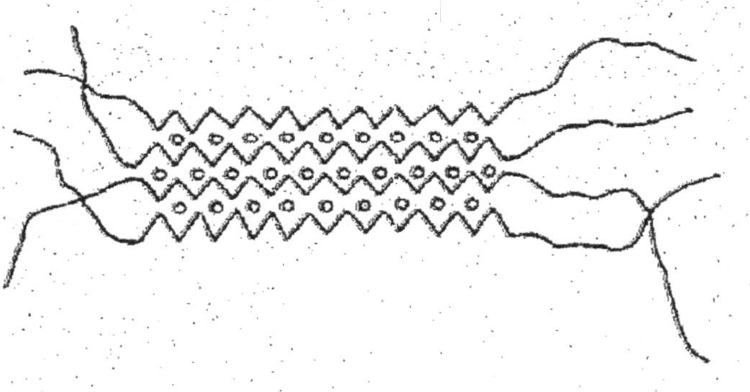

Fig. 10 A two-dimensional model of an "egg box" assembly of chitosan embracing divalent cations (open circles). Grant et al. (1973) (with permission from FEBS Press)

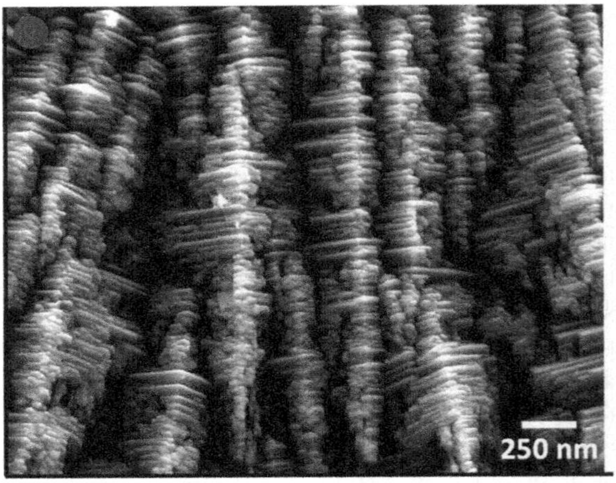

Fig. 11 Stacked layers of Arag hexagonal platelets co-aligned along their c axes. Deposited from a $CaCl_2$ solution (10 mM) with a branched polyamine (1 ppm). Nahi et al. 2023 (an open access paper; Wiley)

Asenath-Smith et al. (2012) provided a good review of the behaviors of hydrogels (hydrogel-like organic matrices) to host crystal growth of CC. They listed several past (< 2012) examples of biomineralization systems and additives in gel matrices. Figure 12 shows the correlation between the Calc growth rate and the strength of the agarose gel matrices. The agarose fibrils embrace the slowly growing Calc particles within a weak matrix. With higher growth rates, Calc is formed across the fibrils, and the same applies to gels with a strong matrix. This shows the importance of a balance between the rates of CC growth and matrix elements.

Zeng et al. (2024) deposited Calc in a chitosan gel layer developed on a glass slide. They used a trick known as the alternate soaking method, which was first attempted by Taguchi et al. (2001). In the first step, the chitosan hydrogel layer was soaked in a 0.1 M $CaCl_2$ solution for 24 h at room temperature, and Ca^{2+}

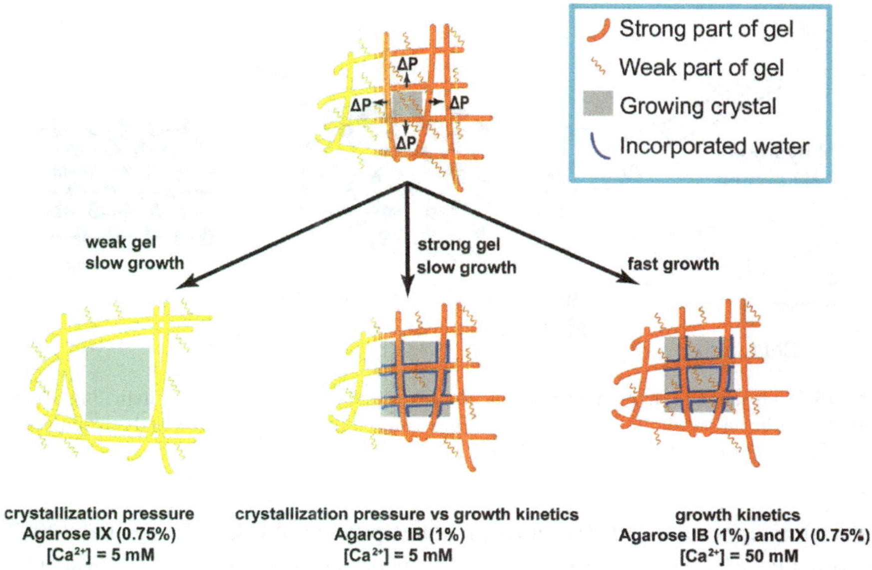

Fig. 12 CC crystallization in agarose hydrogel. Crystal growth causes the pressure (ΔP) to expand the gel matrix. A slow-growing crystal is (left) embedded in the weak gel matrix, whereas (center) it grows across the matrix cells. (right) A fast-growing crystal extends across the matrix cells of an even stronger network. Asenath-Smith et al. (2012). (with permission from Wiley)

ions were trapped in the chitosan network, as shown in Fig. 13. A chitosan gel network was already constructed without forming an eggbox-like structure before the ions diffused into the gel. In the second step, the hydrogel was soaked in a 0.1 M $NaHCO_3$ solution for up to 12 h; then Calc crystallites were precipitated in situ within the chitosan networks. As the precipitation proceeded and the crystallites grew, the elasticity (Young's modulus and tensile strength) increased till 3 h, but then decreased. That is, brittleness was added to the chitosan hydrogel layer by the longer periods of mineralization. Abalymov et al. (2024) reported a similar polymer network of alginate. They prepared ~2 µm size Calc particles by rapidly mixing 0.33 M Na_2CO_3 (1 mL) and 0.33 M $CaCl_2$ (1 mL) and were stirred at 500 rpm for 1 min. The collected Calc microparticles (20 mg) were dispersed in an ALP solution (5 mg/mL) and agitated for 2 h. Calc particles with or without ALP were then dispersed in a sodium alginate solution (1 mass%/v) to obtain mm-sized hybrid spheroid particles. Figure 14 schematically shows the preparation step and the hybrid structure. They expected that drying the as-prepared wet spheroids "would concentrate the Vat particles, giving a spheroid shape suitable for osteoblastic cell growth." However, the MC3T3-E1 cell culture did not indicate that cell viability depended on the presence of alkaline phosphatase (ALP), though hydroxyapatite (HAp) was increasingly deposited during incubation. The chelating interactions between calcium ions and electron-donating groups, such as carboxyl (-COOH), amino (-NH_2), and imino (C=N-) groups, might exhibit either function to promote or inhibit carbonate crystallization. This is an

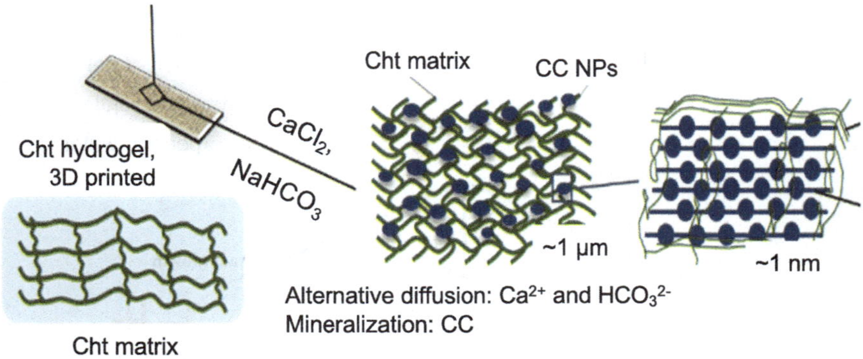

Fig. 13 Chitosan (Cht) hydrogel layer was first developed on a glass slide. In alternating contact with the carbonation solutions, Ca^{2+} and HCO_3^{2-} diffused into the Cht matrix and mineralized to CC (Calc). Zeng et al. (2024) (an open access paper; MDPI)

interesting enzymatic (ALP) route for the precipitation of HAp. Huang et al. (2007) reported in 2007 a step-by-step method for preparing ACC using poly(acrylic acid) (PAA). They first caught the calcium ions (complexation step) by dropwise addition of PAA (Mw: 1.2 k, 2.1 k, 5 k, and 24 k) solution (2 m mol-unit/L) to 5 mL of 0.1 M $CaCl_2$ solution (adjusted to pH 8.3 by aqueous NH_3). Figure 15 shows that the PAA-Ca particle size was controlled by the period of contact under gentle stirring. After an appropriate contact period (3 min ~ 24 h), a $(NH_4)_2CO_3$ solution (0.1 M; pH 10 with aqueous NH_3) was added to the PAA-Ca solution at a rate of 1 mL/min. The collected particles were calcined to yield Calc, Calc + Vat, and X-ray amorphous powders depending on the experimental conditions. The molar ratio of $H_2O/CaCO_3$ of the ACC particles before calcination was 1.33 ~ 1.9. It might be interesting to compare the structure of these PAA-CC amorphous particles with that of the polymer-induced liquid-precursor (PILP) particles, as discussed later.

Cell Membranes and Lipid Bilayers

The cell membranes have a bilayer structure formed by amphiphilic phospholipid molecules. These molecules have a hydrophilic head with a phosphate group and two hydrophobic tails derived from the fatty acids. Therefore, they can form flat bilayers for cell membranes and spherical bilayers for liposomes, with the head outside and the tail inside (see any biology textbook). The head part provides good sites for chelation interactions, and hence, the membranes seem applicable for controlling calcium and carbonate ion arrangements. Wei et al. (2020) used *Yeast*, *S aureus*, and *E coli* as the templates. They first conducted carbonation on gram-negative bacteria and *E. coli* and found that the composition of the cell wall (membrane) strongly affected the polymorphs and morphology of CC. They also conducted carbonation on these three cells after coating their cell membranes with three or four layers of electrolyte via the layer-by-layer deposition route. Figure 16 represents the surface layer structure: β-glucan, mannoprotein, PDDA on *Yeast*, PSS on *S aureus*, and peptidoglycan, lipoteichoic acid, and PDDA on *E coli.* (PDDA: poly(diallyldimethyl ammonium)

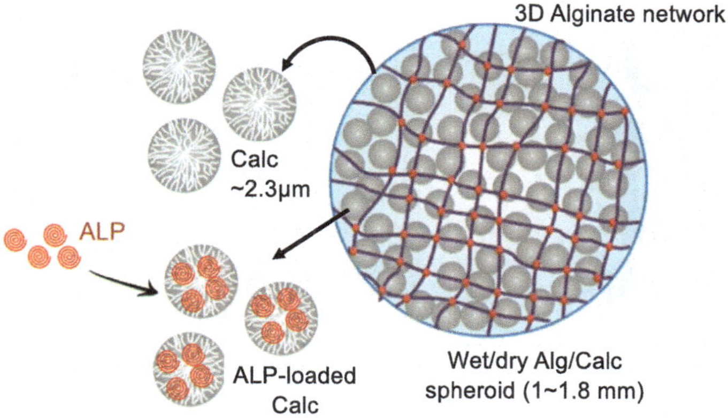

Fig. 14 Vat and ALP-impregnated Calc particles in the Alg network, forming mm-sized composite spheroids. (Dry size: 1 ~1.8 mm with the Alg content: see text.) Calc was converted to Vat during incubation with MC3T3-E1 osteoblastic cells. Abalymov et al. (2024) (with permission from the American Chemical Society)

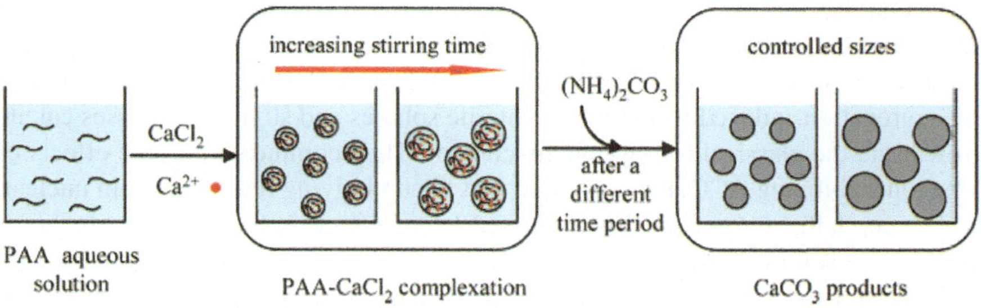

Fig. 15 PAA (Mw: 1.2k ~ 24k) mediated control of ACC and CC particles. The stirring period controlled the size of the PAA-$CaCl_2$ hybrid particles to determine the size of the ACC or CC after calcination. Huang et al. (2007) (with permission from the American Chemical Society)

chloride, PSS: poly(styrene sulfonic acid) sodium salt). Despite the different surface structures (electrolyte layering), the resultant CC consisted of smaller fractions of Calc and larger portions of Vat. From the XRD intensity, the mass ratio Calc:Vat was 14:86 for *S aureus* and *E coli* and 36:64 for *Yeast*. The CC crystallites were distributed mainly on the microorganisms, indicating that less CC was deposited in the solution. Liu et al. (2024) examined the effects of threonine (Thr; an amino acid) and polythreonine (pThr) on CC formation. In an aqueous solution, an equal number of positive and negative charges are on Thr and pThr to be dipolar ions (zwitterions), and seemingly, they have no charge. Liu et al. found that both Thr and pThr stimulated the crystallization of Calc (with no XRD data, the rhombohedral shape of the precipitates (SEM photos) suggested they were Calc). In contrast, their dose did not affect the crystalline morphology. Poly(aspartic acid) (pAsp) is known to retard or inhibit the conversion of ACC to crystalline forms. This indicates that pAsp is one

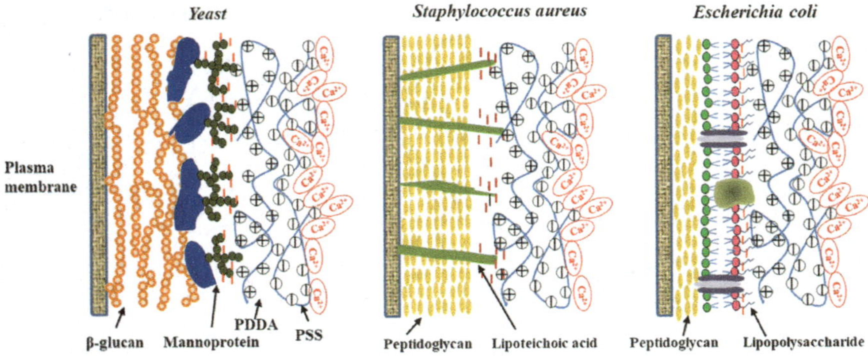

Fig. 16 The cell membrane (denoted as the plasma membrane) of each microbial (Yeast, S. aureus, and E. coli) is modified with three layers of electrolytes, as indicated (see text), on which calcium ions are deposited. Those calcium ions are carbonated when CO_2 is bubbled into the solution. Wei et al. (2020) (with permission from Elsevier)

of the stabilizers of the ACC or ACC nuclei. Recently, Wang et al. (2025) reviewed the crystallization of pAsp and ACC. ACC in the pAsp-free systems transforms into a mixture of Calc and Vat via the classical dissolution-recrystallization (ion-by-ion deposition) mechanism. The presence of deca-mers (10-mers) strongly inhibits the aggregation-induced formation of vaterite spheres and slightly depresses calcite growth via the classical ion-by-ion attachment. They commented on the effects of pAsp on stabilizing ACC, but confessed that the underlying reasons remain unclear.

The crystallization of ACC is discussed later in Sect. 3, focusing on whether it involves conventional nucleation growth or the formation of prenucleation clusters.

Sugawara et al. (Sugawara et al. 2003) derived self-organized relief structures of Calc. The report was published two decades ago, but it demonstrated that the Calc crystallites grew along their c-axis, presenting a beautifully and periodically patterned arrangement, as shown in Fig. 17. They used a complex chemical called pullulans, consisting of glucose units (100-mers) attached to cholesterol branches and poly(acrylic acid) (PAA) as an assisting agent. The CC deposition solution was 10 mM $CaCl_2$ with pullulan and PAA. It was placed in a confined vessel together with $(NH_4)_2CO_3$ and maintained at 10 ~ 50 °C. The solution pH was increased from 4.3 to 9.1 as the solution absorbed ammonia and CO_2 generated from the hydrolytic decomposition of the ammonium salt. Such use of ammonium salt hydrolysis is occasionally denoted as the "gas diffusion" route. Similar conditions were applied, as discussed later in the drug delivery section, to the system in which folic acid was employed as a template to synthesize hollow CC particles.

Fadia et al. (2021) published an elaborate review on the preparation of CC nano- and microparticles with biological applications in 2021.

Liu et al. (2019) were inspired by the "processability of polymeric materials that can be manufactured by crosslinking monomers or oligomers" to construct continuously structured inorganic materials by crosslinking ionic oligomers. They prepared large amounts of $[CaCO_3]_n$ oligomers with controllable molecular weights, where

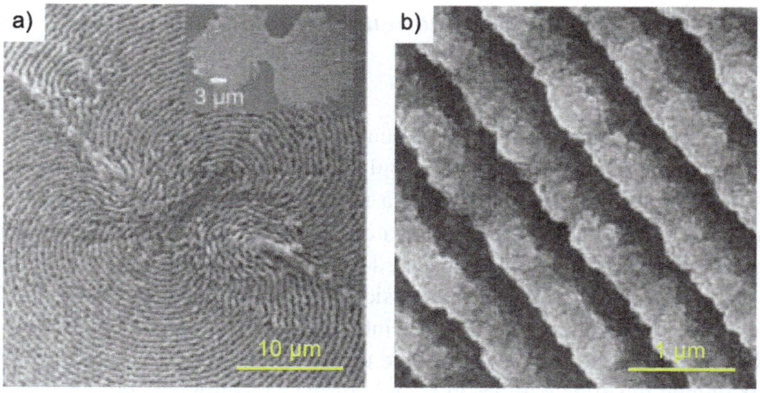

Fig. 17 Periodic patterns of Calc grown on pullulan CHP-3 matrices from 10 mM $CaCl_2$ with 25 ppm PAA (100-mer). The solution and $(NH_4)_2CO_3$ were placed in a closed vessel and maintained at 20 °C for 2 days. Sugawara et al. (2003) (with permission from Wiley)

triethylamine (TEA) stabilized the oligomers as a capping agent. With ethanol in the $CaCl_2 \cdot 2H_2O$ solution, hydrogen bonding between TEA and oligomers was maintained because of its low dielectric constant. As the capping is eliminated in a controlled manner, the oligomers are polymerized to form bulk crystals. Figure 18 shows that they even manipulated and formed an assembly of single-crystal Calc columns in an ordered pattern.

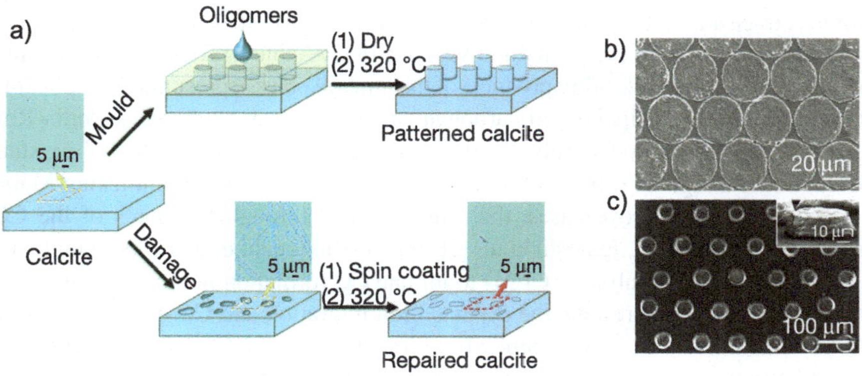

Fig. 18 Calc single crystals from $[CaCO_3]_n$ oligomers. **a** Schemes for pattern construction on single-crystalline Calc (top path) and repair of damaged rough single-crystalline Calc to smooth calcite (bottom path). (**b, c**) Molded Calc with different patterns. The inset shows the single rod. Liu et al. (2019) (with permission from Springer Nature)

2.8 Gel-like Media for Component Diffusion and CC Precipitation

A few interesting kinds of trials are presented in this section. Sánchez-Pastor et al. (2024) set an appropriate amount of waterglass (hydrated sodium silicates containing mainly Na_2SiO_3) in the bottom part of a square cup (⊔)-shaped tube (gel region: 125 mm long, 9 mm in diameter). The waterglass was converted to wet silica gel by adding 1 M HCl, and the pH finally reached 5.5. Note the dry gel is known as a drying agent, "Silica gel." A tube arm on each side was filled either with 0.5 M $CaCl_2$ or 0.5 M Na_2CO_3. Both chemicals diffused into the gel to meet and form CC (although no XRD data were shown, the crystalline morphology suggested that it was Calc). They examined the effects of Na_3PO_4 on hydrogels to form calcium phosphate like octacalcium phosphate (OCP) or HAp. Such a diffusion scheme of chemicals from both sides seems like that found in the alternate soaking technique that Taguchi et al. (2001) used for apatite coating on PAA-grafted poly(ethylene).

Consider the case when the gel part is reduced to an extreme thickness with different salt solutions on either side. This situation resembles that of a process known as chemical garden. A sodium silicate solution is commonly used (e.g., Haudin et al. 2014), and the growing membranes allow bilateral ion diffusion. Getenet et al. (2021) prepared tubular structures of CC (Calc) a few cm long and several mm in diameter by carefully adding 2 M Na_2CO_3 (pH 10.8) to a compact pellet of $CaCl_2{\cdot}2H_2O$. In Fig. 19, the grown Calc membranes show a multilayer structure with a wavy exterior layer and an interior layer of spherical and dumbbell-like Calc crystallites. From the XRD patterns, the tubular membranes consisted only of Calc when incubated for up to 8 h. A trace amount of a mineral named gaylussite ($Na_2Ca(CO_3)_2{\cdot}5H_2O$) appeared after 24 h, and a trace of even NaCl and Vat after 48 h. A table is provided on the acidity of the metal ions and solubility products of the mineral phases, presumably applicable to the formation and ripening of carbonate and silica garden tubes. Escamilla-Roa et al. (2022) grew tiny CC tubes with needles (Arag) and rhombohedral crystals (Calc) under a high CO_2 partial pressure environment (1.05 kPa) mimicking Mars' atmosphere. In the above cases, the ions migrated through the pores of the CC membrane. In contrast, Igarashi et al. (2008) and Takiguchi et al. (2006) employed a cation exchange membrane (CEM) to initiate CC formation in tubular forms. The drawing in Fig. 20 represents the expected ion migration and CC growth. Because the cations, that is, Ca^{2+}, are supplied in one direction, the Ca^{2+} ions are supplied to the bottom of the microtubes, and hence, the tube should grow upward (in this drawing). The SEM images show the morphology of the tubes grown at 50 °C for 1 d (a, b) and 9 d (c, d), respectively. The smaller particles on the tube surface are (a) Vat and (b) Calc. Omran et al. (2023) set up an orthodox chemical garden system with 1 M Na_2SiO_3: they were interested in the Lost City Hydrothermal Field with chimneys of carbonates and hydroxides.

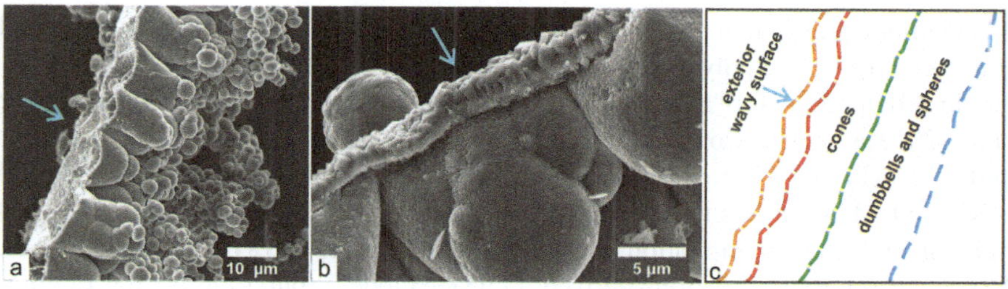

Fig. 19 SEM images of the Calc gardens. Cross-sectional views of the tube wall after **a** 4 h and **b** 24 h of ripening. An exterior wavy surface (blue arrows) comprises a dense layer of interlocked and co-aligned rhombohedral Calc and a less dense interior surface formed by Calc cones, on which open networks of spheres and dumbbells have grown. **c** Schematic illustration of multilayered cross section of the formed Calc membranes. Getenet et al. (2021) (with permission from Wiley)

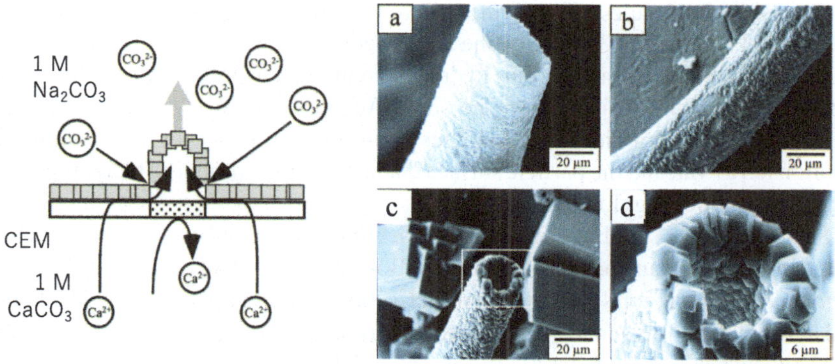

Fig. 20 Vat and Calc microtubes grown in 1M Na_2CO_3 solution. CEM: cation exchange membrane N-117. SEM images of (**a** and **b**) Vat tubes grown at 50 °C for 1 d. Small particles of Vat **a** and Calc **b** are observed on the tube walls. **c**: a Calc tube grown at 50 °C for 9d. **d**: Close-up image of the rectangular part in **c**. Drawing: Igarashi et al. (2008) (with permission from the Ceram Soc Japan); SEM images: Takiguchi et al. (2006) (with permission from the American Chemical Society)

2.9 Surfactants and CC Precipitation

Many types of surfactants have been used for the precipitation of CCs. Typical agents include sodium dodecyl sulfate (SDS), sodium dodecylbenzene sulfonate (SDBS; an anionic surfactant), sodium dodecyl sulfonate (DDS), and the Pluronic® series (product name (BASF) for a series of non-ionic surfactants, for example, F127, triblock copolymers: PEO-PPO-PEO), and cetyltrimethylammonium bromide (CTAB; a cationic surfactant). Here, PEO and PPO are poly(ethylene oxide) and poly(propylene oxide), respectively. It seems to the present author that the real roles of surfactants in the synthesis of CC have not yet been thoroughly clarified. However, many researchers have been able to regulate the morphology, size, and polymorphs of CC. Shen et al. (2023) examined the effects of many additives, such as acids, a chelating agent (ethylenediaminetetraacetic acid EDTA: no Na salts), an alcohol (dipentaerythritol), a polyether (PEG), or an anionic surfactant SDBS, CTAB. They conducted the study for "additive engineering," and the given data are useful. Kanoje et al. (2018) selected two templating agents Pluronics® F98 ($PEO_{118}PPO_{45}PEO_{118}$) and F127 ($PEO_{100}PPO_{65}PEO_{100}$). Simultaneously adding Ca sucrate (1 M) and $NaCO_3$ (1 M) solutions to a mixture of 1.3 mM CTAB and Pluronics® F27 (1 g) immediately led to precipitation of CC, consisting of Calc and a trace amount of Vat. Molecular orbital calculations derived a cluster model around the N^+ ion (ammonium group at the end of CTAB) hydrogen-bonded to a PEO block, with which a few CO_3^{2-} ions interacted. Figure 21 shows a sketch of the clustering and morphology of the CC (Calc> > Vat). Shu et al. (2024) derived microparticles of core-shell structure using a complex system composed of calcium hydroxide, Pluronic F-127, dopamine chloride, and blowing CO_2. They proposed a three-step reaction scheme, as follows: (1) calcium hydroxide and Pluronic® F-127 were assembled to form nanoclusters. (2) The dopamine molecules self-polymerized to form porous cages, embracing calcium hydroxide-F127 units. (3) Finally, the units were carbonated with CO_2 gas to form Calc. That is, some of the calcium hydroxide remained as the core, and the precipitated Calc surrounded it to form the shell. According to Wang et al. (2020), the presence of alkanol amide 6502, another non-ionic surfactant, in the precipitation solution led to Vat, and the particle surface changed from hydrophilic to hydrophobic, preventing particle agglomeration.

Surfactants are suitable agents for fabricating microemulsion systems such as water-in-oil (W/O) and oil-in-water (O/W). Both W/O and O/W phases can coexist to form multiple emulsion systems (Khan et al. (2006)), where lipophilic (hydrophobic) and hydrophilic surfactants are involved. In part of an elaborate and recommendable 2022 review paper, Niu et al. (2022) described a W/O emulsion as one of the systems to derive amorphous and crystalline CC with controlled sizes, morphologies, and inorganic modifications. The resultant CC could then be further engineered with additives such as diethylenetriaminepentaacetic acid (DTPA) via template-induced biomineralization and layer-by-layer assembly into porous, hollow, or core-shell organic-inorganic nanocomposites. Fadia et al. (2021) (Sect. 2.7) touched upon the microemulsion routes to CC using Tween20/80, diaminodiphenyl sulfone (DDS), SDS, or CTAB. They also commented on the O/W/O system (a double emulsion). Liu et al. (2007) were successful in fabricating Calc crystallites from the W/O emulsions with the water phase (Na_2CO_3 and $CaCl_2$), the oil phase (a mixture of 1-butanol/2,2,4-trimethylpentane), and a surfactant tetradecyltrimethylammonium bromide (TTABr).

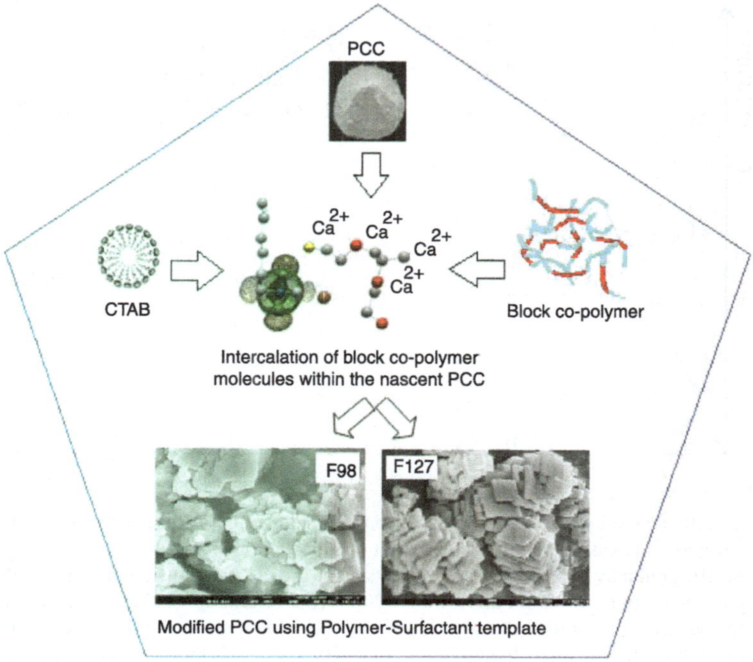

Fig. 21 Schematic representation of the mechanism leading to morphology modification and nucleation of precipitated calcium carbonate (PCC) using a surfactant (CTAB) and block copolymer (PEO–PPO–PEO) template. See text 2.8 for CTAB, PEO, and PPO. Kanoje et al. (2018) (with permission from Elsevier)

3 Crystallization Pathways

3.1 Amorphous Clusters in Solutions

Although they appear uniform or homogenous, solutions and liquids are heterogeneous in micro- to nanoscales owing to their thermal and chemical energy. The classical nucleation-crystal growth theory assumes that each ion or molecule migrates to an appropriate deposition site to form nuclei and contribute to growth. A thermodynamic model depicts this procedure starting from the zeroth stage where some clusters (embryos) repeat formation and dissipation. Occasionally, such embryos live long enough to gather the depositing species, and they grow to the level of nuclei. They are stabilized by the chemical energy (assembly evolves surplus energy; $\Delta H < 0$), surmounting the thermal dispersive energy and decrease in entropy ($T\Delta S < 0$). Thus, a negative free energy change ($\Delta G < 0$) is assured. The nuclei continue to grow and form crystallites. LaMer and Dinegar (1950) and Meldrum and Cölfen (2008) discussed the behavior of the crystallizing components on Fig. 22. Note that this

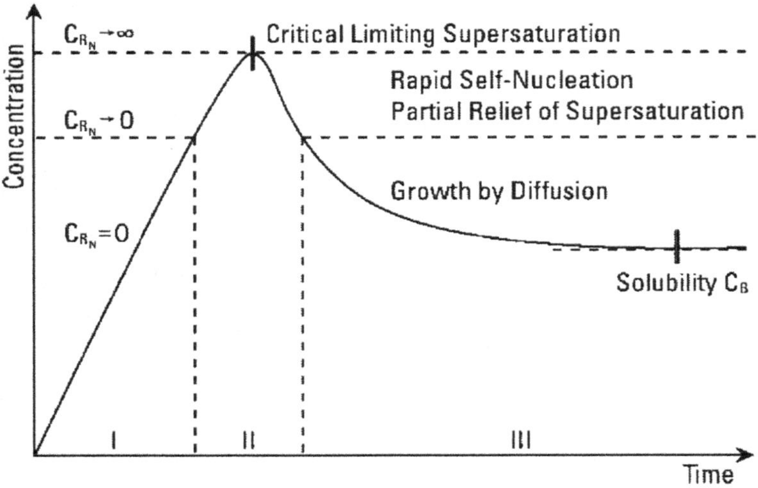

Fig. 22 Schematic representation of solute concentration during crystallization with reaction time. Region I: Rapidly increasing period; II: The limit of supersaturation is relieved by self-nucleation (embryos); III: gradually decreasing period with slower growth by diffusion and approaching the solubility concentration. Meldrum and Cölfen (2008) (the original given by LaMer and Dinegar (1950) represents the preparation of a monodispersed sulfur hydrosol by the slow decomposition of dilute sodium thiosulfate in dilute hydrochloric acid: $2HS_2O_3^- \to 2HSO_3^- + S_2$) (with permission from the American Chemical Society)

figure appears frequently with the modified *x*- or *y*-axis in papers related to the amorphous CC or prenucleation clusters. When the story is applied to CC crystallization, the carbonate ion content steeply increases first because of the reaction between $Ca(OH)_2$ and CO_2 or due to the addition of Na_2CO_3. It soon reached the critical level of supersaturation and then gradually decreased by rapid self-nucleation, followed by approaching the solubility limit by crystal growth. Here, the growth of embryos and their life as prenucleation clusters are the key factors controlling the stability of ACC when the system does not involve crystallization inhibitors (see Fig. 21).

Several decades ago, an interesting case was reported, in which such embryo-like clusters lived long without growing. Posner and Betts, in 1973 and 1975 (Betts 1974), confirmed the presence of stable amorphous precursors, $Ca_9(PO_4)_6$ of 0.95 nm in diameter, within amorphous calcium phosphate (ACP). These are later denoted as Posner or Posner-Betts clusters. Two decades later, Ito-Onuma-Ito-Tateishi (1998) and Oyane et al. (1999) showed that the cluster size was equivalent to the growth step height of hydroxyapatite (HAp) crystallization onto a single-crystal HAp substrate from SBF (introduced above in Sect. 2.5 (Kokubo and Yamaguchi 2019; Kokubo and Takadama 2006; Bohner and Lemaitre 2009). Although SBF itself is supersaturated with respect to HAp and hence is stabilized with an additive, tris (hydroxymethyl)-aminomethane (TRIS)), Oyane et al. (1999) confirmed no effects of TRIS on the cluster or its size in a study on an undersaturated solution. The stability of the Posner-Betts clusters is attributable to no mechanism other than the balance of the dispersion (dissolution) and assembly (deposition) processes. In 2010, Nudelman et al. (2010) observed in situ the behavior of prenucleation clusters of HAp and provided a size 0.87 nm for such clusters.

A similar long research history is present for recognizing ACC and its relevance to the conversion to more stable phases, such as Arag, Vat, or Calc. The existence of ACC was referred to by the 1980s, and its gradual transformation was already pointed out, e.g., by Ogino et al. (1987), as described above in the Introduction. Since 2010, researchers have attempted to understand their inherent stability. Carbonate particles are stabilized by coating with a thin hydrated silica gel (Kellermeier et al. 2010) or organic polymers such as carboxymethylcellulose (Zhang et al. 2024a). "Biogenic calcium carbonate formation is directed by an ordered template of macromolecules," as Pouget et al. (2009) showed from their cryo-TEM study that the prenucleation clusters were ~ 1 nm in size, while the amorphous clusters ranged from 20 to 70 nm in size, and the clusters larger than 70 nm were polycrystalline Vat. They concluded that the formation of prenucleation clusters (PNC) triggers template-directed calcium carbonate formation. Demichelis et al. (2011) proposed a concept of liquid-like ionic polymers for such prenucleation mineral clusters due to their liquid-like flexibility. Thus, they named the stable CC clusters dynamically ordered liquid-like oxyanion polymers (DOLLOP). Moreover, they found that a significant activation barrier existed for dehydration. Kellermeier et al. (2016) proposed that "solute clustering is driven by entropy." The precipitation solution was set at pH 9.5, and the ratio (HCO_3^-)/(CO_3^{2-}) was 6.9 Eq. (5). However, they did not seem to consider the presence of HCO_3^- in their molecular dynamic simulation model. They concluded that the entropy of dehydration ("release of hydration water") is the key factor, and the clusters constitute linear chains. The most important aspect of CC is its high solubility at low temperatures. Moreover, both heat of cluster formation (ΔH_{clst}) and entropy of clustering (ΔS_{clst}) are positive (Kellermeier et al. 2016), indicating that cluster formation is an endothermic process. That is, both enthalpy and entropy changes favor the clustering procedure, different from the classical nucleation concept. Hence, clustering is stimulated also by an increase in the entropy. In other words, the clusters should have a larger degree of randomness than the ionic species in the solution. This is the inverse case for substances, such as sugar, where dissolution in water is endothermic. The positive ΔS_{clst} is probably attributed to the involvement of many water molecules near the inorganic ions in the clusters. The high dehydration barrier may be due to the strong hydrogen bonding among these components. Clark et al. (2022) conducted small and ultra-small angle neutron scattering experiments on deuterated ACC particles. The ACC particles were prepared by mixing 50 mM $CaCl_2$ with 50 mM Na_2CO_3 (pH 13.7) at 4 °C. They have four levels of hierarchical mesostructures due to multi-stage aggregation: the smallest building units have a gyration radius of 3 nm; the second level units are 55 nm; the third and fourth levels are 370 nm and 2.8 μm in size.

In 2008, Gebauer et al. (2008) demonstrated that dissolved calcium carbonate contained stable prenucleation ion clusters that formed even in an undersaturated solution, as discussed above. They found that the amount of Ca^{2+} ions as 10 mM $CaCl_2$ added at a rate of 10 μL/min to a carbonate buffer solution was (dosed Ca^{2+})

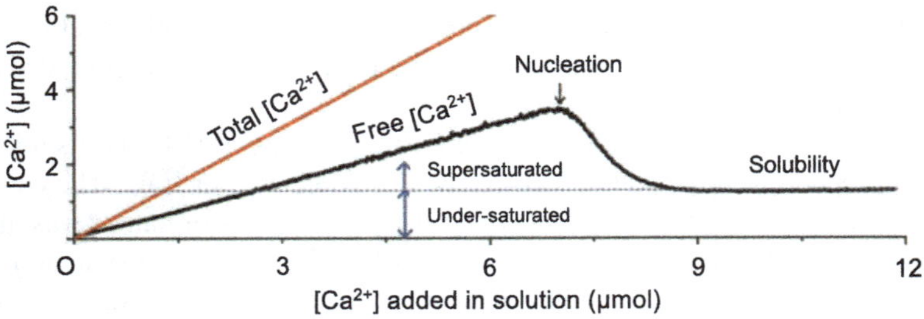

Fig. 23 The amount of free calcium ions (black line) in the carbonate buffer solution (pH 9.25) and the total calcium ions (red line) after the addition of 10 mM $CaCl_2$ at a rate of 10μL/min. Modified from the original where the *x*-axis is assigned to the time of adding the Ca solution. The difference between the red and black lines represents the number of calcium ions bound in the clusters. Gebauer et al. (2008) (with permission from AAAS)

almost 2 times as large as the free Ca^{2+} ions detected in the solution (measured Ca^{2+}), as shown in Fig. 23. The difference between these two is the number of calcium ions involved (bound) within the amorphous clusters. On these bases, they proposed a multiple-binding model to characterize the clusters. Their experiments inspired them to believe that these clusters are thermodynamically stable and not metastable, as classically considered, because an equilibrium constant of cluster formation exists, corresponding to a minimum Gibbs energy. Moreover, they visualized the change in the solubility product (ion activity product (IP)) with the reaction time, and found the presence of ACC I and II with calcitic and vateric short range order, respectively, different in solubilities. Nicholas et al. (2023) conducted a combined study due to a hybrid reverse Monte Carlo (HRMC) and X-ray total scattering but did not touch upon the presence of two ACC phases. In a 2010 paper, Gebauer et al. (2010) reported the results of a ^{13}C magic-angle-spinning Solid-State NMR (MAS NMR) study. They compared the spectra for Calc, Vat, and ACC to find that the NMR spectrum for ACC showed peaks relevant to that of Calc and Vat: they named those ACC phases pc-ACC (pro-calcite) and pv-ACC (pro-vaterite). In addition, the atomic correlations of Ca-O, Ca-Ca, and Ca-O/Ca-CCa K-edge EXAFS supported the presence of pc- and pv-ACC. Following those results, Cartwright et al. (2012) summarized the CC polymorphism and raised a question: "How many amorphous calcium carbonates are there?"

3.2 *Phase Separation in the Carbonate-Related Systems*

Even if we were convinced of the existence of isolated prenucleation clusters or amorphous clusters for CC crystallization, we might not still understand what should stimulate the formation of such stable clusters. Three groups have independently proposed interesting viewpoints: phase separation from a group of D. Gebauer, classical pathway by the group of J. De Yoreo, and polymer-induced liquid precursor

(PILP) from the group of L. Gower. The first and third concepts are introduced in this monograph.

The phenomenon, known as phase separation, was first noticed in the 1940s by engineers working on melts (metals, ceramics, and glass). To the best of our knowledge, Cahn was the first to treat this phenomenon theoretically (for example, J. Chem Phys. 1959, 1965). Enthalpy and entropy changes are involved in phase separation. Figure 24a shows a phase separation diagram of ordinary systems (Nakanishi 1997), such as melts of ceramic oxide mixtures, which would separate into two phases with a decrease in temperature. In contrast, b is a diagram for systems such as some polymer solutions and the present system $CaCO_3$-H_2O (Faatz et al. 2004), which separates into two phases with an increase in temperature. Wallace et al. (2013) shows a similar diagram for a calcium carbonate system. Gower (2008) cited the diagram given by Faatz et al. (2004) in her excellent review paper, whereas Avaro et al. (2020) employed only the left branch, that is, the region of the dilute solution. Figure 24a and b demonstrate an important issue: we have two modes of separation, denoted as binodal and spinodal decompositions. Figure 24b illustrates the resultant microstructures of the system owing to phase separation. The binodal region extends between the solid and broken lines in (a), while the binodal region in (b) is indicated by lines B–C and D–E. In this region, the system is metastable and forms a droplet-dispersed microstructure. The spinodal region in (a) is inside the corn (the broken line, denoted as spinodal) and in (b) the region for line C–D. Within this region, the system is unstable and any density fluctuation leads to phase separation. Therefore, the two separated phases exhibit an entangled microstructure. In both (a) and (b), the vertex of the miscibility gap corns is the critical temperature Tc, and the region outside the miscibility gap corn is a homogeneous solution area. Here, the saturation degree increases as the calcium content approaches the miscibility gap corn. That is, the homogeneous region consists of undersaturated (far from the gap corn) and supersaturated (near the gap corn) subregions. CC exhibits retrograde solubility; hence, it follows the phase separation diagram in Fig. 24b as the polymer solutions. The Flory-Huggins theory interprets the behavior of polymers (see polymer chemistry textbooks). From the viewpoint of enthalpy (interactions among solution components), the following scenario leads to phase separation, according to diagram (a). At temperatures $Tc < T$, the system remains a homogeneous mixture or solution, even if the components are inherently immiscible with each other. Density fluctuations are observed in all liquid systems. Eventually, regions of higher density (embryos for crystallization) are occasionally formed, but they may disappear to homogeneity owing to the dispersion of the thermal energy. As the temperature decreases, the thermal energy cannot dismiss the tendency of the components to aggregate together to form clusters. At $T < Tc$, components of a similar type begin to separate and form individual liquid phases. In contrast, when polymerizing clusters appear and grow in a system, immiscible interactions grow gradually and tend to drive the system to phase separation, even at a constant temperature. The entropy of the system decreases because of the decrease in free monomers (smaller molecules), and at the same time, solvent compatibility is degraded to promote phase separation. This process is called "chemical cooling" and is common in polymer solutions. Nakanishi (1997) provided a typical example

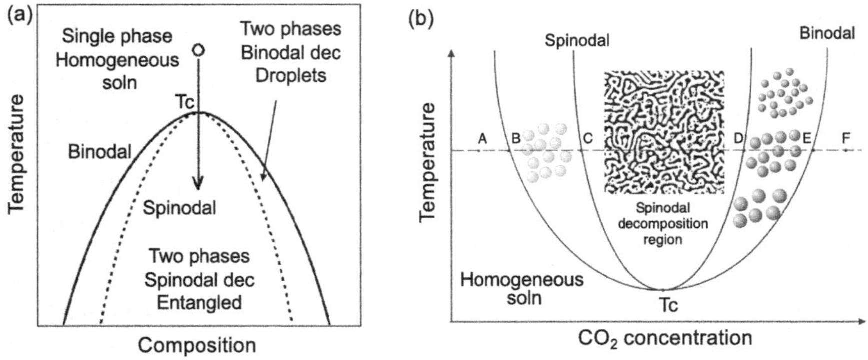

Fig. 24 **a** Phase separation diagram for an ordinary system: a circle with an arrow indicates that the decrease in temperature leads to phase separation at the critical temperature Tc. The inversed-parabola-like immiscibility gap cone (solid line) has a boundary between the binodal and spinodal decomposition regions. Nakanishi (1997) (after modification). (with permission from Springer Nature). **b** The diagram for the system $CaCO_3$-H_2O. The miscibility corns (both binodal and spinodal) are upward, with Tc at the bottom. Microstructures are schematically presented for the binodal (lines B–C and D–E) and spinodal (line C–D) decomposition regions. Homogeneous solutions extend outside the binodal corn (regions A and F). Faats et al. (2004) (with permission from Wiley)

of an inorganic/polymer sol-gel system of $(RO)_4Si$-H_2O-HNO_3-polymer. Here, R: alkyl groups such as CH_3 or C_2H_5, and a polymer such as poly(methyl methacrylate).

Faatz et al. (2004) utilized the diagram (b) for preparing ACC microspheres via the slow hydrolysis of dimethyl carbonate in the presence of $CaCl_2$. The mean sizes of the spheres decreased with increasing temperature: 759 nm (15, 20, and 175 nm (30 °C). Based on the number of particles per unit volume, they elucidated the Tc in this case was approximately 10 °C. Avaro et al. (2013) proposed liquid-liquid phase separation (LLPS) based on stable prenucleation clusters but not on unstable or metastable density fluctuations. Thus, the comments above in this section started with such density fluctuations in the solutions might be incompatible with their LLPS concept. Another paper was published in 2021 by the Gebauer group on phase separation at the nanoscale. Gindele et al. (2021) constructed an ammonia diffusion system (named as AMD process; see Fig. 32a, Sect 4), using a desiccator as the container (2.4 L internal volume) for freshly ground $(NH_4)_2CO_3$ held on a Petri dish and 5 mm^2-sized Si wafers or cover glasses in the wells of a 24-well cell culture plate. They placed a 20 μL droplet of $CaCl_2$ solution (20–40 mM), with or without poly(acrylic acid) (PAA; Mw: 7800; 0.1 ~ 0.5 g/L) on each piece of wafer or cover glass. The cell culture plate and Petri dish were covered with a lid with a 0.5 mm hole and a cap with three 1 mm holes. They proposed that a dense liquid phase deposits on the solution drop surface in the form of a film or droplet, and it solidifies to ACC particles before crystalline CC is precipitated because of the dissolution-redeposition process or via growth to larger ACC particles. They stressed that liquid precursor formation occurred in this system.

In melts of ceramic materials, the components themselves are the solutes and solvents, while in the system $CaCO_3$-H_2O, the calcium and carbonate (or bicarbonate) ions are the solutes in water (the solvent). Actually, Sebastiani et al. (2017) stressed on the significance of ion hydration. Moreover, experiments were conducted by slow addition of a dilute calcium salt and carefull analysis of the behavior of Ca^{2+} within the range of undersaturation to supersaturation. The saturation was determined by the solubility product Ksp of $CaCO_3$ on the order of ~10^{-9} $(mol/L)^2$ (see Table 1). In contrast, it is common to dump either a calcium or carbonate solution into a reaction vessel holding the counterpart solution. Thus, the ion concentration at the reaction front exceeds the supersaturation level. In such cases, the system already reaches Stage II of Fig. 22; hence, the component ions are rapidly assembled to form nuclei, leading to crystal growth.

3.3 CC Growth: A Classical Pathway

It should be fair to refer here to a classic model due to nucleation and crystallization pathways, although Avaro et al. (2020) claimed that "the classical nucleation theory should not be considered for the aqueous calcium carbonate system, or likely any system where homogenous phase self-association is significant." The Posner-Betts clusters for hydroxyapatite crystallization have not been described in terms of phase separation, but in terms of the growth units. Yet, in the context of this claim, the P-B cluster is also a child of the phase separation movement. These clusters form homogenous systems and might be called "homogeneous clustering," analogous to the classic models of crystallization. The two studies to be introduced below take the CC growth under "heterogeneous nucleation and growth" model. Mills et al. (2021) studied the fractionation of the two calcium isotopes, the most and second abundant (^{40}Ca (96.9%) and ^{44}Ca (2.1%), during calcite precipitation. They postulated that fractionation depends on the solution stoichiometry and is driven by Ca exchange at the surface sites during growth. This would directly test the conceptual model of Ca isotope discrimination. They used a mixture system of 0.25 M $CaCl_2$ and 0.25 M K_2CO_3 (pH 8.5 set with 0.1 M KOH), and studied Calc growth on calcite seed crystals. The results confirmed the ion-by-ion attachment/detachment model. In industrial engineering, the scaling of pipe/tube walls is a vital subject. Armstrong et al. (Armstrong et al. 2024) recently correlated the rate of Calc nucleation with nanoscale tomographic surface. The experiments were well designed to clarify the surface topographical effects on the Calc deposition with varied supersaturation σ: $[Ca^{2+}]\cdot[CO_3{}^{2-}]$/Ksp (Calc) (4.44 ~ 4.86). In Fig. 25a, solutions of 0.1 M $CaCl_2$ and Na_2CO_3 were introduced through different syringes into a microfluidic chip reactor to form a laminar flow (channel: height 0.8 mm height width, 1.7 mm) at a rate of 0.25 mL/min (Re <10, Re: the Reynolds number). The mixed solution was placed in an observation zone consisting of upper and lower substrates with smooth or "nano-engineered" microstructures, where the number of nuclei was counted. Figure 25b illustrates that the surfaces of the substrates and pieces of cover glass were lined with

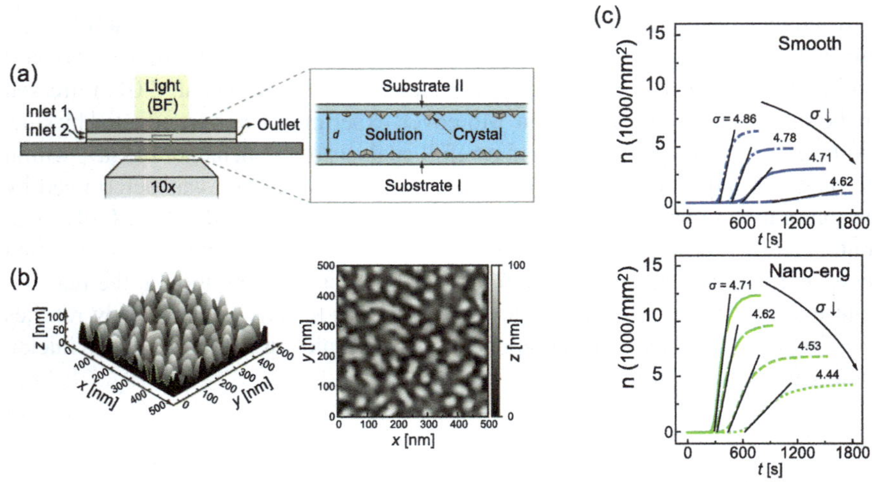

Fig. 25 **a** A setup to observe nucleation of Calc from 0.1M $CaCl_2$ and Na_2CO_3 solutions. **b** Nano-engineered inner surface of the substrate in **a**. **c** the number of nuclei, n, as a function of reaction time. σ is supersaturation (see text). The rate of nucleation (slope) increases with σ. Armstrong et al. (2024) (an open access paper; Wiley)

≈80 nm high and 50 nm thick protrusions. Both substrates were finally coated with a thiol-based self-assembled monolayer (SAM). The SAM surface was terminated with a carboxyl group to provide high calcium ion affinity. Figure 25c shows the number of nuclei n (mm^{-2}) for both substrates. The slope corresponds to the nucleation rate. They claimed that the nanoengineered surface exhibits a nucleation rate 300 times larger than the smooth surface, although the former shows a roughness index of only 2.45 times larger than the latter (smooth one). They concluded that the enhanced nucleation rate is not solely attributable to the surface area, but that the nano-curvature is the key factor, that is, they rationalized the results with the classic nucleation theory.

Darkins et al. (2024) published a short paper claiming that the classical mechanism would interpret CC crystallization, and that the classical nucleation pathway theory could not be translated to the PNC model. Dou et al. (2022) discussed the CC nucleation from the viewpoint of diffusion.

Gebauer et al. (2018) discussed in 2018 both the classical and non-classical pathways.

A recent contribution from the group of JJ De Yoreo is concerned with the behavior of "peptoids" or derivatives of peptides. Zhang et al. (2024b) synthesized peptoid molecules, block-copolymer of two peptides: the hydrophobic parts involve N-(2-phenylethyl)glycine group (Npe), mimicking the hydrophobic phenylalanine residue, and the other hydrophilic parts involve N-(2-carboxyethyl)glycine group (Nce), mimicking aspartic acid or glutamic acid residue. They studied their effects on the step growth rate of Calc, in conjunction with the deprotonation of HCO_3^- and desolvation of Ca^{2+} (Eq. (9); ppt: precipitation).

$$HCO_3^- \rightarrow CO_3{}^{2-} \text{ (ready for ppt)} + H^+ \text{(aq or associated with the peptoids)} \quad (9a)$$

$$Ca^{2+} \text{ (aq) (coordinated to } H_2O) \rightarrow Ca^{2+} \text{ (ready for ppt)} \quad (9b)$$

Both processes are essential for carbonate crystallization. Because the former (8a) is known to be an order of magnitude slower than the latter 8(b) (Schulz et al. 2006), Zhang et al. hypothesized that the deprotonation process enhanced by the peptoids would accelerate step growth. From the standpoint of the step-growth mechanism, it is easily presumed that a high rate of crystal growth should be achieved when both ions come to the deposition sites at a similar frequency (Andersson et al. 2016). That is, the effects of peptoids are to facilitate the dating journey of each ion. As a result, the copolymer 8Nce-4Npe seemed to be the best for balancing electrostatic and hydrophobic interactions.

3.4 ACC Atomic Structures

Extensive studies were conducted before the first decade of the twenty-first century. For example, Michel et al. (2008) applied X-ray absorption fine structure (EXAFS) and X-ray adsorption near-edge spectra (XANES) for the Ca K-edge region, and MAS ^{13}C NMR (400 MHz, 9.4 T, 10 kHz spinning) to study the atomic structures of ACC, derived from two routes: ACC I was prepared by rapidly mixing 20 mM Na_2CO_3 (pH > 14 with 0.5 M NaOH) and 20 mM $CaCl_2$ solutions at room temperature (according to Koga et al. *Thermochim. Acta* 318 (1998) 239). ^{13}C enriched (99%) carbonate was used for NMR analysis. ACC II was derived from the method using dimethyl carbonate and calcium chloride dihydrate (Faatz et al. 2004). The two samples were virtually identical. The pair distribution functions (PDFs) for either ACC gave a predominant peak at 2.41 Å for the Ca-O distance (0.241 nm; for the convention, Å (=0.1 nm) was used). The pre-edge feature at ~4.04 kV, attributable to the 1 s → 3d transition, was more intense for ACC than for other reference materials (Calc, Arag, Vat, or $Ca(OH)_2$) in the XANES profiles. This is a forbidden band in octahedral symmetries; however, they considered that the transition seems slightly allowed owing to thermal disorder. The point is that the weak peak for ACC exhibited a greater intensity than that for Arag, and Calc showed a weak doublet peak around this region. Thus, it may be inferred that "the first shell coordination of the Ca atom is significantly distorted relative to an octahedron, and perhaps also relative to the coordination in Arag." Moreover, PDF confirmed that they were virtually indistinguishable and showed equally a prominent feature at 2.4 Å for Ca-O bond distance, but the most important overall feature is the rapid attenuation of the PDFs: they lose structural coherence beyond ~1.5 Å and have little intermediate-range ordering. In other words, these ACCs exhibit only short-range ordering and can be considered truly amorphous. From the NMR analysis, they claimed that the protons (^1H) in ACC are present as rigid H_2O, coordinated to Ca atoms, and their motions are restricted (not mobile) because they are involved in hydrogen bonding. That is, H_2O stabilizes the ACC structure that is not "a nano-crystalline or disordered form of monohydrocalcite." The fact that the present ACC samples have no HCO_3^- in their structure is acceptable because the solution pH is almost equivalent to that of 1 M NaOH, and the concentration of bicarbonate ions is negligible according to Eq. (5).

Nicholas et al. (2023) recently reported a refining work on the ACC structure. Figure 26 represents that they successfully elucidated an interatomic potential function that can interpret the experimental total X-ray diffraction of ACC (or PDF) structures. Their modeling technique was a hybrid reverse Monte Carlo (HRMC) approach, and the calculation was performed on 12,960 atoms corresponding to 1620 $CaCO_3{\cdot}H_2O$ formula units. The HRMC is believed to provide a suitable compromise between the experiment and the model. The experimental PDF exhibits two large and broad peaks at approximately 4 Å and 6 Å (for the convention: Å = 0.1 nm), corresponding to the Ca···Ca distance illustrated in Fig. 26a. Accordingly, the application potential should have two wells centered around these separations. They commented

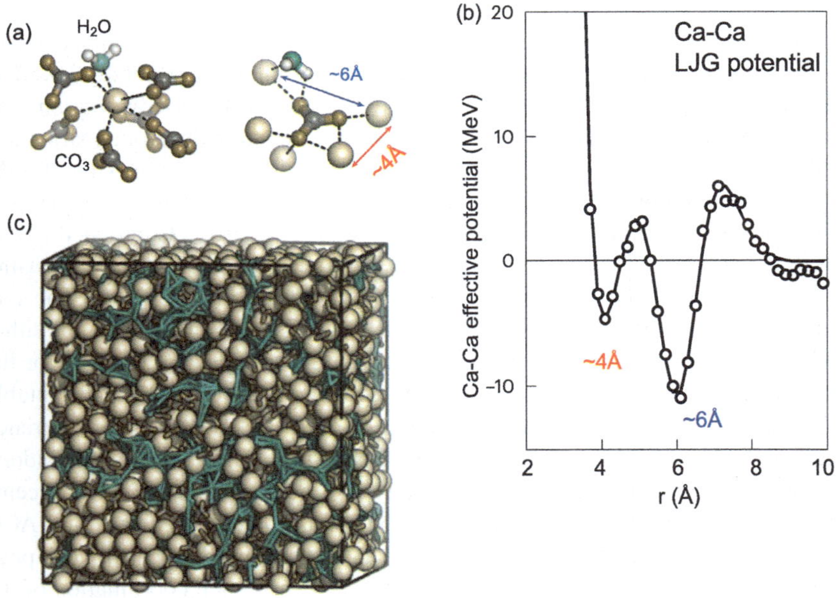

Fig. 26 **a** Representative coordination around Ca^{2+} (beige spheres) and CO_3^{2-} ions from the HTMC simulation. (O: small blue spheres). **b** The Ca-Ca effective potential, extracted from the HRMC runs and best-fitted (solid lines with open circles). Note that the potential wells at the Ca-O-Ca (~ 4 Å; red arrow) and Ca-O-C-O-Ca (~ 6 Å; blue arrow) distances are given in **a**. **c** Representative Monte Carlo configuration of Ca atoms (beige spheres) generated by the LJG (Leonard-Jones-Gauss) potential **b** using the unit distances in **a**. The Ca atoms are not uniformly distributed, but cluster to leave Ca-poor voids, shown as aquamarine surfaces. Nicholas et al. (2024) (an open access paper: Springer Nature)

on the physical meaning of this potential, and Fig. 26b shows the effective Ca···Ca interatomic potential (open circles: HRMC runs; solid line: least-squares fit using a Lenard-Jones-Gaussian model). Figure 26c shows the model from which the atomistic arrangements in (a) are extracted. The Ca atoms were not uniformly distributed but formed clusters, leaving Ca-poor voids (blue regions). Note in (c) that those water molecules connect each other to form filamentary strands (aquamarine strings) that separate calcium carbonate-rich domains (Ca: beige spheres, carbonate ions: stick representation), like "blue cheese." Nicholas et al. (2023) were skeptical of such an interpretation on the role or behavior of water molecules that nearly all H_2O molecules are bound to Ca^{2+}.

3.5 Polymer-Induced Liquid Precursors (PILP)

PILP in Calcium Phosphate (Ca-P) Systems

Almost all organisms employ calcium and organic macromolecules to construct organic-inorganic hybrid skeletons showing beautiful hierarchical microstructures. We have been fascinated by the beauty of the pearly layer of nacre, as shown in Fig. 27 (Bruet et al. 2005), a hybrid of aragonite (Arg) plates and chitin or protein, known as the "brick and mortar" structure. Bone systems consist of nanocrystalline carbonated hydroxyapatite embedded within an organic (mostly collagen) matrix. The microstructure of turkey tendon tissue is shown in Fig. 28a, according to Landis et al. (1993). This illustrates the alignment of collagen fibrils assembled in a complex microstructure with gaps and holes, which is known as a quarter-staggered structure. Bone mineralization has attracted the attention of researchers to clarify its mechanism of action. In the context of bone mineral calcification, the group led by Gower extensively accumulated results on the correlation between non-collagenous proteins

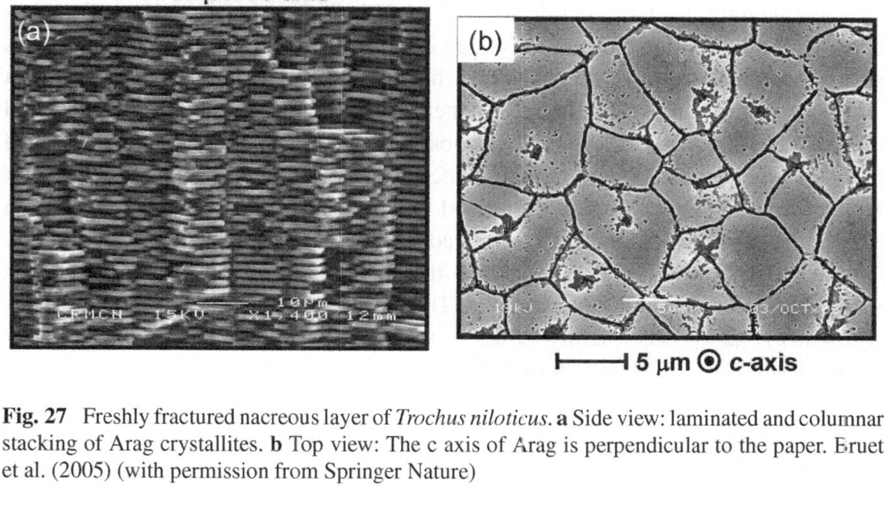

Fig. 27 Freshly fractured nacreous layer of *Trochus niloticus*. **a** Side view: laminated and columnar stacking of Arag crystallites. **b** Top view: The c axis of Arag is perpendicular to the paper. Bruet et al. (2005) (with permission from Springer Nature)

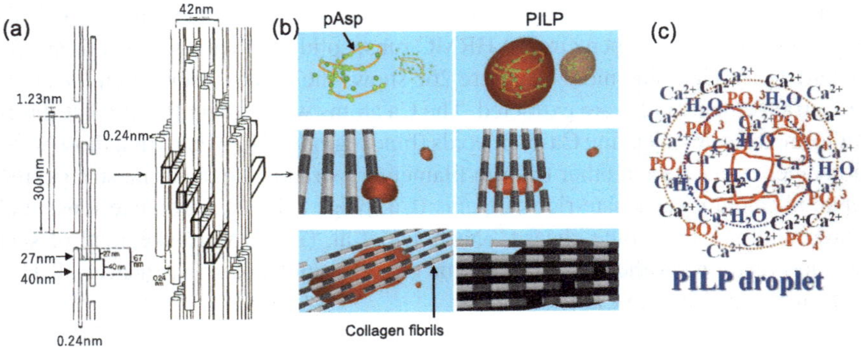

Fig. 28 **a** Schematic drawing of the quarter-staggered structure of 1.2 nm thick and 300 nm long collagen fibrils. The 40 nm holes (thick rectangular cuboids passing through aligned fibrils), 27 nm overlap zones, and 0.24 nm inter-fibril separation are observed. Landis et al. (1993) (with permission from Elsevier). **b** A PILP cluster is generated in the solution, diffused into the hole part of the collagen assembly to grow, and transformed into a new bone system. Cölfen (2010) (with permission from Springer Nature). **c** Molecular assembly model of the PILP droplet. The tangled red line represents an oligomer, for example, pAsp (Courtesy of Dr. L.B. Gower, Univ Florida)

(NCP) and hydroxyapatite formation. Readers may want to access their works and related papers listed in the last part of this monograph, though only a few. The conclusions can be summarized as follows (Olszta et al. 2007): (1) some non-collagenous proteins (NCPs) such as otonecine, osteocalcin, phosphophoryn, aspartic acid, and phosphoserine play an essential role, because (2) they have high affinities for collagen and calcium, and (3) they tend to hold calcium (due to chelation interactions). Item (3) is important for reducing the activity of Ca^{2+} in the solution. If dissolved in plasma supersaturated for HAp nucleation and crystallization, the NCPs stabilize the solution by reducing the apparent $[Ca^{2+}]$ or supersaturation level, working as an inhibitor of HAp crystallization, that is, bone mineralization. From an experiment on the intrafibrillar mineralization of type I collagen, they found that HAp was deposited in spherulitic clusters 15–40 μm in diameter on the scaffold surface. It was suggested that those clusters resulted from heterogeneous nucleation and growth "in a non-specific fashion." In fact, the component crystallites of the spherulites exhibited the characteristic morphology that we observed for hemispherical HAp deposited on bioactive porous silica or titanium oxide surfaces (Kokubo and Yamaguchi 2019; Kokubo and Takadama 2006; Bohner and Lemaitre 2009). In contrast, the solution containing pAsp (15 μg/mL; 15 ppm) led to infiltration with calcium phosphate. Cölfen (2010) drew a cartoon, as shown in Fig. 28b, which schematically demonstrates the infiltration and sedimentation. The molecular model of the PILP droplet is shown in Fig. 28c. Consequently, a PILP droplet is an amorphous assembly with water molecules, and the oligomer promotes the stability of the particles when in solution, yet it allows the embraced pieces to settle on the sites properly for mineralization (crystallization). This concept has been applied to the development of biomedical materials such as bone grafts (Thula et al. 2011). Jee et al. (2010) examined the effects of the length of the polymer additives using pAsp of 10.3 k and 32.2 k (molar weight (Mw)). As a result, the latter pAsp yielded better and quicker mineralization.

PILP in the Carbonate Systems

Figure 29 schematically represents the calcium carbonate crystallization pathways (Gower 2008). The PILP process provided a metastable intermediate amorphous phase. It is to be an issue of interests how the oligomers behave to collect component species and stabilize the clusters or how the cluster releases the ions for further phase transformation. In 2012, Bewernitz et al. (2012) discussed the interactions between pAsp (Mw: 14 k) and calcium carbonate. They analyzed in detail the ^{13}C NMR profiles of the solution (9 mM $CaCl_2$, 30.15 mM bicarbonate buffer; with or without (=control) pAsp. They observed a phase separation in the solution with pAsp or PILP formation in the NMR profile. It is significant that they found the growth of the PILP peak at the bicarbonate ions-related region centered at 161.2 in δ (ppm). That is, the PILPs grew, incorporating bicarbonate ions, whereas the prenucleation cluster (PNC) models denied such inclusion (e.g., Gebauer et al. 2008). Some interpretation was made as to why PNCs would not lead to the presence of the bicarbonates. Homeijer et al. (2010) examined if the PILP process could be expanded to the crystallization of $BaCO_3$ and $SrCO_3$. They obtained nanograined textured <1 mm long $SrCO_3$ or $BaCO_3$ fibers from 15 mL of 6 mM $BaCl_2$ or $SrCl_2$ solution with 100 μg/mL poly(acrylic acid) (PAA; Mw: 5100) held in a vial. The carbonate ions were supplied from $(NH_4)_2CO_3$ wrapped in a film hanging over the solution in the vial. The ammonium salt is spontaneously hydrolyzed to NH_3, H_2O, and CO_2 to be supplied to the solution system for the mineralization of Sr^{2+} and Ba^{2+} and to keep the system alkaline. Depending upon the PAA content (10, 50, and 100 μg/mL), spherulitic aggregates of $BaCO_3$ (typical sheath of wheat morphology), many long fibers thinner than 1 μm, and polycrystalline "horse tails" were yielded. At 500 μg/mL PAA, film-like objects were observed at the solution/air interface. A similar morphology variation was observed for $SrCO_3$ crystallization. They elucidated a possible new mechanism for the formation of the carbonate granule-based fibrils: (1) the formation of PILP droplets embracing M^{2+}, CO_3^{2-}, and H_2O with PAA, (2) PILP-deposition on higher surface energy sites (like a top of a bump: ∩) with charge-matching, (3) continued deposition leading to the fibril growth. On the other hand, Wolf et al. (2011) studied the possibility of another type of polymer, ovalbumin, to be a PILP polymer for the eggshell formation, while Gower and Odom postulated (2000) that some polypeptides should play a role similar to pAsp. In this study, a saturated solution of calcium bicarbonate with ovalbumin and lysozyme (7.5 mg/mL) was used as the starting material, different from the others. They chose a high protein content to provide conditions similar to those in the uterine fluid. As the solution was kept still, water slowly evaporated to stimulate the slow release of CO_2 owing to the decomposition of HCO_3^- (Kitano method, Bull. Chem. Soc. Japan, 1962). Thus, the precipitation of CC proceeds slowly under almost neutral conditions because the system is a bicarbonate buffer solution and the inherent pH is approximately 7.4. The results show that ovalbumin binds calcium, whereas lysozyme does not. However, calcium remained highly coordinated in the presence of ovalbumin. A

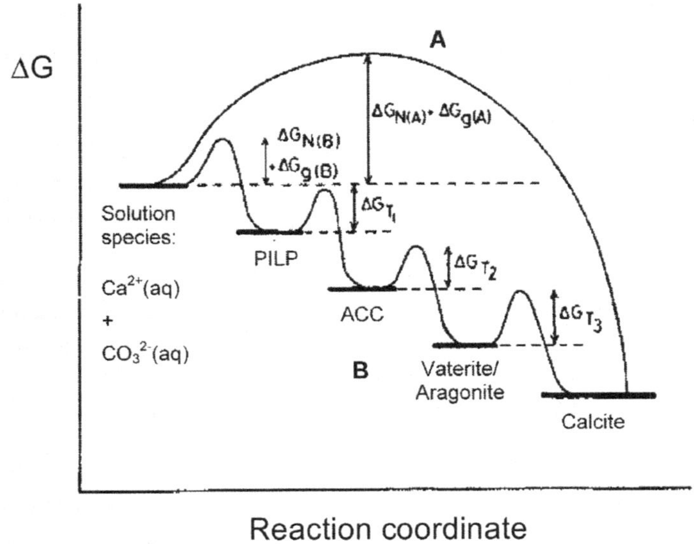

Fig. 29 PILP process within crystallization pathways from solution to Calc (calcite). A: the conventional route without passing through any intermediate phase. B: the route to Calc via metastable crystalline phases (Vat, Arag) and amorphous phases (PILP, ACC). The changes in the free energy ΔG are not drawn to scale. Gower (2008) (with permission from the American Chemical Society)

probable interpretation is that the Ca ions are highly hydrated (H_2O around them), and hence there are no chelating interactions with the protein. In conclusion, ovalbumin stabilizes the liquid precursor phase as a PILP'ing additive for calcium carbonate and contributes to the eggshell formation. In contrast, lysozyme destabilized the emulsified phase, leading to coalescence.

3.6 Glass Transition in Amorphous Calcium Carbonate (ACC)

The correlations between the liquid, supercooled liquid, glass, and crystal states of a substance are schematically represented in Fig. 30, where the enthalpy, volume, and entropy of a substance are plotted as a function of temperature T. Here, Tg is the glass transition temperature of the substance, and Tmp is the melting point if it melts without decomposition at the temperature elevation. The melts of common salts may crystallize catastrophically around Tmp with a decrease in T. Note that glass does not denote a liquid state, but is indicative of an amorphous solid. At Tg, a break may appear in the property-temperature plot. Glass wares in our daily life easily attain the glass state by pouring melts into molds or shaping baths. Many substances can be vitrified by quenching melts at high cooling rates. As discussed above, we have

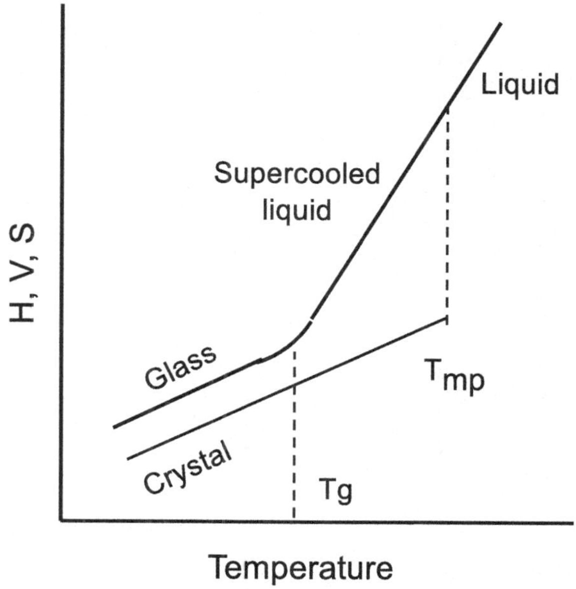

Fig. 30 The enthalpy, volume, or entropy of a substance is plotted as a function of temperature to represent the correlation between the liquid, supercooled liquid, crystal, and glass states. Note that glass is not a liquid but an amorphous solid. Tg: glass transition temperature, Tmp: melting point. (An original drawing)

amorphous calcium carbonate, and we may have a good chance to observe the glass transition when the temperature of the system is varied.

A series of three papers were published by the same research group, all of which employed fast scanning differential scanning calorimetry (DSC) or fast DSC for the analysis. For readers unfamiliar with this field, additional information on the glass transition or DSC principle is provided here. Most of the molecular motions are frozen below Tg during cooling, and a portion contributing to the lattice thermal expansion is retained. Inversely, the lost freedom of motion is revitalized by heating, and this step is an endothermic process. At Tg, a greater amount of energy is necessary to fully activate all freedoms of movement because the state changes from solid to supercooled liquid. DSC machines detect the heat flow accompanying changes in the energetic state. Therefore, precise measurements require slower heating rates (5–10 °C at most) so that the sample temperature and heater control are in equilibrium as much as possible. The fast DSC technique uses tremendously high heating rates (500–2000 °C/s) to separate the glass transition and crystallization events.

The first paper is by Bissort et al. (2024) on the glass transition of an anhydrous ACC. They prepared 0.25 M $CaCl_2$ and 0.25 M Na_2CO_3 solutions (no pH adjusted) and kept them at 10 °C in the refrigerator for at least 4 h before mixing. The precipitations were collected by filtering, freeze-dried for 12 h, and stored in a desiccator until use. They obtained DSC charts (Fig. 31) of heat flow vs. temperature) that resembled the back-head-nose line of an elephant. Tg is assigned to the temperature at the boundary of the back head. Then, they plotted each Tg for the scan rate, and the temperature, due to extrapolation to scan rate = 0 °C, was taken as the Tg of the sample. In fact, it was 339 °C. Hess et al. (2023) studied Tg of anhydrous

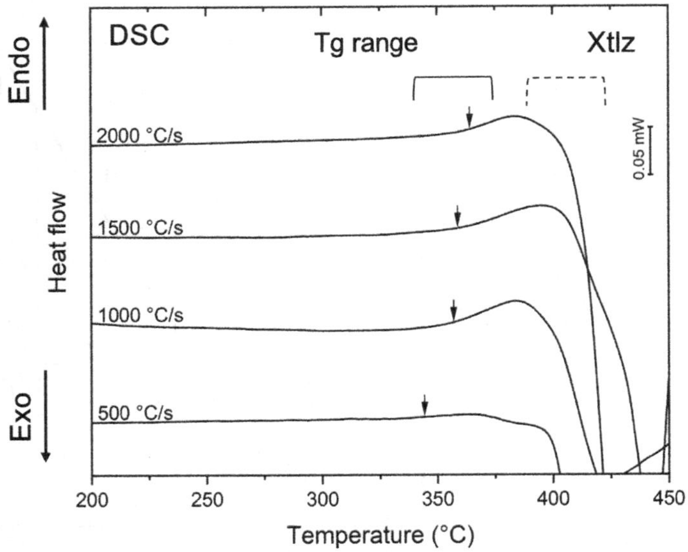

Fig. 31 Fast-scanning DSC charts of anhydrous ACC. The temperature scanning rates are indicated (500~2000°C/s. The arrows indicate the apparent Tg. Xtlz: Deep exothermic peaks due to crystallization. Bissbort et al. (2024) (an open access paper: DeGruyter)

calcium magnesium carbonate $Ca_{0.95}Mg_{0.05}CO_3$. The preparation was mostly the same as above. The precipitates from adding 0.25 M (Ca + Mg)Cl_2 ([Mg]/([Mg] + [Ca]) = 0.12) (80 mL) solution to 0.25 M Na_2CO_3 solution (80 mL) in a container were collected and freeze-dried for 12 h. Final drying at 250 °C for 1 min to 1 h was conducted to examine the drying effects. Fast scanning DSC operations were conducted in the temperature range from 50 to 580 °C at a scanning rate between 2000 K/s and 6000 K/s. Tg for the present sample ACMC (5% Mg substitution) was 376 °C, about 35 °C higher than the pure ACC.

The last paper by Weidendorfer et al. (2023) concerns the melt-quenched glasses in the system K_2CO_3-$MgCO_3$-H_2O. The given content (mol %) of each component is in the range of 31.7 ~ 55.9 (K_2CO_3), 25.9 ~ 44.9 ($MgCO_3$), and 0.1 ~ 42.4 (H_2O). The lowest water content was due to the inevitable uptake of atmospheric humidity. They encapsulated the dry carbonates (30 ~ 50 mg) and a known amount of H_2O in an air-tight Au capsule (<100 mg) and embedded the capsule in a crushable MgO sleeve. The MgO sleeve with a capsule was set in a hot-press cylinder with a MgO piston on either side and heated at 750 °C for 24 h under 1 GPa (a few steps before soaking the system at the top temperature) before the heating power was cut and let the system cool down (the cooling rate was ~200 °C/s). For DSC, they employed a 2–20 mg sample in a Pt crucible at 10 K/min as the heating rate under Ar-purging (30 mL/min). The vitreous carbonates may have a stressed structure that is quenched at a higher temperature. The structure is relaxed when a sample is kept near Tg: this is the process of annealing. In the present case, some samples were rendered to the DSC measurements a few times, that is, the samples may experience stress relaxation. The stress-relaxed structure exhibits a reduction in volume (suppose the case the glass has a reduced volume in Fig. 30). It means that a lower Tg is assigned to the annealed samples. The annealing effects are common to the daily glasses. In the present carbonate glass, however, they found dehydration on each DSC run, or the water content drifted, and Tg varied, accordingly. For example, a glass with an initial H_2O content of 42% [31.7K_2CO_3, 25.9$MgCO_3$, 42.4H_2O] showed 356 K (83 °C) for the first DSC run, while Tg jumped up to 518 K (245 °C) for the composition [55K_2CO_3, 45$MgCO_3$, 0.1H_2O]. The increase in Tg, therefore, is attributed to the decrease in the water content but not to the structure relaxation. A glass specialist may want to further discussion on the structural roles of water molecules and on the constitution of the amorphous network itself.

4 CO_2 as the Source for Carbonate Ions

4.1 On-Site Generation of CO_2

Gas-Diffusion or Ammonia Diffusion Processes for ACC or CC Formation
Some groups employed NH_3 and CO_2, which resulted from the hydrolysis of $(NH_4)_2CO_3$ or NH_4HCO_3 under a humid atmosphere, to precipitate carbonates in a calcium salt solution within a confined space (denoted as the gas diffusion or ammonia diffusion procedure). For example, Nahi et al. (2023) and Homeijer et al. (2010) used this carbonation route, as already introduced above. Ju et al. (2022) followed Chen et al. (2013, Chem. Commn.) for fabricating stable ACC nanospheres without any additive. They first dissolved the $CaCl_2$ solution into a binary solution of 55 H_2O-10,000 EtOH (in volume ratio, EtOH: ethanol) to obtain a 13.6 mM solution. The Ca solution was placed in an air-tight desiccator together with $(NH_4)_2CO_3$ (see Fig. 32a). The ammonium salt was spontaneously hydrolyzed to produce NH_3, CO_2, and H_2O, all of which would migrate into the calcium salt solution to precipitate ACC nanoparticles. The TEM images of their microstructure in Fig. 32b indicate that the ACC particles consisted of nanoclusters of ~2 nm. Figure 32c exhibits that those nanospheres grew with the reaction time (4, 8, and 12 h). Thus, as Gindele et al. (2021), Ju et al. also stated (2022) that this is additional evidence for the liquid-liquid precursor (LLP) for CC crystallization. Moreover, they examined the effects of methanol, 1-propanol, and 1-butanol on the ACC nanosphere formation but found hardly any difference. When they added cellulose fibers into the H_2O-EtOH binary solution, they observed ACC nano-beads deposited on the fibrils. Moreover, they also showed the ACC deposition on a graphene oxide (GO) nano-sheet and fabricated GO-Calc (calcite) composites. Yao et al. (2015) already in 2015 used the gas-diffusion process to challenge the fabrication of a nacre-like carbonate (Calc or Vat) on GO template surface. They concluded that GO is helpful for lateral growth of Calc.

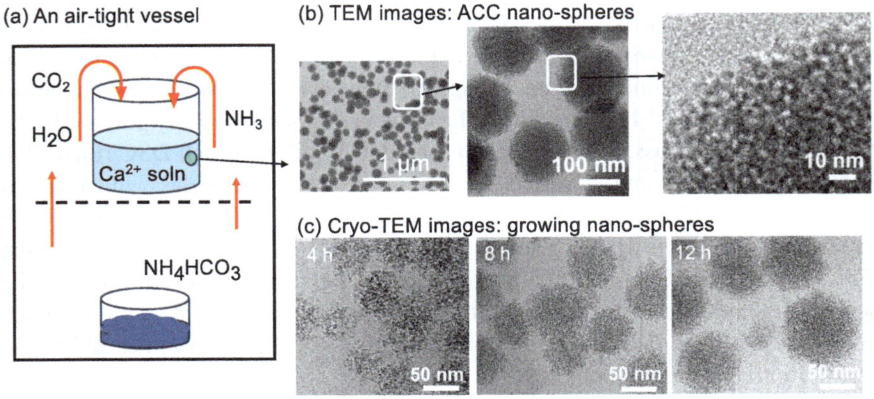

Fig. 32 **a** A schematic drawing of the gas-diffusion route: CO_2 and NH_3 from the hydrolysis of $(NH_4)_2CO_3$ powder were supplied to a calcium salt solution under ambient conditions, leading to ACC precipitation. Enzymatic or microbial activities against urea can generate gaseous components. (original drawing). **b** Nanospheres from nano-clusters (~2 nm) **c** Nano-spheres growth with time. Ju et al. (2022), (with permission from Wiley)

The fabrication of similar cellulose coated with CC beads was reported by Kim et al. (2022b) for paper-filler applications. No other tricks than they simply added Ca-O (44.6 g) into the suspension of cellulose nano-fiber (CF; 2 g/L), into which they injected CO_2 to attain 80 g of CF-$CaCO_3$ suspension (CF/$CaCO_3$ = 1:40).

Because it is a mild and ambient process to produce ACC nanoparticles, the gas or ammonia diffusion is applicable to hybridize CC with precious drugs. Yu et al. (2023) prepared ACC nanoparticles loaded with indocyanine green (ICG) (ICG@ACC) as the photosensitizer by the gas diffusion procedure. ICG is excited to release heat with irradiation of a near infrared beam, and a photothermal tumor therapeutic activity is expected. A $CaCl_2$ (1.0 g) solution in 50 mL absolute ethanol (EtOH; ~9 mM) was held in a flask with an Al foil cap, and the foil was punctured with five pores. This solution was placed in a vacuum desiccator together with 66.5 mg $(NH_4)_2CO_3$ in a beaker for the gas diffusion effects. After the reaction at 25 °C for 18 h, the resultant ACC particles were collected by centrifuging, rinsed with absolute EtOH, and vacuum-dried at room temperature. ICG@ACC nanoparticles were prepared in the same way, except that 3.5 mg ICG was added into the EtOH solution of $CaCl_2$. Later, they encapsulate ICG@ACC and Doxorbicin (DOX; a cancer drug) into poly(lactic-co-glycolic acid)-ss-chondroitin sulfate A (PSC): PSC/ICG@ + DOX nano-particles or nanomedicine. An advantage of ACC is that it neutralizes the acidic environment within a tumor and protects ICG until near-infrared heating is practiced.

A UV-sensitive molecule to generate CO_2 is also applicable to an in-situ CO_2-diffusion process. Menichetti et al. (2021) prepared calcium and barium carbonates in 20 mM MCl_2 (M: Ca, Ba) aqueous solution, dissolved with photo-active Ketoprofen anion K^- (2-(3-benzoylphenyl)propanoate; X-CH(CH_3)COO^-) (20 mM). With the irradiation of a UV light (365 nm), K^- is decomposed to X-CH_2Me (insoluble in water) and bicarbonate ion HCO_3^-. Figure 33 shows the morphology of the deposited

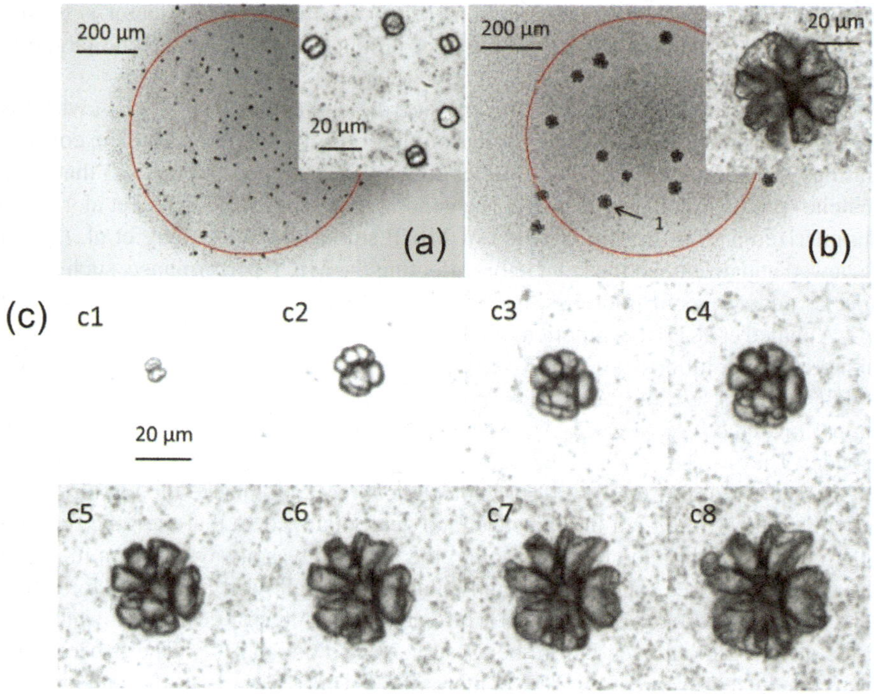

Fig. 33 TEM images: Morphology of $BaCO_3$ deposited by UV irradiation. **a** Irradiation for 900 s (0.9 ks) (red circle: UV spot: 365 nm, 1.3 mW/mm^2). The inset shows the morphologies of the particles. **b** After 150 min (= 9 ks) of irradiation (red circle: UV spot, 365 nm, 0.1 mW/mm^2). Inset: morphology of particle 1. c1–c8) Growth of particle 1 in **c** after irradiation for 1 ks (<10 µm), 2 ks, 3 ks, 4 ks, 5 ks (~30 µm), 6 ks, 7 ks, 8 ks, and 9 ks (~50µm), respectively. Menichetti et al. (2021) (an open access paper; Wiley). (ks: 1000 s)

$BaCO_3$ due to UV irradiation for 900 s (365 nm, 1.3 mM/mm^2), and the growth of a specific particle with the irradiation period from <10 µm (1 ks), ~30 µm (5 ks), ~50 µm (9ks). Note the irradiation power in (b) was reduced by an order of magnitude than in (a). They denoted the assemblies of the $BaCO_3$ crystallites as "Biomorphs" from the morphology. No comments were given on the crystallization mechanism.

Microorganism (Microbe)-Mediated Carbonate Formation: MICP and EICP
Urea is an interesting substance because it is decomposed at lower temperatures (<100 °C) to yield NH_3 and CO_2. When some microbes are present in a Ca-containing environment, the enzymatic activity of urease (urea amidohydrolase) within them secretes NH_3 and CO_2 under ambient conditions to precipitate CC (calcium carbonate). This is the principle of the microbially induced calcium carbonate or calcite (Calc) precipitation, frequently denoted as MICP. You may sometimes encounter confusion on microbes and bacteria. In a derivative way, it is also reasonable to add urease to calcium salt solutions if the pH or other solution conditions are compatible with the enzyme activity. Hence, it is denoted as

enzyme-induced carbonate precipitation (EICP). Therefore, a key factor is to find better bacteria or microbes for the efficient production of CC under the targeting environment.

MICP and EICP are useful in soil engineering and extensively studied, whereas the experimental details, especially the mixing ratio of solutions or their concentrations, are sometimes missing. Boquet et al. (1973) pointed out in 1973 that Calc (calcite) production by soil bacteria is a general phenomenon. Canakci et al. (2015) summarized a short history (<2015) of MICP studies on soils. Tang et al. (2020) reviewed and discussed the key factors affecting the MICP performance, such as the species and strains of microbes, bacterial solution concentration, temperature, and pH. Almajed et al. (2019) reported in 2019 on an EICP treatment of silica sand. They first prepared solutions of 0.67 M $CaCl_2$ and 1.0 M urea, as well as 3 g/L urease: Soln 1. For Soln 2, 4 g/L of non-fat milk powder was added to the Soln 1 recipe, while Soln 3 involved 0.25 M $CaCl_2$, 0.37 M urea, 0.85 g/L urease, and 4 g/l non-fat milk powder. They mixed 75 mL of the solutions and 350 g of silica sand, known as Ottawa 20/30 and commonly employed for geotechnical research, placed the mixture in an acrylic cylinder (5.08 cm in diameter), and gently tamped so that the sand reached 10.16 cm in height. Due to the tamping, the solution was always a few mm above the sand top surface. The packed sand columns were allowed for curing for 3 d at ~20 °C. The specimens were rinsed with one pour volume of de-ionized water and dried at 40 °C in an oven before being subjected to the analysis. The experiments were conducted in threefold. The content of CC (mass%) was in the order of the solutions: Soln 3 < Soln 2 < Soln 1, whereas the compressive strength (MPa) was in the order: Soln 1 (~0.14) < < Soln 3 (~1.1) < Soln 2. (~1.7). They remarked that the addition of non-fat milk powder highly promoted the increase in the compressive strength. Moreover, Chuo et al. (2020) stated that bacterial activity is affected by bacterial strain, bacterial concentration, nutrient concentration, calcium source concentration, addition of other substances, and methods to distribute bacteria. They discussed those from the viewpoint of construction materials and biocementation, listing many microbes.

Anbu et al. (2016) reviewed MICP-related works before 2016, while Seifan and Berenjian, in their 2019 review paper (Seifan and Berenjian 2019), listed many microbes and related metabolic pathways other than ureolysis (mentioned above), such as sulfate reduction, photosynthesis, denitrification, and conversion of organic acid to CC. It is a challenge that we may apply the MICP procedure within hydrogels to provide them with bone repair or bone regeneration ability (Douglas et al. 2017). To mimic the outer shell of crayfish, Nawarathna et al. (2021) prepared fusion proteins having a calcium-binding domain (CaBP) and a chitin-binding domain (ChBD). In hybridizing CC (Calc: calcite) on a chitin surface, they employed ureolysis for the slow formation of CC. Recently, Lv et al. (2024) studied the effects of an electric field on the MICP process. Xiong et al. (2022) indicated that pearl oysters utilize tyrosinase (an EICP process) in the calcium carbonate deposition on the nacre.

An article in Wikipedia USA (https://en.wikipedia.org/wiki/Microbiologically_induced_calcite_precipitation, n.d.) may provide a good briefing on the MICP procedure. Also, a paper by Yi et al. (2021) is a good read to zap the history and examples of applications.

4.2 Behavior of CO_2 Bubbles in Calcium Salt Solutions

CO_2 gas is bubbled into a calcifying solution or suspension to precipitate calcium carbonates, like the cases of (Liendo et al. 2020; Surmeneva et al. 2020a; Polat 2019; Han et al. 2005; Boyjoo et al. 2014; Kezuka et al. 2021; Jimoh et al. 2018; Tanaka et al. 2022; Madhav et al. 2023; Ma et al. 2023; Oral et al. 2020; Yang et al. 2021; Hadiko et al. 2005; Grimes et al. 2020) to name a few. Among those examples, Jimoh et al. (2018), in a 2018 paper, reviewed the effect of various organic and inorganic additives used in the synthesis of the different CC polymorphs. Tanaka et al. (2022) were concerned with the stabilization of concrete sludge, while Madhav et al. (2023) studied carbon oxide capture with calcium salt solutions involving N-methyl diethanolamine (MDEA) and triethanolamine (TEA) as additives to retain the solution basic (pH 10 ~ 11). Ma et al. (2023) prepared hollow Vat (vaterite) spheres (specific surface area: 17 m^2/g) with a spray reactor where $(NH_4)_2CO_3$ and $CaCl_2$ solutions were separately let into the spray tee, and the mixture was sprayed by CO_2. The micro-droplets were composed of the CO_2 core and shell of the mixed solution. Oral et al. (2020) and Yang et al. (2021) prepared CC microspheres for biomedical or medical applications, as described later. Hadiko et al. (2005) were the first, to the knowledge of the present monograph author, to show that the CO_2 bubble surface should be a template of CC (Vat and Calc, depending on the pH of the calcium solution), denoting "bubble templating." They bubbled CO_2 (10 μm in size) at a rate of 3 L/min into 0.05 M $CaCl_2$ held in an Erlenmeyer flask (a conical flask) where the solution was kept at 27‡C and pH was adjusted to 9.7 ~ 12.7 with HCl and NH_4OH. Figure 34a, which illustrates the reaction steps to generate Vat hollow particles. The initial bubble size was set at 10 μm while the SEM image (a-4) indicates the resulting hollow particles were ~ 7 μm in diameter with a ~ 1 μm thick crust. An important suggestion herein (a) is that even at the beginning stage Vat (blue dots) would precipitate in the solution in the region apart from the bubble surface (red-circled). When CO_2 is in contact with an aqueous system, the states of C(IV) are limited to $CO_2(g)$, $CO_2(aq)$, $HCO_3^-(aq)$, and $CO_3^{2-}(aq)$, while, at $9.7 < pH < 12.7$, the ratio of bicarbonate and carbonate $(CO_3^{2-})/(HCO_3^-)$ is 0.23 ~ 224 and favoring the precipitation of CC (the ratio Vat:Calc = 0:~10 (at pH 9.7); 3:5 (pH 10.0); 9:1 (pH 12.7), according to the XRD intensity ratio). Because (a-2) indicates CO_2 diffusion by arrows, Hadiko et al. (2005) might have implicitly considered (a-1) for the situation a little after the initiation of CO_2 bubbling. It is unlikely that they assumed the direct reactions of gaseous CO_2 to yield the CC precipitation because the ionization reactions of CO_2 were indicated in the discussion part. Their results seem to inspire Grimes et al. (2020) who revisited the analysis of the behavior of CO_2

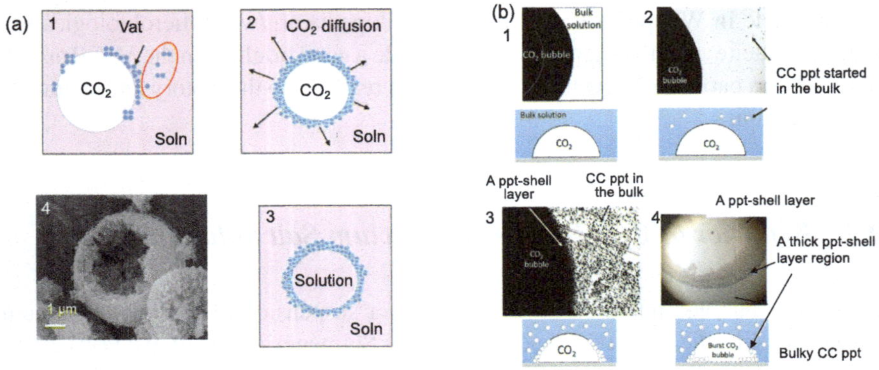

Fig. 34 **a** Clockwise: (1) the beginning stage, showing vaterite (Vat) in the region apart from the bubble surface (red circle), as well as on the bubble-solution (soln) interface. (2) Vat crystallites form a shell around the interface, where CO_2 diffuses into the soln. (3) CO_2 is exhausted to form a hollow Vat crust. (4) An SEM image of dried hollow Vat spherules. Hadiko et al. (2005) (with permission from Elsevier). **b** A single hemispherical CO_2 bubble (<1 mm) is formed on the bottom of a petri dish with 10 mM $CaCl_2$ solution (pH 11). The top figures (b-1~b-4) are optical microscope images of the bubble, and the bottom figures schematically show CC deposition on and near the bubble. The bubble presented at the top of b-4 is already burst due to solution evaporation, leaving a thick, bulky rim of ppt. Grimes et al. (2020) (an open access paper; the American Chemical Society)

bubbles in the static and dynamic modes. From the static bubble study (semispherical CO_2 on a glass substrate in contact with 10 mM $CaCl_2$ solution under pH 12), they derived the same conclusions as Hadiko et al. (2005), approving the calcite particles precipitated in the bulk solution were sedimented on the bubble surface to form a shell. Both ions, Ca^{2+} and $CO_3{}^{2-}$, are similarly mobile in the solutions, because their molar conductivity $\Lambda(10^{-4}\ S\ m^2/mol)$ and diffusion coefficient D ($10^{-5}\ cm^2/s$) were 119 and 1.58 for Ca^{2+} while 138.6 and 1.84 for $CO_3{}^{2-}$, respectively according to CRC Handbook [100th Ed, p. 5–94]. A counter diffusion of out-going carbonate ions and approaching calcium ions is probable as soon as the CO_2 is in contact with the solution. It may postulate that CC could be precipitated far apart from the bubble surface. Yet, it is still perplexing that the carbonate ions would not encounter any calcium ions to be free within a mm distance without forming ACC or CC particles. Grimes et al. (2020) also examined the effects of the flowing CO_2 on the CC particle size, residence time, or other in a cross-flow type cylinder reactor.

5 Templates and Hybridization

Several polymers play important roles as additives to control morphology and polymorphs, while in a few examples, polymeric molecules control the microstructures of the resulting materials. Nacre layers are more than beautiful hybrids of CC (Arag) and chitin, where the polymers control the orientation and screwing angles of the

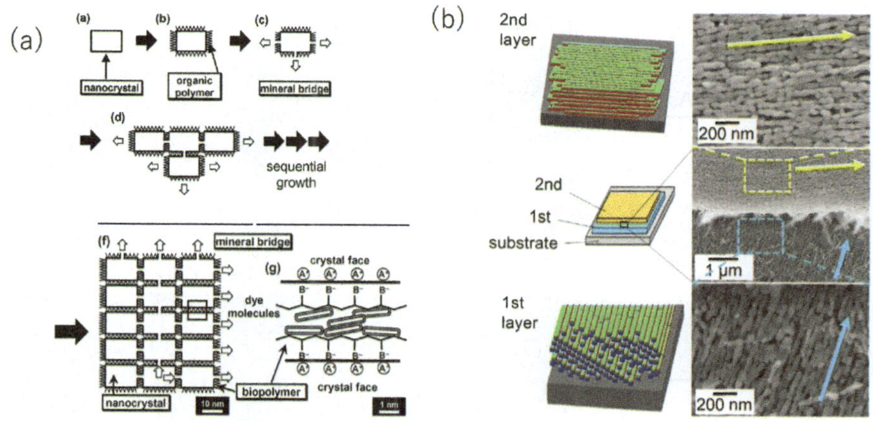

Fig. 35 **a** (top) Each nanocrystallite is surrounded by biopolymers (zigzag lines). (bottom) They are minerally bridged to accomplish nano-assembly structures. Oaki et al. (2006) (with permission from Wiley). **b** Calcite nanorods assembled on Si wafer with a cross-lamellar structure. Takasaki et al. (2016) (with permission from the Royal Society of Chemistry)

CC micro-plates. This is a typical case where a living organism constructs hierarchically organized structures under ambient conditions. A group led by H. Imai has conducted a series of works on organized assemblies of CC blocks. Oaki et al. (2007) first analyzed the nano-structures of the nacreous layer of shells, the sponge skeletons of echinoderms, coral, foraminifera, and eggshells of hens and emus. They elucidated that each component crystallite is surrounded by biopolymers yet they should have a mineral bridge to accomplish those nano-assembly structures. Figure 35a shows their assembling process model (Oaki et al. 2006). In 2016, Takasaki et al. (2016) learned how to elongate CC nanocrystalline blocks with top-to-end bonding and keep the c-axis through the assembly. Takasaki et al. (2018) fabricated an oriented assembly of Calc (calcite) in a cross-lamellar structure (see Fig. 35b). A trick is that they used a high magnetic field (12 T), under which the calcite crystallites aligned their *c*-axis parallel to the field (Takasaki et al. 2018). Moreover, the strings of this 1-dimensional (1 D) assemblies can be thermally fragmented into nano-sized pieces (Takasaki et al. (2020).

In the ACC-related sections above, we have recognized the significance of ACC in many stages of CC formation. Yet, we found only limited discussion about its roles in conjunction to how living organisms utilize or manipulate it in hybridizing polymeric substances. Cantaert et al. (2017) published an inspiring review paper on using ACC to design new materials based on a wide range of tissues and organs. It was published in 2017 but is still a must-read. Jiang et al. (2017) indicated the L- and D-enantiomers of amino acids (Asp and Glu) controlled the morphology of calcite and vaterite (Fig. 36). Their solutions contained 1 mM Na_2CO_3 (50 mL) and 5 mM $CaCl_2$ (50 mL), to which 20 m M of L- or D-Asp (aspartic acid) or 20 mM racemic mixture of Asp, or 20 mM L- or D-Glu (glutamic acid). pH of the solutions was adjusted to 10. The solutions stood still during the mineralization for up to

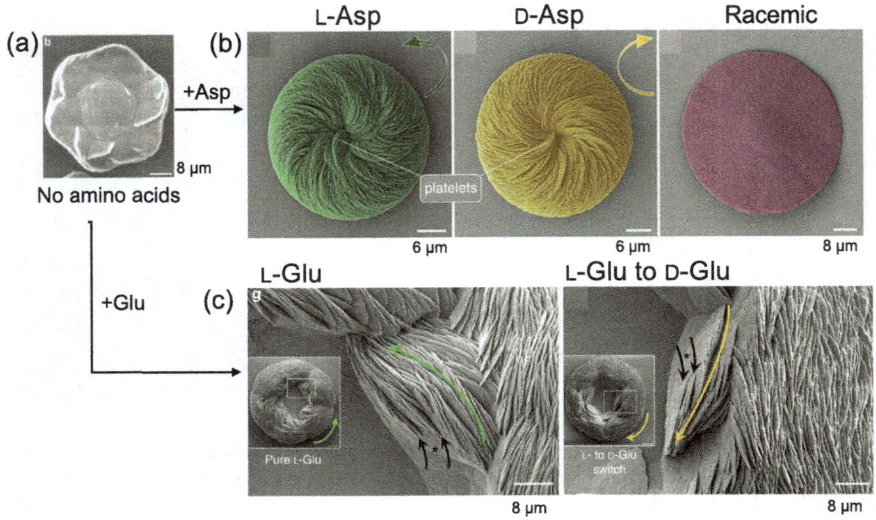

Fig. 36 **a** Vaterite toroids obtained from solutions containing 1 mM Na_2CO_3 and 5 mM $CaCl_2$. A hexagonal Vat (vaterite) crystallite appears from the solution without any amino acid additives. **b** With additives: (left) 20 mM L-Asp, (middle) 20 mM D-Asp, and (right) a 20 mM racemic mixture of Asp. L-Asp produces chiral toroids with a counterclockwise spiraling morphology (green arrow), whereas D-Asp produces chiral toroids with a clockwise spiraling morphology (yellow arrow). The racemic conditions exhibit no chirality effects. **c** With addition of (left) 20 mM L-Glu, and (right) 20 mM D-Glu. L-Glu induces toroids with a counterclockwise spiraling morphology (green arrows), leaving a central core region uncovered by vaterite platelets. The addition of D-Glu alters the spiraling direction clockwise (yellow arrows). Bar for inset: 10 μm. Jiang et al. (2017) (an open access paper; Springer Nature)

24 h. In Fig. 36, the top left SEM image shows a hexagonal Vat (vaterite) crystallite from the solution without any amino acids. The top right image indicates that L-Asp produces chiral toroids with a counterclockwise spiraling morphology (green arrow), and D-Asp produces chiral toroids with a clockwise spiraling morphology (yellow arrow). In contrast, the racemic conditions show no chirality effects. Bottom-right: L-Glu induces toroids of the counterclockwise spiraling morphology (green arrows) with a central core region remaining uncovered by Vat platelets. Chiral switching is observed when D-Glu addition changes the direction of spiraling to clockwise (yellow arrows). Bar for inset: 10 μm. Another paper by Jiang et al. (2018) further supports and discusses chiral-switching phenomena in detail. They observed another few cases of chiral switching involving layer-by-layer rotation of vaterite platelets. A mechanism leading to chiral switching is proposed.

The molecular structures of some marine organisms have been studied because they are potential targets for mimicking. Here, only two will be introduced. Kertmen et al. (Kertmen et al. 2021) studied the skeleton of the giant *Ianthella basta* (a marine demosponge), using chitin as a template to form nano-structured microfibers of a

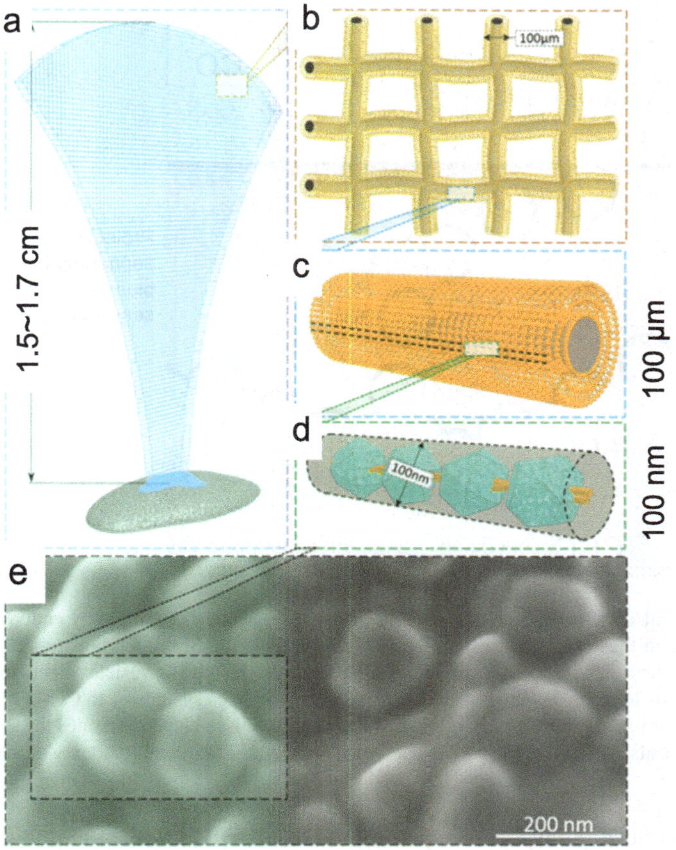

Fig. 37. **a** Hierarchical structure of the mineralized giant network-like skeleton of *I. basta demosponge.* **b** The flat construct comprise highly organized intercalated meshes of microfibers with a diameter of 100 μm. **c** These fibers are made of nanostructured chitin and (d) templates for the formation of calcite nanocrystals. **e** SEM image of the Calc crystallites. Kertmen et al. (2021) (an open access paper; MDPI)

chitin-calcite hybrid. Figure 37 illustrates the hierarchical nanostructure of a network-like skeleton. In Fig. 38, Mass et al. (2017) schematically demonstrate the processes of CC deposition onto a living thing, taking coral as an example. The deposition starts with capturing seawater (calcium and carbonate ions) as vesicles (Stp1); stable ACC precursors are formed inside (Stp 2). ACC grows with carbonate ions injected into the vesicles (Stp 3). Vesicles eject ACC precursors by exocytosis to the growing surface, i.e., CC deposition (Stp 4). ACC crystalizes to CCC (crystalline CC: Arag for coral, and Calc for sea urchin spines or other) (Stp 5). Kijima et al. (2011) were concerned with a repair model of, say, a bivalve shell (*Pinctada Margaritifera*) when damaged. In their in vitro experiments, they first gave damage by acid etching to their prismatic layer consisting of Calc prisms aligned in the c-axis with an intervening

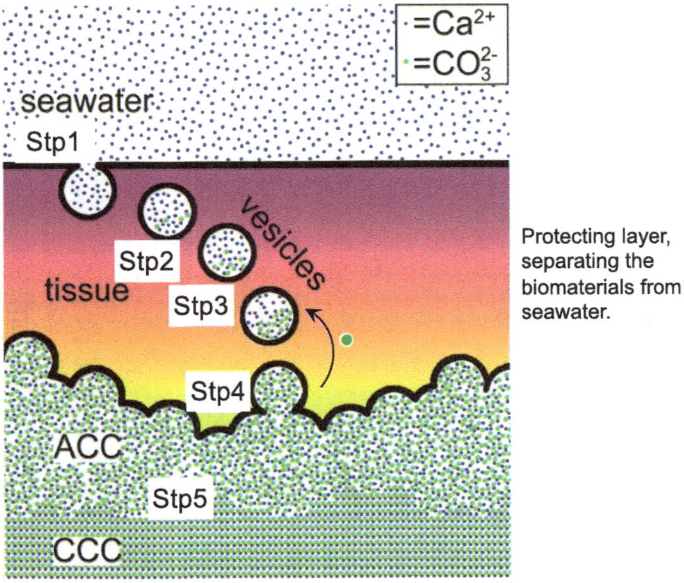

Fig. 38 Coral skeleton formation in five steps. Stp 1: seawater is captured by endocytosis. Stp 2: ACC forms in these vesicles to stabilize the ACC precursors. Stp 3: Carbonate ions (green dots secreted by the living organisms) are injected into the vesicles. Stp 4: Vesicles eject Acc precursors via exocytosis to the growing surface (deposition). Stp 5: Acc crystallizes to CCC (Arag). CCC is Calc found in sea urchin spines, spicules, or teeth. The top tissue layer separates the seawater from the biomaterials. Mass et al. (2017) (an open access paper; the National Academy of Science, USA)

organic framework layer. For repairing the damaged sites, they employed the gas-diffusion method to supply CO_2 due to the hydrolysis of $(NH_4)_2CO_3$. The repair solution comprised of 20 mM $CaCl_2$ and 0.5 mM poly(acrylic acid) (PAA, Mw 2000). When the etched pieces were placed in this repairing solution, the "CO_2" migrated to the damaged site to precipitate calcite crystals on the etched part of the prismatic layer. Here, the migrating C(IV) species are likely bicarbonate ions (HCO_3^-) when the presence of PAA is considered. They pointed out that the presence of PAA is inevitable for the deposition of calcite mesocrystals at the repairing site.

ACC plays some roles also in microbes. Mehta studied ACC in cyanobacteria (Mehta et al. 2023) since they are interested in the calcium sites within the microbe. Bacteriophages may be involved in the CC formation in other ways than the MICP process. Borkowski et al. (2024) studied the effects of Escherichia virus P1 and lipid-enveloped Pseudomonas virus Phi6 on Vat (vaterite) precipitation. They concluded that bacteriophages may selectively bind both ACC and Vat, and indirectly affect the formation of structural defects in calcite crystallites. They further suggested the applicability of these Vat-phage composites for drug-delivering vehicles. An earlier study of this group was concerned also with bacteriophage and CC precipitation (Słowakiewicz et al. 2021). They considered microbes to be infected with the phages before secreting Vat clusters.

6 Biomedical Applications

6.1 *Bone Repair Materials*

We have observed that calcium carbonates (CC) can be controlled in size and porous structures, are tissue-compatible, chemically stable, and moderately unstable, which leads to numerous studies. They are also beneficial for human tissue repair. Liu and Wang (2023) fabricated chitosan-CC scaffolds for bone repair with 90–93% porosity, depending on the calcite content (20–60%). Their scaffold effectively supported cell proliferation and in vivo tests. Lee et al. (2007) initially prepared green compacts of $Ca(OH)_2$ and NaCl (0.1–0.3 mm in size) and carbonated the samples in flowing CO_2 to produce $CaCO_3$-NaCl composites. NaCl was washed out with water at 60 °C, resulting in macroporous CC pieces (80–90% CC). The mechanical properties (tensile strength: <0.15 MPa) and degree of carbonation depended on the pressure applied to the green compacts. Suzawa et al. (2015) prepared hydroxyapatite (HAp) and CC on agarose gel disks using the alternate soaking method developed by Taguchi et al. (2001). Assays for cell culture activity indicated that both biominerals on agarose gel are suitable for use as bone graft substitutes in various in vivo bone defect models (CC/gels showed a slight advantage). Melatonin is known to be effective in preventing and treating osteoporosis (bone degradation in the elderly). Zhu et al. (2018) reported that one out of four groups of rats fed a diet containing melatonin and CC showed significant improvement in bone density of the lumbar vertebra and bilateral femur, with elevated mineral levels and increased serum calcium, as well as activities of SOD (superoxide dismutase) and GSH-Px (glutathione peroxidase). The levels of each marker were improved by 1.3–1.5 times compared to the osteoporosis group, according to the given figures (not provided by the authors). Research by Jee and Thula on bone grafts and related CC formation is discussed in Sect. 3.5 (Thula et al. 2011; Jee et al. 2010). Sumeneva et al. (Surmeneva et al. 2020b) coated CC on a titanium alloy (Ti6Al4V) bone substitute and explored the effectiveness of ultrasound irradiation. Min et al. (Min et al. 2024b) reviewed calcium-based materials for bone regeneration. Unfortunately, they provided no insights into the direct bonding of bone materials.

6.2 *Calcium Carbonates in Drug Delivery Vehicles*

A 2022 review paper by Huang et al. (2022) provides excellent overviews of the drug carriers based on calcium carbonate (CC) and alginate biomaterials. They compared CC and alginate in terms of their similarity and dissimilarity, referring to the "yin-&-yang of CC & alginate," which is a concept of Chinese philosophy and literally means those two show opposite properties but can be interconnected with each other. CC nanoparticles (NPs) are promising candidates for medical diagnostics, including fluorescence imaging (FLI), magnetic resonance imaging (MRI), and ultrasound (US)

Table 2 Few examples of CC-related drug delivery systems

Research group	Year	Drugs	Systems	Comment
Huang et al. (2022)	2022		Alg hgel-ACC*	Host-design: Review
Dai et al. (2016)	2016	MTX*	Chitosan, calc, vat	$CaCl_2$, NH_4HCO_3
Zhou et al. (2016)	2016		CC* on GO*	Ethylene glycol
Wang et al. (2018)	2018	MTX	Chitosan-Calc, vat	$CaCl_2$, $NaHCO_3$ Na_2CO_3
Pan et al. (2018)	2018	Gentamycin	Calc NPs*	CO_2 into 6%ca$(OH)_2$, 1%EDTA*
Vergaro et al. (2018)	2018	NVP-BEZ235*	Porous Calc NPs	2-gun spray ($NaHCO_3$, $CaCl_2$)
Maleki Dizaj et al. (2019)	2019	Drugs, genes	CC NPs as vehicles	
Mo et al. (2022)	2022	Doxorubicin	Hollow Calc	Folic acid as the template, CO_2
Yu et al. (2023)	2023	Doxorubicin	ACC	Photothermal
Ghaffari et al. (2024)	2024	Chlorhexidine	CC NPs	For dental infections

*Abbreviations in this table
Alg hgel: Alginate hydrogel
MTX: Methotrexate, GO: graphene oxide, NVP-BEZ235: A drug for advanced solid tumors
NP(s): Nanoparticle(s), EDTA: Ethylenediamine tetraacetate

imaging. Zhao et al. (2022) briefly reviewed their potential in biomedical applications: diagnosis, drugs and gene carriers, sensitizers in photodynamic therapy, Ca^{2+} generators for immunotherapy, and MRI contrast enhancement, to name a few. Examples of drug delivery are listed in Table 2, along with additional comments.

Calcium carbonates: ACC: amorphous, Calc: calcite, CC: calcium carbonates (phases not described)

Zhou et al. (2016) prepared CC@GO, or calcium carbonate-coated graphene oxide, which they are considering for use in drug delivery vehicles. Yu et al. (2023) prepared ACC nanoparticles for the delivery of Doxorubicin for photothermal cancer therapy. Mo et al. (2022) used folic acid as the template to hold calcium ions, into which CO_2 is added to obtain CC nano-particles after calcination (550 °C). They added light-emitting carbon quantum dots for securing photosensitivity. Ghaffari et al. (2024) prepared CC NPs (nanoparticles) for the prevention of dental infections.

6.3 Carbonates in Medical Imaging Diagnosis

Ultrasound Imaging

Due to their gas-generating properties and sensitivity to physiological conditions, Chuzeville et al. (2024) considered using CC nanoparticles for contrast-enhanced ultrasound imaging (CEUS). They proposed lignin as a coating layer of CC NPs for contrast-enhanced ultrasound imaging.

MRI Imaging

Dong et al. (2022) prepared highly hydrated ACC particles with paramagnetic properties to serve as an MRI contrast-enhancing agent. They highlighted the advantages of Gd-ACC systems over other agents and the necessity of hydration of the carrier systems. Their paramagnetic ACC nanoclusters (ACNCs) achieved a significantly higher water-to-Ca ratio (water/Ca = 7.2) than conventional ACCs (approximately 0.4–1.9). For optimal MRI imaging, the NMR relaxivity, commonly measured by "longitudinal relaxivity (r_1)" should be maximized. Indeed, r_1 of their ACNCs reached 37.21/mM·s, ten times greater than that of a commercially available material known as Gd-DTPA (3.19/mM·s). Although Gd^{3+} is toxic to the human body (causing hemolysis, for example), the ACNCs are found nontoxic. From the in vivo tests, the ACNCs produced well-defined MRI images (MR angiography) of a rat, rabbit, beagle dog, or other animals.

7 Miscellaneous Topics

Ultrasound in CC Formation

Only a few examples will be presented that utilize ultrasound (US) for CC preparation. One example is the study by Sumeneva et al. (2020b), mentioned earlier. Oliveira et al. (2024) employed US to regulate scaling on heating equipment. Juhasz-Bortuzzo et al. (2017) applied US (20 kHz) to the mixtures of 0.1, 0.5, and 1 M $NaHCO_3$ and $Ca(OAc)_2$ (10 mL each) to obtain pure vaterite (Vat) crystallites. They took a pulse sequence: US on (1 s) and off (0.2 s), varying the irradiation duration from 10 s to 10 min. The particle size or yield of the Vat was highly dependent on the US power (pulse height and duration). Luo et al. (2021) applied US to wastewater from an ammonia industry containing $CaCl_2$ and $(NH_4)_2CO_3$ without any additives. They produced spherical Vat particles of 2.78 μm in size (specific surface area, SSA: 20.9 m^2/g) at 100% ultrasound amplitude. An increase in the US amplitude reduced the particle size and consequently increased SSA.

Energy Storage

Carbonates are potential candidates for energy storage. A 2019 review paper by Carrillo et al. (2019) is a little older now but describes well a series of high-temperature storage materials and systems (thermochemical heat storage): Heat decomposes a metal carbonate to produce the metal oxide and CO_2, which are separately stored and recombined to recover heat when necessary.

Crystallization and Mineralization in Narrower Space

In a confined space, the crystallizing species are restricted in their diffusion and supply, and they will readily find surface (substrate) sites to settle in their vicinity, which may stabilize metastable states. Therefore, some processes are likely to differ from those discussed above where open space is available for them. A paper by Zeng et al. (2018) provides us with valuable insight into ion behaviors in smaller pores to enhance our understanding of biomineralization procedures within organisms. Lotsari et al. (2018) focus on the mineralization of calcium phosphate, rather than carbonates, i.e., the transformation of ACC to crystalline bone-like apatite in micellar spaces among confined nanodomains of a hexagonally ordered, polymerized lyotropic liquid crystal (PLLC) matrix. The environment of the amorphous Ca-P might be similar to that discussed above in the section on PILP. According to the authors, PLLC is a soft polymeric matrix composed of nanoscale micellar fibrils (NMF) that are 7–10 nm in diameter, organized in a hexagonal lattice at the submicron scale. He et al. (2019) employed the surface energy of micro-droplets in the crystallization of CC. In contrast, Xue et al. (2022) examined CC dissolution within a microfluidic device to find different species that we expect in an ordinary dissolution reaction.

Conclusive Remarks

As discussed above, calcium carbonate (CC) presents us with various aspects. Whenever we approach it, CC reveals another new aspect. Tens of thousands of papers have been published on this mineral over the past few decades, yet no one has been able to fully clarify its behavior. This monograph focuses on only a portion of the topics covered in the literature. Consequently, many significant works could not be introduced, such as those on the applications of CC in foods or agricultural fields.

Finally, a few papers are listed below for further reading, though some are cited in the text.

- Ultrasound imaging.

Köse, G., et al. (2020), Molecular Ultrasound Imaging, Nanomaterials, 10(10), 1935. https://doi.org/10.3390/nano10101935

- Crystallization inhibitor.

Zhang, H et al. (2024). Inhibition of calcium carbonate nucleation and crystallization by carboxymethyl dextran: Experiments and molecular dynamics simulations. Desalination, 573 (2023) 117205. https://doi.org/10.1016/j.desal.2023.117205

- Controlling extracellular pH: cancer applications.

Rahman, A. et al. (2023). Immunotherapy Enhancement by Targeting Extracellular Tumor pH in Triple-Negative Breast Cancer Mouse Model. Cancers, 15(20) 1924. https://doi.org/10.3390/cancers15204931

Som, A. et al. (2016). Monodispersed calcium carbonate nanoparticles modulate local pH and inhibit tumor growth in vivo. Nanoscale, 8(25) 12639–12,647. https://doi.org/10.1039/C5NR06162H

- Uranium adsorption and separation.

Jinan Parvin, V. M. et al. (2024). Calcium carbonate microparticles show enhanced anti-cancer properties under the influence of a magnetic field. New J. Chem.,48(43) 18465–18,473. https://doi.org/10.1039/D4NJ02757D

- Amorphous calcium carbonate as a basis of new materials.

Cantaert, B., et al. (2017) Use of Amorphous Calcium Carbonate for the Design of New Materials. ChemPlusChem, 82 (1) 107–120. (Ref. (Cantaert et al. 2017)

- Phase separation, clusters.

Prenucleation clusters: ref. (Demichelis et al. 2011; Kellermeier et al. 2016; Clark et al. 2022; Gebauer et al. 2008; Nicholas et al. 2023; Gebauer et al. 2010; Cartwright et al. 2012)

PILP: ref. (Olszta et al. 2007; Cölfen 2010; Thula et al. 2011; Jee et al. 2010; Bewernitz et al. 2012; Homeijer et al. 2010; Wolf et al. 2011; Gower and Odom 2000)

Step growth: ref. (Wallace et al. 2013; Zhang et al. 2024b; Andersson et al. 2016)

Mergelsberg, S. T. et al. (2020). Metastable solubility and local structure of amorphous calcium carbonate (ACC). Geochim. Cosmochim. Acta, 289, 196–206. https://doi.org/10.1016/J.GCA.2020.06.030

Blue, C. R. et al. (2017). Chemical and physical controls on the transformation of amorphous calcium carbonate into crystalline CaCO3 polymorphs. Geochim. Cosmochim. Acta, 196, 179–196. https://doi.org/10.1016/J.GCA.2016.09.004

Pokroya, B. and Aizenberga, J, (2007). Calcite shape modulation through the lattice mismatch between the self-assembled monolayer template and the nucleated crystal face. CrystEngComm, 9, 1219–1225.

- Biomineralization.

Issue 12, 2007 of CrystEngComm

References

#2623 cupric chloride (2013) Merck Index, 15th Ed., RSC Publishing, Cambridge, UK

A.A. Abalymov, N. Asadi Heris, A.G. Skirtach, B.V. Parakhonskiy, Macro-calcium carbonate-hydrogel hybrid spheroids: Design and biomedical applications. ACS Applied Bio Materials **7**, 5201–5210 (2024)

L. Addadi, S. Raz, S. Weiner, Taking advantage of disorder: amorphous calcium carbonate and its roles in biomineralization. Adv. Mater. **15**, 959–970 (2003)

A. Almajed, H.K. Tirkolaei, E. Kavazanjian, N. Hamdan, Enzyme induced Biocementated Sand with high strength at low carbonate content. Scient. Reports **9**, 1–7 (2019)

C.C. Alvarez, G. Quitté, J. Schott, E.H. Oelkers, Nickel isotope fractionation as a function of carbonate growth rate during Ni coprecipitation with calcite. Geochim. Cosmochim. Acta **299**, 184–198 (2021)

P. Anbu, C.H. Kang, Y.J. Shin, J.S. So, Formations of calcium carbonate minerals by bacteria and its multiple applications. Springerplus **5**, 1–26 (2016)

M.P. Andersson, S. Dobberschütz, K.K. Sand, D.J. Tobler, J.J. De Yoreo, S.L.S. Stipp, A microkinetic model of calcite step growth. Angew. Chem. Int. Ed. **55**, 11086–11090 (2016)

T. Armstrong, J. Schmid, J.P. Niemelä, I. Utke, T.M. Schutzius, Nanostructured Surfaces enhance nucleation rate of calcium carbonate. Small **20**(47), 2402690 (2024)

E. Asenath-Smith, H. Li, E.C. Keene, Z.W. Seh, L.A. Estroff, Crystal growth of calcium carbonate in hydrogels as a model of biomineralization. Adv. Funct. Mater. **22**, 2891–2914 (2012)

J.T. Avaro, S.L.P. Wolf, K. Hauser, D. Gebauer, Stable prenucleation calcium carbonate clusters define liquid–liquid phase separation. Angew. Chem. Int. Ed. **59**, 6155–6159 (2020)

A. Becker, U. Bismayer, M. Epple, H. Fabritius, B. Hasse, J. Shi, A. Ziegler, Structural characterisation of X-ray amorphous calcium carbonate (ACC) in sternal deposits of the crustacea Porcellio scaber. RSC. Dalton Trans. **3**, 551–555 (2003)

E. Beniash, J. Aizenberg, L. Addadi, S. Weiner, Amorphous calcium carbonate transforms into calcite during sea urchin larval spicule growth. Proc Royal Soc. B: Biologi Sci. **264**, 461–465 (1997)

F. Betts, A.S. Posner, An X-ray radial distribution study of amorphous calcium phosphate. Mater. Res. Bull. **9**, 353–361 (1974)

M.A. Bewernitz, D. Gebauer, J. Long, H. Cölfen, L.B. Gower, A metastable liquid precursor phase of calcium carbonate and its interactions with polyaspartate. Faraday Discuss. **159**, 291–312 (2012)

T. Bissbort, K.U. Hess, M. Wilding, J.E.K. Schawe, B. Purgstaller, K.E. Goetschl, S. Sturm, K. Müller-Caspary, E.V. Sturm, W. Schmahl, E. Griesshaber, D. Weidendorfer, M. Dietzel, D.B. Dingwell, The glass transition temperature of anhydrous amorphous calcium carbonate. Am. Mineral. **109**(7), 1303–1306 (2024)

M. Bohner, J. Lemaitre, Can bioactivity be tested in vitro with SBF solution? Biomaterials **30**, 2175–2179 (2009)

E. Boquet, A. Boronat, A. Ramos-Cormenzana, Production of calcite (calcium carbonate) crystals by soil bacteria is a general phenomenon. Nature **246**(5434), 527–529 (1973)

A. Borkowski, P. Działak, K. Berent, M. Gajewska, M.D. Syczewski, M. Słowakiewicz, Mechanism of bacteriophage-induced vaterite formation. Sci. Rep. **14**(1), 1–17 (2024)

Y. Boyjoo, V.K. Pareek, J. Liu, Synthesis of micro and nano-sized calcium carbonate particles and their applications. J. Mat. Chem. A **2**(35), 14270–14288 (2014)

B.J.F. Bruet, H.J. Qi, M.C. Boyce, R. Panas, K. Tai, L. Frick, C. Ortiz, Nanoscale morphology and indentation of individual nacre tablets from the gastropod mollusk Trochus niloticus. J. Mat. Res. **9**, 2400–2409 (2005)

H. Canakci, W. Sidik, I. Halil Kilic, Effect of bacterial calcium carbonate precipitation on compressibility and shear strength of organic soil. Soils Found. **55**, 1211–1221 (2015)

B. Cantaert, D. Kuo, S. Matsumura, T. Nishimura, T. Sakamoto, T. Kato, Use of amorphous calcium carbonate for the design of new materials. ChemPlusChem **82**(1), 107–120 (2017)

A.J. Carrillo, J. Joségonzaíez-Aguilar, M. Romero, J.M. Coronado, Solar energy on demand: a review on high temperature thermochemical heat storage systems and materials. Chem. Rev. **119**(2019), 4777–4816 (2019). https://doi.org/10.1021/acs.chemrev.8b00315

J.H.E. Cartwright, A.G. Checa, J.D. Gale, D. Gebauer, I. Sainz-Díaz, D. Gebauer, Biomineral Polyamorphism calcium carbonate Polyamorphism and its role in biomineralization: how many amorphous calcium carbonates are there? Angew. Chem. Int. Ed. **51**, 11960–11970 (2012)

S.C. Chuo, S.F. Mohamed, S.H.M. Setapar, A. Ahmad, M. Jawaid, W.A. Wani, A.A. Yaqoob, M.N.M. Ibrahim, Insights into the current trends in the utilization of bacteria for microbially induced calcium carbonate precipitation. Materials **13**(21), 1–28 (2020)

L. Chuzeville, A. Aissani, A. Manisekaran, Y. Fleming, P. Grysan, S. Contal, A. Chary, D. Duday, O. Couture, R. Anand, J.S. Thomann, Size and phase preservation of amorphous calcium carbonate nanoparticles in aqueous media using different types of lignin for contrast-enhanced ultrasound imaging. J. Colloid Interface Sci. **658**, 584–596 (2024)

S.M. Clark, B. Colas, D.E. Jacob, J.C. Neuefeind, H.W. Wang, K.L. Page, A.K. Soper, P.I. Schodder, P. Duchstein, B.A. Zubiri, T. Yokosawa, V. Pipich, D. Zahn, E. Spiecker, S.E. Wolf, The nano-

and meso-scale structure of amorphous calcium carbonate. Sci. Rep. **12**(1), 1–12 (2022). https://doi.org/10.1038/s41598-022-10627-9

H. Cölfen, Biomineralization A Crystal View. Nature Mater. **9**, 960–963 (2010)

J. Courtois, C. Li, C. Wang, H. Zhang, H. Jin, W. Feng, Calcium carbonate/ε-poly(lysine) hybrid microparticles for uranium seawater extraction: An eco-compatible emergency response to marine nuclear disasters. Colloids Surf A: Physicochem Eng Aspects **703**, 135339 (2024)

C.F. Dai, W.Y. Wang, L. Wang, L. Zhou, S.P. Li, X.D. Li, Methotrexate intercalated calcium carbonate nanostructures: synthesis, phase transformation and bioassay study. Mat. Sci. Eng.: C **69**, 577–583 (2016)

R. Darkins, D.M. Duffy, I.J. Ford, Prenucleation cluster pathway is inconsistent with $CaCO_3$ kinetics. C. Cryst. Growth Des. **24**, 4013–4016 (2024)

Y. Dauphin, A brief history of biomineralization studies. ACS Biomater. Sci. Eng. **9**, 1774–1790 (2023)

R. Demichelis, P. Raiteri, J.D. Gale, D. Quigley, D. Gebauer, Stable prenucleation mineral clusters are liquid-like ionic polymers. Nat. Commun. **2**(1), 1–8 (2011)

L. Dong, Y.J. Xu, C. Sui, Y. Zhao, L.B. Mao, D. Gebauer, R. Rosenberg, J. Avaro, Y.D. Wu, H.L. Gao, Z. Pan, H.Q. Wen, X. Yan, F. Li, Y. Lu, H. Cölfen, S.H. Yu, Highly hydrated paramagnetic amorphous calcium carbonate nanoclusters as an MRI contrast agent. Nat. Commun. **13**(1), 1–13 (2022)

F.C. Donnelly, F. Purcell-Milton, V. Framont, O. Cleary, P.W. Dunne, Y.K. Gun'ko, Synthesis of $CaCO_3$ nano—and micro-particles by dry ice carbonation. Chem. Commun. **53**, 6657–6660 (2017)

F.C. Donnelly, F. Purcell-Milton, P.W. Dunne, A. Rulikowska, V. Alguacil, Y.K. Gun'ko, Luminescent calcium carbonate micro 'bow ties.'. Mater. Today Commun. **20**, 00590 (2019). https://doi.org/10.3390/nano14010100

X. Dou, H. Huang, Y. Han, The role of diffusion in the nucleation of calcium carbonate. Chin. J. Chem. Engi. **43**, 275–281 (2022)

T.E.L. Douglas, A. Łapa, S.K. Samal, H.A. Declercq, D. Schaubroeck, A.C. Mendes, P. der Voort, van, Dokupil, A., Plis, A., de Schamphelaere, K., Chronakis, I. S., Pamuła, E., Skirtach, A. G., Enzymatic, urease-mediated mineralization of gellan gum hydrogel with calcium carbonate, magnesium-enriched calcium carbonate and magnesium carbonate for bone regeneration applications. J. Tissue Eng. Regen. Med. **11**, 3556–3566 (2017)

I. Erceg, J. Kontrec, V. Strasser, S. Atida, D. Domazet Jurasin, M. Curlin, B.N. Dzakula, N. Matijakovic Mlinaric, S. Segota, D.M. Lyons, D. Kralj, M. Dutour Sikiric, Precipitation of calcium phosphates and calcium carbonates in the presence of differently charged liposomes. Minerals **12**(2), 208 (2022)

E. Escamilla-Roa, M.P. Zorzano, J. Martin-Torres, C.I. Sainz-Díaz, J.H.E. Cartwright, Self-assembled structures formed in CO2-enriched atmospheres: A case-study for Martian biomimetic forms. Astrobiology **22**, 863–879 (2022)

D. Evans, W.R. Gray, J.W.B. Rae, R. Greenop, P.B. Webb, K. Penkman, R. Kröger, N. Allison, Trace and major element incorporation into amorphous calcium carbonate (ACC) precipitated from seawater. Geochim. Cosmochim. Acta **290**, 293–311 (2020)

M. Faatz, F. Gröhn, G. Wegner, Amorphous calcium carbonate: Synthesis and potential intermediate in biomineralization. Adv. Mater. **16**, 996–1000 (2004)

P. Fadia, S. Tyagi, S. Bhagat, A. Nair, P. Panchal, H. Dave, S. Dang, S. Singh, Calcium carbonate nano- and microparticles: Synthesis methods and biological applications. 3 Biotech **11**, 457 (2021) (30 pages)

Z. Fang, W. Liu, T. Yao, G. Zhou, S. Wei, L. Qin, Experimental study of chromium (III) coprecipitation with calcium carbonate. Geochim. Cosmochim. Acta **322**, 94–108 (2022)

W. Feng, Z.Y. Ng, H. Chen, J. Zhang, D. Xu, Y. He, H. Wei, L. Dang, Calcium ion deposition with precipitated calcium carbonate: influencing factors and mechanism exploration. PRO **12**, 629 (2024)

X. Feng, Z. Steiner, S.A.T. Redfern, Fluorine incorporation into calcite, aragonite and vaterite $CaCO_3$: computational chemistry insights and geochemistry implications. Geochim. Cosmochim. Acta **308**, 384–392 (2021)

E. Fiorito, G.E. Porcedda, L. Brundu, C. Passiu, D. Atzei, G. Ennas, B. Elsener, M. Fantauzzi, A. Rossi, Calcium carbonate as sorbent for lead removal from wastewaters. Chemosphere **296**, 133897 (2022)

B. Gao, K.M. Poduska, Tracking amorphous calcium carbonate crystallization products with far-infrared spectroscopy. Minerals **13**, 110 (2023)

D. Gebauer, A. Völkel, H. Cölfen, Stable prenucleation calcium carbonate clusters. Science **322**(5909), 1819–1822 (2008)

D. Gebauer, P.N. Gunawidjaja, J.Y.P. Ko, B. Zolt, B. Aziz, L. Liu, Y. Hu, L. Bergström, C.-W. Tai, M. Tsun-Kong Sham, N.H. Edén, Proto-calcite and proto-Vaterite in amorphous calcium carbonates. Angew. Chem. Int. Ed. **49**, 8889–8891 (2010)

D. Gebauer, P. Raiteri, J.D. Gale, H. Cölfen, On classical and non-classical views on nucleation. Amer. J. Sci. **318**(9), 969–988 (2018)

M. Getenet, J. Rieder, M. Kellermeier, W. Kunz, J. Manuel García-Ruiz, Tubular structures of calcium carbonate: Formation, characterization, and implications in natural mineral environments. Chem. Eur. J. **27**, 16135–16144 (2021)

T. Ghaffari, P. Daneshfar, A. Mosayebzadeh, S. Maleki Dizaj, S. Sharifi, S/4 inhibitory effects of chlorhexidine-loaded calcium carbonate nanoparticles against dental implant infections. BMC Oral Health **24**(1), 1–11 (2024)

M.B. Gindele, L.V. Steingrube, D. Gebauer, Generality of liquid precursor phases in gas diffusion-based calcium carbonate synthesis. CrystEngComm **23**(45), 7938–7943 (2021)

L.B. Gower, Biomimetic model systems for investigating the amorphous precursor pathway and its role in biomineralization. Chem. Rev. **108**(11), 4551–4627 (2008). https://doi.org/10.1021/CR800443H/ASSET/IMAGES/MEDIUM/CR-2008-00443H_0046.GIF

L.B. Gower, D.J. Odom, Deposition of calcium carbonate films by a polymer-induced liquid-precursor (PILP) process. J. Cryst. Growth **210**, 719–734 (2000)

G.T. Grant, E.R. Morris, D.A. Reeds, P.J.C. Smith, D. Thom, Biological interactions between polysaccharides and divalent cations: The egg-box model. FEBS Lett. **32**, 195–200 (1973)

C.J. Grimes, T. Hardcastle, M.S. Manga, T. Mahmud, D.W. York, Calcium carbonate particle formation through precipitation in a stagnant bubble and a bubble column reactor. Cryst. Growth Des. **20**(8), 5572–5582 (2020). https://doi.org/10.1021/acs.cgd.0c00741

J.D. Guerrero, E.R. Arias, L.B. Gutierrez, Enhancing copper and lead adsorption in water by in-situ generation of calcium carbonate on alginate/chitosan biocomposite surfaces. Int. J. Biol. Macromol. **266**, 131110 (2024)

G. Hadiko, Y.S. Han, M. Fuji, M. Takahashi, Synthesis of hollow calcium carbonate particles by the bubble templating method. Mater. Lett. **59**(19–20), 2519–2522 (2005). https://doi.org/10.1016/J.MATLET.2005.03.036

Y.S. Han, G. Hadiko, M. Fuji, M. Takahashi, Effect of flow rate and CO_2 content on the phase and morphology of $CaCO_3$ prepared by bubbling method. J. Cryst. Growth **276**(3–4), 541–548 (2005)

F. Haudin, J.H.E. Cartwright, F. Brau, A. de Wit, Spiral precipitation patterns in confined chemical gardens. Proc. Nat. Acad. Sci. **111**, 17363–17367 (2014)

Z. He, Z. Xia, M. Zhang, J. Wu, W. Wen, Calcium carbonate mineralization in a surface-tension-confined droplets array. Crystals **9**(6), 284 (2019). https://doi.org/10.3390/CRYST9060284

K.U. Hess, J.E.K. Schawe, M. Wilding, B. Purgstaller, K.E. Goetschl, S. Sturm, K. Müller-Caspary, E.v. Sturm, W. Schmahl, E. Griesshaber, T. Bissbort, D. Weidendorfer, M. Dietzel, D.B. Dingwell, Glass transition temperatures and crystallization kinetics of a synthetic, anhydrous, amorphous calcium-magnesium carbonate. Phil. Trans. R. Soc. A **381**, 20220356 (2023)

S.J. Homeijer, R.A. Barrett, L.B. Gower, Polymer-induced liquid-precursor (PILP) process in the non-calcium based systems of barium and strontium carbonate. Cryst. Growth Design **10**(3), 1040–1052 (2010)

https://en.wikipedia.org/wiki/Microbiologically_induced_calcite_precipitation (Wikepedia USA)
S.C. Huang, K. Naka, Y. Chujo, A carbonate controlled-addition method for amorphous calcium carbonate spheres stabilized by poly(acrylic acid)s. Langmuir **23**(24), 12086–12095 (2007)
Y. Huang, L. Cao, B.V. Parakhonskiy, A.G. Skirtach, Hard, soft, and hard-and-soft drug delivery carriers based on $CaCO_3$ and alginate biomaterials: synthesis, properties, pharmaceutical applications. Pharmaceutics **14**, 909 (2022)
K. Igarashi, M. Takiguchi, H. Ooshima, Growth mechanism of the calcium carbonate tubes on a cation-exchange membrane. J. Ceram. Soc. Japan. **118**, 111–114 (2008)
S.S. Jee, T.T. Thula, L.B. Gower, Development of bone-like composites via the polymer-induced liquid-precursor (PILP) process. Part 1: Influence of polymer molecular weight. Acta Biomater. **6**, 3676–3686 (2010)
T. Jeon, Y.-E. Na, D. Jang, I.W. Kim, Stabilized amorphous calcium carbonate as a precursor of microcoating on calcite. Materials **13**, 3762 (2020)
W. Jiang, M.S. Pacella, D. Athanasiadou, V. Nelea, H. Vali, R.M. Hazen, J.J. Gray, M.D. McKee, Chiral acidic amino acids induce chiral hierarchical structure in calcium carbonate. Nat. Commun. **8**, 15066 (2017)
W. Jiang, M.S. Pacella, H. Vali, J.J. Gray, M.D. McKee, Chiral switching in biomineral suprastructures induced by homochiral l-amino acid. Sci. Adv. **4**(8), 9819–9820 (2018)
O.A. Jimoh, K.S. Ariffin, H.b. Hussin, A.E. Temitope, Synthesis of precipitated calcium carbonate: a review. Carbon. Evaporites **33**(2), 331–346 (2018)
Y. Jing, X. Nai, L. Dang, D. Zhu, Y. Wang, Y. Dong, W. Li, Reinforcing polypropylene with calcium carbonate of different morphologies and polymorphs. Sci. Eng. Composite Mater. **25**, 745–751 (2018)
Y.-M. Ju, Y. Zhao, Q.F. Guan, S.Y. Yang, W. Wang, B.B. Yan, Y.F. Meng, S.C. Li, P.P. Tang, L.B. Mao, S.H. Yu, Amorphous calcium carbonate cluster Nanospheres in water-deficient organic solvents. Angew. Chem. Intl. Ed. **61**, e202211254 (2022)
J.A. Juhasz-Bortuzzo, B. Myszka, R. Silva, A.R. Boccaccini, Sonosynthesis of Vaterite-type calcium carbonate. Cryst. Growth Des. **17**(5), 2351–2356 (2017)
B. Kanoje, J. Parikh, K. Kuperkar, Crystallization study and morphology behaviour of calcium carbonate crystals in aqueous surfactant-Pluronics® prototype. J. Mater. Res. Tech. **7**, 508–514 (2018)
M. Kellermeier, E. Melero-García, F. Glaab, R. Klein, M. Drechsler, R. Rachel, J.M. García-Ruiz, W. Kunz, Stabilization of amorphous calcium carbonate in inorganic silica-rich environments. J. Am. Chem. Soc. **132**, 17859–17866 (2010)
M. Kellermeier, P. Raiteri, J.K. Berg, A. Kempter, J.D. Gale, D. Gebauer, Entropy drives calcium carbonate ion association. ChemPhysChem **17**, 3535–3541 (2016)
A. Kertmen, I. Petrenko, C. Schimpf, D. Rafaja, O. Petrova, V. Sivkov, S. Nekipelov, A. Fursov, A.L. Stelling, K. Heimler, A. Rogoll, C. Vogt, H. Ehrlich, Calcite nanotuned chitinous skeletons of giant ianthella basta marine demosponge. Int. J. Molec. Sci. **22**(22), 12588 (2021)
Y. Kezuka, K. Kawai, K. Eguchi, M. Tajika, Fabrication of single-crystalline calcite needle-like particles using the aragonite-calcite phase transition. Minerals **7**, 133 (2017)
Y. Kezuka, Y. Kuma, S. Nakai, K. Matsubara, M. Tajika, Calcium carbonate chain-like nanoparticles: synthesis, structural characterization, and dewaterability. Powd. Tech. **335**, 195–203 (2018)
Y. Kezuka, M. Yoshida, M. Tajika, Template-free fabrication of single-crystalline calcite nanorings during crystal growth in water. Cryst Eng Comm **22**, 9–13 (2020). https://doi.org/10.1039/C9CE01403A
Y. Kezuka, E. Tochigi, H. Murata, M. Yoshida, A. Nakahira, Y. Ikuhara, M. Tajika, Fabrication of calcite-core/Mg-calcite-shell nanorods for better thermal stability. Adv. Powd. Techn. **32**(7), 2577–2584 (2021). https://doi.org/10.1016/J.APT.2021.05.033
Y. Kezuka, H. Murata, M. Yoshida, K. Eguchi, A. Nakahira, M. Tajika, Effects of trace Si impurities in water on the growth of calcite nanoparticles. CrystEngComm **24**(4), 747–754 (2022)
A.Y. Khan, S. Talegaonkar, Z. Iqbal, F.J. Ahmed, R.K. Khar, Multiple emulsions: an overview. Curr. Drug Deliv. **3**, 429–443 (2006)

M. Kijima, Y. Oaki, H. Imai, In vitro repair of a biomineral with a mesocrystal structure. Chem. Eur. J. **17**(10), 2828–2832 (2011)

H.M. Kim, F. Miyaji, T. Kokubo, T. Nakamura, Preparation of bioactive Ti and its alloys via simple chemical surface treatment. J. Biomed. Mater. Res. **32**, 409–417 (1996)

S. Kim, J. Jeon, M.J. Kim, Vaterite production and particle size and shape control using seawater as an indirect carbonation solvent. J. Environ. Chem. Eng. **10**, 107296 (2022a)

S.Y. Kim, Y.B. Seo, J.S. Han, Effect of Calendering on the properties of paper containing flexible calcium carbonate with a cellulose Nanofibril Core. ACS Omega **7**, 35305–35315 (2022b)

T. Kokubo, H. Takadama, How useful is SBF in predicting in vivo bone bioactivity? Biomaterials **27**, 2907–2915 (2006)

T. Kokubo, S. Yamaguchi, Simulated body fluid and the novel bioactive materials derived from it. J. Biomed. Mater. Res., Part A **107**, 968–977 (2019)

D. Konopacka-Łyskawa, Synthesis methods and favorable conditions for spherical vaterite precipitation: a review. Crystals **9**, 223 (2019)

V.K. LaMer, R.H. Dinegar, Theory, production and mechanism of formation of monodispersed hydrosols. J. Am. Chem. Soc. **72**, 4847–4854 (1950)

W.J. Landis, M.J. Song, A. Leith, L. McEwen, B.F. McEwen, Mineral and organic matrix interaction in normally calcifying tendon visualized in three dimensions by high-voltage electron microscopic tomography and graphic image reconstruction. J. Structu. Biol. **110**, 39–54 (1993)

Y. Lee, Y.M. Hahm, S. Matsuya, M. Nakagawa, K. Ishikawa, Development of macropores in calcium carbonate body using novel carbonation method of calcium hydroxide/sodium chloride composite. J. Mat. Sc. **42**(14), 5728–5735 (2007)

F. Liendo, M. Arduino, F.A. Deorsola, S. Bensaid, Optimization of $CaCO_3$ synthesis through the carbonation route in a packed bed reactor. Powder Technol. **377**, 868–881 (2020). https://doi.org/10.1016/J.POWTEC.2020.09.038

F. Liendo, M. Arduino, F.A. Deorsola, S. Bensaid, Factors controlling and influencing polymorphism, morphology and size of calcium carbonate synthesized through the carbonation route: a review. Powder Technol. **398**, 117050 (2022)

P.Y. Lin, H.M. Wu, S.L. Hsieh, J.S. Li, C. Dong, C.W. Chen, S. Hsieh, Preparation of vaterite calcium carbonate granules from discarded oyster shells as an adsorbent for heavy metal ions removal. Chemosphere **254**, 126903 (2020). https://doi.org/10.1016/J.CHEMOSPHERE.2020.126903

C. Liu, W. Zhang, H. Liu, Threonine and Polythreonine accelerate calcium carbonate formation. Cryst. Growth Des. **24**(3), 892–898 (2024)

L. Liu, D. Fan, H. Mao, X. Fang, J. Hao, Multi-phase equilibrium microemulsions and synthesis of hierarchically structured calcium carbonate through microemulsion-based routes. J. Colloid Interface Sci. **306**, 154–160 (2007)

X. Liu, Z. Wang, Chitosan-calcium carbonate scaffold with high mineral content and hierarchical structure for bone regeneration. Smart Mater. Medi. **4**, 552–561 (2023). https://doi.org/10.1016/J.SMAIM.2023.04.006

Z. Liu, C. Shao, B. Jin, Z. Zhang, Y. Zhao, X. Xu, R. Tang, Crosslinking ionic oligomers as conformable precursors to calcium carbonate. Nature **574**, 394–398 (2019)

A. Lotsari, A.K. Rajasekharan, M. Halvarsson, M. Andersson, Transformation of amorphous calcium phosphate to bone-like apatite. Nat. Commun. 2018 9:1 **9**(1), 1–11 (2018). https://doi.org/10.1038/s41467-018-06570-x

Luo, X., Song, X., Lai, C., Wang, J., Cao, Y. Sonochemical synthesis of vaterite-type calcium carbonate using steamed ammonia liquid waste without additives. ACS Omega, 6 (2021) (37) 23846–23854. (2011) https://doi.org/10.1021/acsomega.1c02774

C. Lv, C.-S. Tang, J.-Z. Zhang, H. Liu, X.-H. Pan, Regulating the process of microbially induced calcium carbonate precipitation through applied electric fields: evidence and insights using microfluidics. J. Geotechn. Geoenviron. Eng. **150**(10), 12534 (2024). https://doi.org/10.1061/JGGEFK.GTENG-12534

J. Ma, Y. Tang, M. Yaseen, L. Qin, X. Chen, S. Xiong, D. Liao, Z. Tong, Hollow spherical vaterite calcium carbonate prepared by spray-bubble template method for immobilization of papain. Separat. Purificat. Techn. **322**, 124278 (2023)

D. Madhav, B. Buffel, F. Desplentere, P. Moldenaers, Vandeginste., Bio-inspired mineralization of CO2 into $CaCO_3$: single-step carbon capture and utilization with controlled crystallization. Fuel **345**, 128157 (2023)

S. Maleki Dizaj, S. Sharifi, E. Ahmadian, A. Eftekhari, K. Adibkia, F. Lotfipour, An update on calcium carbonate nanoparticles as cancer drug/gene delivery system. Expert Opini. Drug Deliv. **16**(4), 331–345 (2019)

T. Mass, A.J. Giuffre, C.Y. Sun, C.A. Stifler, M.J. Frazier, M. Neder, N. Tamura, C.v. Stan, M.A. Marcus, P.U.P.A. Gilbert, Amorphous calcium carbonate particles form coral skeletons. Proc. Natl. Acad. Sci. USA **114**(37), E7670–E7678 (2017). https://doi.org/10.1073/pnas.1707890114

V. Mavromatis, J.M. Brazier, K.E. Goetschl, Controls of temperature and mineral growth rate on Mg incorporation in aragonite. Geochim. Cosmochim. Acta **317**, 53–64 (2022). https://doi.org/10.1016/J.GCA.2021.10.015

Mayorga, I. C., Astilleros, J. M., Fernández-Díaz, L. Precipitation of $CaCO_3$ polymorphs from aqueous solutions: The role of pH and sulphate groups. Minerals, 9 (2019) 178

M.T. McCulloch, J.P. D'Olivo, J. Falter, M. Holcomb, J.A. Trotter, Coral calcification in a changing world and the interactive dynamics of pH and DIC upregulation. Nat. Commun. **8**, 1–8 (2017)

N. Mehta, D. Vantelon, J. Gaëtan, A. Fernandez-Martinez, L. Delbes, C. Travert, K. Benzerara, Calcium speciation and coordination environment in intracellular amorphous calcium carbonate (ACC) formed by cyanobacteria. Chem. Geol. **641**, 121765 (2023)

F.C. Meldrum, H. Cölfen, Controlling mineral morphologies and structures in biological and synthetic systems. Chem. Rev. **108**, 4332–4432 (2008)

A. Menichetti, A. Mavridi-Printezi, G. Falini, P. Besirske, J.M. García-Ruiz, H. Cölfen, M. Montalti, Local light-controlled generation of calcium carbonate and barium carbonate biomorphs via photochemical stimulation. Chem. Eur. J. **7**(49), 12521–12525 (2021)

F.M. Michel, J. MacDonald, J. Feng, B.L. Phillips, L. Ehm, C. Tarabrella, J.B. Parise, R.J. Reeder, Structural characteristics of synthetic amorphous calcium carbonate. Chem. Mater. **20**, 4720–4728 (2008)

J.v. Mills, D.J. DePaolo, L.N. Lammers, The influence of ca: CO_3 stoichiometry on ca isotope fractionation: Implications for process-based models of calcite growth. Geochim. Cosmochim. Acta **298**, 87–111 (2021)

K.H. Min, D.H. Kim, K.H. Kim, J.-H. Seo, S.P. Pack, Biomimetic scaffolds of calcium-based materials for bone regeneration. Biomimetics **9**, 511 (2024a)

K.H. Min, D.H. Kim, K.H. Kim, J.-H. Seo, S.P. Pack, Biomimetic scaffolds of calcium-based materials for bone regeneration. Biomimetics **9**(9), 511 (2024b)

F. Mo, Q. Chen, X. Zhang, Synthesis of hollow calcium carbonate microspheres by a template method for DOX loading and release with carbon dots photosensitivity. Materials **15**(24), 8768 (2022)

Z. Molnár, I. Dódony, M. Pósfai, Transformation of amorphous calcium carbonate in the presence of magnesium, phosphate, and mineral surfaces. Geochim. Cosmochim. Acta **345**, 90–101 (2023)

O. Nahi, A.N. Kulak, S. Zhang, X. He, Z. Aslam, M.A. Ilett, I.J. Ford, R. Darkins, F.C. Meldrum, Polyamines promote aragonite nucleation and generate biomimetic structures. Adv. Sci. **10**, 2203759 (2023). https://doi.org/10.1002/advs.202203760

K. Nakanishi, Pore structure control of silica gels based on phase separation. J. Porous Mat. **4**, 67–112 (1997)

N. Nassrallah-Aboukaïs, A. Boughriet, J. Laureyns, L. Gengembre, A. Aboukaïs, Stabilization of the vaterite structure in the presence of copper (II): Thermodynamic and spectroscopic studies. Chem. Mater. **11**, 44–51 (1999)

T.H.K. Nawarathna, K. Nakashima, T. Kawabe, W. Mwandira, K. Kurumisawa, S. Kawasaki, Artificial fusion protein to facilitate calcium carbonate mineralization on insoluble polysaccharide for efficient biocementation. ACS Sustain. Chem. Eng. **9**(34), 11493–11502 (2021)

T.T.M. Nguyen, S. Hazoor, T. Vuong, L.M. Kydd, I. Shortt, F.W. Foss, E. la Plante, Synthesis of metastable calcium carbonate using Long-chain bisphosphonate molecules. ACS Appl. Mater. Interfaces **16**, 30567–30579 (2024)

T.C. Nicholas, A.E. Stones, A. Patel, F.M. Michel, R.J. Reeder, D.G.A.L. Aarts, V.L. Deringer, A.L. Goodwin, Geometrically frustrated interactions drive structural complexity in amorphous calcium carbonate. Nat. Chem. **16**, 36–41 (2023)

Y.Q. Niu, J.H. Liu, C. Aymonier, S. Fermani, D. Kralj, G. Falini, C.H. Zhou, Calcium carbonate: controlled synthesis, surface functionalization, and nanostructured materials. Chem. Soc. Rev. **51**(18), 7883–7943 (2022)

F. Nudelman, K. Pieterse, A. George, P.H.H. Bomans, H. Friedrich, L.J. Brylka, P.A.J. Hilbers, G. de With, N.A.J.M. Sommerdijk, The role of collagen in bone apatite formation in the presence of hydroxyapatite nucleation inhibitors. Nature Mat. **9**, 1004–1009 (2010). https://doi.org/10.1038/nmat2875

Y. Oaki, A. Kotachi, T. Miura, H. Imai, Bridged nanocrystals in biominerals and their biomimetics: classical yet modern crystal growth on the nanoscale. Adv. Funct. Mater. **16**(12), 1633–1639 (2006)

Y. Oaki, S. Hayashi, H. Imai, A hierarchical self-similar structure of oriented calcite with association of an agar gel matrix: Inheritance of crystal habit from nanoscale. Chem. Commun. **2**(27), 2841–2843 (2007)

T. Ogino, T. Suzuki, K. Sawada, The formation and transformation mechanism of calcium carbonate in water. Geochim. Cosmochim. Acta **51**(10), 2757–2767 (1987)

L.R. Oliveira, L.G. Pereira, L.d.R. Teixeira, et al., Calcium carbonate scaling control on heat plate exchange surfaces using ultrasound. J. Braz. Soc. Mech. Sci. Eng. **46**, 111 (2024)

M.J. Olszta, X. Cheng, S.S. Jee, R. Kumar, Y.Y. Kim, M.J. Kaufman, E.P. Douglas, L.B. Gower, Bone structure and formation: A new perspective. Mat. Sci. Eng. R **58**, 77–116 (2007)

A. Omran, A. Gonzalez, C. Menor-Salvan, M. Gaylor, J. Wang, J. Leszczynski, T. Feng, Serpentinization-associated mineral catalysis of the Protometabolic Formose system. Life **13**, 1297 (2023) (13 pages)

K. Onuma, A. Ito, Cluster growth model for hydroxyapatite. Chem. Mat. **10**, 3346–3351 (1998)

Ç.M. Oral, A. Çalışkan, Y. Göçtü, D. Kapusuz, B. Ercan, Synthesis of calcium carbonate microspheres via inert gas bubbling for orthopedic applications. Ceram. Int. **46**(3), 3513–3522 (2020)

Ç.M. Oral, B. Ercan, D. Kapusuz, Calcium carbonate polymorph dictates in vitro osteoblast proliferation. J. Austral. Ceram. Soc. **56**, 1421–1426 (2020a)

Y. Ota, S. Inui, T. Iwashita, T. Kasuga, Y. Abe, Preparation of aragonite whiskers. J. Amer. Ceram. Soc. **78**, 1983–1984 (1995)

A. Oyane, K. Onuma, T. Kokubo, A. Ito, Clustering of calcium phosphate in the system CaCl2-H3PO4-KCl-H2O. J. Phys. Chem. B **103**, 8230–8235 (1999)

X. Pan, S. Chen, D. Li, W. Rao, Y. Zheng, Z. Yang, L. Li, X. Guan, Z. Chen, The synergistic antibacterial mechanism of gentamicin-loaded $CaCO_3$ nanoparticles. Front. Chem. **5**, 130 (2018)

F. Persano, C. Nobile, C. Piccirillo, G. Gigli, S. Leporatti, Monodisperse and Nanometric-sized calcium carbonate particles synthesis optimization. Nano **12**, 1494 (2022)

S. Polat, Evaluation of the effects of sodium laurate on calcium carbonate precipitation: Characterization and optimization studies. J. Cryst. Growth **508**, 8–18 (2019)

E.M. Pouget, P.H.H. Bomans, J.A.C.M. Goos, P.M. Frederik, G. de With, N.A.J.M. Sommerdijk, The initial stages of template-controlled $CaCO_3$ formation revealed by Cryo-TEM. Science **323**(5920), 1455–1458 (2009)

R.J. Qi, Y.J. Zhu, Microwave-assisted synthesis of calcium carbonate (vaterite) of various morphologies in water—Ethylene glycol mixed solvents. J. Phys. Chem. B **110**, 8302–8306 (2006). https://doi.org/10.1021/jp060939s

N. Sánchez-Pastor, A.J. Pinto, P. del Buey Fernández, J.M. Astilleros, Crystallization of calcium carbonate and calcium phosphate phases in silica hydrogel: Morphological and compositional characterization. Crystals **14**, 635 (2024)

H. Saulat, M. Cao, M.M. Khan, M. Khan, M.M. Khan, A. Rehman, Preparation and applications of calcium carbonate whisker with a special focus on construction materials. Construc. Build. Mater., 236 (2020)

K. Sawada, The mechanisms of crystallization and transformation of calcium carbonates. Pure Appl. Chem. **69**, 921–928 (1997). https://doi.org/10.1351/pac199769050921

K.G. Schulz, U. Riebesell, B. Rost, S. Thoms, R.E. Zeebe, Determination of the rate constants for the carbon dioxide to bicarbonate inter-conversion in pH-buffered seawater systems. Mar. Chem. **100**, 53–65 (2006)

F. Sebastiani, S.L.P. Wolf, B. Born, T.Q. Luong, H. Cölfen, D. Gebauer, M. Havenith, Water dynamics from THz spectroscopy reveal the locus of a liquid–liquid binodal limit in aqueous $CaCO_3$ solutions. Angew. Chem. Int. Ed. **56**, 490–495 (2017)

M. Seifan, A. Berenjian, Microbially induced calcium carbonate precipitation: A widespread phenomenon in the biological world. Appl. Microbiol. Biotech. **103**(12), 4693–4708 (2019)

Y. Seo, T. Goto, S. Cho, T. Sekino, Densification of transparent hydroxyapatite ceramics via cold sintering process combined with biomineralization. J. Eur. Ceram. Soc. **44**(2024), 4285–4293 (2024)

Y. Shen, S. Hao, A. Suonan, Y. Liu, H. Li, W. Ma, L. Zhao, Y. Zhang, Controllable synthesis of Nano-micro calcium carbonate mediated by additive engineering. Crystals **13**, 1432 (2023)

W. Shu, J. Gong, H. Zhang, F. Zheng, J. Zeng, X. Wang, S. Qin, C. Zhang, H. Xue, B. Dai, Nano-calcium carbonate with Core-Shell structure was prepared by dopamine chelation using Pluronic F-127 as template. Part. Part. System Charact. **41**, 230019 (2024)

Y. Shuseki, S. Kohara, K. Ohara, T. Ohkubo, K. Takei, M.G. Tucker, A.I. Kolesnikov, M.T. McDonnell, R.L. Sacci, J.C. Neuefeind, K. Takeuchi, Structural analyses of amorphous calcium carbonate before and after removing strontium ions from an aqueous solution. J. Ceram. Soc. Jpn. **130**, 225–231 (2022)

T. Siva, S. Muralidharan, S. Sathiyanarayanan, E. Manikandan, M. Jayachandran, Enhanced polymer induced precipitation of polymorphous in calcium carbonate: Calcite aragonite Vaterite phases. J. Inorg. Organometal. Polym. Mater. **27**, 770–778 (2017)

M. Słowakiewicz, A. Borkowski, M.D. Syczewski, I.D. Perrota, F. Owczarek, A. Sikora, A. Detman, E. Perri, M.E. Tucker, Newly-discovered interactions between bacteriophages and the process of calcium carbonate precipitation. Geochim. Cosmochim. Acta **292**, 482–498 (2021)

Sugawara, A., Ishii, T., Kato, T. Self-organized calcium carbonate with regular surface-relief structures. Angew. Chem. Int., 42 (2003) 52995303

M. Sun, H. Jin, X. Guo, S. Wang, J. Bi, Z. Ji, Y. Zhao, Precipitation and in-situ surface modification of calcium carbonate in synthetic seawater: Polymorph control, crystallization kinetics, and hydrophobic vaterite preparation. J. Environm. Chem. Eng. **11**, 110019 (2023)

M.A. Surmeneva, E.A. Chudinova, R.V. Chernozem, A. Lapanje, A.V. Koptyug, T. Rijavec, K. Loza, O. Prymak, M. Epple, A. Wittmar, M. Ulbricht, R.A. Surmenev, Development of a bone substitute material based on additive manufactured Ti6Al4V alloys modified with bioceramic calcium carbonate coating: characterization and antimicrobial properties. Ceram. Int. **46**, 25661–25670 (2020a)

M.A. Surmeneva, E.A. Chudinova, R.v. Chernozem, A. Lapanje, A.v. Koptyug, T. Rijavec, K. Loza, O. Prymak, M. Epple, A. Wittmar, M. Ulbricht, R.A. Surmenev, Development of a bone substitute material based on additive manufactured Ti6Al4V alloys modified with bioceramic calcium carbonate coating: Characterization and antimicrobial properties. Ceram. Int. **46**(16), 25661–25670 (2020b)

Y. Suzawa, N. Kubo, S. Iwai, Y. Yura, H. Ohgushi, M. Akashi, Biomineral/agarose composite gels enhance proliferation of mesenchymal stem cells with osteogenic capability. Int. J. Molec Sci **16**, 14245–14258 (2015)

T. Taguchi, Y. Muraoka, H. Matsuyama, A. Kishida, M. Akashi, Apatite coating on hydrophilic polymer-grafted poly(ethylene) films using an alternate soaking process. Biomaterials **22**, 53–58 (2001)

M. Takasaki, Y. Kimura, T. Yamazaki, Y. Oaki, H. Imai, 1D oriented attachment of calcite nanocrystals: formation of single-crystalline rods through collision. RSC Adv. **6**, 61346–61350 (2016)

M. Takasaki, T.S. Suzuki, Y. Oaki, H. Imai, Biomimetic macroscopic mesocrystalline films produced by oriented assembly of nanorods under magnetic field. Nanoscale **10**, 22161 (2018). https://doi.org/10.1039/C8NR07853J

M. Takasaki, M. Tago, Y. Oaki, H. Imai, Thermally induced fragmentation of nanoscale calcite. RSC Adv. **10**(10), 6088–6091 (2020)

S. Takasaki, K.I. Parsiegla, J.L. Katz, Calcite growth and the inhibiting effect of iron(III). J. Cryst. Growth **143**, 261–268 (1994)

M. Takiguchi, K. Igarashi, M. Azuma, H. Ooshima, Tubular structure agglomerates of calcium carbonate crystals formed on a cation-exchange membrane. Cryst. Growth Design **6**, 1611–1614 (2006)

S. Tanaka, K. Takahashi, M. Abe, M. Noguchi, A. Yamasaki, Preparation of high-purity calcium carbonate by mineral carbonation using concrete sludge. ACS Omega **7**(23), 19600–19605 (2022)

C.S. Tang, L.Y. Yin, N.J. Jiang, C. Zhu, H. Zeng, H. Li, B. Shi, Factors affecting the performance of microbial-induced carbonate precipitation (MICP) treated soil: a review. Environ. Earth Sci. **79**(5), 79.94 (2020)

Z. Tao, X. Cheng, C. Huo, The precipitation of calcium carbonate via a bubbling method in the presence of Mg^{2+} and glucose. Molec. Cryst. Liq. Cryst. **703**, 52–66 (2020)

C. Tas, A., Aragonite coating solutions (ACS) based on artificial seawater. Appl. Surface Sci. **330**, 262–269 (2015)

T.T. Thula, D.E. Rodriguez, M.H. Lee, L. Pendi, J. Podschun, L.B. Gower, In vitro mineralization of dense collagen substrates: a biomimetic approach toward the development of bone-graft materials. Acta Biomat. **7**(8), 3158–3169 (2011). https://doi.org/10.1016/j.actbio.2011.04.014

S. Umemoto, T. Furusawa, H. Unuma, M. Tajika, T. Sekino, In vivo bioresorbability and bone formation ability of sintered highly pure calcium carbonate granules. Dent. Mater. J. **40**, 1202–1207 (2021)

V. Vergaro, M. Civallero, C. Citti, M. Cosenza, F. Baldassarre, G. Cannazza, S. Pozzi, S. Sacchi, F.P. Fanizzi, G. Ciccarella, Cell-penetrating $CaCO_3$ nanocrystals for improved transport of NVP-BEZ235 across membrane barrier in T-cell lymphoma. Cancer **10**, 31 (2018)

A.F. Wallace, L.O. Hedges, A. Fernandez-Martinez, P. Raiteri, J.D. Gale, G.A. Waychunas, S. Whitelam, J.F. Banfield, J.J. de Yoreo, Microscopic evidence for liquid-liquid separation in supersaturated CaCO3 solutions. Science **341**(6148), 885–889 (2013)

J. Wang, Y. Kong, F. Liu, D. Shou, Y. Tao, Y. Qin, Construction of pH-responsive drug delivery platform with calcium carbonate microspheres induced by chitosan gels. Ceram. Int. **44**(7), 7902–7907 (2018)

J. Wang, J. Song, Z. Ji, J. Liu, X. Guo, Y. Zhao, J. Yuan, The preparation of calcium carbonate with different morphologies under the effect of alkanolamide. Colloids Surf. A Physicochem. Eng. Asp. **588**, 124392 (2020)

Q. Wang, W. Huang, J. Wang, F. Long, Z. Fu, J. Xie, Z. Zou, Stabilization and crystallization mechanism of amorphous calcium carbonate. J. Colloid Interface Sci. **680**, 24–35 (2025)

Y. Wei, H. Xu, S. Xu, H. Su, R. Sun, D. Huang, L. Zhao, Y. Hu, K. Wang, X. Lian, Synthesis and characterization of calcium carbonate on three kinds of microbial cells templates. J. Cryst. Growth **547**, 128755 (2020)

D. Weidendorfer, K.U. Hess, R.M. Ruhekenya, J.E.K. Schawe, M.C. Wilding, D.B. Dingwell, Effect of water on the glass transition of a potassium-magnesium carbonate melt. Phil. Trans. R. Soc. A **381**, 20220355 (2023)

T. Wen, Y. Zhao, T. Zhang, B. Xiong, H. Hu, Q. Zhang, S. Song, Selective recovery of heavy metals from wastewater by mechanically activated calcium carbonate: Inspiration from nature. Chemosphere **246**, 125842 (2020)

S.E. Wolf, J. Leiterer, V. Pipich, R. Barrea, F. Emmerling, W. Tremel, Strong stabilization of amorphous calcium carbonate emulsion by ovalbumin: Gaining insight into the mechanism of "polymer-induced liquid precursor" processes. J. Am. Chem. Soc. **133**(32), 12642–12649 (2011)

L. Xiang, Y. Wen, Q. Wang, Y. Jin, Formation and characterization of dispersive Mg substituted $CaCO_3$. Mater. Lett. **60**, 1719–1723 (2006)

X. Xiong, Y. Cao, Z. Li, R. Huang, Y. Jiao, L. Zhao, X. Du, Z.X. Zheng, Insights from tyrosinase into the impacts of modified morphology of calcium carbonate on the nacre formation of pearl oysters. Front. Marine Sci. **9**, 935609 (2022)

J. Xu, M.T. Balhoff, Novel regimes of calcium carbonate dissolution in micron-scale confined spaces. Adv. Water Resour. **164**, 104200 (2022). https://doi.org/10.1016/J.ADVWATRES.2022.104200

K. Yamaguchi, S. Hashimoto, Mechanism of densification of calcium carbonate by cold sintering process. J. Eur. Ceram. Soci. **42**, 6048–6055 (2022)

T. Yang, Y. Ao, J. Feng, C. Wang, J. Zhang, Biomineralization inspired synthesis of $CaCO_3$-based DDS for pH-responsive release of anticancer drug. Mater. Today Commun. **27**, 102256 (2021)

C. Yao, A. Xie, Y. Shen, J. Zhu, H. Li, Nacre-like calcium carbonate controlled by ionic liquid/graphene oxide composite template. Mat. Sci. Eng. C **51**, 274–278 (2015)

H. Yi, T. Zheng, Z. Jia, T. Su, C. Wang, Study on the influencing factors and mechanism of calcium carbonate precipitation induced by urease bacteria. J. Cryst. Growth **564**, 126113 (2021)

J. Yu, L. Wang, X. Xie, H. Yu, J. Xu, J. Ren, W. Zhu, Z. Lei, L. Lv, Multifunctional nanoparticles Codelivering doxorubicin and amorphous calcium carbonate preloaded with Indocyanine green for enhanced chemo-Photothermal cancer therapy. Int. J. Nanomedicine **18**, 323–337 (2023)

L. Yu, S. Sun, D. Hao, X. Hou, Preparation and characterization of organic modified calcium carbonate by sodium stearate (or sodium Oleate) using wet method. Surface Rev. Lett. **27**, 1950224 (2020)

M. Zeng, Y.Y. Kim, C. Anduix-Canto, C. Frontera, D. Laundy, N. Kapur, H.K. Christenson, F.C. Meldrum, Confinement generates single-crystal aragonite rods at room temperature. Proc. Natl. Acad. Sci. USA **115**(30), 7670–7675 (2018). https://doi.org/10.1073/PNAS.1718926115/-/DCSUPPLEMENTAL

H. Zhang, Z. Xu, Y. Zhao, J. Wang, B. Wang, Inhibition of calcium carbonate nucleation and crystallization by carboxymethyl dextran: Experiments and molecular dynamics simulations. Desalination **573**, 117205 (2024a)

M. Zhang, Y. Chen, C. Wu, R. Zheng, Y. Xia, E.G. Saccuzzo, T.K.H. Trinh, E.A.Q. Mondarte, E. Nakouzi, B. Rad, B.A. Legg, W.J. Shaw, J. Tao, J.J. de Yoreo, C.L. Chen, A molecular view of peptoid-induced acceleration of calcite growth. Proc. Nat. Acad. Sci. USA **121**(45), e2412358121 (2024b)

P. Zhao, Y. Tian, J. You, X. Hu, Y. Liu, Recent advances of calcium carbonate nanoparticles for biomedical applications. Bioengineering **9**(11), 110693 (2022). https://doi.org/10.3390/BIOENGINEERING9110691

X. Zhou, W. Liu, C. Tian, S. Mo, X. Liu, H. Deng, Z. Lin, Mussel-inspired functionalization of biological calcium carbonate for improving Eu(III) adsorption and the related mechanisms. Chem. Eng. J. **351**, 816–824 (2018)

Z. Zhou, Y. Li, S. Yao, H. Yan, Preparation of calcium carbonate@graphene oxide core–shell microspheres in ethylene glycol for drug delivery. Ceram. Int. **42**(2), 2281–2288 (2016)

F. Zhu, Z. Liu, Y. Ren, Mechanism of melatonin combined with calcium carbonate on improving osteoporosis in aged rats. Experim. Therap. Med. **16**(1), 192–196 (2018)

Zeng, XY., Zhu, Z., Chang, W., Wu, B., Huang, W. Biomineralization process inspired in situ growth of calcium carbonate nanocrystals in chitosan hydrogels. Appl. Sci. (Switzerland) 14 (2024) 9193

Ion-Substituted Nano-hydroxyapatite: A Multifunctional Biomaterial with Anticancer, Antibacterial, and Osteogenic Properties

Antonia Ressler

Abstract Bone tissue engineering increasingly employs biomimetic calcium phosphate systems to develop biomaterials for bone regeneration. Ionic substitution within calcium phosphates, mainly hydroxyapatite, allows precise tuning of physicochemical properties and enables antibacterial and anticancer functionality without relying on growth factors or drugs. This chapter outlines the structural features of hexagonal hydroxyapatite, whose lattice can accommodate biologically relevant cationic and anionic substitutions. In vitro safety and efficacy depend on the controlled, sustained release of ions from the lattice. Antibacterial performance can be achieved with Ag^{+} and other therapeutic ions, while dose-controlled $SeO_3{}^{2-}$ substitution provides selective cytotoxicity toward osteosarcoma cells. Parallel regenerative benefits arise from Sr^{2+} and Mg^{2+}, which stimulate osteogenesis and reduce osteoclast activity. In addition to the effects of substituted ions, the surface charge of biomaterials further influences cell attachment. Mono- and multi-substituted calcium phosphate powders enhance stem-cell proliferation and osteogenic marker expression while simultaneously providing antibacterial and anticancer properties. Cutting-edge fabrication technologies, such as additive manufacturing, now open new avenues to replicate bone-like porosity and achieve trabecular-scale mechanical properties after high-temperature sintering. Together, co-/multi-substituted calcium phosphates and advanced fabrication techniques offer promising pathways toward personalized scaffolds without relying on pharmacological agents.

Keywords Anticancer properties · Antimicrobial resistance · Bone tissue engineering · Ion-substituted hydroxyapatite · Osteogenic differentiation

---

A. Ressler (✉)
Faculty of Engineering and Natural Sciences, Tampere University, Tampere, Finland
e-mail: antonia.ressler@tuni.fi

Tampere Institute for Advanced Study, Tampere University, Tampere, Finland

R. Narayan (ed.), *Nanostructured Biomaterials and Their Applications*,
https://doi.org/10.1007/978-3-032-16316-5_9

1 Introduction

Bone tissue engineering (BTE) is a rapidly evolving field that aims to develop biomaterials and methods to repair, replace, or regenerate damaged bone tissue. This interdisciplinary field combines principles from biology, materials science, medicine, physics, and engineering to create biomaterials (e.g., powders, grains, porous scaffolds) that support cell growth and tissue formation. The current state of the art in BTE includes using biomimetic biomaterials (e.g., calcium phosphates, CaPs) that are known for their biocompatibility with biological systems and regenerative role in the bone healing process (Maji and Mondal 2020). However, new challenges have arisen, and CaP ceramics offer possibilities to tackle these problems via ionic substitutions within chemical structures. Developments in this direction hold promise for enhancing antibacterial and anticancer properties, while using biomimetic strategies to improve bone regeneration. Important challenges where the ionic substitution can be applied include:

(i) Growth factors have often been used with CaPs to improve the osteogenic properties of artificial biomaterials. However, concerns about the safety of growth factors, especially the risk of ectopic or unwanted bone formation, have emerged. Because of this, studies have started to explore alternative methods for stimulating bone growth. One promising approach involves the substitution of ions such as sodium (Na^+), magnesium (Mg^{2+}), zinc (Zn^{2+}), strontium (Sr^{2+}), and selenite ($SiO_4{}^{4-}$) into CaPs, primarily hydroxyapatite (HAp), to achieve the desired osteogenic effects (Bose et al. 2013; Minardi et al. 2015).

(ii) A major global health issue is bacterial resistance, primarily caused by the misuse of antibacterial drugs and antibiotics. The World Health Organization (WHO) has reported an increase in bacterial infections that are difficult to treat due to the decreasing efficacy of key antibiotics. While bacterial resistance occurs naturally, its rapid rise is mainly due to improper drug use, which leads to prolonged hospital stays, higher costs, treatment failures, and increased mortality. Pre-surgery antibiotics, taken orally or via biomaterials, often fail to provide sufficient protection against bacterial infections. Incorrect antibiotic selection or inadequate doses can also promote resistant bacterial strains, complicating future treatments. While specific ion substitutions in CaPs enhance bone regeneration, the substitution of antibacterial ions can lead to biomaterials with antibacterial properties that are less prone to misuse and only pose risks at high ion concentrations. With the increasing occurrence of antibiotic resistance, there is growing demand in alternative antibacterial strategies to effectively combat pathogenic microorganisms, particularly in hospital-acquired infections associated with orthopedic implants (Martínez-Gracida et al. 2020; Choe et al. 2022; Vasiliadis et al. 2021; Vila et al. 2016).

(iii) Cancer remains the second leading cause of mortality worldwide, despite extensive therapeutic developments. Traditional therapies, such as chemotherapy and radiotherapy, often face significant challenges, including systemic toxicity and painful procedures that require long recovery periods (Kargozar et al. 2022).

Cancer cells in the bone create a feedback loop by stimulating bone-resorbing cells (osteoclasts) through the action of Receptor Activator of Nuclear factor Kappa-B Ligand (RANKL), which leads to increased bone resorption and the release of growth factors that support further cancer growth. This vicious cycle contributes to the progression of bone metastasis, as shown in Fig. 1. Metastasized cancer cells in the bone stimulate osteoblasts (bone formation cells) to produce a RANKL. RANKL binds to RANK receptor on the surface of osteoclasts, further promoting their activity. The increased activity of osteoclasts leads to enhanced bone resorption. As bone is resorbed, growth factors stored in the bone matrix are released, promoting the growth and survival of cancer cells. This creates a favorable environment for cancer cells, further perpetuating the cycle (Wu et al. 2020; Guise 2002; Cappariello and Capulli 2018; Zhang and Zhang 2020). Therefore, finding alternative solutions is of great interest. CaPs in powder or scaffoldScaffold form have emerged as a promising approach for treating bone cancers. CaPs are biocompatible, support bone regeneration, and can serve as carriers for anticancer drugs. In addition to their potential use as drug carriers, CaPs can be enhanced by substituting therapeutic ions with anticancer properties into their lattice structure. Given the increasing threat of bone cancer and the limitations of current treatments, the development and application of CaPs substituted with anticancer therapeutic ions represent a promising strategy for cancer treatment.

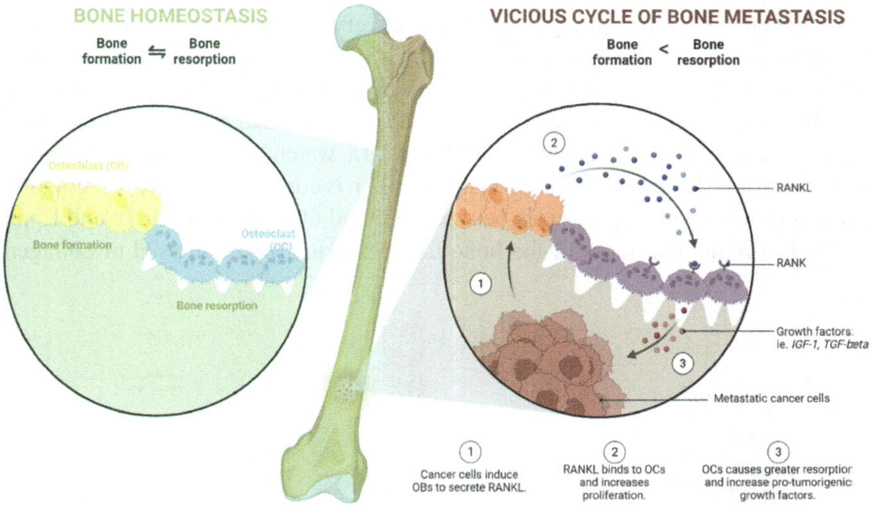

Fig. 1 Schematic representation of the feedback loop in bone metastasis. Cancer cells in the bone stimulate osteoblasts to produce RANKL, which binds to RANK on osteoclasts, promoting their proliferation and activity. Increased bone resorption and the release of growth factors from the bone matrix further support cancer cell growth and survival, perpetuating the cycle (Von Moos and Haynes 2013). Created in BioRender.com

1.1 Why biomimetic approach in bone tissue engineering?

To implement a biomimetic approach in BTE, it is essential to understand the chemical composition and lattice structure of HAp, the substitution mechanisms, and their effects on physicochemical properties and the bone formation process. Two crystal forms of HAp are known: monoclinic ($P2_1/b$ space group) and hexagonal ($P6_3/m$ space group). The hexagonal form is more commonly used because the monoclinic form is easily destabilized by impurities and foreign ions. The hexagonal structure features two calcium sites, Ca1 and Ca2, and a phosphate assembly intersected by parallel channels filled with OH^- ions aligned along the crystallographic *c*-axis. The Ca2 sites are arranged in a staggered triangular pattern, while the Ca1 sites are positioned in columns parallel to the OH^- channels (Fig. 2a). The hexagonal form is characterized by lattice parameters: $a = b = 9.418$ Å, $c = 6.884$ Å, $\alpha = \beta = 90°$, $\gamma = 120°$, with a Ca/P molar ratio of 1.67 and the chemical formula $Ca1_4Ca2_6(PO1O2O3_2)_6(OH)_2$. This flexible hexagonal structure of HAp can accommodate a wide range of cationic (Sr^{2+}, Na^+, K^+, Mg^{2+}, Zn^{2+}, Ag^+, etc.) and anionic (${CO_3}^{2-}$, ${SiO_4}^{4-}$, ${SeO_3}^{2-}$, ${SeO_4}^{2-}$, F^-, Cl^-, Br^-, etc.) substitutions (Boanini et al. 2010; Matsunaga 2008; Wopenka and Pasteris 2005). In natural bone tissue, various ionic substitutions are crucial for apatite solubility in bone, dentin, and enamel (Table 1). Each of these apatites requires different solubility properties depending on their environment and role in the body (Dorozhkin and Epple 2002).

In biological systems, apatite serves as the primary inorganic component in bones, teeth, and enamel, with varying percentages and crystal sizes: enamel contains 97% inorganic material, 1.5% organic material, and 1.5% water, with crystal dimensions of $100 \times 50 \times 50$ μm; dentin comprises 70% inorganic material, 20% organic material, and 10% water, with crystal sizes of $35 \times 25 \times 4$ nm; and bone consists of 65% inorganic material, 25% organic material, and 10% water, with crystal sizes ranging from $50 \times 25 \times 2$–4 nm. In contrast, synthetic HAp is composed entirely of inorganic material (100%) with crystal sizes between 200 and 600 nm (Dorozhkin and Epple 2002). The remaining mass of the bone tissue is primarily composed of collagen,

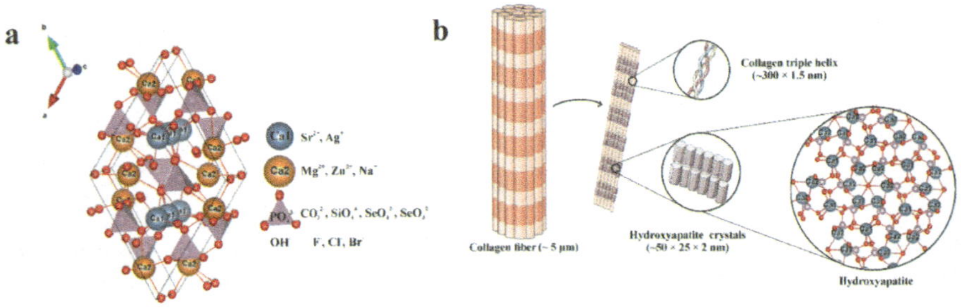

Fig. 2 **a** HAp lattice with Ca sites and substituting ion positions. **b** The hierarchical structure of collagen and HAp as main constituents of natural bone tissue (Ressler et al. 2021a). Reprinted from Ressler et al. (2021a), with permission from Elsevier.

Table 1 Chemical composition of human enamel, dentin, bone, and synthetic HAp (Dorozhkin and Epple 2002)

Composition (wt%)	Enamel	Dentin	Bone	Synthetic HAp
Ca^{2+}	36.5	35.1	34.8	39.6
PO_4^{3-}	17.7	16.9	15.2	18.5
Na^+	0.5	0.6	0.9	–
Mg^{2+}	0.44	1.23	0.72	–
K^+	0.08	0.05	0.03	–
CO_3^{2-}	3.5	5.6	7.4	–
F^-	0.01	0.06	0.03	–
Cl^-	0.30	0.01	0.13	–

various proteins (such as glycoproteins, proteoglycans, sialoproteins, and bone "gla" proteins), and water (Cordonnier et al. 2011). Bone tissue in the human body serves multiple functions: (i) mechanical, providing strength for the locomotor system; (ii) synthetic, acting as a site for cell production; and (iii) metabolic, regulating Ca^{2+} and PO_4^{3-} levels, storing minerals, and maintaining acid–base balance (Ansari 2019). Bone is a complex biomaterial with a hierarchical structure at various scales. Its building blocks are mineralized collagen fibers, composites of biological apatite and type I collagen molecules (Fig. 2b). The collagen matrix in natural bone tissue provides elasticity and serves as a matrix for the deposition and growth of apatite crystals (Dorozhkin and Epple 2002; Sadat-Shojai et al. 2013). These crystals align parallel to the collagen fibers and are formed through the self-assembly of the collagen triple helix (Ansari 2019).

Bone serves as a biomineralized matrix that provides a structural and functional support for essential cell types, including stem cells, osteoblasts, osteocytes, and osteoclasts. Stem cells are multipotent progenitors capable of differentiating into diverse lineages such as chondrocytes, adipocytes, tenocytes, myoblasts, and osteoblasts (Cordonnier et al. 2011). Osteoblasts, bone-forming cells, play a key role in the synthesis, deposition, and mineralization of the bone matrix by producing osteoid, a proteinaceous mixture. Osteocytes, the most abundant cells in bone tissue, exhibit a stellate morphology and represent terminally differentiated osteoblasts embedded within the mineralized matrix. They are crucial for several biochemical signaling pathways. Bone-lining cells (inactive osteoblasts) are found on the bone surface. Osteoclasts, derived from the hematopoietic lineage, control bone resorption by secreting enzymes and acids that dissolve bone minerals (Ansari 2019; Florencio-Silva et al. 2015). The bone remodeling process, in which old bone is replaced by new bone, is highly complex and involves the coordinated actions of all bone cell types (Mavrogenis et al. 2009). A schematic representation of the bone remodeling cycle, including various cell types, is shown in Fig. 3. Trace elements in bone tissue are essential for the normal function of each cell type. Deficiency in specific elements can enhance osteoclast activity, leading to reduced bone density and osteoporosis

(Bose et al. 2013; Mavrogenis et al. 2009). Bose et al. (2013) provide a comprehensive review of the role of trace elements in bone metabolism and the remodeling process.

In our previous studies, we investigated the potential of a biomimetic approach in BTE by incorporating ionic substitutions such as SeO_3^{2-} (Ressler et al. 2021b), Zn^{2+} (Ressler et al. 2023), Mg^{2+} (Ressler et al. 2023), Sr^{2+} (Ressler et al. 2020, 2022a), and Ag^+ (Ressler et al. 2022a; Ivankovic et al. 2023) with in CaPs crystal structures. These studies aimed to develop biomaterials with antibacterial, anticancer, and osteogenic properties. CaP phases with ionic substitutions were synthesized using a wet precipitation method, typically with substitution levels ranging from 0 to 5 mol%. In vitro cytocompatibility assessments confirmed non-cytotoxic effects and that substituted ions (Zn^{2+}, Mg^{2+}, and Sr^{2+}) promoted the proliferation of human embryonic kidney (HEK 293) cells (Ressler et al. 2020, 2022a, 2023). However, a 0.029 mol% substitution with SeO_3^{2-} ions induced apoptosis of HEK 293 cells, while a 0.007 mol% substitution was non-cytotoxic. Notably, the 0.007 mol% of SeO_3^{2-} substitution exhibited selective anticancer activity, inducing apoptosis in osteosarcoma cells while supporting healthy cell viability (Ressler et al. 2021b). In a study focused on Ag^+ substitution (Ressler et al. 2022a), HEK 293 cell viability significantly decreased after three days of culture in extracts of HAp substituted with 2.5 and 5 mol% Ag^+ ions. However, no significant difference in viability was observed for the 1 mol% Ag^+ substitution compared to non-substituted HAp. To further evaluate cytocompatibility, human mesenchymal stem cells were cultured in extracts of HAp samples substituted with 1 and 2.5 mol% Ag^+ ions. After three days, non-cytotoxicity was confirmed, with an increase in cell viability observed in the tested samples (Ressler et al. 2022a). Studies have demonstrated that the substitution levels of SeO_3^{2-} and Ag^+ in HAp must be carefully optimized to prevent cytotoxic effects on healthy human cells. Substitution levels below 0.007 mol% for

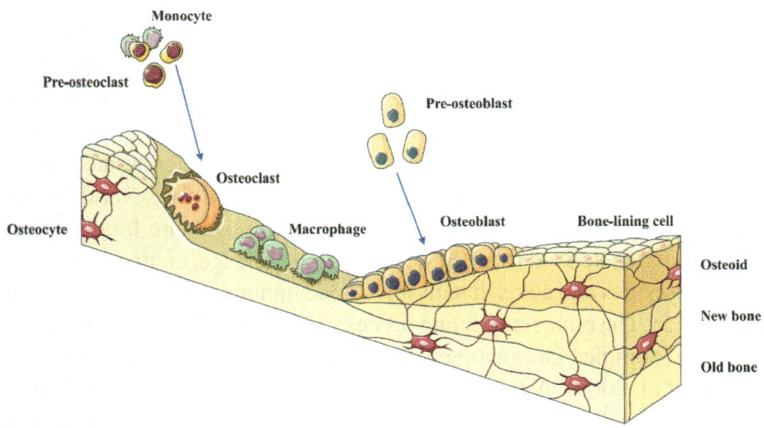

Fig. 3 Bone remodeling cycle including various cell types (Smart Servier Medical Art).

SeO_3^{2-} and below 2.5 mol% for Ag^+ are considered favorable for maintaining cell viability and promoting positive biological responses (Ressler et al. 2021b, 2022a).

The multi-substituted HAp powder substituted with 0.5 mol% of SeO_3^{2-}, Zn^{2+}, Mg^{2+}, Sr^{2+}, and Ag^+ ions, resulted in a multifunctional biomaterial that is non-cytotoxic to human cells and exhibits antibacterial properties with potential anticancer properties. HAp mono-substituted with Ag^+, as well as a mixture of mono-substituted HAps with Ag^+, Sr^{2+}, Mg^{2+}, Zn^{2+}, and SeO_3^{2-} ions, demonstrated antibacterial efficacy against drug-resistant clinical isolates of *Acinetobacter baumannii.* A lower substitution level of Ag^+ ions (0.5 mol%) compared to the higher level (2.5 mol%) resulted in a reduced antibacterial effect in the bacterial suspension. However, both concentrations exhibited comparable antibacterial activity in a 24-h disc-diffusion assay, with similar inhibition zones and bacterial adhesion on the biomaterial surface. Clinical isolates of *A. baumannii* were affected by silver in both mono-substituted HAp and the mixture of mono-substituted HAps, likely to a similar extent as other commercially available Ag-doped materials. Additionally, determined time-dependent reduction in the bactericidal activity of silver against *A. baumannii* should be considered (Ivankovic et al. 2023).

Study on composite scaffolds demonstrated that multi-ion substitutions can enhance the osteogenic properties of biomaterials for BTE applications (Ressler et al. 2022b). The study shows that composite scaffolds composed of chitosan and multi-substituted CaPs (primarily HAp) provide a three-dimensional structure that supports the proliferation and osteogenic differentiation of human mesenchymal stem cells. The expression of key osteogenic markers (alkaline phosphatase, bone sialoprotein, collagen type I, and dentin matrix protein I) along with the presence of phosphate deposits and newly-formed bone tissue indicates extracellular matrix mineralization over 21 days of culture. Differences in bone cell growth, collagen type I expression, and mineral formation capacity among the scaffolds followed the trend: SC_5MIX (5 mol% multi-substituted) > SC_1MIX (1 mol% multi-substituted) > SC_0 (non-substituted). These findings suggest that multiple ion substitutions (Sr^{2+}, Mg^{2+}, Zn^{2+}, and SeO_3^{2-}) in CaPs positively affect cells and tissue (Ressler et al. 2022b). A schematic illustration summarizing the antibacterial and biological properties of HAp substituted with Sr^{2+}, Zn^{2+}, Mg^{2+}, SeO_3^{2-}, and Ag^+, based on our previous studies, is presented in Fig. 4. Collectively, these studies highlight the potential of various elements and their combinations to create multifunctional biomaterials. Such biomaterials can closely mimic the chemical composition of natural bone tissue, potentially reducing or eliminating the need for growth factors, antibiotics, and other pharmacological agents.

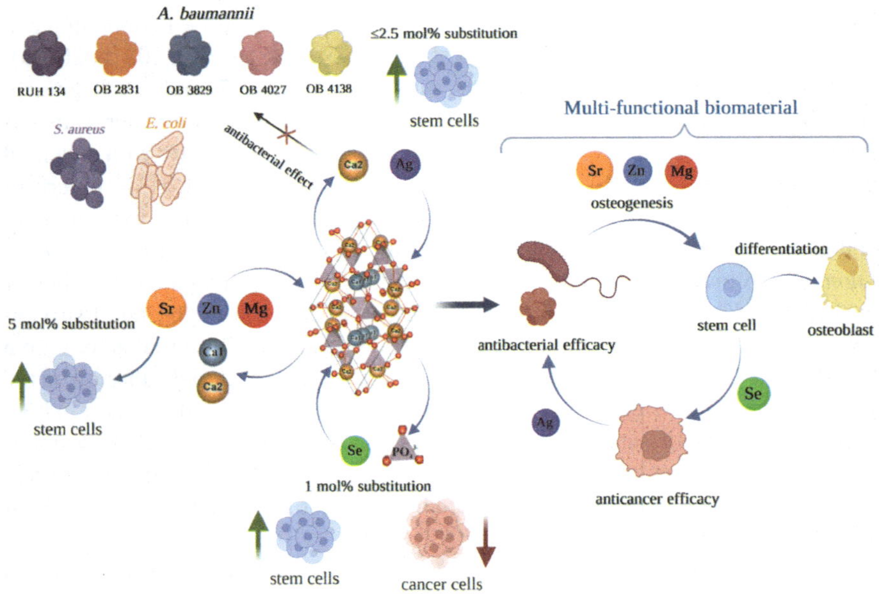

Fig. 4 Illustration of antibacterial and biological properties of HAp substituted with Sr^{2+}, Zn^{2+}, Mg^{2+}, $SeO_3{}^{2-}$, and Ag^{+} according to our previous studies (Ressler et al. 2020, 2021b, 2022a, b, 2023; Ivankovic et al. 2023). Reprinted from Ivankovic et al. (2023), with permission from Elsevier.

2 Impact of trace elements on antibacterial, anticancer, and osteogenic properties

2.1 *Antibacterial properties*

Antimicrobial resistance presents a critical global health challenge, largely driven by the widespread and inappropriate use of antibacterial agents, including antibiotics. According to the WHO, there has been a rise in bacterial infections due to the weakened efficacy of essential antibiotics. Different scientific fields are developing alternatives for bacterial treatments by creating new antibacterial molecules and materials to prevent the rapid growth of bacterial resistance worldwide. The use of synthetic materials substituted with metal ions may offer a more effective strategy than conventional drug-based approaches, posing cytotoxic risks only at elevated metal ion concentrations (Martínez-Gracida et al. 2020). Drug-resistant bacteria represent a major concern in hospital-acquired infections, particularly those associated with orthopedic implants such as prosthetic joints within the context of BTE (Choe et al. 2022; Vasiliadis et al. 2021; Vila et al. 2016). The ESKAPE pathogens (*Enterococcus faecium*, *Staphylococcus aureus*, *Klebsiella pneumoniae*, *Acinetobacter baumannii*, *Pseudomonas aeruginosa*, and *Enterobacter* spp.) demand urgent attention and the development of novel antimicrobial therapies (Moubareck and Halat 2020; Weinberg et al. 2020; McNeilly et al. 2023). Silver nanoparticles are now among the most commercialized nanomaterials, and they have applications in various fields where antibacterial properties are needed. However, several review articles have explored the toxicological properties of silver nanoparticles when utilized as antimicrobial agents. Given the potential health risks associated with using nanoparticle in the human body, the development of alternative antibacterial materials and treatment approaches is essential (Ferdous and Nemmar 2020; Riaz Ahmed et al. 2017; Maurer and Meyer 2016; Bapat et al. 2018).

When ions are adsorbed onto or dispersed within biomaterials without incorporation into the crystal lattice, rapid ion release may occur, potentially resulting in toxic effects on the surrounding tissue. Ionic incorporation into the crystal lattice enables sustained release, ensuring prolonged biological activity of the ions during the bone regeneration process (Li et al. 2018). To obtain HAp with antibacterial properties, ions such as Ag^+, Zn^{2+}, Cu^{2+}, Ce^{3+}, Ga^{3+}, $SeO_3{}^{2-}$, Ti^{4+}, and Sr^{2+} are substituted within the lattice (Ghosh et al. 2022; Kolmas et al. 2014). The antibacterial activity of Ag-substituted HAp is well established and is typically evaluated using standard model organisms (e.g., *Escherichia coli*, *Staphylococcus aureus*). In our previous study (Ivankovic et al. 2023), HAp mono-substituted with various ions was examined against clinical isolates of the multidrug-resistant bacteria. The clinical isolates of *A. baumannii* demonstrated sensitivity to Ag^+ ions when substituted into HAp (Ivankovic et al. 2023). Ag^+ ions exhibit antimicrobial activity through multiple mechanisms that ultimately lead to cell death. The mechanisms include the denaturation of proteins and nucleic acids, disruption of the respiratory electron chain, interference with DNA replication components, and increased membrane permeability. Ag^+ binds to sulfhydryl (thiol) groups in amino acids, inactivating enzymes and proteins. A key target is the cell respiration system, where Ag^+ uncouples the respiratory chain from oxidative phosphorylation at the cytoplasmic membrane, resulting in cell death. Silver also inactivates enzymes essential for peptidoglycan synthesis and binds to nitrogen, oxygen, or sulfur atoms in DNA, inhibiting cell replication. Additionally, Ag^+ triggers the release of iron from damaged organic molecules, forming reactive oxygen species that disrupt proteins, enzymes, and DNA, culminating in cell death. Furthermore, Ag^+ accumulates in the periplasmic space, where it inactivates proteins and enzymes, disrupts efflux and uptake molecular pumps, and causes plasma membrane disintegration. Gram-negative bacteria may be more susceptible to silver due to their thinner peptidoglycan layer, allowing more significant accumulation of ions in the periplasm. Silver's diverse mechanisms of action reduce the likelihood of microbial resistance, while silver exhibits low cytotoxicity toward human cells at appropriate concentrations (Ressler et al. 2022a; Ivankovic et al. 2025; Ishida 2018; Jung et al. 2008; Randall et al. 2015). A schematic illustration of the antibacterial mechanism of Ag^+ ions on bacteria is shown in Fig. 5.

In addition to the well-documented antibacterial properties of Ag^+ ions, Gopi et al. (2014) and Predoi et al. (2020) reported that Ce-substituted HAp also exhibits antibacterial activity, as determined by measured inhibition zones obtained by the disc diffusion method and assay of bacteria suspension with developed biomaterial (Gopi et al. 2014, Predoi et al. (2020). Both studies employed laboratory

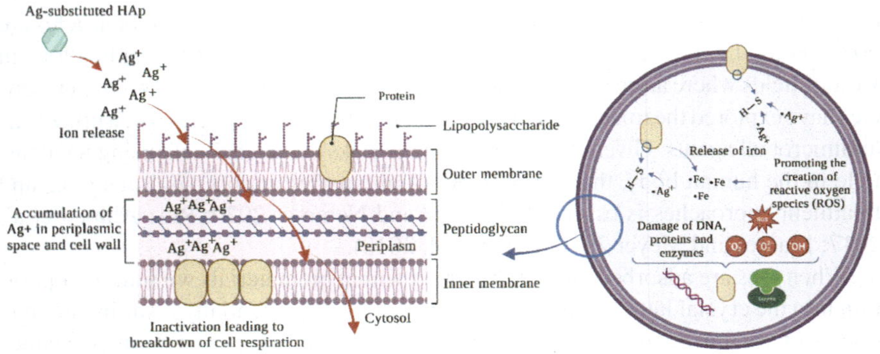

Fig. 5 Schematic illustration of antibacterial mechanism of Ag^+ ions on bacteria (Ressler et al. 2022a). Reprinted from Ressler et al. (2022a), with permission from Elsevier

bacteria strains, likely lacking antibiotic resistance; therefore, evaluating antibacterial efficacy against clinical isolates would provide deeper insights into the comparative performance of Ce^{3+} versus Ag^+ ions. Further, a study by Muthusamy et al. (2021) showed that Mn-substituted HAp samples have no significant difference in antibacterial effect against *E. coli* compared to non-substituted HAp. However, *S. aureus* bacterial colonies were reduced with increasing Mn-substitution levels (Muthusamy et al. 2021). Bootchanont et al. (2022) reported inhibition zones for Mn-substituted HAp against Gram-positive bacteria, whereas no inhibition zones were observed for Gram-negative bacteria. Contrary to these studies, by analyzing the scanning electron microscopy images, Wang et al. (2021) determined that Mn-substituted HAp exhibits antibacterial activity against both *E. coli* and *S. aureus*, even with trace amounts of Mn^{2+} ions at ppm levels. Mn^{2+} ions and redox-active centers within Mn-substituted HAp are believed to play a critical role in the antibacterial mechanism. These centers facilitate redox cycling, leading to the accumulation of reactive oxygen species, which is considered the primary factor underlying the observed antibacterial activity of Mn-substituted HAp (Wang et al. 2021).

Further, the antibacterial mechanism of gallium (Ga^{3+}) is primarily attributed to its ability to mimic iron, enabling bacterial uptake, a process known as the Trojan Horse strategy (Lapa et al. 2020). As a redox-inert metal that cannot be reduced under physiological conditions, gallium disrupts iron-dependent enzymes essential for bacterial growth, leading to metabolic failure and cell death (Kelson et al. 2013). Bacteria can intake iron through specific receptors for ferric complexes with siderophores, ferrous iron, transferrin, lactoferrin, hemoglobin, and heme (Fig. 6). Once internalized, iron supports protein synthesis and regulates Fur gene expression. In iron-rich conditions, the Fur protein binds Fe^{3+} and attaches to Fur sites on bacterial DNA, repressing iron transport genes. In iron-depleted conditions, Fur no longer represses these genes, allowing their expression (Seyoum et al. 2021; Li et al. 2022). The challenge for bacteria to develop resistance to gallium arises from the fact that reducing gallium uptake would also diminish iron uptake, which is essential for their survival.

Consequently, Ga-based compounds show promise as next-generation of biomaterials for treating resistant bacteria (Kircheva and Dudev 2020). Beyond antibacterial activity, Ga^{3+} ions localize in metabolically active bone tissue, reducing bone resorption by lowering osteocalcin mRNA and protein levels, similar to TGF mechanisms (Vukomanovic et al. 2022).

When designing biomaterials, it is important to consider that high concentrations of antibacterial ions may induce apoptosis in human healthy cells. Therefore, cytotoxicity, biocompatibility, and optimal substitution levels should be evaluated alongside antibacterial performance (Ivankovic et al. 2025). Surface charge is a critical factor in the antibacterial performance of biomaterials, as it strongly influences bacterial adhesion. Bacterial cells generally exhibit a net negative charge due to the presence of carboxyl, amine, and phosphate groups (Mediaswanti 2016). Gram-negative bacteria typically display a more pronounced negative surface charge compared to Gram-positive species. This difference is primarily attributed to the presence of lipopolysaccharides in the outer membrane of Gram-negative bacteria, which markedly increase their negative surface charge. In contrast, Gram-positive bacteria, although negatively charged due to teichoic acids in their thick peptidoglycan layer, generally exhibit a less negative overall charge (Sára and Sleytr 2000). As a result, the negatively charged surface of HAp creates a repulsive electrostatic effect, which inhibits bacterial adhesion (Halder et al. 2015). The results of our study have shown that clinical isolates of multidrug-resistant Gram-positive bacteria (*Methicillin-Sensitive Staphylococcus aureus*, MSSA; *Methicillin-Resistant Staphylococcus epidermidis*, MRSE; *Methicillin-Resistant Staphylococcus aureus*, MRSA) adhered in more significant numbers to the non-substituted HAp surface (negative zeta potential) than Gram-negative bacteria (*Multidrug-Resistant Acinetobacter baumannii*, MRAB; *Non-Resistant Escherichia coli*, NREC; *Klebsiella pneumoniae Carbapenemase*, KPC; *Carbapenem-Resistant Pseudomonas aeruginosa*, CRPA). The obtained results suggest that Gram-positive bacteria with a less-negative surface charge reduce the repulsive electrostatic effect, leading to increased attachment. In

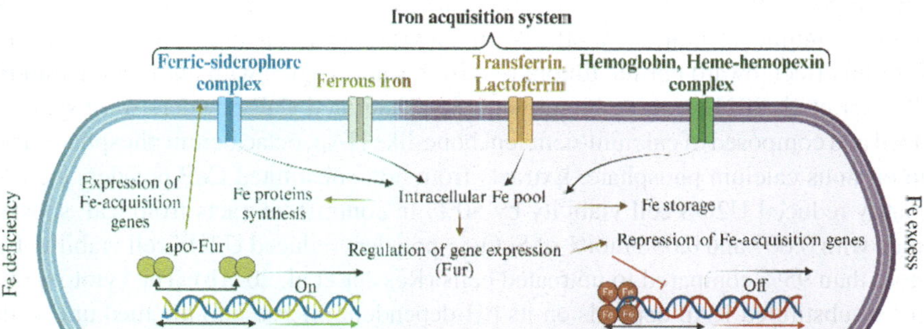

Fig. 6 Schematic of general iron uptake system and ferric uptake regulator (fur)-mediated iron uptake regulation in bacteria. Adapted from Kelson et al. (2013). Created in BioRender.com

contrast, Gram-negative bacteria with a more-negative surface charge enhance the repulsive electrostatic effect, resulting in fewer cells attaching to the surface of HAp biomaterial (Ivankovic et al. 2025).

2.2 Anticancer properties

The standard treatments for osteosarcoma (a highly malignant bone tumor) include surgery, radiotherapy, and chemotherapy (Wang et al. 2018). HAp has demonstrated strong apoptosis-inducing effects on various cancer cells. To improve the anticancer properties of CaPs, research has focused on modifying their structure by substituting specific ions with anticancer effects (Wei et al. 2019). Selenium (SeO_3^{2-}), one of the essential elements for healthy bone tissue, has strong antioxidant properties and beneficial effects on cardiovascular diseases, cancers, brain function, reproduction, viral infections, and bone tissue. Selenium may be crucial in protecting against osteoarthritis, rheumatoid arthritis, and osteoporosis (Pajor et al. 2018). Deficiencies in selenium can hinder growth and affect bone tissue metabolism. The mechanisms behind these processes involve selenoproteins, with at least nine expressed in human fetal osteoblasts, which protect bones from oxidative stress and regulate inflammation and bone cell differentiation (Zeng et al. 2013). Appropriate selenium levels in the human body are believed to help prevent various cancers, including lung, colorectal, and prostate. However, despite its importance to human health, the range between selenium's nutritional and toxic doses is very narrow (Rayman 2005; Kieliszek et al. 2017; Bai et al. 2025).

SeO_3^{2-} has gained attention as a CaP substituent not only due to its ability to induce tumor cell apoptosis but also due to its beneficial effect on healthy cells (Ressler et al. 2021b; Wei et al. 2019). A study by Wang et al. (2016) confirmed that Se-substituted HAp exhibits antitumor activity and can induce apoptosis in human osteosarcoma cells (Wang et al. 2016). These findings are further supported by the study reported by Uskoković et al. (2017), where HAp substituted with SeO_3^{2-} ions showed significant inhibitory effects on osteosarcoma cell lines while having no harmful effect toward normal fibroblasts. Both studies agree with our previous study (Ressler et al. 2021b) where biomimetic Se-substituted CaP powders were synthesized and composed of calcium-deficient bone-like HAp, octacalcium phosphate, and amorphous calcium phosphate. Extracts from non-substituted CaP powders significantly reduced U2OS cell viability by 50%. In contrast, extracts from CaP substituted with 0.007 and 0.058 mol% of SeO_3^{2-} powders reduced U2OS cell viability by more than 95% compared to untreated cells (Ressler et al. 2021b). The cytotoxicity of Se-substituted HAp depends on its pH-dependent release into the medium, with high SeO_3^{2-} concentrations potentially causing non-selective cytotoxicity (apoptosis of osteosarcoma and healthy cells). In a study by Uskoković et al. (2017), high SeO_3^{2-} content (3.0 wt%) was reported to induce cell death in non-cancerous Mouse Calvaria-derived 3 T3-E1 cells, causing abnormal morphological changes within 24 h of treatment and reducing the expression of bone γ-carboxyglutamate protein 3 (Uskoković et al. 2017). Therefore, it can be concluded that the responses of cancer cells to selenite and its metabolites vary depending on the dose and form (Breuer et al. 2023; Bao et al. 2015).

As previously mentioned, the negative effects of metal nanoparticles on the human body are well known. However, studies on specific metal nanoparticles can provide valuable insights into the mechanisms by which these metals affect healthy human and osteosarcoma cells. A study by Bao et al. (2015) was the first study to demonstrate protein-assisted self-assembly of Se-nanoparticles in Se-treated cancer cells. Se-nanoparticles were found within 24 h of exposure in all tested cell lines, with cell viability inversely correlating with Se-nanoparticle levels. The study showed that Se-nanoparticles sequester glycolytic enzymes, leading to inhibition of glycolysis, ATP depletion, and mitochondrial dysfunction. This process causes the translocation of BAX to mitochondria, loss of mitochondrial membrane integrity, and release of cytochrome c, ultimately disrupting mitochondrial function. This pathway is distinct from other known mechanisms of Se-induced cytotoxicity. Additionally, Se-nanoparticles sequester tubulin, leading to microtubule depolymerization in cancer cells. This affects cell division, organelle positioning, and shape, making microtubules important targets for antitumor agents. Se-nanoparticles also decrease heat shock proteins 90 (HSP90) expression, leading to a switch from autophagy to apoptosis in cancer cells. HSP90 typically stabilizes proteins and protects cells from stress, but its inhibition by Se-nanoparticles results in the degradation of these proteins. Furthermore, Se-nanoparticles induce oxidative stress, causing DNA strand breaks and nuclear fragmentation. The study highlights the potential toxicity of high selenium intake and the need for further research to improve the clinical effectiveness of Se-nanoparticles and Se-based materials. Understanding the interactions between Se-nanoparticles and cellular processes opens new avenues for interdisciplinary cancer therapy and human health research (Bao et al. 2015). The mechanism of selenite-induced cytotoxicity in cancer cells according to the findings of the study (Bao et al. 2015) is shown in Fig. 7.

Further, a study by Barbanente et al. (2021) successfully prepared Se-substituted HAp with a substitution level up to 13 wt%. Selenium release from Se-substituted HAp was 1.5 times faster under slightly acidic conditions (pH 6.5) than under physiological conditions (pH 7.4), due to the pH-dependent solubility of HAp and the degradation-mediated release pattern of selenium. In vitro cell tests showed that Se-substituted HAp nanoparticles with low SeO_3^{2-} concentrations were biocompatible with cells. In contrast, high selenium concentrations exhibited strong cytotoxic activity against cancer cells but increased toxicity in human bone marrow stromal cells (Barbanente et al. 2021). The results of the biological characterization further support the findings that achieving selective anticancer properties with Se-substituted HAp requires careful selection of the appropriate substitution level. The study by Shoueir et al. (2020) obtained an interesting co-substitution combination where thallium (Tl) and selenium were substituted in HAp with varying Tl concentrations. The Tl/Se-substituted HAp cell viability tests on normal and cancerous human lung cells demonstrated selective behavior, with normal cells being significantly preserved

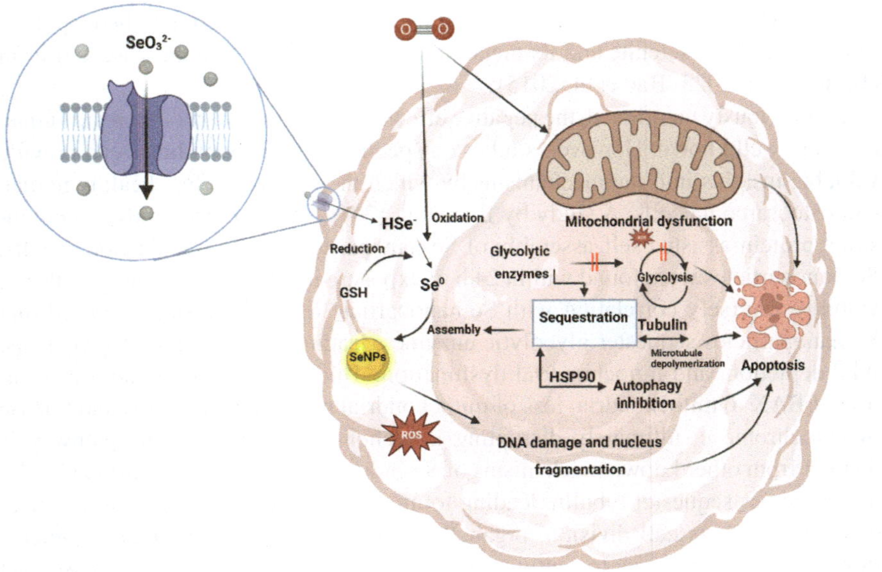

Fig. 7 Mechanism of Se-induced cytotoxicity in cancer cells. Adapted from Bao et al. (2015). Created in BioRender.com

compared to cancer cells. Tl/Se-substituted HAp revealed that it induced a prominent arrest in the G2/M phase compared to the control cells. This arrest is linked to DNA damage, activating checkpoint kinase 1 and inactivating Cdc25C, leading to apoptosis. Thallium ions, known to cause DNA damage, are believed to contribute to this effect (Shoueir et al. 2020). In the study by Dhatchayani et al. (2020), the anticancer properties of Se-substituted HAp were investigated against human bone cancer cells (MG-63). This research provides valuable insights into the effects of SeO_3^{2-} ions on bone cancer cells. An increase in the selenite ratio enhanced the anticancer activity, with a 63% activity observed at a selenite ratio of $Se/(Se + P) = 5\%$ at a concentration of 300 μg/mL. Furthermore, an innovative approach was used and selenite was combined with curcumin. This combination further increased the anticancer activity to 71% at the same concentration against MG-63. Therefore, the combined effect of selenite and curcumin shows promise for treating bone cancer cells (Dhatchayani et al. 2020). Although Se-substituted HAp particles are generally not considered to have negative side effects at low concentrations of selenite as metal nanoparticles, Zhou et al. (2023a) highlighted the importance of detecting their in vivo distribution. Europium (Eu) substituted HAp can be used as a fluorescence bioimaging tool for non-destructive observation in vitro and in vivo, though its application in osteosarcoma therapy remains rare. Study aimed to develop a new material to address osteosarcoma inhibition and bioimaging by Se/Eu-co-substitution of HAp. The results showed that Se-substituted HAp inhibited osteosarcoma cells by up to 80%, while Eu-substituted HAp emitted red light under 396 nm excitation. The

Se/Eu-co-substitution HAp demonstrated enhanced anticancer activity and fluorescence, with an osteosarcoma cell inhibition rate exceeding 90%, enabling cancer cell imaging. These findings indicate that Se/Eu-co-substitution HAp nanoparticles offer both osteosarcoma inhibition and bioimaging capabilities, making them promising candidates for postoperative treatment and imaging of osteosarcoma resection (Zhou et al. 2023a).

Another innovative approach in the field was reported by Park et al. (2022), where Mn-substituted HAp conjugated with counter folic acid (FA) and IR-783 fluorescence dye (Mn-HAp/FA-IR-783) was developed as a nanostructured system. In a cancer-bearing mouse model, the system demonstrated excellent contrast and enhanced photothermal/photodynamic therapy efficacy. The Mn-HAp/FA-IR-783 nanoparticles exhibit broad near-infrared absorbance, along with high biosafety, biocompatibility, and photostability. Both in vitro and in vivo experiments showed significant anticancer effects, with fluorescence imaging guiding the photothermal/photodynamic therapy treatment. Photothermal therapy uses ablation agents that convert light into heat, while photodynamic therapy generates ROS to cause cancer cell apoptosis. For fluorescence-guided treatment in an in vivo cancer model, a standardized dose of 200 μg/ml of 2.0 mol% Mn-HAp/FA-IR-783 nanoparticles, combined with 0.75 W cm^{-2} laser irradiation for 7 min, proved to be a practical and targeted theranostic approach (Park et al. 2022). Further, Jebapriya et al. (2023) combined iron and silver to obtain multifunctional HAp with antibacterial and anticancer properties. Antibacterial tests demonstrated that the synthesized samples effectively inhibited three types of bacteria: *S. aureus* (Gram-positive), *S. typhi* (Gram-negative), and *E. coli* (Gram-negative). The cell structure damage ratio on healthy (L929) and cancer cells (HT29) primarily depended on the concentration of the substituted trace elements. Consequently, higher concentrations of Ag^{+}/Fe^{2+} co-substituted HAp may be the most effective option for targeting cancer cells (Jebapriya et al. 2023). To further confirm the potential of substitutions for obtaining multifunctional biomaterials, Al-Shahrablee and Jaber (2022) prepared Nd-Ce-Mg-Zn-substituted HAp, which significantly altered the biological properties of HAp, enhancing its resistance to various bacteria and fungi. Additionally, it was found to be safe for healthy cells while exhibiting anticancer effects on bone cancer cells (Al-Shahrablee and Jaber 2022).

2.3 *Osteogenic properties*

A biomimetic approach in BTE was initially implemented to enhance the bone regeneration and osteogenic properties of biomaterials. This approach aims to develop biomaterials that closely resemble the natural composition of bone to promote their integration and functionality. Ionic substitutions can introduce beneficial properties such as enhanced bioactivity, improved mechanical strength, and targeted therapeutic effects. Our previous review paper (Ressler et al. 2021a) mainly focused on cationic (e.g., Na^{+}, Mg^{2+}, Zn^{2+}, Sr^{2+}) and anionic (e.g., F^{-}, $CO_3{}^{2-}$) substitutions, explaining how these ions substitute into the HAp lattice and their specific roles in improving biological performance and their synthesis methods, including the use of synthetic precursors and biogenic sources (Ressler et al. 2021a). This section solely focuses on the mechanisms through which these ionic substitutions enhance osteogenic properties and bone regeneration. Table 2 lists the most common ions used as substitutes to enhance osteogenic properties and their mechanisms of action. By understanding the specific roles and mechanisms of these ions, researchers can design more effective biomaterials for clinical applications with multifunctional applications.

The two highly explored, understood and most promising ions for promoting osteogenic differentiation and bone regeneration are Sr^{2+} and Mg^{2+}. The mechanism of action of these ions is well explored in the literature (Stipniece et al. 2021; Yan et al. 2022; Côrtes et al. 2024; Jiang et al. 2021; Gu et al. 2019). The stimulatory effect of Sr^{2+} on osteoblast cells is mediated through the activation of the calcium-sensing receptor (CaSR), promoting osteoblast proliferation, differentiation, and survival. In contrast, the same CaSR activation in osteoclast cells by Sr^{2+} induces apoptosis, thereby decreasing bone resorption (Fig. 8a) (Bose et al. 2013; Saidak and Marie 2012). Sr^{2+} ion enhances osteoblastogenesis by stimulating the replication and differentiation of osteoblastic cells and reducing apoptosis. This is achieved through mechanisms involving the nuclear factor of activated T-cells (NFATc)/Wnt signaling, increased production of prostaglandin E2 (PGE2), and activation of fibroblast growth factor receptors (FGFR) in osteoblastic cells. Additionally, Sr reduces the expression of sclerostin, a Wnt antagonist, in osteocytes (Fig. 8b) (Saidak and Marie 2012).

In a study by Xu et al. (2022), it was reported that bone formation is stimulated, and bone fracture healing is improved in cystic fibrosis transmembrane conductance regulator (CFTR) mutant mice by the implantation of Mg-containing implants. Although the study did not investigate Mg-substituted HAp, it explains the mechanism of action of Mg^{2+} ions. The magnesium implants enhance Wnt/β-catenin signaling in the bone, and the beneficial effects on fracture healing in CFTR-mutant mice are blocked by the inhibition of this pathway with iCRT14. It is further demonstrated that Mg^{2+} ions enter osteocytes, intracellular cAMP levels increase, and ATF4 is activated. ATF4 is a key transcription factor known to regulate Wnt/β-catenin signaling pathway. The in vivo downregulation of ATF4 results in the abolition of the magnesium implant-activated β-catenin in bones and the reversal of the improved fracture healing in CFTR-mutant mice. Additionally, the oral supplementation of magnesium results in the activation of ATF4 and β-catenin, and the enhancement of bone volume and density in CFTR-mutant mice. Together, these results suggest that magnesium implantation or supplementation may be a potential anabolic therapy for cystic fibrosis-related bone disease (Xu et al. 2022). Further, the MAPK/ERK pathway is a key signaling pathway that governs the osteogenic differentiation of stem cells. It has been reported that Mg^{2+} selectively activates the MAPK/ERK pathway, inducing stem cell differentiation. During this process, magnesium transporter 1 (MagT1) influences the osteoinductive effect of Mg^{2+} by mediating the influx of Mg^{2+} (Zhou et al. 2021).

Table 2 Common ions used as substitutes to increase osteogenic properties and their mechanisms of action (↑ increase, ↓ decrease, ¬ inhibition)

Ion	Role and mechanism of action	References
Sr^{2+}	(i) ↑ differentiation and activity of osteoblasts → increased bone matrix production and mineralization. (ii) ¬ the differentiation and activity of osteoclasts. Osteoblast stimulation (i) and osteoclast inhibition (ii) helps maintain a balance between bone formation and resorption, favoring bone regeneration. (iii) ↑ angiogenesis, the formation of new blood vessels, crucial for nutrients and oxygen supply	Harrison et al. (2021), Ran et al. (2023), Liu et al. (2023), Côrtes et al. (2024) and Neves et al. (2017)
Mg^{2+}	(i) ↑ osteoblasts' proliferation, migration, and differentiation, primarily mediated through the TRPM/PI3K signaling pathway. (ii) ¬ the formation and activity of osteoclasts, mainly through the nuclear factor-κB (NF-κB) signaling pathway. (iii) Mg^{2+} ions regulate the immune response in the bone environment by transforming macrophage phenotypes, promoting the secretion of bone growth factors, and reducing inflammatory cytokines. This creates a favorable environment for bone regeneration. (iv) ↑ proliferation, migration, and adhesion of vascular endothelial cells, contributing to angiogenesis	Zhou et al. (2023b), Wu et al. (2022) and Antoniac et al. (2023)
Zn^{2+}	↑ osteoblasts' proliferation, differentiation, and mineralization, through the activation of various signaling pathways (e.g., MAPK and Wnt/β-catenin pathways)	O'Connor et al. (2020)
Li^{+}	(i) ↑ proliferation, differentiation, and mineralization of osteoblasts, through the activation of the Wnt/β-catenin signaling pathway. (ii) Li^{+} ions regulate the immune response in the bone environment by promoting the polarization of macrophages towards the M2 phenotype, which is associated with anti-inflammatory and tissue repair functions	Lin et al. (2025) and Zhang et al. (2024)
SiO_4^{4-}	(i) ↑ osteoblasts' proliferation, differentiation, and mineralization, through the activation of various signaling pathways. (ii) ↑ angiogenesis, facilitated by the upregulation of vascular endothelial growth factor (VEGF) expression. (iii) SiO_4^{4-} ions can modulate the immune response by ↑ the polarization of macrophages towards the M2 phenotype, which is associated with anti-inflammatory and tissue repair functions	Sun et al. (2024) and Yang et al. (2021)
Cu^{+}	(i) ↑ proliferation and differentiation of osteoblasts, by activating various signaling pathways. (ii) ↑ angiogenesis, formation of new blood vessels, facilitated by the upregulation of VEGF expression. (iii) Cu^{+} ions can modulate the immune response by promoting the polarization of macrophages towards the M2 phenotype, which is associated with anti-inflammatory and tissue repair functions	Xu et al. (2021) and Shen et al. (2021)
$Mn^{2+/3+}$	(i) ↑ proliferation, differentiation, and mineralization of osteoblasts, through the activation of various signaling pathways. (ii) $Mn^{2+/3+}$ ions are a component of the enzyme manganese superoxide dismutase, which protects osteoclasts from oxidative damage	Taskozhina et al. (2024)

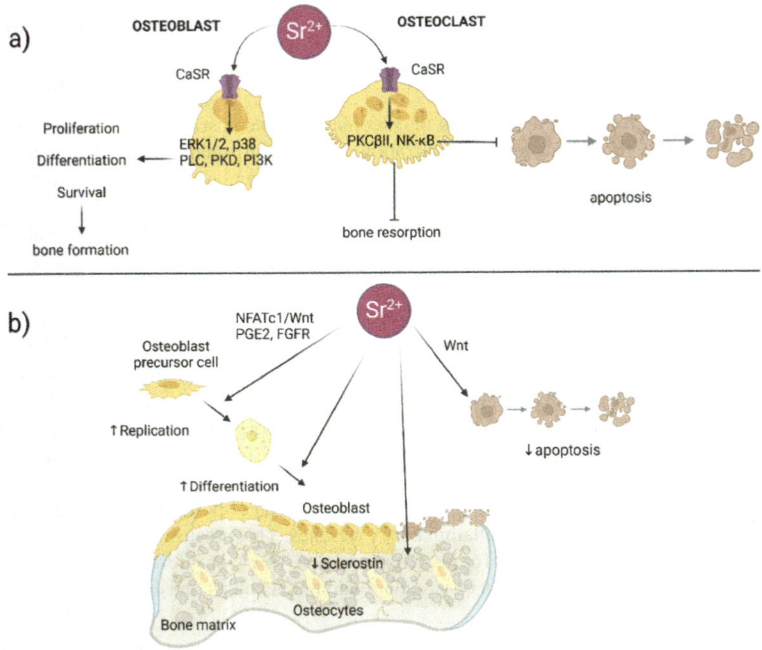

Fig. 8 **a** A visual representation of the dual action of Sr^{2+} ions: (i) positive impact on osteoblast cells and (ii) negative impact on osteoclast cells. **b** A schematic showing how Sr^{2+} activates osteoblastogenesis. Adapted with permission from Bose et al. (2013). Created in BioRender.com. *Abbreviations ERK ½* extracellular-signal-regulated kinase ½, *PI3K* phosphatidylinositide 3-kinases, *P38* a mitogen-activated protein kinases, *PLC* phospholipase C is a class of enzymes that cleave phospholipids, *PKD* protein kinase D, *PKCβII* protein kinase C βII, *NF-κB* nuclear factor kappa beta, *NFATc* nuclear factors of activated T-cells, *PGE2* prostaglandin E2, *FGFR* fibroblast growth factor receptor.

3 The future of trace elements in bone tissue engineering

Single-substituted HAp bone grafts have demonstrated improved biological performance both in vitro and in vivo. However, single substitutions in CaPs often lack the multifunctionality required for clinical applications. Therefore, it is reasonable to hypothesize that co/multi-substituted HAp could further enhance the beneficial effects of individual substituents (Bose et al. 2013). The simultaneous influence of two or three substituents on the physicochemical and biological properties of HAp has been extensively researched. Co-substituted HAp can be synthesized from synthetic precursors with added trace elements and/or biogenic sources. The introduction of ionic impurities can serve as internal antibacterial agents (Ag^+, Zn^{2+}, Cu^{2+}, and F^-), bone metabolism stimulators (Mg^{2+}, Sr^{2+}, Mn^{2+}), or anticancer factors ($SeO_3{}^{2-}$, $SeO_4{}^{2-}$, Fe^{3+}) (Ressler et al. 2021a; Laskus et al. 2019). The desired material properties for specific bone applications can be fine-tuned by combining key ions. Further studies should explore different combinations of substituted elements and the mechanisms by which certain elements affect cells and bone regeneration. At the same time, researchers should focus on the applications of these substituted CaP and explore the forms in which they can be used for the best results. In our recent study (Ressler et al. 2024), an Sr, Mg, Zn-substituted CaP system was used to fabricate scaffolds that fully mimic the chemical composition and microstructure of natural bone tissue (Fig. 9). Scaffolds were fabricated via vat photopolymerization from photosensitive ceramic suspensions and examined to explore trace element substitutions and sintering temperatures and their effects on scaffold properties. The scaffolds showed uniform trace element distribution, 3D-designed porosity similar to natural bone, and mechanical properties comparable to trabecular bone at higher sintering temperatures. This research highlights the potential of custom-made bioactive HAp powders and advanced manufacturing techniques to tailor bone scaffolds for specific defects. This study is an example of how the multi-substituted CaPs can be used and the possibilities for combining this material with novel methods.

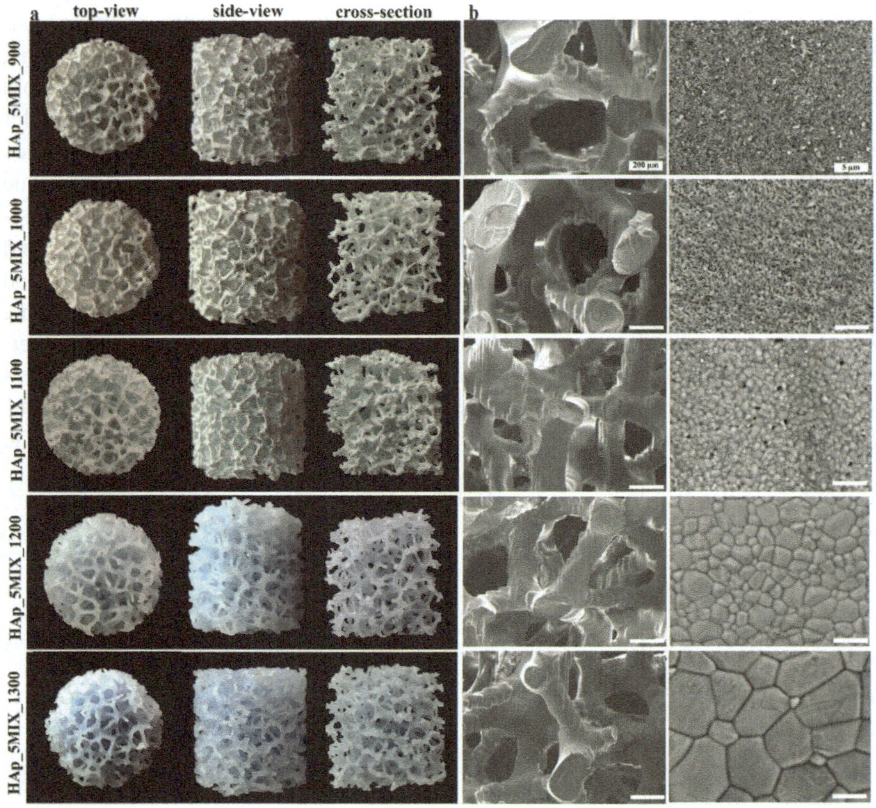

Fig. 9 **a** Morphology and **b** microstructure of fabricated scaffolds based on HAp substituted with Sr^{2+}, Mg^{2+} and Zn^{2+} ions, sintered at different temperatures. Scale bar: 200 and 5 μm. With permission from Ressler et al. (2024)

References

S.Q. Al-Shahrablee, H.A. Jaber, Investigation of the Nd-Ce-Mg-Zn/substituted hydroxyapatite effect on biological properties and osteosarcoma cells. J. Renew. Mater. **11**, 1485–1498 (2022). https://doi.org/10.32604/jrm.2023.025011

M. Ansari, Bone tissue regeneration: biology, strategies and interface studies. Prog. Biomater. **8**, 223–237. https://doi.org (2019). https://doi.org/10.1007/s40204-019-00125-z

I. Antoniac, V. Manescu, A. Antoniac, G. Paltanea, Magnesium-based alloys with adapted interfaces for bone implants and tissue engineering. Regen. Biomater. **10**, rbad095 (2023). https://doi.org/10.1093/rb/rbad095

S. Bai, M. Zhang, S. Tang, M. Li, R. Wu, S. Wan, L. Chen, X. Wie, S. Feng, Effects and impact of selenium on human health, a review. Molecules **30**(1), 50 (2025). https://doi.org/10.3390/molecules30010050

P. Bao, Z. Chen, R.-Z. Tai, H.-M. Shen, F.L. Martin, Y.-G. Zhu, Selenite-induced toxicity in cancer cells is mediated by metabolic generation of endogenous selenium nanoparticles. J. Proteome Res. **14**(6), 2876–2884 (2015). https://doi.org/10.1021/pr501086e

R.A. Bapat, T.V. Chaubal, C.P. Joshi, P.R. Bapat, H. Choudhury, M. Pandey, B. Gorain, P. Kesharwani, An overview of application of silver nanoparticles for biomaterials in dentistry. Mater. Sci. Eng. C **91**, 881–898 (2018). https://doi.org/10.1016/j.msec.2018.05.069

A. Barbanente, B. Palazzo, L.D. Esposti, A. Adamiano, M. Iafisco, N. Ditaranto, D. Migoni, F. Gervaso, R. Nadar, P. Ivanchenko, S. Leeuwenburgh, N. Margiotta, Selenium-doped hydroxyapatite nanoparticles for potential application in bone tumor therapy. J. Inorg. Biochem. **215**, 111334 (2021). https://doi.org/10.1016/j.jinorgbio.2020.111334

E. Boanini, M. Gazzano, A. Bigi, Ionic substitutions in calcium phosphates synthesized at low temperature. Acta Biomater. **6**, 1882–1894 (2010). https://doi.org/10.1016/j.actbio.2009.12.041

A. Bootchanont, T. Wechprasit, N. Isran, J. Theangsunthorn, N. Chaosuan, N. Chanlek, P. Kidkhunthod, R. Yimnirun, A. Jiamprasertboon, T. Eknapakul, T. Siritanon, W. Sailuam, T. Saisopa, Materialia **26**, 101586 (2022). https://doi.org/10.1016/j.mtla.2022.10158

S. Bose, G. Fielding, S. Tarafder, A. Bandyopadhyay, Understanding of dopant-induced osteogenesis and angiogenesis in calcium phosphate ceramics. Trends Biotechnol. **31**, 594–605 (2013). https://doi.org/10.1016/j.tibtech.2013.06.005

O. Breuer, O. Brodin, A. Razaghi, D. Brodin, B. Gammelgaard, M. Björnstedt, Intravenous infusion of high dose selenite in end-stage cancer patients: analysis of systemic exposure to selenite and seleno-metabolites. Biomedicine **11**(2), 295 (2023). https://doi.org/10.3390/biomedicines110 20295

A. Cappariello, M. Capulli, The vicious cycle of breast cancer-induced bone metastases, a complex biological and therapeutic target. Curr. Mol. Biol. Rep. **4**, 123–131 (2018). https://doi.org/10.1007/s40610-018-0099-5

H. Choe, J.M. Tatro, B.S. Hausman, K.M. Hujer, S.H. Marshall, O. Akkus, P.N. Rather, Z. Lee, R.A. Bonom, E.M. Greenfied, *Staphylococcus aureus* and *Acinetobacter baumannii* inhibit osseointegration of orthopedic implants. Infect. Immun. **90**, e0066921 (2022). https://doi.org/10.1128/iai.00669-21

T. Cordonnier, J. Sohier, P. Rosset, P. Layrolle, Biomimetic materials for bone tissue engineering—state of art and future trends. Adv. Eng. Mater. **13**, B135–B150 (2011). https://doi.org/10.1002/adem.201080098

J.A. Côrtes, J. Dornelas, F. Duarte, M.R. Messora, C.F. Mourão, G. Alves, The effects of the addition of strontium on the biological response to calcium phosphate biomaterials: a systematic review. Appl. Sci. **14**(17), 7566 (2024). https://doi.org/10.3390/app141775662

S. Dhatchayani, S. Vijaykumar, N. Sarala, B. Vaseeharan, K. Sankaranarayanan, Effect of curcumin sorbed selenite substituted hydroxyapatite on osteosarcoma cells: an in vitro study. J. Drug Deliv. Sci. Technol. **60**, 101963 (2020). https://doi.org/10.1016/j.jddst.2020.101963

S.V. Dorozhkin, M. Epple, Biological and medical significance of calcium phosphates. Angew. Chem. Int. Ed. Engl. **41**, 3130–3146 (2002). https://doi.org/10.1002/1521-3773(20020902)41:17<3130::AID-ANIE3130>3.0.CO;2-1

Z. Ferdous, A. Nemmar, Health impact of silver nanoparticles: a review of the biodistribution and toxicity following various routes of exposure. Int. J. Mol. Sci. **21**, 2375 (2020). https://doi.org/10.3390/ijms21072375

R. Florencio-Silva, G.R. da Silva Sasso, E. Sasso-Cerri, M.J. Simoes, P.S. Cerri, Biology of bone tissue: structure, function, and factors that influence bone cells. Biomed. Res. Int. 421746 (2015). https://doi.org/10.1155/2015/421746

R. Ghosh, S. Das, S.P. Mallick, Z. Beyene, A review on the antimicrobial and antibiofilm activity of doped hydroxyapatite and its composites for biomedical applications. Mater. Today Commun. **31**, 103311 (2022). https://doi.org/10.1016/j.mtcomm.2022.103311

D. Gopi, S. Ramya, D. Rajeswari, P. Karthikeyan, L. Kavitha, Strontium, cerium co-substituted hydroxyapatite nanoparticles: synthesis, characterization, antibacterial activity towards prokaryotic strains and in vitro studies. Colloids Surf. A Physicochem. Eng. Asp. **451**, 172–180 (2014). https://doi.org/10.1016/j.colsurfa.2014.03.035

Y. Gu, J. Zhang, X. Zhang, G. Liang, T. Xu, W. Niu, Three-dimensional printed Mg-doped β-TCP bone tissue engineering scaffolds: effects of magnesium ion concentration on osteogenesis and angiogenesis in vitro. Tissue Eng. Regen. Med. **16**, 415–429 (2019). https://doi.org/10.1007/s13770-019-00192-0

T.A. Guise, The vicious cycle of bone metastases. J. Musculoskelet. Neuronal Interact. **2**(6), 570–572 (2002)

S. Halder, K.K. Yadav, R. Sarkar, S. Mukherjee, P. Saha, S. Haldar, S. Karmakar, T. Sen, Alteration of zeta potential and membrane permeability in bacteria: a study with cationic agents. SpringerPlus **4**, 672 (2015). https://doi.org/10.1186/s40064-015-1476-7

C.J. Harrison, P.V. Hatton, P. Gentile, C.A. Miller, Nanoscale strontium-substituted hydroxyapatite pastes and gels for bone tissue regeneration. Nano **11**(6), 1611 (2021). https://doi.org/10.3390/nano11061611

https://www.who.int/docs/default-source/antimicrobial-resistance/amr-factsheet.pdf

https://www.who.int/news/item/17-05-2024-who-updates-list-of-drug-resistant-bacteria-most-threatening-to-human-health

https://www.who.int/news-room/fact-sheets/detail/antimicrobial-resistance

T. Ishida, Antibacterial mechanism of Ag^{+} ions for bacteriolyses of bacterial cell walls via peptidoglycan autolysins, and DNA damages. MOJ Toxicol. **4**, 345–350 (2018). https://doi.org/10.15406/mojt.2018.04.00125

T. Ivankovic, H. Turk, J. Hrenovic, Z. Schauperl, M. Ivankovic, A. Ressler, Antibacterial activity of silver doped hydroxyapatite toward multidrug-resistant clinical isolates of *Acinetobacter baumannii*. J. Hazard. Mater. **458**, 131867 (2023). https://doi.org/10.1016/j.jhazmat.2023.131867

T. Ivankovic, A. Zuzic, I. Urlic, V.A. Gobbo, B. Dadic, T. Sandblom, S. Zakeri, M. Virpinen, I. Goic-Barisic, J. Hrenovic, J. Massera, E. Levänen, A. Ressler, Cerium, copper, gallium, manganese and silver substituted hydroxyapatite: cytotoxicity and antibacterial activity toward multidrug-resistant clinical isolates. J. Hazard. Mater. Adv. **18**, 100731 (2025). https://doi.org/10.1016/j.hazadv.2025.100731

M. Jebapriya, R. Venkatesan, S. Ansan, S.C. Kim, Enhancement of physicochemical characterization of nanocomposites on Ag^{+}/Fe^{2+} codoped hydroxyapatite for antibacterial and anticancer properties. Colloids Surf. B Biointerfaces **229**, 113463 (2023). https://doi.org/10.1016/j.colsurfb.2023.113463

Y. Jiang, S. Tan, J. Hu, X. Chen, F. Chen, Q. Yao, Z. Zhou, X. Wang, Z. Zhou, Y. Fan, J. Liu, Y. Lin, L. Liu, S. He, Amorphous calcium magnesium phosphate nanocomposites with superior osteogenic activity for bone regeneration. Regen. Biomater. **8**(6), rbab068 (2021). https://doi.org/10.1093/rb/rbab068

W.K. Jung, H.C. Koo, K.W. Kim, S. Shin, S.H. Kim, Y.H. Park, Antibacterial activity and mechanism of action of the silver ion in *Staphylococcus aureus* and *Escherichia coli*. Appl. Environ. Microbiol. **74**, 7 (2008). https://doi.org/10.1128/AEM.02001-07

S. Kargozar, S. Mollazadeh, F. Kermani, T.J. Webster, S. Nazarnezhad, S. Hamzehlou, F. Baino, Hydroxyapatite nanoparticles for improved cancer theranostics. J. Funct. Biomater. **13**(3), 100 (2022). https://doi.org/10.3390/jfb13030100

A.B. Kelson, M. Carnevali, V. Truong-Le, Gallium-based anti-infectivnes: targeting microbial iron-uptake mechanisms. Curr. Opin. Pharmacol. **13**, 707–716 (2013). https://doi.org/10.1016/j.coph.2013.07.001

M. Kieliszek, B. Lipinski, S. Błażejak, Application of sodium selenite in the prevention and treatment of cancers. Cells **6**(4), 39 (2017). https://doi.org/10.3390/cells6040039

N. Kircheva, T. Dudev, Gallium as an antibacterial agent: a DFT/SMD study of the Ga^{3+}/Fe^{3+} competition for binding bacterial siderophores. Inorg. Chem. **59**, 6242–6254 (2020). https://doi.org/10.1021/acs.inorgchem.0c00367

J. Kolmas, E. Groszyk, D. Kwiatkowska-Rozycka, Substituted hydroxyapatite with antibacterial properties. Biomed. Res. Int. **2014**, 178123 (2014). https://doi.org/10.1155/2014/178123

A. Lapa, M. Cresswell, I. Campell, P. Jackson, W.H. Goldmann, R. Detsch, A.R. Boccaccini, Gallium- and cerium-doped phosphate glasses with antibacterial properties for medical applications. Adv. Eng. Mater. **22**, 1901577 (2020). https://doi.org/10.1002/adem.201901577

A. Laskus, A. Zgadzaj, J. Kolmas, Zn^{2+} and $SeO_3{}^{2-}$ co-substituted hydroxyapatite: physicochemical properties and biological usefulness. Ceram. Int. **48**, 22707–22715 (2019). https://doi.org/10.1016/j.ceramint.2019.07.308

P. Li, Z. Jia, Q. Wang, P. Tang, M. Wang, K. Wang, J. Fang, C. Zhao, F. Ren, X. Ge, X. Lu, A resilient and flexible chitosan/silk cryogel incorporated Ag/Sr co-doped nanoscale hydroxyapatite for osteoinductivity and antibacterial properties. J. Mater. Chem. B **6**, 7427–7438 (2018). https://doi.org/10.1039/C8TB01672K

F. Li, F. Liu, K. Huang, S. Yang, Advanced of gallium and gallium-based compounds as antimicrobial agents. Front. Bioeng. Biotechnol. **10**, 827960 (2022). https://doi.org/10.3389/fbioe.2022.827960

Y.-H. Lin, C.-Y. Chen, K.-H. Chen, T.-Y. Kuo, T.-L. Lin, M.-Y. Shie, Lithium-doped calcium silicate cement regulates the immune microenvironment and promotes M2 macrophage polarization for enhancing bone regeneration. J. Biol. Eng. **19**(1), 3 (2025). https://doi.org/10.1186/s13036-024-00467-8

X. Liu, H. Huang, J. Zhang, T. Sun, W. Zhang, Z. Li, Recent advance of strontium functionalized in biomaterials for bone regeneration. Bioengineering **10**(4), 414 (2023). https://doi.org/10.3390/bioengineering100404141

K. Maji, S. Mondal, Calcium phosphate biomaterials for bone tissue engineering: properties and relevance in bone repair, in *Racing for the Surface* (Springer, 2020), pp. 535–555

N.O. Martínez-Gracida, S.C. Esparza-González, N.A. Castillo-Martínez, A. Serrano-Medina, I. Olivas-Armendariz, L.G. Campos-Múzquiz, E.M. Múzquiz-Ramos, Synergism in novel silver-copper/hydroxyapatite composites for increased antibacterial activity and biocompatibility. Ceram. Int. **46**, 20215–20225 (2020). https://doi.org/10.1016/j.ceramint.2020.05.102

K. Matsunaga, First-principles study of substitutional magnesium and zinc in hydroxyapatite and octacalcium phosphate. J. Chem. Phys. **128**, 245101 (2008). https://doi.org/10.1063/1.2940337

L.L. Maurer, J.N. Meyer, A systematic review of evidence for silver nanoparticle-induced mitochondrial toxicity. Environ. Sci. Nano **3**, 311–322 (2016). https://doi.org/10.1039/C5EN00187K

A.F. Mavrogenis, R. Dimitriou, J. Parvizi, G.C. Babis, Biology of implant osseointegration. J. Musculoskelet. Neuronal Interact. **9**, 61–71 (2009)

O. McNeilly, R. Mann, M.L. Cummins, S.P. Djordjevic, M. Hamidian, C. Gunawan, Development of nanoparticle adaptation phenomena in *Acinetobacter baumannii*: physiological change and defense response. Bacteriol. Spectr. **11**, e02857–e02822 (2023). https://doi.org/10.1128/spectrum.02857-22

K. Mediaswanti, Influence of physicochemical aspects of substratum nanosurface on bacterial attachment for bone implant applications. J. Nanotechnol. **2016**, 1–6 (2016). https://doi.org/10.1155/2016/5026184

S. Minardi, B. Corradetti, F. Taraballi, M. Sandri, J. Van Eps, F.J. Cabrera, B.K. Weiner, A. Tampieri, Evaluation of the osteoinductive potential of a bio-inspired scaffold mimicking the osteogenic niche for bone augmentation. Biomaterials **62**, 128–137 (2015). https://doi.org/10.1016/j.biomaterials.2015.05.011

C.A. Moubareck, D.H. Halat, Insights into *Acinetobacter baumannii*: a review of microbiological, virulence, and resistance traits in a threatening nosocomial pathogen. Antibiotics **9**, 119 (2020). https://doi.org/10.3390/antibiotics9030119

M.S. Mulani, E.E. Kamble, S.N. Kumkar, M.S. Tawre, K.R. Pardesi, Emerging strategies to combat ESKAPE pathogens in the era of antimicrobial resistance: a review. Front. Microbiol. **10**, 539 (2019). https://doi.org/10.3389/fmicb.2019.00539

S. Muthusamy, B. Mahendiran, S. Sampath, S.N. Jaisankar, S.K. Anandasadagopan, G.S. Krishnakumar, Hydroxyapatite nanophases augmented with selenium and manganese ions for bone regeneration: physiochemical, microstructural and biological characterization. Mater. Sci. Eng. C **126**, 112149 (2021). https://doi.org/10.1016/j.msec.2021.112149

N. Neves, D. Linhares, G. Costa, C.C. Ribeiro, M.A. Barbosa, In vivo and clinical application of strontium-enriched biomaterials for bone support or regeneration. Bone Joint Res. **6**(6), 311 (2017). https://doi.org/10.1302/2046-3758.66.BJR-2016-0311.R13

J.P. O'Connor, D. Kanjilal, M. Teitelbaum, S.S. Lin, J.A. Cottrell, Zinc as a therapeutic agent in bone regeneration. Materials **13**(10), 2211 (2020). https://doi.org/10.3390/ma13102211

K. Pajor, L. Pajchel, B. Kolodziejska, J. Kolmas, Selenium-doped hydroxyapatite nanocrystals—synthesis, physicochemical properties and biological significance. Crystals **8**, 188 (2018). https://doi.org/10.3390/cryst8050188

S. Park, J. Choi, V.H. Minh Doan, O.S. Hwi, Biodegradable manganese-doped hydroxyapatite antitumor adjuvant as a promising photo-therapeutic for cancer treatment. Front. Mol. Biosci. **9**, 1085458 (2022). https://doi.org/10.3389/fmolb.2022.1085458

D. Predoi, S.L. Iconaru, M.V. Predoi, A. Groza, S. Gaiaschi, K. Rokosz, S. Raaen, C.C. Negrila, A.-M. Prodan, A. Costescu, M.L. Badea, P. Chapon, Development of cerium-doped hydroxyapatite coatings with antimicrobial properties for biomedical applications. Coatings **10**, 516 (2020). https://doi.org/10.3390/coatings10060516

L. Ran, L. Liu, J. Gao, Y. Pan, M. Ramalingam, X. Du, Y. Liu, L. Cheng, Z. Shi, Strontium-doped hydroxyapatite and its role in osteogenesis and angiogenesis. Int. J. Dev. Biol. **67**(4), 137–146 (2023). https://doi.org/10.1387/ijdb.230091lc

C.P. Randall, A. Gupta, N. Jackson, D. Busse, A.J. O'Neill, Silver resistance in gram-negative bacteria: a dissection of endogenous and exogenous mechanisms. J. Antimicrob. Chemother. **70**, 1037–1046 (2015). https://doi.org/10.1093/jac/dku523

M.P. Rayman, Selenium in cancer prevention: a review of the evidence and mechanism of action. Proc. Nutr. Soc. **64**(4), 527–542 (2005). https://doi.org/10.1079/pns2005467

A. Ressler, M. Cvetnic, M. Antunovic, I. Marijanovic, M. Ivankovic, H. Ivankovic, Strontium substituted biomimetic calcium phosphate system derived from cuttlefish bone. J. Biomed. Mater. Res. B Appl. Biomater. **108**, 1697–1709 (2020). https://doi.org/10.1002/jbm.b.34515

A. Ressler, A. Zuzic, I. Ivanisevic, N. Kamboj, H. Ivankovic, Ionic substituted hydroxyapatite for bone regeneration applications: a review. Open Ceram. **6**, 100122 (2021a). https://doi.org/10.1016/j.oceram.2021.100122

A. Ressler, M. Antunovic, M. Cvetnic, M. Ivankovic, H. Ivankovic, Selenite substituted calcium phosphates: preparation, characterization, and cytotoxic activity. Materials **14**(12), 3436 (2021b). https://doi.org/10.3390/ma14123436

A. Ressler, T. Ivankovic, B. Polak, I. Ivanisevic, M. Kovacic, I. Urlic, I. Hussainova, H. Ivankovic, A multifunctional strontium/silver-co-substituted hydroxyapatite derived from biogenic source as antibacterial biomaterial. Ceram. Int. **48**, 18361–18373 (2022a). https://doi.org/10.1016/j.ceramint.2022.03.095

A. Ressler, M. Antunovic, L. Teruel-Biosca, G. Gallego Ferrer, S. Babic, I. Urlic, M. Ivankovic, H. Ivankovic, Osteogenic differentiation of human mesenchymal stem cells on substituted calcium phosphate/chitosan composite scaffold. Carbohydr. Polym. **277**, 118883 (2022b). https://doi.org/10.1016/j.carbpol.2021.118883

A. Ressler, T. Ivankovic, I. Ivanisevic, M. Cvetnic, M. Antunovic, I. Urlic, H. Ivankovic, M. Ivankovic, Multiphase zinc and magnesium mono-substituted calcium phosphates derived from cuttlefish bone: a multifunctional biomaterials. Ceram. Int. **49**, 11005–11017 (2023). https://doi.org/10.1016/j.ceramint.2022.11.295

A. Ressler, S. Zakeri, J. Dias, M. Hannula, J. Hyttinen, H. Ivanković, M. Ivanković, S. Miettinen, M. Schwentenwein, E. Levänen, E.J. Frankberg, Vat photopolymerization of biomimetic bone scaffolds based on Mg, Sr, Zn-substituted hydroxyapatite: effect of sintering temperature. Ceram. Int. **50**, 27403–27415 (2024). https://doi.org/10.1016/j.ceramint.2024.05.038

K.B. Riaz Ahmed, A.M. Nagy, R.P. Brown, Q. Zhang, S.G. Malghan, P.L. Goering, Silver nanoparticles: significance of physicochemical properties and assay interference on the interpretation of in vitro cytotoxicity studies. Toxicol. Vitr. **38**, 179–192 (2017). https://doi.org/10.1016/j.tiv.2016.10.012

M. Sadat-Shojai, M.T. Khorasani, E. Dinpanah-Khoshdargi, A. Jamshidi, Synthesis methods for nanosized hydroxyapatite with diverse structures. Acta Biomater. **9**, 7591–7621 (2013). https://doi.org/10.1016/j.actbio.2013.04.012

Z. Saidak, P.J. Marie, Strontium signaling: molecular mechanisms and therapeutic implications in osteoporosis. Pharmacol. Ther. **136**, 216–226 (2012). https://doi.org/10.1016/j.pharmthera.2012.07.009

M. Sára, U.B. Sleytr, S-layer proteins. J. Bacteriol. **182**, 859–868 (2000). https://doi.org/10.1128/JB.182.4.859-868.2000

Y. Seyoum, K. Bay, C. Humblot, Iron homeostasis in host and gut bacteria—a complex interrelationship. Gut Microbes **13**, e1874855 (2021). https://doi.org/10.1080/19490976.2021.1874855

Q. Shen, Y. Qi, Y. Kong, H. Bao, Y. Wang, A. Dong, H. Wu, Y. Xu, Advances in copper-based biomaterials with antibacterial and osteogenic properties. Front. Bioeng. Biotechnol. **9**, 2021 (2021). https://doi.org/10.3389/fbioe.2021.795425

K. Shoueir, M.K. Ahmed, S.A.A. Gaber, M. El-Kemary, Thallium and selenite doped carbonated hydroxyapatite: microstructural features and anticancer activity assessment against human lung carcinoma. Ceram. Int. **46**, 5201–5212 (2020). https://doi.org/10.1016/j.ceramint.2019.10.268

L. Stipniece, S. Wilson, J.M. Curran, R. Chen, K. Salma-Ancane, P.K. Sharma, B.J. Meenan, A.R. Boyd, Strontium substituted hydroxyapatite promotes direct primary human osteoblast maturation. Ceram. Int. **47**, 3368–3379 (2021). https://doi.org/10.1016/j.ceramint.2020.09.182

G. Sun, T. Shu, S. Ma, M. Li, Z. Qu, A. Li, A submicron forest-like silicon surface promotes bone regeneration by regulating macrophage polarization. Front. Bioeng. Biotechnol. **12**, 2024 (2024). https://doi.org/10.3389/fbioe.2024.1356158

G. Taskozhina, G. Batyrova, G. Umarova, Z. Issanguzhina, N. Kereyeva, The manganese–bone connection: investigating the role of manganese in bone health. J. Clin. Med. **13**(16), 4679 (2024). https://doi.org/10.3390/jcm13164679

V. Uskoković, M. Adiraj Iyer, V.M. Wu, One ion to rule them all: the combined antibacterial, osteoinductive and anticancer properties of selenite-incorporated hydroxyapatite. J. Mater. Chem. B **5**, 1430–1445 (2017). https://doi.org/10.1039/C6TB03387C

A.V. Vasiliadis, F. Poutoglidou, V. Chatziravdeli, D. Metaxiotis, A. Beletsiotis, Acute periprosthetic hip joint infection caused by multidrug-resistant *Acinetobacter baumannii*: is debridement, antibiotics, irrigation, and implant retention a viable treatment option? Cureus **13**, e13090 (2021). https://doi.org/10.7759/cureus.13090

A. Vila, H. Pagella, C. Amadio, A. Leiva, *Acinetobacter* prosthetic joint infection treated with debridement and high-dose tigecycline. Infect. Chemother. **48**, 324–329 (2016). https://doi.org/10.3947/ic.2016.48.4.324

R. Von Moos, I. Haynes, Where do bone-targeted agents RANK in breast cancer treatment? J. Clin. Med. **2**(3), 89–102 (2013). https://doi.org/10.3390/jcm2030089

M. Vukomanovic, L. Gazvoda, N. Anicic, M. Rubert, D. Suvorov, R. Muller, S. Hofmann, Multi-doped apatite: strontium, magnesium, gallium and zinc ions synergistically affect osteogenic stimulation in human mesenchymal cells important for bone tissue engineering. Biomater. Adv. **140**, 213051 (2022). https://doi.org/10.1016/j.bioadv.2022.213051

Y. Wang, J. Wang, H. Hao, M. Cai, S. Wang, J. Ma, Y. Li, C. Mao, S. Zhang, In vitro and in vivo mechanism of bone tumor inhibition by selenium-doped bone mineral nanoparticles. ACS Nano **10**, 9927–9937 (2016). https://doi.org/10.1021/acsnano.6b03835

Y. Wang, W. He, H. Hao, J. Wu, N. Qin, Eggshell derived Se-doped HA nanorods for enhanced antitumor effect and curcumin delivery. J. Sol-Gel Sci. Technol. **87**, 600–607 (2018). https://doi.org/10.1007/s10971-018-4765-0

M. Wang, M. Li, Y. Wang, Y. Shao, Y. Zhu, S. Yang, Efficient antibacterial activity of hydroxyapatite through ROS generation motivated by trace Mn(III) coupled H vacancies. J. Mater. Chem. B **9**, 3401–3411 (2021). https://doi.org/10.1039/D1TB00098E

L. Wei, H. Yang, J. Hong, Z. He, C. Deng, Synthesis and structure properties of Se and Sr co-doped hydroxyapatite and their biocompatibility. J. Mater. Sci. **54**, 2514–2525 (2019). https://doi.org/10.1007/s10853-018-2951-7

S.E. Weinberg, A. Villedieu, N. Bagdasarian, N. Karah, L. Teare, W.F. Elamin, Control and management of multidrug resistant *Acinetobacter baumannii*: a review of the evidence and proposal of novel approaches. Infect. Prev. Pract. **2**, 100077 (2020). https://doi.org/10.1016/j.infpip.2020.100077

B. Wopenka, J.D. Pasteris, A mineralogical perspective on the apatite in bone. Mater. Sci. Eng. C **25**, 131–143 (2005). https://doi.org/10.1016/j.msec.2005.01.008

Y. Wu, L. Woodbine, A.M. Carr, A.R. Pillai, A. Nokhodchi, M. Maniruzzaman, 3D printed calcium phosphate cement (CPC) scaffolds for anti-cancer drug delivery. Pharmaceutics **12**(11), 1077 (2020). https://doi.org/10.3390/pharmaceutics12111077

J. Wu, F. Liu, Z. Wang, Y. Liu, X. Zhao, C. Fang, F. Leung, K.W.K. Yeung, The development of a magnesium-releasing and long-term mechanically stable calcium phosphate bone cement possessing osteogenic and immunomodulation effects for promoting bone fracture regeneration. Front. Bioeng. Biotechnol. **11**(9), 803723 (2022). https://doi.org/10.3389/fbioe.2021.803723

D. Xu, J. Qian, X. Guan, L. Ren, K. Yang, X. Huang, S. Zhang, Y. Chai, X. Wu, H. Wu, X. Zhang, B. Yu, Copper-containing alloy as Immunoregulatory material in bone regeneration via mitochondrial oxidative stress. Front. Bioeng. Biotechnol. **8**, 620629 (2021). https://doi.org/10.3389/fbioe.2020.620629

J. Xu, P. Hu, X. Zhang, J. Chen, J. Wang, J. Zhang, Z. Chen, M.K. Yu, Y.W. Chung, Y. Wang, X. Zhang, Y. Zhang, N. Zheng, H. Yao, J.G. Yue, H.C. Chan, L. Qin, Y.C. Ruan, Magnesium implantation or supplementation ameliorates bone disorder in CFTR-mutant mice through an ATF4-dependent Wnt/β-catenin signaling. Bioact. Mater. **8**, 95–108 (2022). https://doi.org/10.1016/j.bioactmat.2021.06.034

M.D. Yan, Y.J. Ou, YJ. Lin, R.M. Liu, Y. Fang, W.L. Wu, L. Zhou, X. Yao, J. Chen, Does the incorporation of strontium into calcium phosphate improve bone repair? A meta-analysis. BMC Oral Health **22**, 62 (2022). https://doi.org/10.1186/s12903-022-02092-7

Y. Yang, A. Kulkarni, G.D. Soraru, J.M. Pearce, A. Motta, 3D printed SiOC(N) ceramic scaffolds for bone tissue regeneration: improved osteogenic differentiation of human bone marrow-derived mesenchymal stem cells. Int. J. Mol. Sci. **22**(24), 13676 (2021). https://doi.org/10.3390/ijms222413676

H. Zeng, J.J. Cao, G.F. Combis, Selenium in bone health: roles in antioxidant protection and cell proliferation. Nutrients **5**(1), 97–110 (2013). https://doi.org/10.3390/nu5010097

X. Zhang, Y. Zhang, Calcium homeostasis: a potential vicious cycle of bone metastasis in breast cancer. Front. Oncol. **10**, 293 (2020). https://doi.org/10.3389/fonc.2020.00293

X. Zhang, K. Nan, Y. Zhang, K. Song, Z. Geng, D. Shang, L. Fan, Lithium and cobalt co-doped mesoporous bioactive glass nanoparticles promote osteogenesis and angiogenesis in bone regeneration. Front. Bioeng. Biotechnol. **11**, 2023 (2024). https://doi.org/10.3389/fbioe.2023.1288393

H. Zhou, B. Liang, H. Jiang, Z. Deng, K. Yu, Magnesium-based biomaterials as emerging agents for bone repair and regeneration: from mechanism to application. J. Magnes. Alloy **9**, 779–804 (2021). https://doi.org/10.1016/j.jma.2021.03.004

S. Zhou, J. Ren, L. Wang, L. Liu, C. Deng, A report on Se/Eu-doped hydroxyapatite: crystal structure analysis, biological property assessment, and applications in osteosarcoma inhibition and bioimaging. Mater. Adv. **4**, 2147–2161 (2023a). https://doi.org/10.1039/D3MA00046J

Y. Zhou, A. Zhang, J. Wu, S. Guo, Q. Sun, Application and perspectives: magnesium materials in bone regeneration. ACS Biomater. Sci. Eng. **10**(6), 3514–3527 (2023b). https://doi.org/10.1021/acsbiomaterials.3c01713

The Biological Activity of Iron Oxide Nanoparticles

Wencheng Zhu and Xujun Zheng

Abstract Iron oxide nanoparticles (IONs) have gained significant attention in biomedical research due to their biocompatibility, biodegradability, and versatile applications, particularly as magnetic resonance imaging (MRI) contrast agents for non-invasive tissue imaging in clinical diagnosis and in vivo cell tracking and integrated therapeutics in basic research. The undesired cellular effects of labeling with IONs, such as altered cell migration, reduced differentiation potential, and bystander uptake by immune cells, complicate the interpretation of tracking results. While ION labeling may induce undesired cellular effects, ION-induced cellular responses such as ferroptosis and autophagy also offer therapeutic and regenerative opportunities. This chapter summarizes both unintended biological effects of ION labeling and their therapeutic potential, underscoring the need for careful evaluation for ION-based applications. Further exploration of the molecular mechanisms driving these cellular responses is essential to optimize ION-based strategies for clinical diagnostic and therapeutic purposes.

Keywords Iron oxide nanoparticles · Cell death · Autophagy · Cell differentiation · Immune response · Theranostics

1 Introduction

Iron oxide nanoparticles (IONs) consist of maghemite (γ-Fe_2O_3) and/or magnetite (Fe_3O_4) particles with diameters ranging from 1 to 150 nm. The biocompatibility, biodegradability, and diverse applications of IONs have led to extensive research

W. Zhu (✉)
Institute of Molecular Physiology, Shenzhen Bay Laboratory, Shenzhen, China
e-mail: wzhu@szbl.ac.cn

X. Zheng (✉)
School of Chemistry, Sun Yat-Sen University, Guangzhou, China
e-mail: zhengxj65@mail.sysu.edu.cn

Department of Chemistry, Duke University, Durham, United States

R. Narayan (ed.), *Nanostructured Biomaterials and Their Applications*,
https://doi.org/10.1007/978-3-032-16316-5_10

and development in both preclinical and clinical settings over the past decades, positioning them among the most widely studied nanomaterials. Historically, the first iron–dextran complex was reported in 1954 as an analog of ferritin, a major iron storage protein in humans (Fletcher and London 1954). This complex, IMFERON (Fison™), had been applied to treat hypochromic anemia in humans by intravenously administer iron. Subsequent studies proposed its nanoscale structure with an iron core wrapped in a colloidal sheath (London 2004). The first application of small iron oxide particles as magnetic contrast agents was realized in 1957 (Gilchrist et al. 1957). Notably, several formulations of IONs have been approved for human use in imaging and the treatment of iron-deficiency anemia by the U.S. Food and Drug Administration (FDA) and European Union health authorities (Jin et al. 2022; Alphandery 2019; Bulte 2019). The stability of IONs in colloidal form is of great importance during the preparation and storage. Surface modifications are often used to enhance the colloidal stability, which also crucially influences their biodistribution and blood circulation half-life in vivo (Gupta and Gupta 2005). Currently, most clinically approved SPIONs are composed of inorganic iron oxide cores with hydrophilic coating polymers, such as polysaccharide (e.g. dextran and its derivatives) or poly (ethylene glycol) (PEG) (Alphandery 2019; Jin et al. 2014).

The synthesis, characterization, and applications of IONs have been reviewed and discussed before (Gupta and Gupta 2005; Thorek et al. 2006; Liu et al. 2013; Ling et al. 2015; Teja and Koh 2009). In this chapter, we summarize findings regarding unexpected biological activities of IONs in diversified biological contexts.

2 Undesired Cellular Effects Toward IONs After Cell Labeling

MRI has long been a cornerstone of clinical diagnostics, transforming the landscape of non-invasive imaging with its remarkable ability to visualize soft tissues in unprecedented detail. Among the many advancements in MRI technology, IONs, particularly superparamagnetic iron oxide nanoparticles (SPIONs), have emerged as highly effective contrast agents. As a subset of IONs, SPIONs exhibit superparamagnetism, where they function as magnets only in the presence of an external magnetic field. By altering the local magnetic field, SPIONs cause a loss of signal in MRI images, a property that has made them valuable for a wide range of applications, including the non-invasive tracking of transplanted or injected cells. This capability is especially crucial in fields like stem cell therapy and tissue engineering, where understanding the movement and fate of introduced cells is vital for assessing treatment efficacy. More recently, magnetic particle imaging (MPI), a cutting-edge imaging modality, has further expanded the utility of IONs (Bulte et al. 2022). MPI offers a new frontier in in vivo imaging, providing high-resolution, real-time tracking of cells with minimal background interference. This has opened up exciting possibilities for dynamic and precise cell monitoring in various therapeutic and research contexts. However, while IONs are generally regarded as biodegradable and biocompatible, some studies have raised concerns about their potential unintended effects on cellular behavior when used for cell labeling.

Dendritic cells (DCs) are antigen presenting cells and essential for immune responses, particularly in vaccine therapies. The ability to track DC migration in vivo could provide valuable insights into the effectiveness of DC-based immunotherapies. Inspired by previous in vivo tracking of ION-labeled immune cells, Ahrens et al. first reported the labeling of DCs with dextran–SPIO conjugated to an anti-CD11c monoclonal antibody (mAb) for in vivo MRI (Ahrens et al. 2003). The mAb conjugation enabled efficient labeling through a receptor-mediated endocytosis mechanism. Initial assessments indicated that SPIO labeling did not adversely affect the immunological function of DCs. However, a later study found that SPIO (Feridex®) labeling reduced the overall migration capacity of DCs, likely due to the size of the nanoparticles (de Chickera et al. 2011). Notably, magnetic separation of SPIO-labeled DCs prior to injection has been shown to enhance their migration to lymph nodes and improve the alignment between MRI data and DC presence in vivo.

Our previous study suggested that labeling DCs with polyethylenimine (PEI)-coated SPIONs (PEI–SPIONs) could promote DC maturation (Xu et al. 2015). Fluorescence activated cell sorting (FACS) analysis revealed that the labeling induced increased levels of maturation markers, including antigen presentation (MHC-II), migration (Ccr7), and co-stimulation (Cd80 and Cd86). In contrast, labeling performed after DC maturation induction did not show this maturation-promoting effect. PEI, as a cationic macromolecule, is widely regarded as an autophagy inducer (Gao et al. 2011). Autophagy is an intracellular degradation process that delivers cytoplasmic materials to the lysosome for degradation and recycling, including damaged cellular contents or foreign species like microbes or nanomaterials. In DCs, autophagy is essential for processing engulfed antigens and promoting cell maturation (Lee et al. 2007). Therefore, PEI–SPION-induced DC maturation could be mediated by autophagy. Our data demonstrated that lactosylated PEI-SPIONs could induce protective autophagy in DCs, as autophagy inhibition with wortmannin led to apoptotic cell death (Shen et al. 2018). FACS data also suggested that autophagy inhibition using 3-Methyladenine (3-MA) reduced DC maturation under both lipopolysaccharide (LPS)-induced and nanoparticle-induced conditions. Liu et al. further provided evidence that SPION-labeled DCs promoted the maturation and migration of DCs in vitro (Liu et al. 2018). Additionally, their data showed that SPIONs coated with 3-aminopropyltrimethoxysilane (APTS, positive charge) exhibited better adjuvant potentials for the promotion of antigen cross-presentation and T cell activation compared to SPIONs coated with meso-2,3-dimercaptosuccinic acid (DMSA, negative charge).

The cellular impact of SPION labeling on macrophage function has also been investigated. Hsiao et al. labeled mouse macrophages (RAW 264.7) with the clinically used SPION, ferucarbotran (Resovist®), and found that SPIO labeling did not affect macrophage viability or proliferation, suggesting the nanoparticles were nontoxic at the concentrations used (Hsiao et al. 2008). However, macrophage functions were differentially influenced by the SPIO concentration. At lower concentrations

(10 mg Fe/mL), phagocytic activity was reduced, whereas at higher concentrations (100 mg Fe/mL), macrophage migration and the production of pro-inflammatory cytokines, including tumor necrosis factor-alpha (TNF-α) and nitric oxide, were enhanced. Our work further demonstrated that lactosylation of PEI could reduce autophagy and cell death in RAW 264.7 cells labeled with PEI-coated SPIONs (Du et al. 2016).

Apart from the intentional labeling of macrophages with IONs, there is a possibility of bystander uptake of these particles by macrophages when tracking other cell types using IONs. This could lead to inaccurate interpretation of tracking results, particularly when using MRI to monitor cell migration. Pawelczyk et al. demonstrated that activated macrophages (AMs), exposed to dextran–SPION (Feridex)-labeled cells in a Boyden chamber model of inflammation, could internalize SPIONs from dead labeled cells (Pawelczyk et al. 2008). After 96 h of incubation, up to 20% of AMs were found to be dextran-positive, indicating uptake of released SPIONs. The extent of SPIONs uptake by AMs depended on the ratio of labeled cells to inflammatory cells and the surrounding microenvironment, suggesting that factors such as inflammation or tissue injury could exacerbate this bystander effect.

Mesenchymal stem cells (MSCs) are stromal cells known for their self-renewal and multilineage differentiation capabilities, making them a prominent focus in regenerative medicine. Unlike the above-discussed immune cells, which have strong phagocytic capabilities, labeling MSCs with IONs typically requires transfection agents. Arbab et al. first established a protocol for labeling human MSCs using a ferumoxides (Feridex)–poly-L-lysine (PLL) complex for in vivo MR tracking (Arbab et al. 2003a). Labeled cells showed no short- or long-term toxicity, no changes in the differentiation capacity of the stem cells, or alterations in phenotype when compared with unlabeled cells (Arbab et al. 2003b). However, a later study suggested that PLL–Feridex-labeling significantly inhibited chondrogenesis in MSCs (Kostura et al. 2004). Notably, this inhibition was not solely attributed to the PLL transfection agent, indicating that either PLL or the combination of PLL and Feridex may play a role in the observation. Although the inhibitory effects of SPIO labeling on differentiation remains debated (Bulte et al. 2004), further study revealed that PLL–SPION labeling has a dose-dependent detrimental effect on chondrogenic differentiation (Roeder et al. 2014). Additionally, chondrogenic gene expression (*COL2A2*, *ACAN*, *SOX9*, *COL10* and *COMP*) was significantly reduced in labeled cells in a dose-dependent manner.

Kim et al. conducted a study comparing the labeling efficiencies of three iron oxide-based MRI contrast agents—Feridex, Resovist, and monocrystalline iron oxide (MION)—in human MSCs (Kim et al. 2010). The results indicated that Feridex and Resovist achieved higher labeling efficiencies than MION when paired with a PLL transfection agent. Despite these differences, cell viability and proliferation remained unaffected by labeling. Notably, *OCT4* mRNA expression increased at day 1 after labeling, and by day 7, the cellular phenotype shifted from $CD45^-$ $CD44^+$ $CD29^+$ to $CD45^{low}$ $CD44^+$ $CD29^+$, resembling freshly isolated bone marrow-derived human MSCs. These findings further highlighted that IONs labeling could lead to changes in gene expression and cell surface markers.

In terms of tissue regenerative potential, neural precursor cells (NPCs) are like MSCs, which have the potential to restore injured tissues. For NPCs, they can be transplanted for the treatment of central nervous system injuries and neurodegenerative disorders. Lepore et al. first demonstrated that PLL-coated SPIONs (Feridex) could successfully label NPCs, including neuronal-restricted precursors and glial-restricted precursors, for MRI tracking following transplantation into the adult spinal cord of rats (Lepore et al. 2006). The study further showed that labeled NPCs retained their ability to differentiate into neurons, astrocytes, and oligodendrocytes, suggesting that SPION labeling did not inhibit NPC differentiation. However, an interesting observation was the induction of an influx of ED1-positive macrophages and microglia in response to the labeled cells. These immune cells internalized small amounts of iron from the grafted NPCs, although the majority of the SPION signal remained within the transplanted cells. Bystander uptake of released IONs has also been observed during long-term monitoring of labeled NSCs. Berman et al. labeled C17.2 NSCs with SPIONs (Molday ION Rhodamine B™) and transplanted the cells into immunodeficient Rag2 mice (graft-accepting) and immunocompetent Balb/c mice (graft-rejecting) for monitoring over a 93-day period (Berman et al. 2011). As expected, the transplanted cells increased in the graft-accepting mice but disappeared in the graft-rejecting mice, as indicated by bioluminescence imaging. However, the hypointense MR signal persisted for a longer period in the rejecting Balb/c mice, while the signal in Rag2 mice cleared more rapidly. They further found that the prolonged MR signal in the graft-rejecting mice was due to the internalization of SPIONs by infiltrating leukocytes and microglia, which surrounded and phagocytosed dead cells. The study emphasized that signal changes observed in long-term MRI tracking may not solely reflect cell death but could also be influenced by live cell proliferation, which leads to dilution of the contrast agent. A study on the long-term monitoring of SPION (Resovist and Endorem)-labeled microglial cells reached a similar conclusion. Cianciaruso et al. transplanted labeled microglial cells, engineered to undergo controlled cell death via a suicide gene, into mouse brains, and monitored them for 90 days using MRI and bioluminescence (Cianciaruso et al. 2014). While MRI successfully detected the presence of the labeled cells, no significant changes in SPION signal voids were observed after the cells underwent controlled death. Ex vivo analyses confirmed that iron nanoparticle deposits persisted at the transplantation site, suggesting that the SPION signal may not accurately reflect the actual presence of live cells. This persistence of the SPION signal could lead to misinterpretations of the fate of labeled cells, particularly when studying cell death or turnover.

Soenen et al. further evaluated the cytotoxicity and labeling efficiency of more types of IONs, including Endorem, Resovist, lipid-coated magnetoliposomes (MLs), and citrate-coated very small iron oxide particles (VSOP) (Soenen et al. 2011). Various cell types, including C17.2 cells, were tested. VSOP induced higher levels of reactive oxygen species (ROS) in C17.2 cells compared to the other three types of IONs. Overall, the study demonstrated that MLs allowed for the highest concentrations of iron per cell without causing toxicity, whereas VSOP were found to be the most toxic. Cromer Berman et al. further demonstrated that the motility of mouse neural stem cells (NSCs, C17.2 cell line) labeled with SPIONs (Molday

ION Rhodamine B) was reduced in vitro (Cromer Berman et al. 2013). Upon transplantation of these labeled NSCs into the mouse brain, rapid exocytosis of SPIO by living cells was observed as early as 48 h post-engraftment. More importantly, SPIO-depleted cells exhibited better migration than those without exocytosis of SPIO. The inhibitory effect on migration was also observed in neural progenitors derived from human induced pluripotent stem cells.

Therefore, while IONs are generally biocompatible, their impact on cell behaviors, including migration, differentiation, and function, needs further exploration. Future research should focus on optimizing IONs to minimize any functional impacts on cells, addressing dose-dependent effects, and improving their accuracy in tracking, particularly in immune cell applications such as stem cell and macrophage tracking.

3 Harnessing ION-Induced Cellular Responses for Therapeutic Purposes

Different cell types exhibit distinct cellular functions and fates. For example, immune cells such as DCs and primary macrophages are terminally differentiated and lack the ability to proliferate or survive long-term. In contrast, MSCs and NPCs possess the capacity for self-renewal and can differentiate into various cell lineages. As a result, certain cellular responses, such as differentiation, may be specific to particular cell types. This distinction in cellular characteristics results in varying responses to IONs, such as differentiation and autophagy, which can be modulated for biomedical applications, including cancer therapy, immune modulation, and tissue regeneration.

Khan et al. found that lab-synthesized IONs selectively induced autophagy in human lung adenocarcinoma cells (A549) while showing minimal toxicity to normal human lung fibroblast cells (IMR-90) (Khan et al. 2012). The autophagy induced by IONs was correlated with ROS production and mitochondrial damage in cancer cells. The use of *N*-acetylcysteine (NAC), an antioxidant, was found to protect cells against ROS-induced damage. 3-MA-prevented autophagy could promote cell viability in cancer cells. Therefore, ION-induced autophagy could offer a selective treatment for killing certain types of cancer cells. Further mechanistic studies revealed that SPIONs disrupt the mitochondrial electron transport chain (METC) in cancer cells, impairing ATP production, mitochondrial membrane potential, and calcium microdistribution, ultimately leading to cell apoptosis (He et al. 2016). Additionally, SPIONs generate mitochondria ROS, resulting in cancer-specific cytotoxicity due to the lower antioxidative capacity of cancer cells.

The application of IONs in cellular research extends beyond tracking and imaging, as they can also influence cellular behavior through controlled magnetic forces. In a study by Shen et al., SPIONs were used to label human umbilical vein endothelial cells (HUVECs), and their responses to intracellular force were analyzed under different magnetic fields (Shen et al. 2014). The nanoparticles were internalized via endocytosis and localized to lysosomes, where they could be repositioned using external magnetic forces. The magnetic manipulation not only repositioned intracellular nanoparticles but also enhanced cell migration, highlighting the potential of SPIONs in manipulating cellular mechanics. Our previous work suggested that lysosomal relocation triggered by pro-inflammatory cytokine stimulus acts as a protective cellular response in various cancer cells (Yu et al. 2022). Therefore, magnetic manipulation of lysosomal relocation could be a promising strategy for cancer cell killing, especially when combined with other therapeutic agents.

After being internalized by cells, IONs trigger a variety of cellular responses, with autophagy being one of the most prominent. Our previous study found that two clinically used SPIONs, Resovist and ferumoxytol (Feraheme®), specifically induced autophagy in macrophages (both primary and cell lines) through the activation of Toll-like receptor 4 (TLR4) on the macrophage membrane (Jin et al. 2019). This activation led to the phosphorylation of p38 and nuclear translocation of Nrf2, which together promoted the expression of autophagy-related genes such as *p62/SQSTM1* and the macrophage scavenger receptor *SR-AI*. Overexpressed p62 in macrophages conjugated with LC3 to form aggresome-like induced structures (ALIS), which subsequently fused with SPION-containing endosomes and lysosomes to create autolysosomes. In vivo studies further demonstrated that intravenously administrated SPIONs induced autophagy in macrophages (Kupffer cells) in mouse liver, the primary imaging target. In addition to autophagy, SPIONs also stimulated the production of inflammatory cytokines through TLR4 signaling in macrophages. Deng et al. further revealed that the carboxylated dextran–SPIONs induced a reduction in macrophage autophagy compared to the unmodified nanoparticles, resulting in a milder inflammatory response (Deng et al. 2022). The reduced autophagy observed with carboxylated dextran–SPIONs was linked to increased albumin adsorption on the nanoparticle surface. Consequently, pro-inflammatory activation of macrophages was effectively reduced, as evidenced by the lower expression of TNF-α, IL-1β, and IL-6. These findings underscore how surface properties of nanoparticles can significantly influence their immune interactions, offering valuable insights for biomedical applications.

We demonstrated that surface modification with glucose significantly enhanced the immunostimulatory efficacy of IONs compared to mannose and galactose (Liu et al. 2024). In vitro studies showed that glucosylation enhanced the pro-inflammatory efficacy of IONs by up to 300-fold, even surpassing that of LPS under certain conditions. In vivo investigations revealed that glucosylated IONs elicited increased anticancer immunity and achieved favorable therapeutic outcomes in multiple mouse tumor models. Mechanistically, glucosylation was found to amplify the immunostimulatory effect of IONs by enhancing TLR4 activation. Specifically, glucosylated IONs directly interacted with the TLR4-MD2 complex, resulting in M1 macrophage polarization and enhanced anticancer immunity via activation of the NF-κB, MAPK, and STAT1 signaling pathways. These findings highlight the potential of IONs as a promising tool for augmenting immune responses and advancing cancer therapy.

In addition to autophagy activation, Zhang et al. showed that SPIO-nanoworms pre-incubated with human serum (SPIO–Serum) induced ferroptosis in human ovarian cancer cells (SKOV3 and A2780). SPIO-Serum effectively triggered lipid peroxidation and generated abundant toxic ROS (Zhang et al. 2021). It also downregulated *GPX4* and *xCT*, resulting in iron-dependent oxidative cell death. Furthermore, SPIO-Serum disrupted intracellular iron homeostasis by regulating iron uptake, and the cells exhibited missing mitochondrial cristae and ruptured outer mitochondrial membranes. This study suggests that leveraging ferroptosis through SPIO–Serum could offer a promising approach for ovarian cancer treatment, overcoming the limitations of conventional therapeutic.

The unexpected biological activity of IONs extends beyond cancer treatment. We found that both Feraheme and Resovist intrinsically inhibit receptor activator NF-κB ligand (RANKL)-induced osteoclastogenesis in bone marrow-derived monocytes/macrophages (BMMs) (Liu et al. 2020). IONs significantly suppressed the formation of tartrate-resistant acid phosphatase (TRAP)-positive multinuclear osteoclasts and functional actin ring structures. More importantly, this inhibitory effect was verified in vivo, as intravenous injection of IONs effectively mitigated bone loss in ovariectomized (OVX) mice. Mechanistically, IONs upregulated p62, leading to the recruitment of CYLD and enhanced deubiquitination of TRAF6, a master controller of RANKL signaling. Consequently, downstream activation of NF-κB and MAPK signaling pathways was attenuated, reducing expression of osteoclastogenesis-related genes. Taken together, clinically used IONs can inhibit osteoclastogenesis through regulation of the TRAF6-p62-CYLD signaling complex, highlighting their potential as alternative therapeutic agents for osteoporosis.

Li et al. designed a core-shell nanostructure featuring SPIONs as the core and hydroxyapatite (HA) as the shell (Li et al. 2021). The dual-functional nanomaterial not only inhibited osteoclastogenesis but also promoted osteogenesis. Mechanistic studies suggested that the SPIONs suppressed the differentiation of osteoclasts from bone marrow monocytes by modulating the TRAF6-p62-CYLD signaling complex. Simultaneously, SPIONs enhanced the osteogenic differentiation of MSCs by regulating the TGF-β, PI3K-AKT, and calcium signaling pathways. In vivo experiments demonstrated that SPIONs significantly prevented bone loss in OVX mice and increased bone mineral density (BMD) by 9.4%. Additionally, Zheng et al. developed bone-targeting antioxidative IONs (Zheng et al. 2022). They demonstrated that daily administration of the IONs alleviated estrogen deficiency-induced osteoporosis in vivo by scavenging ROS, a key contributor to bone loss in osteoporotic conditions. The IONs also promoted osteogenic differentiation of bone marrow MSCs and inhibited osteoclast differentiation from monocytes in treated mice.

Autophagy activation is generally regarded as a cellular protective process. Duan et al. showed that lab-synthesized dextran–SPIONs could be internalized by HUVECs without causing obvious cytotoxicity while effectively triggering autophagy (Duan et al. 2019). Notably, dextran–SPIONs enhanced HUVEC survival under oxidative stress conditions induced by H_2O_2. This protective effect was attributed to autophagy activation, which was suppressed by the autophagy inhibitor 3-MA. Further investigation revealed that dextran–SPIONs induced autophagy by reducing the phosphorylation of PRAS40, a key upstream regulator of autophagy initiation. These findings highlight the potential of dextran–SPIONs as a therapeutic agent for enhancing cellular resilience against oxidative stress via autophagy activation.

ION-triggered cellular responses in one cell type can be utilized to affect another cell type. Xu et al. found that lab-synthesized SPIONs promoted the survival of MSCs by upregulating *HO-1* expression under inflammatory conditions (Xu et al. 2021). SPION-labeled MSCs (SPION-MSCs) significantly improved cecal ligation and puncture (CLP)- or LPS-induced sepsis and liver injury in mice after infusion, enhancing macrophage polarization to the M2 type, an anti-inflammatory phenotype. This regulation of macrophage polarization was dependent on MSC-expressed TRAF1. Additionally, they showed that SPION-MSCs homed to the lungs and liver after infusion, staying longer in injured organs, and provided long-term protection in sepsis (Pan et al. 2022). SPIO-induced ferroptosis of MSCs promoted the efferocytosis of macrophages, reprogramming them to the M2 type, which further protected mice against sepsis. Consequently, inhibition of ferroptosis using Ferrostatin-1 or Liproxtatin-1 impaired the therapeutic benefits of SPION-MSCs. Therefore, ION labeling can modify MSCs to alter macrophage function. This cross-cell communication provides protective effects during bacterial infection, contributing to improved outcomes in sepsis.

The above findings demonstrate that IONs have significant therapeutic potential by inducing cellular responses such as autophagy, ferroptosis, and differentiation, which can be tailored for tumor, immune modulation, and tissue regeneration therapies. Surface modifications and controlled exposure enhance their effectiveness in specific therapeutic contexts. However, further research is needed to optimize biocompatibility, targeting, and controlled release to improve their clinical applicability.

4 Conclusions

Together, these findings highlight both the undesired biological effects of ION labeling and the emerging therapeutic effects associated with their controlled use (Fig. 1). While originally developed as MRI contrast agents, IONs are increasingly recognized as versatile regulators of cellular behavior. The ability of IONs to induce specific cellular responses, such as autophagy and ferroptosis, presents new avenues for therapeutic interventions. An important insight into the therapeutic potential of IONs is their ability to manipulate cellular mechanisms that are critical in disease progression and recovery. This includes their role in enhancing cell differentiation or triggering cell death pathways, which could be harnessed to target cancer cells or boost immune responses. The need for finely tuned surface modifications and controlled delivery systems to precisely manage their biological effects becomes apparent, as improper regulation could lead to unwanted side effects like immune activation or impaired cell function. The challenge going forward lies in understanding how IONs induce cellular responses across various cell types and

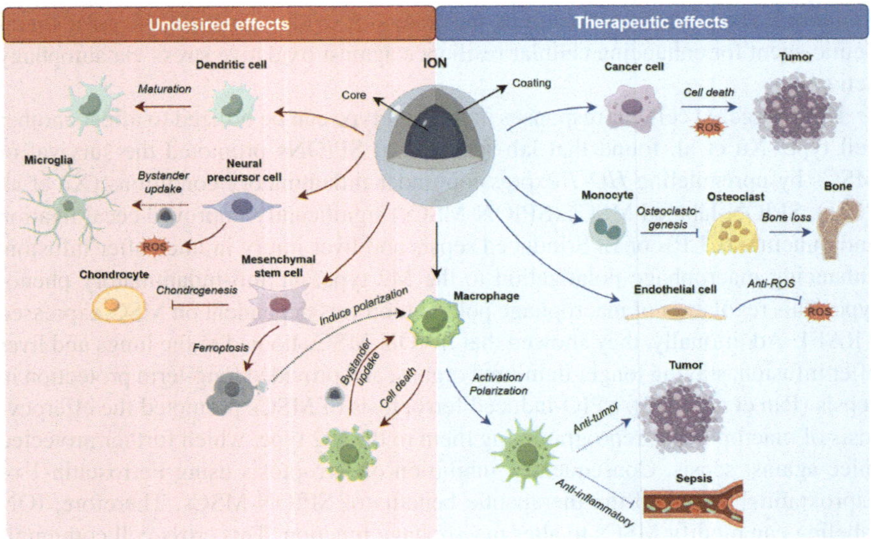

Fig. 1 Dual biological impacts of IONs on diverse cell types. Schematic overview illustrating the undesired (left) and therapeutic (right) cellular effects of IONs. Created by FigDraw (Figdraw.com)

the mechanisms behind these interactions. Questions remain: 1) How do IONs trigger distinct responses across different cell types and physiological states? 2) Are there specific receptors or sensing mechanisms that directly recognize IONs or their surface properties? 3) How do variations in size, composition, and surface chemistry dictate intracellular trafficking and downstream signaling pathways? 4) How do long-term accumulation, degradation, and metabolic processing of IONs influence cellular homeostasis and organismal health? 5) Can the balance between beneficial and deleterious effects be predictively controlled through rational nanoparticle design?Answering these questions could enable the modulation of ION's effects for targeted therapeutic outcomes. With their MRI visibility, IONs have the potential to evolve into theranostic agents, combining diagnostic and therapeutic functions in a single nanomaterial for future clinical applications.

Acknowledgements None.

Conflicts of Interest The authors declare no competing interests.

References

E.T. Ahrens, M. Feili-Hariri, H. Xu, G. Genove, P.A. Morel, Receptor-mediated endocytosis of iron-oxide particles provides efficient labeling of dendritic cells for in vivo MR imaging. Magn. Reson. Med. **49**, 1006–1013 (2003). https://doi.org/10.1002/mrm.10465

E. Alphandery, Biodistribution and targeting properties of iron oxide nanoparticles for treatments of cancer and iron anemia disease. Nanotoxicology **13**, 573–596 (2019). https://doi.org/10.1080/17435390.2019.1572809

A.S. Arbab et al., Intracytoplasmic tagging of cells with ferumoxides and transfection agent for cellular magnetic resonance imaging after cell transplantation: methods and techniques. Transplantation **76**, 1123–1130 (2003a). https://doi.org/10.1097/01.TP.0000089237.39220.83

A.S. Arbab et al., Characterization of biophysical and metabolic properties of cells labeled with superparamagnetic iron oxide nanoparticles and transfection agent for cellular MR imaging. Radiology **229**, 838–846 (2003b). https://doi.org/10.1148/radiol.2293021215

S.C. Berman, C. Galpoththawela, A.A. Gilad, J.W. Bulte, P. Walczak, Long-term MR cell tracking of neural stem cells grafted in immunocompetent versus immunodeficient mice reveals distinct differences in contrast between live and dead cells. Magn. Reson. Med. **65**, 564–574 (2011). https://doi.org/10.1002/mrm.22613

J.W.M. Bulte, Superparamagnetic iron oxides as MPI tracers: a primer and review of early applications. Adv. Drug Deliv. Rev. **138**, 293–301 (2019). https://doi.org/10.1016/j.addr.2018.12.007

J.W. Bulte, D.L. Kraitchman, A.M. Mackay, M.F. Pittenger, Chondrogenic differentiation of mesenchymal stem cells is inhibited after magnetic labeling with ferumoxides. Blood **104**, 3410–3412; author reply 3412–3413 (2004). https://doi.org/10.1182/blood-2004-06-2117

J.W. Bulte, C. Wang, A. Shakeri-Zadeh, In vivo cellular magnetic imaging: labeled versus unlabeled cells. Adv. Funct. Mater. **32**, 2207626 (2022)

C. Cianciaruso et al., Cellular magnetic resonance with iron oxide nanoparticles: long-term persistence of SPIO signal in the CNS after transplanted cell death. Nanomedicine (Lond.) **9**, 1457–1474 (2014). https://doi.org/10.2217/nnm.14.84

S.M. Cromer Berman et al., Cell motility of neural stem cells is reduced after SPIO-labeling, which is mitigated after exocytosis. Magn. Reson. Med. **69**, 255–262 (2013). https://doi.org/10.1002/mrm.24216

S.N. de Chickera et al., Labelling dendritic cells with SPIO has implications for their subsequent in vivo migration as assessed with cellular MRI. Contrast Media Mol. Imaging **6**, 314–327 (2011). https://doi.org/10.1002/cmmi.433

D. Deng et al., Surface carboxylation of iron oxide nanoparticles brings reduced macrophage inflammatory response through inhibiting macrophage autophagy. Regener. Biomater. **9**, rbac018 (2022). https://doi.org/10.1093/rb/rbac018

J. Du et al., Reduction of polyethylenimine-coated iron oxide nanoparticles induced autophagy and cytotoxicity by lactosylation. Regener. Biomater. **3**, 223–229 (2016). https://doi.org/10.1093/rb/rbw023

J. Duan et al., Iron oxide nanoparticles promote vascular endothelial cells survival from oxidative stress by enhancement of autophagy. Regener. Biomater. **6**, 221–229 (2019). https://doi.org/10.1093/rb/rbz024

F. Fletcher, E. London, Intravenous iron. Br. Med. J. **1**, 984 (1954)

X. Gao et al., The association of autophagy with polyethylenimine-induced cytotoxicity in nephritic and hepatic cell lines. Biomaterials **32**, 8613–8625 (2011). https://doi.org/10.1016/j.biomaterials.2011.07.047

R.K. Gilchrist et al., Selective inductive heating of lymph nodes. Ann. Surg. **146**, 596–606 (1957). https://doi.org/10.1097/00000658-195710000-00007

A.K. Gupta, M. Gupta, Synthesis and surface engineering of iron oxide nanoparticles for biomedical applications. Biomaterials **26**, 3995–4021 (2005). https://doi.org/10.1016/j.biomaterials.2004.10.012

C. He et al., Mitochondrial electron transport chain identified as a novel molecular target of SPIO nanoparticles mediated cancer-specific cytotoxicity. Biomaterials **83**, 102–114 (2016). https://doi.org/10.1016/j.biomaterials.2016.01.010

J.K. Hsiao et al., Macrophage physiological function after superparamagnetic iron oxide labeling. NMR Biomed. **21**, 820–829 (2008). https://doi.org/10.1002/nbm.1260

R. Jin, B. Lin, D. Li, H. Ai, Superparamagnetic iron oxide nanoparticles for MR imaging and therapy: design considerations and clinical applications. Curr. Opin. Pharmacol. **18**, 18–27 (2014). https://doi.org/10.1016/j.coph.2014.08.002

R. Jin et al., Iron oxide nanoparticles promote macrophage autophagy and inflammatory response through activation of toll-like receptor-4 signaling. Biomaterials **203**, 23–30 (2019). https://doi.org/10.1016/j.biomaterials.2019.02.026

R. Jin et al., Clinical translational barriers against nanoparticle-based imaging agents. Adv. Drug Deliv. Rev. **191**, 114587 (2022). https://doi.org/10.1016/j.addr.2022.114587

M.I. Khan et al., Induction of ROS, mitochondrial damage and autophagy in lung epithelial cancer cells by iron oxide nanoparticles. Biomaterials **33**, 1477–1488 (2012). https://doi.org/10.1016/j.biomaterials.2011.10.080

H.S. Kim et al., The effects of clinically used MRI contrast agents on the biological properties of human mesenchymal stem cells. NMR Biomed. **23**, 514–522 (2010). https://doi.org/10.1002/nbm.1487

L. Kostura, D.L. Kraitchman, A.M. Mackay, M.F. Pittenger, J.W. Bulte, Feridex labeling of mesenchymal stem cells inhibits chondrogenesis but not adipogenesis or osteogenesis. NMR Biomed. **17**, 513–517 (2004). https://doi.org/10.1002/nbm.925

H.K. Lee, J.M. Lund, B. Ramanathan, N. Mizushima, A. Iwasaki, Autophagy-dependent viral recognition by plasmacytoid dendritic cells. Science **315**, 1398–1401 (2007). https://doi.org/10.1126/science.1136880

A.C. Lepore, P. Walczak, M.S. Rao, I. Fischer, J.W. Bulte, MR imaging of lineage-restricted neural precursors following transplantation into the adult spinal cord. Exp. Neurol. **201**, 49–59 (2006). https://doi.org/10.1016/j.expneurol.2006.03.032

M. Li et al., Dual regulation of osteoclastogenesis and osteogenesis for osteoporosis therapy by iron oxide hydroxyapatite core/shell nanocomposites. Regener. Biomater. **8**, rbab027 (2021). https://doi.org/10.1093/rb/rbab027

D. Ling, N. Lee, T. Hyeon, Chemical synthesis and assembly of uniformly sized iron oxide nanoparticles for medical applications. Acc. Chem. Res. **48**, 1276–1285 (2015). https://doi.org/10.1021/acs.accounts.5b00038

G. Liu, J. Gao, H. Ai, X. Chen, Applications and potential toxicity of magnetic iron oxide nanoparticles. Small **9**, 1533–1545 (2013). https://doi.org/10.1002/smll.201201531

H. Liu et al., SPIO enhance the cross-presentation and migration of DCs and anionic SPIO influence the nanoadjuvant effects related to interleukin-1beta. Nanoscale Res. Lett. **13**, 409 (2018). https://doi.org/10.1186/s11671-018-2802-0

L. Liu et al., Bioactive iron oxide nanoparticles suppress osteoclastogenesis and ovariectomy-induced bone loss through regulating the TRAF6-p62-CYLD signaling complex. Acta Biomater. **103**, 281–292 (2020). https://doi.org/10.1016/j.actbio.2019.12.022

L. Liu et al., Glucosylation endows nanoparticles with TLR4 agonist capability to trigger macrophage polarization and augment antitumor immunity. Biomaterials **304**, 122424 (2024). https://doi.org/10.1016/j.biomaterials.2023.122424

E. London, The molecular formula and proposed structure of the iron-dextran complex, imferon. J. Pharm. Sci. **93**, 1838–1846 (2004). https://doi.org/10.1002/jps.20093

Y. Pan et al., Ferroptotic MSCs protect mice against sepsis via promoting macrophage efferocytosis. Cell Death Dis. **13**, 825 (2022). https://doi.org/10.1038/s41419-022-05264-z

E. Pawelczyk et al., In vitro model of bromodeoxyuridine or iron oxide nanoparticle uptake by activated macrophages from labeled stem cells: implications for cellular therapy. Stem Cells **26**, 1366–1375 (2008). https://doi.org/10.1634/stemcells.2007-0707

E. Roeder et al., Dose-response of superparamagnetic iron oxide labeling on mesenchymal stem cells chondrogenic differentiation: a multi-scale in vitro study. PLoS One **9**, e98451 (2014). https://doi.org/10.1371/journal.pone.0098451

H. Shen, S. Tong, G. Bao, B. Wang, Structural responses of cells to intracellular magnetic force induced by superparamagnetic iron oxide nanoparticles. Phys. Chem. Chem. Phys. **16**, 1914–1920 (2014). https://doi.org/10.1039/c3cp51435h

T. Shen et al., Lactosylated N-alkyl polyethylenimine coated iron oxide nanoparticles induced autophagy in mouse dendritic cells. Regener. Biomater. **5**, 141–149 (2018). https://doi.org/10.1093/rb/rbx032

S.J. Soenen, U. Himmelreich, N. Nuytten, M. De Cuyper, Cytotoxic effects of iron oxide nanoparticles and implications for safety in cell labelling. Biomaterials **32**, 195–205 (2011). https://doi.org/10.1016/j.biomaterials.2010.08.075

A.S. Teja, P.-Y. Koh, Synthesis, properties, and applications of magnetic iron oxide nanoparticles. Prog. Cryst. Growth Charact. Mater. **55**, 22–45 (2009)

D.L. Thorek, A.K. Chen, J. Czupryna, A. Tsourkas, Superparamagnetic iron oxide nanoparticle probes for molecular imaging. Ann. Biomed. Eng. **34**, 23–38 (2006). https://doi.org/10.1007/s10439-005-9002-7

Y. Xu et al., Superparamagnetic MRI probes for in vivo tracking of dendritic cell migration with a clinical 3 T scanner. Biomaterials **58**, 63–71 (2015). https://doi.org/10.1016/j.biomaterials.2015.04.016

Y. Xu et al., SPION-MSCs enhance therapeutic efficacy in sepsis by regulating MSC-expressed TRAF1-dependent macrophage polarization. Stem Cell Res. Ther. **12**, 531 (2021). https://doi.org/10.1186/s13287-021-02593-2

K. Yu et al., Visualizing lysosomal positioning with a fluorescent probe reveals a new synergistic anticancer effect. ACS Sens. **7**, 1867–1873 (2022). https://doi.org/10.1021/acssensors.2c00375

Y. Zhang et al., p53 promoted ferroptosis in ovarian cancer cells treated with human serum incubated-superparamagnetic iron oxides. Int. J. Nanomedicine **16**, 283–296 (2021). https://doi.org/10.2147/IJN.S282489

L. Zheng et al., Bone targeting antioxidative nano-iron oxide for treating postmenopausal osteoporosis. Bioact. Mater. **14**, 250–261 (2022). https://doi.org/10.1016/j.bioactmat.2021.11.012

Carbon Biomaterials for Sensing

Tharini Jeyapragasam, Sridhar Jayavel, Meena Devi J, Lakshmi Narayanan, Prathingara Subramanian, and Rasu Ramachandran

Abstract The extensive use of pesticides in modern agriculture has resulted in severe contamination of food, water, and soil, posing significant risks to human health and the environment. Although conventional analytical techniques such as high-performance liquid chromatography (HPLC), gas chromatography–mass spectrometry (GC–MS) and spectrophotometry provide excellent sensitivity and reliability, they are constrained by expensive instrumentation, complex sample preparation, and the need for skilled personnel. The carbon based nanomaterials have emerged as promising alternatives due to their high surface area, excellent electrical conductivity, mechanical stability, biocompatibility, and ease of functionalization. This chapter reviews the application of carbon biomaterials, particularly Carbon nanomaterials such as carbon nanotubes, graphene-based nanomaterials, and carbon dots for the sensitive detection of organophosphates, carbamate, pyrethroids, and organochlorine pesticides. The various sensing approaches including electrochemical, colorimetric, fluorometric, surface enhanced Raman scattering (SERS) based and enzyme based biosensors are comprehensively discussed. These carbon-based sensing platforms

T. Jeyapragasam (✉) · S. Jayavel
Department of Biotechnology (CDOE), Madurai Kamaraj University, Madurai, Tamil Nadu, India
e-mail: tharinichem@gmail.com

S. Jayavel
e-mail: jsridharbiotech@mkuniversity.ac.in

M. D. J (✉)
Department of Physics, School of Electrical and Electronics Engineering (SEEE), SASTRA Deemed University, Thanjavur, Tamil Nadu, India
e-mail: jmeenadevi@sastra.ac.in

L. Narayanan
Department of Science and Humanities, Sethu Institute of Technology, Kariapatti, Tamil Nadu, India
e-mail: lkrithick@gmail.com

P. Subramanian · R. Ramachandran
Department of Chemistry, Madura College, Madurai, Tamil Nadu, India
e-mail: brindhachemi18@gmail.com

R. Ramachandran
e-mail: ultraramji@gmail.com

R. Narayan (ed.), *Nanostructured Biomaterials and Their Applications*,
https://doi.org/10.1007/978-3-032-16316-5_11

provide rapid, selective, portable, and highly sensitive detection, often achieving nanomolar to picomolar-level detection limits, making them promising candidates for real-time food safety monitoring and environmental surveillance.

Keywords Carbon nanomaterials · Carbon nanotubes · Electrochemical sensors · Graphene

1 Introduction

In the developing countries, there is a decline in the agricultural land due to the increase in the human population, industrialization and urban sprawl. Hence, the usages of pesticides have been increased tremendously throughout the world. A pesticide is a chemical used to prevent, destroy or repel pests. The pests can be the insects, mice and other animals, weeds, fungi or microorganisms such as bacteria and viruses. Some examples of the pests are termites causing the damage to our homes, dandelions in the lawn and fleas on our dogs and cats. The pesticides are also used to kill the organisms such as mosquitoes, ticks, rats and mice that can cause diseases. The pesticides are mainly used in the agriculture to boost the productivity, crop quality and combat diseases. The pesticides can be classified based on the mode of biological target, chemical structure or safety profile (Krieger 2001). Pesticide is the general term used to describe groups of insecticides, fungicides, herbicides, nematicides, rodenticides, miticides, molluscicides, bactericides and algaecides.

However, the presence of pesticide residues in the food, water and soil has become a major issue in environmental chemistry. Even the low levels of contaminants can cause adverse effects on humans, plants, animals and ecosystems. Over 98% of the sprayed insecticides and 95% of the herbicides reach a destination other than their target species. The pesticides enter the environment either through an application, spill, adsorption, transfer, breakdown and degradation which remain persistent in the environment and ultimately pollute the environment. When a pesticide is applied directly to a target pest (plant or animal), the whole site is affected including crop plants, soil organisms, potentially humans and wild life in the immediate area. In addition, part of it goes to the air or to surface water, due to emission or drift and other part may drain into surface water or volatilize into the air. From the air, it may get transmitted to humans, wild life or plants or the soil. During this process, the pesticides may also leach into ground water. The pesticides in surface water may go into aquatic organisms and by sedimentation into other organisms that remain in the sediment. The persistence of the pesticide depends on its physical, chemical properties and the characteristics of the environment. There are several mechanisms for acute toxicity such as irritation, allergic sensitization, enzyme inhibition, oxidative damage, inhibition of neurotransmission and uncoupling of oxidative phosphorylation. The short-term exposure leads to the abnormal growth and development, impaired neurobehavioral development/functions, cancer, increased susceptibility to infections. The acute toxicity of pesticides leads to dermal and ocular irritation, upper and lower respiratory tract irritation, allergic responses/asthma, gastrointestinal symptoms, chronic illnesses such as cancer, fertility issues, endocrine disruptors,

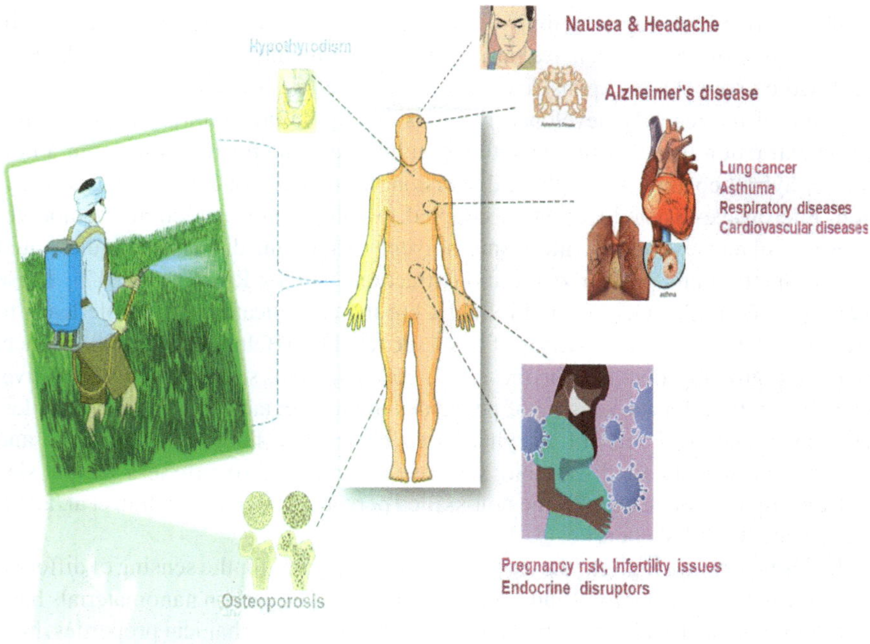

Fig. 1 Short and long-term exposure of pesticides

neurological symptoms, cholinergic crisis, osteoporosis, bleeding, caustic lesions and pulmonary fibrosis. The exposure of pesticide before or during pregnancy has increased the risks such as prenatal death, spontaneous abortion, premature birth, foetal growth retardation, congenital malformations and early childhood cancer (Aragay et al. 2012). The exposure of pesticide during the brain growth has the permanent effects on the brain structure and function, neuronal and axonal differentiation, serotoninergic system, synaptogenesis, programming of synaptic function. Figure 1 illustrates the short-term and long-term exposure of pesticides on human beings (Fig. 1). All this information clearly points out the need for control in the use of pesticides and also for developing suitable methods for their simple and effective analysis.

2 Methods for Pesticides Detection

In the current scenario, there are several methods available for monitoring and sensing of pesticides and their residue in different matrices. The most commonly used methods are high-performance liquid chromatography, gas chromatography with different detectors such as nitrogen phosphorous detector, pulsed flame photometry, mass spectrometry, large volume injection, microwave emission and spectrophotometry (Alvarez-Rodriguez et al. 1997; Moreno-Camacho et al. 2019). These methods offer high reproducibility, lower detection limits, require extraction of large volume of water, extensive purification, often include derivatization, demand qualified personnel and expensive equipment (Luo et al. 2019).

Some of the recently developed methods of sample preparation includes solid-phase extraction using carbon nanotubes, solid-phase microextraction using a new sol-gel hybrid coating, solid-phase dispersion, headspace-solid-phase microextraction, microwave-assisted extraction coupled to solid-phase extraction, membrane-assisted solvent extraction, ultrasonic solvent extraction, dispersive liquid-liquid microextraction and pressurized liquid extraction (Gómez-Ríos et al. 2017). These methods are highly sensitive and reliable, but the complication of sample leads to the delayed detection and analysis of pesticide residues (Beltrán et al. 2000). Hence, there is a growing demand for the rapid, cost-effective, simple, highly sensitive, selective method for the sensing of pesticides in the vegetables and fruits' samples. The electrochemical sensors, enzyme-based biosensors, fluorescence sensors and colorimetric sensors are disposable, selective and reliable, require less sample size and are easy to operate even by the non-skilled personnel (Ramachandran et al. 2019; Picci et al. 2024; Eskandari et al. 2022).

In this review, we higlight the usage of carbon materials for the sensing of different pesticide residues in the food and vegetable samples. The carbon nanomaterials have extraordinary electrical conductivity, thermal properties, mechanical properties, high stability, low toxicity, biocompatibility and higher surface area. Therefore, it is a suitable and promising material for the sensing of pesticides in the food samples. Furthermore, we discuss the classification of pesticides and their structure.

3 Classification of Pesticides

The pesticides can be classified based on their use, chemical nature, formation, toxicity and mode of action. The most common way of classifying pesticide based on their chemical composition and nature of active ingredients. This classification gives the information about the physical and chemical properties of the respective pesticides. The information about the physical and chemical properties of the pesticides is important in determining the mode of application. It is classified into organochlorines, organophosphates, carbamates and pyrethroid (Hoffman et al. 2002) (Fig. 2). The other way of classification pesticides is based on pest target organisms, and pesticides are given specific names to reflect their action. The pesticides worldwide are divided into different categories according to their target organisms, and pesticides are given specific names to reflect their action. Depending on the target, pesticides are divided into insecticides (that kill insect), rodenticides (that kill rate and mice), avicides (that kill birds), fungicides (that kill fungi), herbicides (that kill weeds and other plants), virucides (that kill virus), molluscicides (that kill molluscs) and nematicides (that kill nematodes) (Garcia et al. 2012; Dhuldhaj et al. 2023) (Fig. 3). The excessive use of the pesticides has raised serious concerns about the human health and biodiversity (Pumera 2011; Chen et al. 2012).

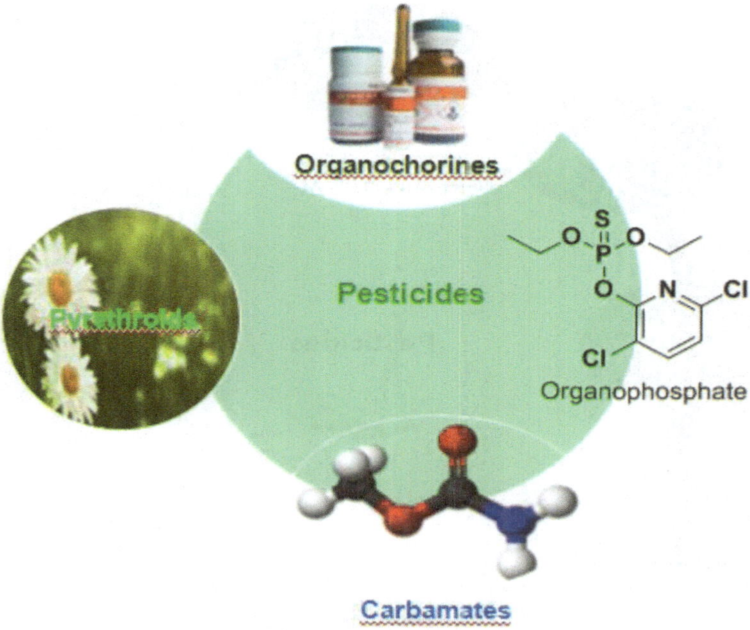

Fig. 2 Classification of pesticides based on mode of application

4 Organophosphates Pesticides

The highly toxic *acetylcholinesterase* (AChE)-inhibiting organophosphates (OP) and carbamate compounds are intensively used as pesticides in the world. OP is known to be highly neurotoxic and commonly used as the chemical warfare agents and pesticides. More than 70% of the pesticides used over the entire world are OP pesticides and their derivatives (Du et al. 2006). Some of the OP compounds are also used as parasiticides in veterinary medicine and as warfare agents. The synthesis of an OP pesticide was first reported in 1854 by Philippe de Clermont. The first insecticide bladan was made commercially available in 1940. The OP pesticides are esters of phosphoric acid (P=O) or phosphorothioic (P=S) acid. The general structure of OP pesticide is given in Fig. 4 (Table 1).

5 Carbamate Pesticides

The carbamate pesticides are esters of carbamic acid and they are classified into *N*-methyl carbamate, thiocarbamate and dithiocarbamate. *N*-methyl carbamate has an oxygen moiety attached at the R_3 position and whose carbamate cation is double bonded to oxygen (Fig. 5). R_1 and R_2 may both be methyl groups (*N*-methylcarbamates—e.g. pirimicarb, Fig. 6) or R_1 may be hydrogen and R_2 a methyl group (*N*-methylcarbamates—e.g. aldicarb, Fig. 7). Carbamates' pesticides whose

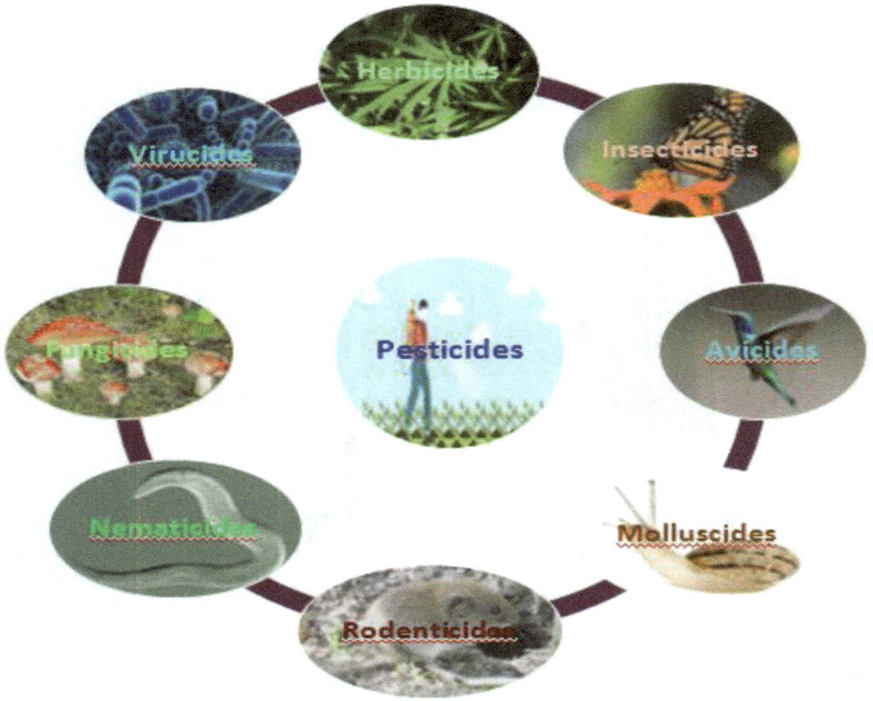

Fig. 3 Classification of pesticides based on pest target organism

Fig. 4 General structure of OP

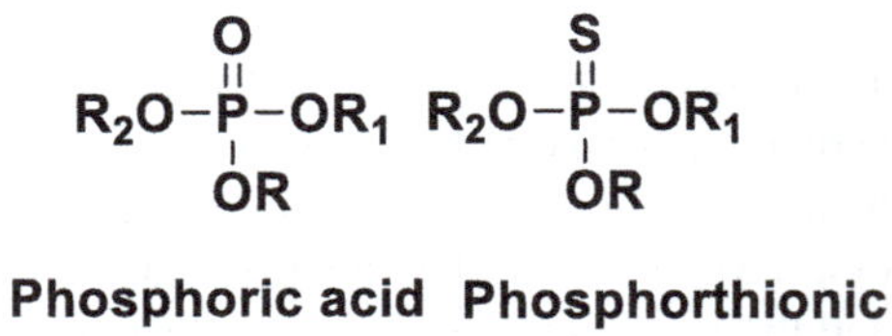

R_1 and R_2 groups are generally larger than hydrogen or a methyl group tend to possess a much reduced anticholinesterase activity and are marketed as herbicides or fungicides.

Thiocarbamates have a sulphur atom attached at the R_3 position and whose carbamate cation is double bonded to oxygen (Fig. 8). Thiocarbamates (e.g. thiobencarb—Fig. 9) are used as herbicides and possess the structural properties required to cause acetylcholine inhibition. Thiocarbamates are far less potent AChE inhibitors than the group *N*-methyl carbamate.

Dithiocarbamates have a sulphur atom attached at the R_3 position and whose carbamate cation is double bonded to sulphur (Fig. 10). Dithiocarbamates (e.g. thiram—Fig. 11) are also used as fungicides and capable of causing AChE inhibition at higher doses.

Table 1 Chemical structure of important organophosphates pesticides

Name of the pesticides	Structure of pesticides
Dichlorvos	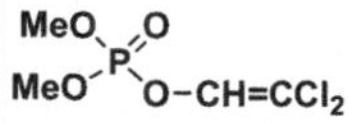
Dimethoate	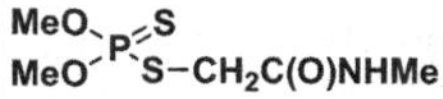
Methamidophos	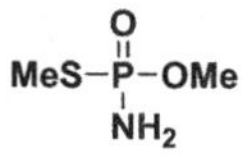
Parathion-methyl	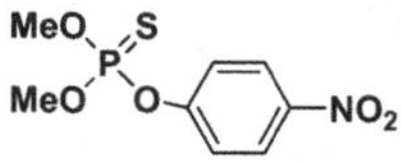
Chlorpyrifos	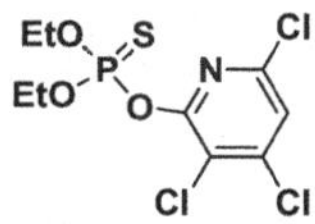
Malathion	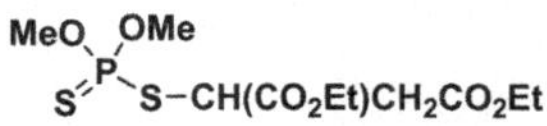
Glyphosate	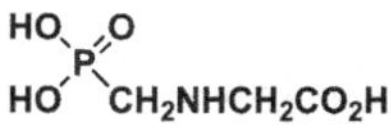
Glufosinate	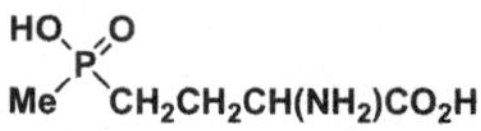
Acephate	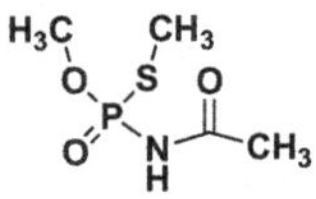

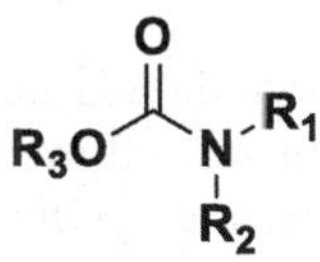

Fig. 5 General structure of carbamate pesticide

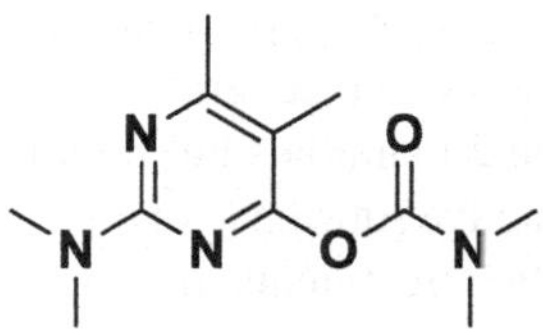

Fig. 6 Structure of pirimicarb

Fig. 7 Structure of aldicarb

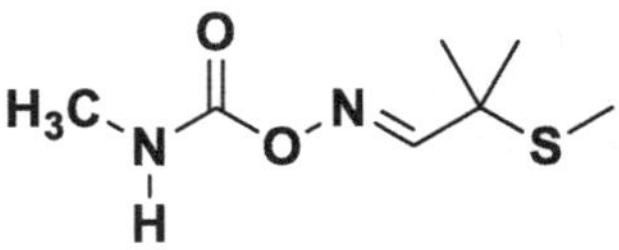

Fig. 8 Structure of thiocarbamate

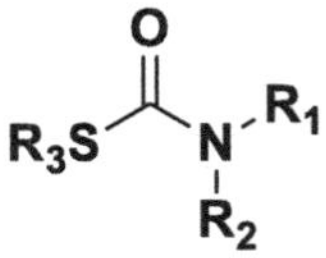

Fig. 9 Structure of thiobencarb

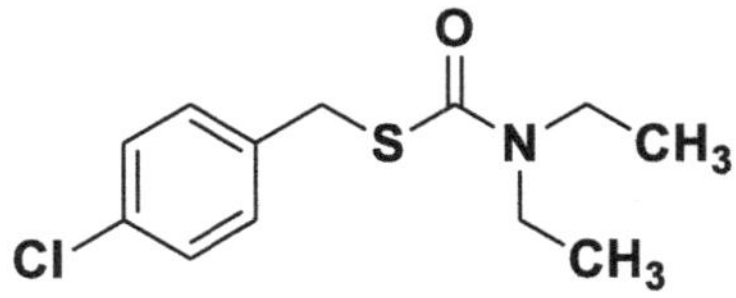

Fig. 10 Structure of dithiocarbamate

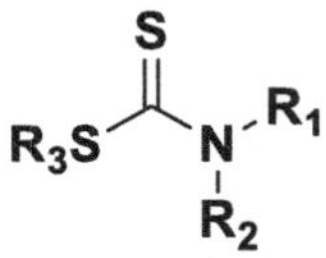

Fig. 11 Structure of thiram

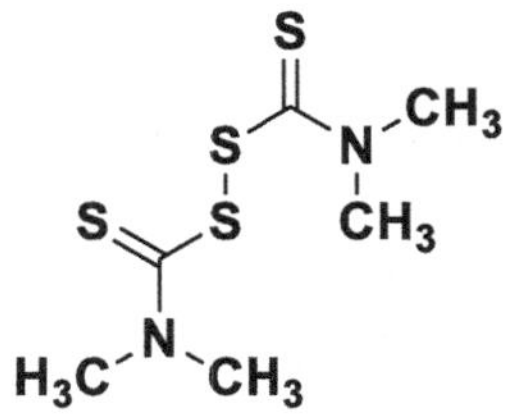

6 Pyrethroid Pesticides

Pyrethroids are natural insecticides derived from the pyrethrum extracts of chrysanthemum flowers known as pyrethrin found in Kenya. By duplicating the structure of natural pyrethrins, synthetic pyrethroid pesticides can be synthesized, which is the group of organic pesticides. The most commonly used synthetic pyrethroid pesticides are cypermethrin and permethrin (Hassaan and El Nemr 2020). Figure 12 shows the general structure of pyrethroid pesticides. They have low toxicity to birds and mammals but high toxicity to arthropods (Narahashi et al. 1992). They are the active substance in many commercial products including pet shampoos, human head lice treatments, pet sprays and topical mosquito repellents.

7 Organochlorine Pesticides (OCPs)

The organochlorine pesticides are chlorinated hydrocarbons used in agriculture and mosquito control. They are stable chemicals that are persistent in the environment and have the tendency to affect the enzymatic nerve membranes and electrophysiological properties (Narahashi et al. 1992). Figures 13 and 14 show the structure of some of the important OCPs pesticides.

8 Carbon Nanomaterials

The rapid advancement of nanoscience and nanotechnology has enchanced significant progress in the tailored synthesis of nanomaterials and the understanding of their unique physical and chemical properties. of nanotechnology The carbon nanomaterials belong to the family of carbon allotropes which includes zero-dimensional materials fullerenes and carbon quantum dots, two-dimensional carbon nanotubes, two-dimensional graphene and three-dimensional nanodiamonds and nanohorns (Geim and Novoselov 2007) (Fig. 15). The carbon nanomaterials are available with the varied arrangement of sp^2 and sp^3 hybridized carbon atoms and hence resulting in the extensive applications in the field of materials science, technology, biology and others. The one-dimensional properties of carbon nanotubes have excellent advantages such as large surface-to-volume ratio, water solubility, electrical properties, mechanical properties, biocompatibility, higher immobilization efficiency and strong photo-luminescence. The fullerenes are the closed cage-type nanomaterials consisting of 20 hexagonal and 12 pentagonal rings. The spherical form of the fullerene nanomaterial contributes to the large surface area (Onyancha et al. 2022; Aguilar 2013). The carbon quantum dots have tuneable physical, chemical, optical

Fig. 12 Structure of pyrethroid

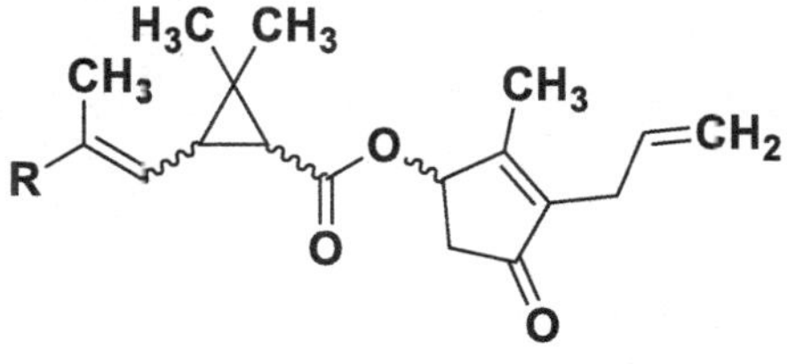

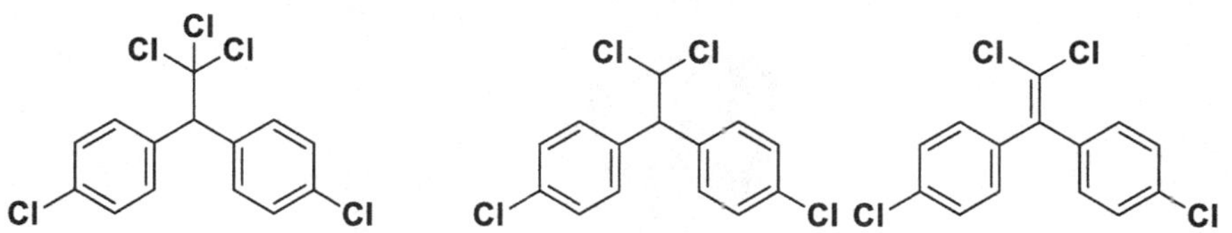

Fig. 13 Structure of dichloro diphenyl trichloroethane (DDT), 2, 2-bis(p-chlorophenyl)ethane (DDD), dichloro diphenyl dichloroethylene (DDE)

Fig. 14 Structure of hexa chloro cyclohexane (HCH) and lindane

properties, non-toxicity, biocompatibility and low cost paving the way to a wide range of applications (Ferrier and Honeychurch 2021).

Single-walled carbon nanotubes (SWCNTs) and multi-walled carbon nanotubes (MWCNTs) display fascinating electronic and catalytic properties which are distinct from C_{60}. Particularly the good conductivity, mechanical stability, ease of functionalization and excellent biocompatibility make CNT as a unique and desirable electrode modifier. The literature on CNT electrochemistry is rather overflowing due to the explosive research on its application in electrochemical super capacitors, sensors and biosensors. Several exclusive reviews on CNT-based electrochemical sensors, biosensors and energy storage devices have been published (Ferrier and Honeychurch 2021; Gupta et al. 2018).

Graphene has been making a profound impact in electrochemistry due to its remarkable physicochemical properties. These include a high specific surface area (theoretically 2630 m^2/g for single-layer graphene), extraordinary electronic properties and electron transport capabilities, unprecedented liability and impermeability,

Fig. 15 Allotrope of carbon

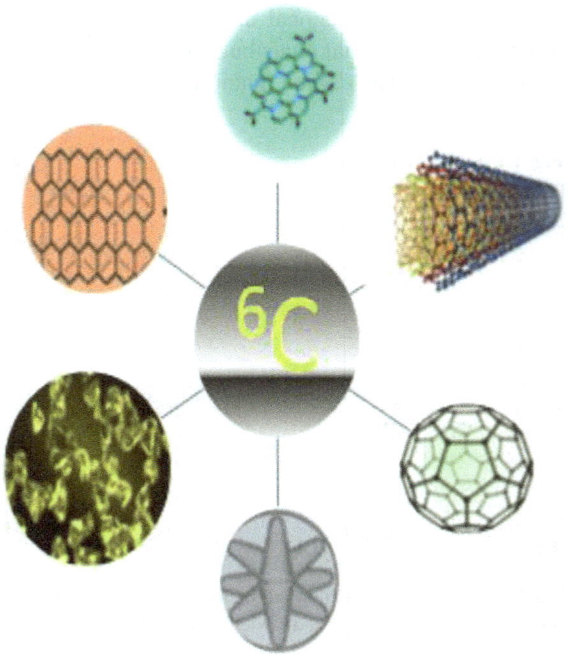

strong mechanical strength and excellent thermal and electrical conductivities. These unique physicochemical properties suggest that it has great potential for providing new approaches and critical improvements in the field of electrochemistry. Several excellent reviews are available on graphene (Bai et al. 2020; Kulakova and Lisichkin 2022).

9 Pesticide Sensors in Various Food Samples and Water Samples Using Different Carbon Nanomaterials

The food samples such as various vegetables, fruits, oil seeds, water samples and others are in direct exposures to the pesticides and hence affect the environment, aqueous being and human health. The Carbon nanomaterials and their nanocomposites have been proven to be superior to other composite for pesticide residue analysis due to various reasons. The carbon nanomaterials have a wide range of excellent properties such as high porosity, excellent conductivity, good adsorption capacity, unique shape, size, high surface area, good electron transfer reaction, several functional groups, inimitable optoelectronic and physio-chemical properties (Lazarević-Pašti 2023; Mishra et al. 2022).

In this review, we discuss rapid, cost-effective, sensitive, selective method, namely electrochemical sensor, photoluminescence sensor, electrochemiluminescence sensor, colorimetric sensor, fluorescence resonance energy, surface-enhanced Raman scattering and enzyme-based sensor for the sensing of pesticides in the food matrices and water samples. In the recent years, several reviews have been published for the sensing of pesticides using carbon nanomaterials and its corresponding nanocomposites (Paul et al. 2023; Mirres et al. 2022; Moreno-Camacho et al. 2019; Ozcelikay et al. 2022; Gowthaman et al. 2023; Souza et al. 2020; Zhao et al. 2018; Gupta et al. 2024; Zhang et al. 2022; Wahyudi et al. 2023; Zhou et al. 2023; Krasley et al. 2024).

10 Carbon Nanotubes

Carbon nanotubes (CNTs) are the best examples of one-dimensional nanostrucutured materials with a very high aspect ratio. It composed of hexagonal shapes with sp^2 hybridized network of carbon which is rolled into a cylindrical form. They can contain single, double or multiple layers resulting in either single-walled (SWCNTs) or multi-walled carbon nanotubes (MWCNTs). They exhibit unique nature, improved thermal and electrical conductivity and high surface-to-volume ratio, adjustable length and high stability (Zhou et al. 2017). We will discuss the role of CNTs for pesticide residue analysis in the further section. Table 2 summarizes the application of carbon nanotube and its composite for the sensing of pesticide residue in the commonly used real sample such as water, fruits and vegetables. Carbon nanotubes have been considered as the promising materials for the sensor application due to their high active surface area, excellent electron transfer reaction, good sensitivity, lower limit of detection and help to immobilize biological recognition elements (Ranjbari et al. 2024). Figure 16 summarizes the rapid, cost-effective, simple methods such as electrochemical sensor, acetyl cholinesterase biosensor, butyrylcholinesterase (BChe), organophosphorus hydrolase (OPH), solid-phase extraction method, colorimeter and immunosensor for the sensing of pesticides. Table 2 summarizes the various methods for the sensing of pesticides using carbon nanotubes and its nanocomposites.

Methyl viologen (1,1′-Dimethyl-4,4′-bipyridinium dichloride) is a widely used herbicide in the world which is used as weed control in plantation crops and fruit orchards. Paraquat is a desiccant for pineapples, sugarcane, soybeans and sunflower. It is highly toxic and has been classified under Level I—extremely hazardous pesticides with a lethal dose of 35 mg/kg (Bismuth et al. 1982). Orlando Fatibello-Filho et al. developed highly sensitive square-wave voltammetric method for the sensing of methyl viologen in natural water samples. They fabricated glassy carbon electrodes with functionalized multi-walled carbon nanotubes immobilized within a dihexadecyl hydrogen phosphate film (Imran et al. 2016).

Flexible electronics is the latest technology for preparing organic or inorganic materials on flexible substrates. Flexible electronics can be bent, folded, stretched, compressed, and changed into different shapes. (Liu et al. 2024). The flexible electrodes are functional materials that possess excellent electrical conductivity, tenability, higher reaction rate, low energy consumption, environmental benefits and with stand large deformation. Low-cost flexible acetylcholinesterase biosensor was fabricated on electrolyte gated carbon nanotube field effect transistor using 3-mercapto propionic acid as the linker molecule. The device was developed using a low-cost spray deposition technique on a flexible polyimide substrate and successfully applied for the sensing of malathion pesticides in real samples, namely water and strawberry juice (Bhatt et al. 2017).

Fipronil (FP) is an effective insecticide that belongs to phenylpyrazole chemical family. It is used to control ants, cockroaches, fleas, tick, termites, mole crickets, thrips, rootworms, weevils and other insects. The excessive use of FP can cause their residue to accumulate in the soil, water, food sample and in the human body. Huang et al. (2023) designed a modified electrochemical immunosensor based on an screen-printed electrode (SPCE) modified with carboxylated multi-walled carbon nanotubes (cMWCNTs), silver nanoparticles (AgNPs), chitosan (CS) and incorporated with anti-FP polyclonal antibodies (FAb). These cMWCNTs-AgNPs-CS-Fab (anti-fipronil)-bovine serum albumin/SPCE would be prepared by the freeze-drying technique for the sensing of FP in leafy vegetables, corn, rice, mango, cucumber, eggplant, red beans, egg and tea.

Very few literatures are reported on the sensing of pesticides using the colorimetric method. Recently, colorimetric nanozyme sensor was developed based on metal nanoparticle-decorated carbon nanotubes (MDCs) for quantification of carbendazim (CBZ) and isoproturon (ISP) in real water and soil samples. The fabricated MDC nanozyme produces different non-covalent interactions when pesticides were adsorbed on the MDCs and hence resulting in their peroxidase-mimicking activities. This can be utilized for the colorimetric sensing of chemically similar structure

Table 2 Application of carbon nanotube and its composite for detection of pesticides

Carbon nanomaterials	Technique	Analyte	Type of pesticides	Linear range	Limit of detection	References
[1]CNTf and [2]AgNPs/ [3]PGE	[4]BIA-MPA	Tap water, orange juice, apple fruit	[5]OPs ([6]DZN, [7]MLT, [8]CLPF)	0.1–20 μM (DZN) 1.0 –30 μM (MLT) 0.25–50 (CLPF)	0.35 μM (DZN) 0.89 μM (MLT) 0.53 μM (CLPF)	Porto et al. (2022)
[9]UZMWCNT and [10]rGO/AuNPs	[11]SWV	Rice and soil sample	Herbicide (picloram)	$0.05–6 \times 10^5$ nM	2.31 pM	Dkhar et al. (2023)
[12]Zr-MOF/[13]ZrO_2/ [14]MWCNT	[15]EIS	Apple, cabbage and soil samples	[5]OPs (malathion, dimethoate, chlorpyrifos, monocrotophos, glyphosate) Fungicide (thiophanate methyl, carbendazim) Herbicide (atrazine, [16]2,4, D)	–	2.02 nM (malathion) 2.8 nM (chlorpyrifos) 2.5 nM (dimethoate) 1.11 nM (monocrotophos) 2.01 nM glyphosate	Gokila et al. (2024)
[14]MWCNT/[17]BSA	Immunosensor	Water, animal feed, root, and leaf extract samples	[18]OCs endosulfan	–	0.184 ppt	Shah et al. (2023)
[19]MIP@[20]SnS_2 QDs/ pg-C_3N_4/MWCNTs	[19]MIP	River water and apple	Oxadiazine (indoxacarb)	20.0 nm–10.0 μM	7.1 nM	Khosropour et al. (2023)
[21]MDC	Colorimetric nanozyme	Soil and water samples	[22]CBZ, [23]DTM, [24]ISP	1–8 μM	10.8 nM (CBZ) 28.8 nM (DTM) 16.8 nM (ISP)	Kumar et al. (2024)

(continued)

Table 2 (continued)

Carbon nanomaterials	Technique	Analyte	Type of pesticides	Linear range	Limit of detection	References
[25]VNSWCNTs/ [26]AuNPs/[27]AChE	AChE biosensor	Water sample	[5]OPs methyl parathion, malathion, chlorpyrifos	10^{-5}–1 ppb (methyl parathion, malathion, chlorpyrifos)	3.04×10^{-6} ppb (methyl parathion) 1.96×10^{-6} ppb (malathion) 2.06×10^{-6} ppb (chlorpyrifos)	Xu et al. (2019)
[14]MWCNTs/ [28]GS-PEI-Au and [26]AuNPs-antibody conjugate	Amperometric immunosensor	Cabbages, green peppers, tomatoes, Chinese chives and peaches	Carbamate (carbofuran)	0.5–500 ng/mL	0.03 ng/mL	Zhu et al. (2013)
MXene/[29]CNTs/ [30]AuPd-[27]AChE	[27]AChE biosensor	Spinach and orange	[5]OPs chlorpyrifos	2.85×10^{-12}–2.85×10^{-6} M	1.98 pM	Hou et al. (2023)
[29]CNT/[31]OPH	[31]OPH biosensor	–	[5]OPs paraoxon, methyl parathion	–	0.15 μM paraoxon 0.8 μM methyl parathion	Deo et al. (2005)
Conducting polythiophene copolymer/[14]MWCNTs	[19]MIP	Vegetable samples	[5]OPs chlorpyrifos	–	4.0×10^{-12} M	Anirudhan et al. (2022)

[1]Functionalized carbon nanotubes, [2]AgNPs, [3]pyrolytic graphite electrode, [4]batch injection analysis system-multiple pulse amperometric, [5]organophosphorus compounds, [6]diazinon, [7]malathion, [8]chlorpyrifos, [9]unzipped multi-walled carbon nanotube, [10]reduced graphene oxide, [11]square-wave voltammetry, [12]zirconium-metal-organic framework, [13]zirconium dioxide, [14]multi-walled carbon nanotube, [15]electrochemical impedance spectroscopy, [16](2,4-dichlorophenoxyacetic acid), [17]bovine serum albumin, [18]organochlorines, [19]molecularly imprinted polymers, [20]tin disulphide quantum dots-carbon nitride-multi-walled carbon nanotubes, [21]metal nanoparticle-decorated carbon nanotube, [22]carbendazim, [23]deltamethrin, [24]isoproturon, [25]vertical nitrogen-doped single-walled carbon nanotubes, [26]gold nanoparticles, [27]acetylcholinesterase, [28]graphene sheets-ethyleneimine polymer-gold, [29]carbon nanotubes, [30]silver-palladium, [31]organophosphorus hydrolase

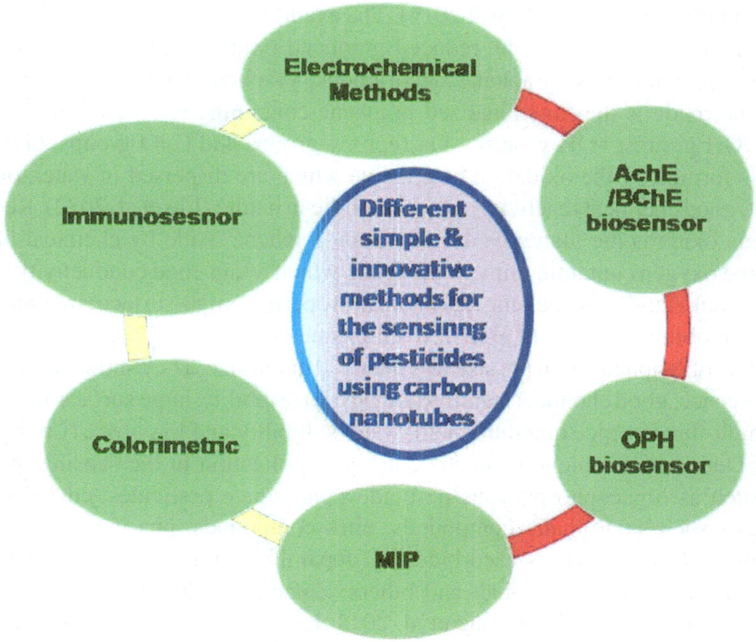

Fig. 16 Different simple and innovative methods for the sensing of pesticides using carbon nanotubes

pesticides namely CBZ and ISP in the real water and soil samples (Kumar et al. 2024).

The novel three-dimensional molecularly imprinted polymer-coated carbon nanotubes were prepared by coating the surface of carboxylated carbon nanotubes with SiO_2 and then terminating with molecularly imprinted polymer (MIP) shells. MIP was grafted to the CNT cores using methacrylic acid monomer, ethylene glycol dimethacrylate as cross linker, and 2,2′-azobisisobutyronitrile (AIBN) as initiator. The designed sensor was successfully applied to the detection of organic thiophosphate namely profenofos in vegetable samples. The fabricated three-dimensional imprinted sensor provides a linear calibration plot within the range of 0.01–200 μM ($r^2 = 0.995$) with a low detection limit of 0.002 μM (3σ) (Amatatongchai et al. 2019).

11 Graphene-Based Nanomaterials

Graphene-based nanomaterials are the special class of materials that combine the unique physical, chemical and biological properties of graphene with other nanomaterials with enhanced physical, chemical and biological properties. Graphene is a two-dimensional material made of sp^2 hybridized carbon atoms arranged in the honeycomb-shaped lattice (Lawal 2019). The examples of graphene-based nanomaterials include graphene oxide, reduced graphene oxide, graphene quantum dots, graphene nanoplatelets, graphene nanoribbons, graphene-based nanocomposites. Graphene oxide is the functionalized graphene-containing functional groups such as –COOH groups, –OH groups, –O– (epoxy) groups and C=O groups. Graphene oxide is formed by the oxidation of graphite which are dispersed in water, organic solvent, good chemical reactivity and hydrophilic in nature (Liu et al. 2022). Reduced graphene oxide is the materials derived from graphene oxide by chemical or heat removing oxygen containing functional group which retain good conductivity, excellent thermal stability, excellent mechanical properties, high surface area and high electron mobility (Ahmed et al. 2023). Graphene quantum dots are tiny, nanoscale fragments of graphene with the size less than 100 nm in size. They show stable photoluminescence, good chemical stability and physical stability, large surface-to-volume ratio, high-fluorescence quantum yield, water solubility and low-toxic (Chung et al. 2021). Due to their unique properties, it finds application in the sensing of pesticides such as organophosphorous pesticides, carbamate pesticides, environmental pollutants such as aromatic compounds, nitro compounds, pharmaceutical pollutants, biomolecules such as ascorbic acid, dopamine, antibiotics and heavy metal such as nickel, cadmium, cobalt and others (Zafar et al. 2023; Lang et al. 2023; Benjamin and Júnior 2022; Chang et al. 2014; Kurniawan et al. 2022; Kalkal et al. 2021; Chung et al. 2021; Sharma et al. 2016; Bai et al. 2020). Table 3 summarizes the various methods for the sensing of pesticides using graphene-based nanomaterials.

Wu et al. developed N-doped-reduced graphene oxide supported Pd-doped lanthanum vanadate for simultaneous detection of carbendazim (CBZ) and methyl parathion (MP) in water sample and vegetable sample namely cabbages and spinach. The presence of N-doping in the reduced graphene oxide could enhance the electron transport reaction and catalytic activity of reduced graphene oxide and prevent the aggregation of Pd-doped lanthanum vanadate. In addition to that, palladium could enhance the insufficient conductivity of lanthanum vanadate. In individual detection, limit of detection of CBZ and MP was found to be 2.42 nmol/L and 1.85 nmol/L, respectively, and for the simultaneous detection, limit of detection of CBZ and MP was 1.94 nmol/L and 1.71 nmol/L, respectively (Li et al. 2023).

Acetylcholinesterase (AChE) is an important enzyme present in the neuromuscular junctions, synapses, red blood cells, that helps in the breaking down the acetylcholine (ATCh) into choline and acetate, terminating the signal transmission at the synapse (the gap between two neurons) and regulating the amount of ACh available for neurotransmission. Both pesticides, namely organophosphates and carbamates, could act as the AChE inhibitors. These chemicals can act in three major ways. (1) Binding to the active site of AChE and preventing the breakdown of Ach. (2) Increasing the amount of ACh in the synapse and hence leading to overstimulation of neurons. (3) Disrupting normal neurotransmission and hence causing various toxic effects (Colovic et al. 2013). For the biosensor studies, we exploit the inhibit action of AChE for the sensing of organophosphate and carbamate pesticides.

Patramanon research group of Thailand fabricated electrochemical biosensor based on cellulose nanofibers/graphene oxide and acetylcholinesterase for the

Table 3 Application of reduced graphene oxide and its composite for detection of pesticides

S. No.	Type of carbon nanomaterials	Method used	Food matrices	Type of pesticides	Linear range	LOD	References
1.	[1]SnS_2/[2]NS-RGO	[3]CV	River water and black grapes	[4]OPs ([5]MP)	–	0.17 nM	Shanmugam et al. (2020)
2.	[6]Gd_2S_3-RGO	[7]EIS, [3]CV	River water and potato	[8]CBMs [9]CF	0.001–1381 μM	0.0128 μM	Mariyappan et al. (2021)
3.	[10]Ag-RGO	Colorimetric	Water	[8]CBMs carbaryl pesticide	0.1–50 μM	42 nM	Minh et al. (2020)
4.	[11]p(Arg)-GO	[12]EC sensor	Water and cucumber	[4]OPs [13]FNT	0.69–20.2 μM	0.173 μM	Bolat et al. (2023)
5.	[14]CMO/B-RGO	[12]EC sensor	Food samples	[9]CF	0.01–365 μM	0.002 μM	Alagarsamy et al. (2023)
6.	[15]GR/[16]AuNPs/[17]AChE/Nafion	[17]AChE biosensor	Tap water and cucumber	[4]OPs [18]ICP	0.1–2000 μg/L	0.012 μg/L	Wen et al. (2023)
7.	[19]CD-[20]GO	Enzyme/fluorescent biosensor	Crops	[21]CPF, [22]PF	–	0.14 and 2.05 ppb	Gaviria et al. (2022)
8.	[23]S-GQ Ds, [24]PVA	Fluorescent sensor	Fruits and vegetables	Carbamate pesticides	–	60 ppb	Nair et al. (2020)
9.	[25]GQDs, [26]MN	Fluorescent sensor	–	Carbamate pesticide, carbofuran	–	0.05–4 μM	Lekshmi et al. (2023)

[1]Tin sulphide nanosheets supported, [2]N, S-codoped reduced graphene oxide nanocomposite, [3]cyclic voltammetry, [4]organophosphorus pesticides, [5]methyl Parathion, [6]gadolinium sulphide rod-embedded reduced graphene oxide, [7]electrochemical impedance spectroscopy, [8]carbamate pesticides, [9]carbofuran, [10]reduced graphene oxide-wrapped silver nanoparticles, [11]poly-arginine/graphene oxide, [12]electrochemical, [13]fenitrothion, [14]cerium molybdate wrapped boron doped reduced graphene oxide, [15]graphene, [16]gold nanoparticles, [17]AChE, [18]isocarbophos, [19]carbon quantum dot, [20]graphene oxide, [21]chlorpyrifos, [22]profenofos, [23]sulphur-doped graphene quantum dots, [24]poly (vinyl alcohol), [25]graphene quantum dots, [26]α-mangostin, [27]1,2-bis[4-(3-sulfonatopropoxyl) phenyl]-1,2-diphenylethene

sensing of highly dangerous organophosphates pesticide namely chlorpyrifos in drinking water and lychee juice (Tun et al. 2023). We prepare cellulose nanofibers from the sugarcane bagasse using the alkaline hydrogen peroxide hydrolysis method. Chlorpyrifos inhibits the catalytic activity of AChE on ATCh, and this inhibition can be measured using square-wave voltammetry. The modified biosensor shows good performance for the detection of chlorpyrifos over a linear calibration range of 25–1000 nM, and the limits of detection and quantification were found to be 2.2 nM and 73 nM, respectively.

The colorimetric method has attracted much attention due to its cheap, simple operation, visual detection results and rapid response. It has been widely developed to achieve rapid and real time sensing of real samples (Wu et al. 2023). Graphene and its derivatives have unique layered structure, large surface area, excellent catalytic performance, large functional group on the surface for loading other nanomaterials. It shows extraordinary physicochemical, optical, electrical properties, extremely high density of surface-active sites for binding analytes to increase the sensitivity of colorimetric sensors (Minh et al. 2020; Deosarkar et al. 2021).

The nanozyme sensors have attracted increased attention over natural enzymes due to their improved stability, increased activity, low cost and ease of preparation (Tai et al. 2023). A simple colorimetric sensor array was developed based on nano ceria crosslinked and heteroatom-doped graphene oxide nanoribbons for the sensing of carbaryl, fluroxypyr-mepthyl, thiophanate-methyl, thiram, diafenthiuron and fomesafen in lake water and apple samples. Herein, nano ceria crosslinked graphene oxide nanoribbons and heteroatom-doped graphene oxide nanoribbons were prepared which exhibit excellent peroxidase-like activities and help in the identification and quantitative analysis of six pesticides.

The dual responsive magnetic Fe_3O_4–TiO_2/reduced graphene oxide nanocomposite (RGO) was developed as an artificial nanozyme for the colorimetric detection and photodegradation of atrazine in an aqueous medium (Boruah and Das 2020). The Fe_3O_4–TiO_2/RGO nanocomposite showed excellent peroxidase-like catalytic activity throughout the oxidation of 3,3′,5,5′-tetramethylbenzidine to the blue-coloured oxidized product in the presence of H_2O_2. In addition to that, Fe_3O_4–TiO_2/RGO nanocomposite was also successfully utilized towards efficient photocatalytic degradation of atrazine molecule under irradiation of natural sunlight.

Tomapatanaget et al. (2020) fabricated fluorescent sulphur-doped graphene quantum dots (S-GQDs) in colloidal and film forms for the ultrasensitive and selective detection of carbofuran and thiram in the real sample. The green fluorescent S-GQDs in aqueous phase give the detection limit of 0.45 ppb for carbofuran and 1.6 ppb for thiram, respectively. Further, S-GQD was added to poly (vinyl alcohol) matrix for the fabrication of flexible solid-state fluorescent sensing platform.

12 Carbon Dots (CDs)

Carbon dots (CDs) can be generally defined as quasi-zero-dimensional carbon-based materials ranging from 2 to 10 nm in size. They are basically carbon-based nanomaterials with fluorescence properties with quasi-spherical structures. They have attracted much attention in the carbon family due to their excellent, tunable photoluminescence, high quantum yield, low toxicity, small size, biocompatibility, unique optical properties, abundant functional groups, high stability and electron mobility (Liu et al. 2020). CDs were accidentally obtained from the purification of single-walled carbon nanotubes (Xu et al. 2004). CDs can be functionalized using a variety of functional groups including amino, epoxy, hydroxyl and carboxyl groups irrespective of their core structures. The surface functionalities contribute to the hydrophilic or hydrophobic nature of the CDs and hence enabling them to readily disperse and stabilized in different solvents (Ozyurt et al. 2023). The electrical and photo luminescent properties of CDs could be fine tuned by incorporating the hetero atoms namely sulphur, nitrogen, boron, phosphorus and gadolinium. CDs belong to the carbon-based fluorescent nanomaterials with varying size, different chemical functional group and different electrical and optical properties. They can be classified into four categories (Fig. 17): (1) graphene quantum dots (GQDs), (2) carbon quantum dots (CQDs), (3) carbon polymer dots (CPDs) and (4) carbon nanoparticles (CNPs) (Đorđević et al. 2022). Table 4 summarizes the literature for the sensing of pesticides using carbon dots.

Kamlesh Shrives et al. prepared nitrogen-doped carbon quantum dots (N-CQDs) for the determination of methiocarb in vegetables by fluorescent paper sensor. The fluorescent paper sensor serves as the instrument free, portable and user-friendly approach. The fluorescent paper sensor is developed by changing the fluorescence of the N-CQDs with the addition of methiocarb using a smartphone and Image J software. The good linear range was found in the range of 700–10,000 μg L^{-1} with the detection limit of 500 μg L^{-1}. The fluorescent paper sensor was used and its response was analyzed using fluorimetry. The developed fluorescent paper sensor shows good recovery in the range from 92 to 95% with excellent selectivity (Patel et al. 2023).

Carbon quantum dots stabilized silver nanoparticles (Ag/C dots) act as the effective colorimetric sensor for the detection of three different pesticides, namely herbicide (atrazine), insecticide (imidacloprid) and organophosphate pesticide (chlorpyrifos) (Imran et al. 2016). Here, we adopt hydrothermal approach for the synthesis of Ag/C dots from gelatin. Then physicochemical properties such as morphology, phase structure, chemical composition and optical and structural were characterized. The AgNPs functionalized C-dots act as the sensing platform for the detection of imidacloprid in water and vegetables' samples with the recovery of 96% and 95%, respectively.

The novel fluorometric sensor (Mahmoudi et al. 2023) was developed for the sensing of malathion and chlorpyrifos using S-doped carbon quantum dots (CQDs)/ Cu^{2+}/acetylcholinesterase (AChE)/acetylthiocholine (ATCh). Fluorescent S-doped carbon quantum dots (CQD) are hydrothermally prepared from two main precursors, namely trisodium citrate dihydrate and sodium thiosulfate. The detection mechanism

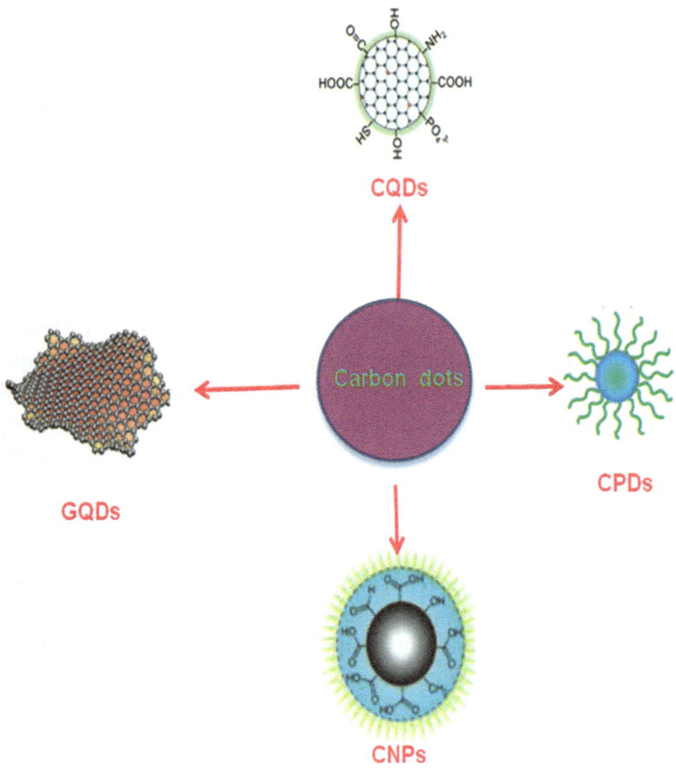

Fig. 17 Different types of carbon dots

for the proposed S-doped CQD-based sensor was well documented by the strong binding of Cu^{2+} ions to carboxyl groups of S-doped CQD and further reaction. Both malathion and chlorpyrifos act as the excellent AchE inhibitors. The designed sensor showed the detection limits of 1.70 ppb and 1.50 ppb for malathion and chlorpyrifos, respectively.

13 Conclusions

This chapter comprehensively reviews the major classes of pesticides used in agriculture, including their classification, chemical structures, toxicity and methods employed for their detection. The unique properties of carbon biomaterials particularly carbon nanomaterials, including carbon nanotubes, graphene-based nanomaterials, and carbon dots, are discussed in relation to their sensing performance. The recent advances in carbon nanomaterial based sensing platforms are summarized, highlighting electrochemical, colorimetric, fluorometric, surface enhanced Raman scattering (SERS) based, and enzyme based biosensors for pesticide detection.

Table 4 Application of carbon dots for detection of pesticide residue

S. No.	Type of carbon nanomaterials	Method used	Food matrices	Type of pesticides	Linear range	LOD	References
1.	[1]CDs	Fluorescence	River water	Atrazine, chlorpyrifos, imidacloprid, lindane, and tetradifon	–	0.013 μM—imidacloprid 04 μM—tetradifon	Mandal et al. (2019)
2.	CDs	Colorimetric	Water samples	Fenitrothion	1.0–250.0 ng m/L	0.2 ng mL^{-1}	Larki (2017)
3.	[2]N and S-CDs	Fluorescence	Apple	Carbaryl	5 ppb	3.2 ppb—dichlorvos 13 ppb—[3]MP	Li et al. (2016)
4.	[4]B, N-CDs	Fluorescence	Tap water, lake water, semen coicis	[3]MP	0.015–1.5 mM	24.7 ng mL^{-1}	Luo et al. (2020)
5.	[5]NC-dots	[6]FRET	–	Paraoxon	10^{-4}–10^{-9} g/L	3.6×10^{-12} mol L^{-1}	Gong et al. (2016)
6.	[7]CQDs/[8]AgNPs	[6]FRET	Rice, carrot, orange and pepper	Propanyl, parathion, dimethoate, chlorpyrifos and pirimicarb	–	–	Carneiro et al. (2019)

[1]Carbon dots, [2]nitrogen and sulphur-doped carbon dots, [3]methyl parathion, [4]boron-nitrogen-doped carbon dots, [5]nitrogen-doped carbon dots, [6]fluorescence resonance energy transfer, [7]carbon quantum dot, [8]silver nanoparticle

Carbon nanotubes and their metal, metal oxide, and polymer-based nanocomposites exhibit excellent electrocatalytic activity toward a broad range of pesticides. Graphene-based nanomaterials and their nanocomposites provide superior electrical conductivity, large surface area, and excellent catalytic properties, making them suitable materials for pesticide sensing and environmental monitoring. Carbon dots have emerged as promising fluorescent probes owing to their exceptional optical properties, high photostability, low toxicity, and tunable surface chemistry, enabling highly sensitive detection of pesticide residues. Carbon nanomaterials, carbon nanotubes, graphene. Carbon nanotubes, graphene.

References

Z.P. Aguilar, Types of nanomaterials and corresponding methods of synthesis. Nanomater. Med. Appl. **50**, 15–29 (2013)

A. Ahmed, A. Singh, S.J. Young, V. Gupta, M. Singh, S. Arya, Synthesis techniques and advances in sensing applications of reduced graphene oxide (rGO) composites: a review. Compos. A Appl. Sci. Manuf. **165**, 107373 (2023)

S. Alagarsamy, R. Sundaresan, S.M. Chen, R. Rasu, M.A. Mohammed, An ultrasensitive carbamate pesticide detection sensor based on metal molybdate encapsulated with boron doped reduced graphene oxide nanocomposite. Colloids Surf. A Physicochem. Eng. Asp. **673**, 131830 (2023)

L. Alvarez-Rodriguez, L. Monferrer-Pons, J.S. Esteve-Romero, M.C. García-Alvarez-Coque, G. Ramis-Ramos, Spectrophotometric determination of carbamate pesticides with diazotized trimethylaniline in a micellar medium of sodium dodecyl sulfate. Analyst **122**(5), 459–463 (1997)

M. Amatatongchai, W. Sroysee, P. Sodkrathok, N. Kesangam, S. Chairam, P. Jarujamrus, Novel three-dimensional molecularly imprinted polymer-coated carbon nanotubes (3D-CNTs@ MIP) for selective detection of profenofos in food. Anal. Chim. Acta **1076**, 64–72 (2019)

T.S. Anirudhan, V.S. Athira, S.S. Nair, Detection of chlorpyrifos based on molecular imprinting with a conducting polythiophene copolymer loaded on multi-walled carbon nanotubes. Food Chem. **381**, 132010 (2022)

G. Aragay, F. Pino, A. Merkoçi, Nanomaterials for sensing and destroying pesticides. Chem. Rev. **112**(10), 5317–5338 (2012)

Y. Bai, T. Xu, X. Zhang, Graphene-based biosensors for detection of biomarkers. Micromachines **11**(1), 60 (2020)

J. Beltrán, F.J. López, F. Hernández, Solid-phase microextraction in pesticide residue analysis. J. Chromatogr. A **885**(1–2), 389–404 (2000)

S.R. Benjamin, E.J.M.R. Júnior, Graphene-based electrochemical sensors for detection of environmental pollutants. Curr. Opin. Environ. Sci. Health **29**, 100381 (2022)

V.D. Bhatt, S. Joshi, M. Becherer, P. Lugli, Flexible, low-cost sensor based on electrolyte gated carbon nanotube field effect transistor for organo-phosphate detection. Sensors **17**(5), 1147 (2017)

C. Bismuth, R. Garnier, S. Dally, P.E. Fournier, J.M. Scherrmann, Prognosis and treatment of paraquat poisoning: a review of 28 cases. J. Toxicol. Clin. Toxicol. **19**(5), 461–474 (1982)

G. Bolat, Y.T. Yaman, S. Abacı, S. Seyyar, Poly-arginine/graphene oxide functionalized disposable sensor for monitoring fenitrothion pesticide residues in water and cucumber samples. Mater. Today Chem. **30**, 101517 (2023)

P.K. Boruah, M.R. Das, Dual responsive magnetic Fe_3O_4-TiO_2/graphene nanocomposite as an artificial nanozyme for the colorimetric detection and photodegradation of pesticide in an aqueous medium. J. Hazard. Mater. **385**, 121516 (2020)

S.V. Carneiro, V.H.R. De Queiroz, A.A.C. Cruz, L.M.U.D. Fechine, J.C. Denardin, R.M. Freire, et al., Sensing strategy based on carbon quantum dots obtained from riboflavin for the identification of pesticides. Sens. Actuators B Chem. **301**, 127149 (2019)

J. Chang, G. Zhou, E.R. Christensen, R. Heideman, J. Chen, Graphene-based sensors for detection of heavy metals in water: a review. Anal. Bioanal. Chem. **406**, 3957–3975 (2014)

X. Chen, C. Li, M. Grätzel, R. Kostecki, S.S. Mao, Nanomaterials for renewable energy production and storage. Chem. Soc. Rev. **41**(23), 7909–7937 (2012)

S. Chung, R.A. Revia, M. Zhang, Graphene quantum dots and their applications in bioimaging, biosensing, and therapy. Adv. Mater. **33**(22), 1904362 (2021)

M.B. Colovic, D.Z. Krstic, T.D. Lazarevic-Pasti, A.M. Bondzic, V.M. Vasic, Acetylcholinesterase inhibitors: pharmacology and toxicology. Curr. Neuropharmacol. **11**(3), 315–335 (2013)

R.P. Deo, J. Wang, I. Block, A. Mulchandani, K.A. Joshi, M. Trojanowicz, et al., Determination of organophosphate pesticides at a carbon nanotube/organophosphorus hydrolase electrochemical biosensor. Anal. Chim. Acta **530**(2), 185–189 (2005)

T. Deosarkar, N. Chandrasekaran, A. Mukherjee, An ultra-sensitive and selective AChE based colorimetric detection of malathion using silver nanoparticle-graphene oxide (Ag-GO) nanocomposite. Anal. Chim. Acta **1142**, 73–83 (2021)

U.P. Dhuldhaj, R. Singh, V.K. Singh, Pesticide contamination in agro-ecosystems: toxicity, impacts, and bio-based management strategies. Environ. Sci. Pollut. Res. **30**(4), 9243–9270 (2023)

D.S. Dkhar, R. Kumari, P. Chandra, Chemically engineered unzipped multiwalled carbon nanotube and rGO nanohybrid for ultrasensitive picloram detection in rice water and soil samples. Sci. Rep. **13**(1), 9899 (2023)

L. Đorđević, F. Arcudi, M. Cacioppo, M. Prato, A multifunctional chemical toolbox to engineer carbon dots for biomedical and energy applications. Nat. Nanotechnol. **17**(2), 112–130 (2022)

B.A. Du, Z.P. Li, C.H. Liu, One-step homogeneous detection of DNA hybridization with gold nanoparticle probes by using a linear light-scattering technique. Angew. Chem. Int. Ed. **45**(47), 8022–8025 (2006)

V. Eskandari, H. Sahbafar, L. Zeinalizad, A. Hadi, A review of applications of surface-enhanced Raman spectroscopy laser for detection of biomaterials and a quick glance into its advances for COVID-19 investigations. ISSS J. Micro Smart Syst. **11**(2), 363–382 (2022)

D.C. Ferrier, K.C. Honeychurch, Carbon nanotube (CNT)-based biosensors. Biosensors **11**(12), 486 (2021)

F.P. Garcia, S.C. Ascencio, J.C.G. Oyarzún, A.C. Hernandez, P.V. Alavarado, Pesticides: classification, uses and toxicity. Measures of exposure and genotoxic risks. J. Res. Environ. Sci. Toxicol. **1**(11), 279–293 (2012)

M.I. Gaviria, K. Barrientos, J.P. Arango, J.B. Cano, G.A. Peñuela, Highly sensitive fluorescent biosensor based on acetylcholinesterase and carbon dots–graphene oxide quenching test for analytical and commercial organophosphate pesticide detection. Front. Environ. Sci. **10**, 825112 (2022)

A.K. Geim, K.S. Novoselov, The rise of graphene. Nat. Mater. **6**(3), 183–191 (2007)

N. Gokila, Y. Haldorai, P. Saravanan, R.T.R. Kumar, Non-enzymatic electrochemical impedance sensor for selective detection of electro-inactive organophosphate pesticides using Zr-MOF/ZrO_2/MWCNT ternary composite. Environ. Res. **251**, 118648 (2024)

G.A. Gómez-Ríos, E. Gionfriddo, J. Poole, J. Pawliszyn, Ultrafast screening and quantitation of pesticides in food and environmental matrices by solid-phase microextraction–transmission mode (SPME-TM) and direct analysis in real time (DART). Anal. Chem. **89**(13), 7240–7248 (2017)

N.C. Gong, Y. Le Li, X. Jiang, X.F. Zheng, Y.Y. Wang, S.Y. Huan, Fluorescence resonance energy transfer-based biosensor composed of nitrogen-doped carbon dots and gold nanoparticles for the highly sensitive detection of organophosphorus pesticides. Anal. Sci. **32**(9), 951–956 (2016)

N.S.K. Gowthaman, M. Amalraj, S. Kesavan, K. Rajalakshmi, S. Shankar, B. Sinduja, et al., Zero-, one- and two-dimensional carbon nanomaterials as low-cost catalysts in optical and electrochemical sensing of biomolecules and environmental pollutants. Microchem. J. **109291** (2023)

S. Gupta, C.N. Murthy, C.R. Prabha, Recent advances in carbon nanotube based electrochemical biosensors. Int. J. Biol. Macromol. **108**, 687–703 (2018)

T. Gupta, M. Dutt, B. Kaur, S. Punia, S. Sharma, P.K. Sahu, L. Saya, Graphene-based nanomaterials as potential candidates for environmental mitigation of pesticides. Talanta 125748 (2024)

M.A. Hassaan, A. El Nemr, Pesticides pollution: classifications, human health impact, extraction and treatment techniques. Egypt. J. Aquat. Res. **46**(3), 207–220 (2020)
D.J. Hoffman, B.A. Rattner, G.A. Burton Jr., J. Cairns Jr. (eds.), *Handbook of Ecotoxicology* (CRC Press, 2002)
X. Hou, R. Ding, W. Jiang, Q. Yang, X. Mao, Detection of chlorpyrifos via carbon nanotubes and AuPd nanoparticles-enhanced MXene electrode-based acetylcholinesterase biosensor. Microchem. J. **195**, 109319 (2023)
W.C. Huang, Y.N. Hsiung, C.L. Li, An electrochemical immunosensor based on a carboxylated multiwalled carbon nanotube-silver nanoparticle-chitosan functional layer for the detection of fipronil. Nanoscale Adv. **5**(23), 6548–6559 (2023)
S.M. Imran, G.N. Shao, H. Kim, https://www.sciencedirect.com/science/article/abs/pii/S092633731500346X (2016)
A. Kalkal, S. Kadian, R. Pradhan, G. Manik, G. Packirisamy, Recent advances in graphene quantum dot-based optical and electrochemical (bio) analytical sensors. Mater. Adv. **2**(17), 5513–5541 (2021)
H. Khosropour, M. Saboohi, M. Keramat, B. Rezaei, A.A. Ensafi, Electrochemical molecularly imprinted polymer sensor for ultrasensitive indoxacarb detection by tin disulfide quantum dots/carbon nitride/multiwalled carbon nanotubes as a nanocomposite. Sens. Actuators B Chem. **385**, 133652 (2023)
A.T. Krasley, E. Li, J.M. Galeana, C. Bulumulla, A.G. Beyene, G.S. Demirer, Carbon nanomaterial fluorescent probes and their biological applications. Chem. Rev. **124**(6), 3085–3185 (2024)
R. Krieger (ed.), *Handbook of Pesticide Toxicology: Principles and Agents* (Academic Press, 2001)
I.I. Kulakova, G.V. Lisichkin, Biosensors based on graphene nanomaterials. Mosc. Univ. Chem. Bull. **77**(6), 307–321 (2022)
M. Kumar, N. Kaur, N. Singh, Colorimetric nanozyme sensor array based on metal nanoparticle-decorated CNTs for quantification of pesticides in real water and soil samples. ACS Sustain. Chem. Eng. **12**(2), 728–736 (2024)
D. Kurniawan, R.J. Weng, Y.Y. Chen, M.R. Rahardja, Z.C. Nanaricka, W.H. Chiang, Recent advances in the graphene quantum dot-based biological and environmental sensors. Sens. Actuators Rep. **4**, 100130 (2022)
T. Lang, M. Xiao, W. Cen, Graphene-based metamaterial sensor for pesticide trace detection. Biosensors **13**(5), 560 (2023)
A. Larki, A novel application of carbon dots for colorimetric determination of fenitrothion insecticide based on the microextraction method. Spectrochim. Acta A Mol. Biomol. Spectrosc. **173**, 1–5 (2017)
A.T. Lawal, Graphene-based nanocomposites and their applications. A review. Biosens. Bioelectron. **141**, 111384 (2019)
T. Lazarević-Pašti, Carbon materials for organophosphate pesticide sensing. Chemosensors **11**(2), 93 (2023)
C.L. Lekshmi, U.S. Swathy, K. Vijayan, H. Simimole, S. Sumalekshmy, Graphene quantum dots derived from honey and mangostin as sustainable materials to construct fluorescence turn-on molecular switches for pesticide detection. Chem. Select **8**(13), e202204869 (2023)
H. Li, C. Sun, R. Vijayaraghavan, F. Zhou, X. Zhang, D.R. MacFarlane, Long lifetime photoluminescence in N, S co-doped carbon quantum dots from an ionic liquid and their applications in ultrasensitive detection of pesticides. Carbon **104**, 33–39 (2016)
W. Li, T. Xie, X. Chen, J. Lu, R. Qiu, J. Chu, et al., N-doped reduced graphene oxide supported Pd-doped lanthanum vanadate constructs an electrochemical sensing platform for simultaneous detection of carbendazim and methyl parathion in food. J. Food Compos. Anal. **124**, 105647 (2023)
J. Liu, R. Li, B. Yang, Carbon dots: a new type of carbon-based nanomaterial with wide applications. ACS Cent. Sci. **6**(12), 2179–2195 (2020)
J. Liu, S. Bao, X. Wang, Applications of graphene-based materials in sensors: a review. Micromachines **13**(2), 184 (2022)
K. Liu, T. Duan, F. Zhang, X. Tian, H. Li, M. Feng, et al., Flexible electrode materials for emerging electronics: materials, fabrication and applications. J. Mater. Chem. A (2024)

P. Luo, X. Liu, F. Kong, L. Chen, Q. Wang, W. Li, et al., Simultaneous determination of 169 veterinary drugs in chicken eggs with EMR-lipid clean-up using ultra-high performance liquid chromatography tandem mass spectrometry. Anal. Methods **11**(12), 1657–1662 (2019)

M. Luo, J. Wei, Y. Zhao, Y. Sun, H. Liang, S. Wang, P. Li, Fluorescent and visual detection of methyl-paraoxon by using boron- and nitrogen-doped carbon dots. Microchem. J. **154**, 104547 (2020)

N. Mahmoudi, F. Fatemi, M. Rahmandoust, F. Mirzajani, S.O.R. Siadat, Development of a carbon quantum dot-based sensor for the detection of acetylcholinesterase and the organophosphate pesticide. Heliyon **9**(9) (2023)

P. Mandal, D. Sahoo, P. Sarkar, K. Chakraborty, S. Das, Fluorescence turn-on and turn-off sensing of pesticides by carbon dot-based sensor. New J. Chem. **43**(30), 12137–12151 (2019)

V. Mariyappan, M. Keerthi, S.M. Chen, Highly selective electrochemical sensor based on gadolinium sulfide rod-embedded RGO for the sensing of carbofuran. J. Agric. Food Chem. **69**(9), 2679–2688 (2021)

P.N. Minh, V.T. Hoang, N.X. Dinh, O. Van Hoang, N. Van Cuong, D.T.B. Hop, et al., Reduced graphene oxide-wrapped silver nanoparticles for applications in ultrasensitive colorimetric detection of Cr(VI) ions and the carbaryl pesticide. New J. Chem. **44**(18), 7611–7620 (2020)

A.C.D.M. Mirres, B.E.P.D.M.D. Silva, L. Tessaro, D. Galvan, J.C.D. Andrade, A. Aquino, et al., Recent advances in nanomaterial-based biosensors for pesticide detection in foods. Biosensors **12**(8), 572 (2022)

S. Mishra, S. Mishra, S.S. Patel, S.P. Singh, P. Kumar, M.A. Khan, et al., Carbon nanomaterials for the detection of pesticide residues in food: a review. Environ. Pollut. **310**, 119804 (2022)

C.A. Moreno-Camacho, J.R. Montoya-Torres, A. Jaegler, N. Gondran, Sustainability metrics for real case applications of the supply chain network design problem: a systematic literature review. J. Clean. Prod. **231**, 600–618 (2019)

R.V. Nair, R.T. Thomas, A.P. Mohamed, S. Pillai, Fluorescent turn-off sensor based on sulphur-doped graphene quantum dots in colloidal and film forms for the ultrasensitive detection of carbamate pesticides. Microchem. J. **157**, 104971 (2020)

T. Narahashi, J.M. Frey, K.S. Ginsburg, M.L. Roy, Sodium and GABA-activated channels as the targets of pyrethroids and cyclodienes. Toxicol. Lett. **64**, 429–436 (1992)

R.B. Onyancha, K.E. Ukhurebor, U.O. Aigbe, O.A. Osibote, H.S. Kusuma, H. Darmokoesoemo, A methodical review on carbon-based nanomaterials in energy-related applications. Adsorp. Sci. Technol. **2022**, 4438286 (2022)

G. Ozcelikay, L. Karadurmus, S. Bilge, A. Sınağ, S.A. Ozkan, New analytical strategies amplified with 2D carbon nanomaterials for electrochemical sensing of food pollutants in water and soils sources. Chemosphere **296**, 133974 (2022)

D. Ozyurt, M. Al Kobaisi, R.K. Hocking, B. Fox, Properties, synthesis, and applications of carbon dots: a review. Carbon Trends **12**, 100276 (2023)

S. Patel, K. Shrivas, D. Sinha, I. Karbhal, T.K. Patle, A portable smartphone-assisted digital image fluorimetry for analysis of methiocarb pesticide in vegetables: nitrogen-doped carbon quantum dots as a sensing probe. Spectrochim. Acta A Mol. Biomol. Spectrosc. **299**, 122824 (2023)

S. Paul, P. Daga, N. Dey, Exploring various photochemical processes in optical sensing of pesticides by luminescent nanomaterials: a concise discussion on challenges and recent advancements. ACS Omega **8**(47), 44395–44423 (2023)

G. Picci, R. Montis, A.M. Gilchrist, P.A. Gale, C. Caltagirone, Fluorescent and colorimetric sensors for anions: highlights from 2020 to 2022. Coord. Chem. Rev. **501**, 215561 (2024)

L.S. Porto, L.F. Ferreira, W.T.P. Dos Santos, A.C. Pereira, Determination of organophosphorus compounds in water and food samples using a non-enzymatic electrochemical sensor based on silver nanoparticles and carbon nanotubes nanocomposite coupled with batch injection analysis. Talanta **246**, 123477 (2022)

M. Pumera, Graphene-based nanomaterials for energy storage. Energy Environ. Sci. **4**(3), 668–674 (2011)

R. Ramachandran, T.W. Chen, S.M. Chen, T. Baskar, R. Kannan, P. Elumalai, et al., A review of the advanced developments of electrochemical sensors for the detection of toxic and bioactive molecules. Inorg. Chem. Front. **6**(12), 3418–3439 (2019)

S. Ranjbari, M. Bolourinezhad, P. Kesharwani, M. Rezayi, A. Sahebkar, Applications of carbon nanotube biosensors: sensing the future. J. Drug Delivery Sci. Technol. **105747** (2024)

M. Shah, P. Kolhe, S. Gandhi, Nano-assembly of multiwalled carbon nanotubes for sensitive voltammetric responses for the determination of residual levels of endosulfan. Chemosphere **321**, 138148 (2023)

R. Shanmugam, S. Manavalan, S.M. Chen, M. Keerthi, L.H. Lin, Methyl parathion detection using SnS_2/N, S–Co-doped reduced graphene oxide nanocomposite. ACS Sustain. Chem. Eng. **8**(30), 11194–11203 (2020)

D. Sharma, S. Kanchi, M.I. Sabela, K. Bisetty, Insight into the biosensing of graphene oxide: present and future prospects. Arab. J. Chem. **9**(2), 238–261 (2016)

A.L.T.D. Souza, M.E. Batalhão, E.C. Cárnio, Study of thermo-regulation as a worsening marker of experimental sepsis in an animal model. Rev. Lat.-Am. Enferm. **28**, e3290 (2020)

S. Tai, J. Wang, F. Sun, Q. Pan, C. Peng, Z. Wang, A colorimetric sensor array based on nanoceria crosslinked and heteroatom-doped graphene oxide nanoribbons for the detection and discrimination of multiple pesticides. Anal. Chim. Acta **1283**, 341929 (2023)

W.S.T. Tun, A. Saenchoopa, S. Daduang, J. Daduang, S. Kulchat, R. Patramanon, Electrochemical biosensor based on cellulose nanofibers/graphene oxide and acetylcholinesterase for the detection of chlorpyrifos pesticide in water and fruit juice. RSC Adv. **13**(14), 9603–9614 (2023)

S. Wahyudi, A. Bahtiar, C. Panatarani, Recent advanced carbon dots derived natural products and aptasensor-based carbon dots for detection of pesticides. Sens. Bio-Sens. Res. **41**, 100576 (2023)

L. Wen, J. Wang, Z. Liu, C.A. Tao, J. Rao, J. Hang, Y. Li, A portable acetylcholinesterase-based electrochemical sensor for field detection of organophosphorus. RSC Adv. **13**(10), 6389–6395 (2023)

X. Wu, P. Wang, S. Hou, P. Wu, J. Xue, Fluorescence sensor for facile and visual detection of organophosphorus pesticides using AIE fluorogenic-SiO_2-MnO_2 sandwich nanocomposites. Talanta **198**, 8–14 (2019)

Y. Wu, J. Feng, G. Hu, E. Zhang, H.H. Yu, Colorimetric sensors for chemical and biological sensing applications. Sensors **23**(5), 2749 (2023)

X. Xu, R. Ray, Y. Gu, H.J. Ploehn, L. Gearheart, K. Raker, W.A. Scrivens, Electrophoretic analysis and purification of fluorescent single-walled carbon nanotube fragments. J. Am. Chem. Soc. **126**(40), 12736–12737 (2004)

M. Xu, S. Jiang, B. Jiang, J. Zheng, Organophosphorus pesticides detection using acetylcholinesterase biosensor based on gold nanoparticles constructed by electroless plating on vertical nitrogen-doped single-walled carbon nanotubes. Int. J. Environ. Anal. Chem. **99**(10), 913–927 (2019)

M.A. Zafar, D. Waligo, O.K. Varghese, M.V. Jacob, Advances in graphene-based electrochemical biosensors for on-site pesticide detection. Front. Carbon **2**, 1325970 (2023)

X. Zhang, X. Liao, Y. Hou, B. Jia, L. Fu, M. Jia, et al., Recent advances in synthesis and modification of carbon dots for optical sensing of pesticides. J. Hazard. Mater. **422**, 126881 (2022)

F. Zhao, J. Wu, Y. Ying, Y. She, J. Wang, J. Ping, Carbon nanomaterial-enabled pesticide biosensors: design strategy, biosensing mechanism, and practical application. TrAC Trends Anal. Chem. **106**, 62–83 (2018)

M. Zhou, Z. Wang, X. Wang, Carbon nanotubes for sensing applications, in *Industrial Applications of Carbon Nanotubes* (Elsevier, 2017), pp. 129–150

C. Zhou, J. Feng, Y. Tian, Y. Wu, Q. He, G. Li, J. Liu, Non-enzymatic electrochemical sensors based on nanomaterials for detection of organophosphorus pesticide residues. Environ. Sci. Adv. **2**(7), 933–956 (2023)

Y. Zhu, Y. Cao, X. Sun, X. Wang, Amperometric immunosensor for carbofuran detection based on MWCNTs/GS-PEI-Au and AuNPs-antibody conjugate. Sensors **13**(4), 5286–5301 (2013)

Graphene-Based Heterostructures and Their Applications as Bionanomaterial

Alejandra Garcia-Garcia, Huma Sadiq, and Rene Hernández-Delgadillo

Abstract Graphene-based heterostructures represent a frontier in bionanomaterials, combining the exceptional electrical, mechanical, and chemical properties of graphene with the complementary functionalities of zero-, one-, two-, and three-dimensional nanostructures. This chapter presents an overview of recent progress in the synthesis, properties, and biomedical applications of graphene heterostructures. It discusses key fabrication strategies, including chemical vapor deposition, hydrothermal, and microwave-assisted routes, as well as layer-by-layer assembly, that enable the formation of vertical and lateral architectures with tailored interfaces and controlled defect structures. Emphasis is given to their use in biosensing, drug delivery, tissue engineering, and antibacterial systems, where graphene's tunable surface chemistry, high conductivity, and biocompatibility offer multifunctional performance. The chapter also examines surface functionalization approaches (covalent, non-covalent, green chemistry, and inorganic hybridization) that enhance biointerface interactions and enable targeted therapeutic delivery. Emerging evidence on graphene selenium nanoparticle hybrids highlights their synergistic antimicrobial mechanisms and potential for clinical translation. Finally, the challenges of toxicity, biocompatibility, and large-scale synthesis are addressed, outlining future perspectives for integrating graphene-based heterostructures into next-generation biomedical devices and theragnostic systems.

Keywords Graphene-based heterostructures · Biomedical applications · Functionalization techniques · Drug delivery · Biosensing

A. Garcia-Garcia (✉) · H. Sadiq
Centro de Investigación en Materiales Avanzados S.C., Subsede Monterrey, Apodaca, Nuevo León, México
e-mail: alejandra.garcia@cimav.edu.mx

R. Hernández-Delgadillo
Facultad de Odontología, Universidad Autónoma de Nuevo León , Monterrey, México

R. Narayan (ed.), *Nanostructured Biomaterials and Their Applications*,
https://doi.org/10.1007/978-3-032-16316-5_12

1 General Introduction

Graphene is the fundamental building block of graphite with a single layer of carbon atoms arranged in a honeycomb lattice (Mirtaghavi et al. 2020). It is easy to create a tunable work function using chemical and electrostatic doping, allowing adjustment of various properties of this structure, including mechanical flexibility and strength, as well as higher charge mobility and excellent transparency (Sharma et al. 2022). Until 2004, it was not possible to separate a single graphene layer from graphite (Novoselov et al. 2004). However, a method was developed that enables the separation of layers using adhesive tape (Taghizadeh et al. 2022). Shortly after, another research team independently developed a method to grow ultrathin graphite films on silicon carbide (SiC), paving the way for large-scale graphene synthesis (Torres-Pinto et al. 2023). These pioneering studies highlighted graphene as the first-ever 2D material, spurring the development of more advanced techniques for its production. These techniques now include more advanced methods, such as metal catalysts via chemical vapor deposition with a wide range of precursors (Jakus et al. 2015), reduction and exfoliation of GO (Faria et al. 2014), and liquid-phase exfoliation (Geim et al. 2013).

Over the last few decades, graphene's limitations have become apparent. One of the most significant drawbacks is the absence of a bandgap in the graphene electronic structure, which limits its effectiveness for various applications. The focus has now shifted toward exploring novel categories of two-dimensional (2D) layered materials for various bionanomaterial applications (Geim et al. 2007). Mixed-dimensional heterostructures, created by integrating graphene or graphene analogs with materials of different dimensions, offer a range of multifunctional properties that cannot be achieved by separate 0D, 1D, 2D, or 3D materials. The sharp variations in the energy dependence of the density of states and electrostatic screening across these mixed-dimensional interfaces significantly modify their electrical, magnetic, optical, and thermal characteristics, leading to novel and enhanced functionalities for technological applications. Among the heterostructures, most prominent are hexagonal boron nitride (h-BN) (Maestro et al. 2010), an insulating substance with a lattice structure like graphene, and transition metal dichalcogenides (TMDs) from group VI (Erol et al. 2018), which are semiconductors possessing band gaps in the range of 1–2 eV. Notably, these 2D/2D structures can be synthesized by integrating graphene with these materials, providing a means to address the intrinsic limitations of each material while facilitating the emergence of new properties through their deliberate combination. In this context, the term "heterostructure" refers to a composite material consisting of graphene or a two-dimensional material combined with other materials.

Graphene and graphene oxide, along with their unique structures, have numerous applications in the biomedical field (Erol et al. 2018). These structures are valuable for various applications, including antimicrobial (Allard et al. 2024), biosensing (Radisavljevic et al. 2011), antibacterial (Li 2017), and drug delivery (Murjani et al. 2022). The purpose of this chapter is to introduce recent advancements made, with a particular focus on applications in the field of bionanomaterials and the construction of heterostructures. This chapter will also discuss the fabrication of these materials, their properties, and future trends.

2 Graphene-Based Heterostructures: An Overview

As graphene possesses remarkable properties, it faces challenges, particularly due to its lack of an intrinsic bandgap (Bullock and Bussy 2019). Given the wide range of available two-dimensional (2D) materials, many of which exhibit complementary characteristics, the integration of these materials into 2D/2D heterostructures offers promising and innovative possibilities (Castiello et al. 2023). The formation of these structures can substantially augment the capabilities of these materials, providing thin films with novel functionalities. By leveraging the unique properties of different materials in structures, it is possible to develop entirely 2D devices with enhanced and desirable characteristics, including cutting-edge biomaterial applications.

A key advantage of incorporating graphene into heterostructures is that it serves as a substrate with exceptional electrical conductivity and high carrier mobility (Shuai et al. 2023). In 2D materials, the layered structure, a practical approach to constructing such heterostructures, is achieved by intentionally stacking different layers of materials (Corbet et al. 2016). Van der Waals forces dominate between these layers, and this weak interlayer bonding facilitates the isolation of individual layers through exfoliation, allowing the stacking of diverse materials without the limitations imposed by lattice mismatches. This capability enables the creation of various types of vertical structures by strategically assembling layers in a specific order (Dean et al. 2010). As explored in the following section, recent advancements in 2D material processing have enabled the fabrication of complex vertical structures with a wide range of functionalities. Additionally, ongoing efforts focus on developing methods to synthesize such structures, aiming to achieve the high output required for large-scale production (Corbet et al. 2016).

Over time, significant progress has been made in the techniques for stacking these materials. One of these methods is the dry transfer method, which leverages the van der Waals forces between the stacked layers. In this transfer process, an exfoliated flake is used to sequentially take an additional exfoliated layer, which together forms the final heterostructure (Iannazzo et al. 2017; Mudusu et al. 2021; Debmalya Roy 2024). This process yields a cleaner product without direct contact with polymers and solvents. Nevertheless, these surfaces are exposed to ambient conditions during exfoliation and layer stacking. For materials that are unstable in the atmosphere, transfer can be performed under an inert atmosphere, as observed for $NbSe_2$ (Cadamuro et al. 2023).

A novel approach for exfoliating and transferring single layers of TMDs onto various substrates has been developed. This is done by evaporating a thin film of gold (Au) on a bulk TMD using thermal tape, which is then peeled off, leaving the Au film behind. It is easy to compare the properties of these structures with those of materials synthesized by a wide range of methods, while achieving orders-of-magnitude improvements in size and uniformity (Zhang et al. 2019).

Bulk materials composed of exfoliated layers are particularly suitable for rapid prototyping technologies based on layered structures, as they eliminate the need for direct growth processes. Using these strategies, different two-dimensional materials can be stacked with virtually no intrinsic limitations. Moreover, the relative rotation between adjacent layers can be precisely controlled with sub-degree accuracy, enabling the tuning of interlayer interactions (Liu et al. 2023). These approaches have enabled the fabrication of a wide variety of van der Waals heterostructures, including graphene combined with transition metal dichalcogenides such as molybdenum disulfide and tungsten disulfide (Reina et al. 2017) as well as systems incorporating hexagonal boron nitride (Hashemzadeh et al. 2020) and other layered materials such as TMDs (Sun et al. 2013). However, factors like lattice and energetic mismatches may arise depending on the specific material combination. While mechanically stacked designs offer significant flexibility and advantages for fundamental studies, they remain difficult to scale and are therefore not practical for many industrial applications of graphene-based heterostructures.

3 Nanomaterials Classified by Dimension and Heterostructures

3.1 0D Materials

Zero-dimensional (0D) materials, e.g., quantum dots (QDs) (Sun et al. 2013), nanoparticles (Xu et al. 2018), and so forth, are a kind of nanostructures where the size in each direction (x, y, and z) is at the nanoscale. These materials exhibit unique optical, electrical, and magnetic properties resulting from quantum confinement effects, which occur when electrons are confined to minuscule dimensions. 0D materials also open new frontiers in various bionanomaterials fields, such as drug and gene payloads (Zhang et al. 2022), bioimaging probes (Hauke et al. 2018), and biosensors that exhibit improved properties when incorporated into heterostructures with graphene. Cadmium selenide (CdSe) is of special interest in research on quantum dots due to its well-characterized optical properties, in particular, size-dependent fluorescence (Chia et al. 2021). Quantum dots can be surface-functionalized on graphene or embedded between (or within) the layers of graphene in a heterostructure to enhance the electronic and optical properties (Chen et al. 2016). Their design enables high resolution and sensitivity, making them an ideal platform for bioimaging applications (Heo et al. 2022).

0D materials and graphene provide efficient energy-transfer platforms like Förster resonance energy-transfer FRET (Hu et al. 1999) or field effect transistor FET (Li et al. 2021). This is extremely helpful in biosensing, where the interaction of a target molecule with the heterostructure can be manifested as fluorescence or a change in electrical signals. For instance, GQDs modified with antibodies or aptamers can sense specific pathogens or cancer markers by monitoring changes in fluorescence intensity upon binding (Lin et al. 2018).

Restorative applications of these materials with GO are the most encouraging to date, particularly for drug delivery and related heterogeneous nanocomposites comprising 0D nanostructures. Chemically, the high surface area and biocompatibility of GO platforms confer them an outstanding property for the development of multifunctional nanocomposites from poisonous nanoparticle additives. A potentially effective strategy is to combine it with gold nanoparticles (AuNPs)-reduced graphene oxide (rGO). In this sense, the GO-AuNP hybrid was found to be more effective for drug delivery due to its improved binding and ability to modulate release at the site. GO also provides a functionalized platform for drug attachment, whereas AuNPs serve as vehicles for targeted delivery and photothermal therapy, making the system highly effective in cancer therapy (Park et al. 2013). Apart from drug delivery, GO interacts with different nanomaterials, which make its own antimicrobial properties. For example, it has been demonstrated that when GO is used in conjunction with silver nanoparticles (AgNPs), biofilm inhibition on surfaces exposed to Pseudomonas aeruginosa can be achieved at rates exceeding 100%. These nanocomposites also demonstrated enhanced cell adhesion and tissue compatibility, making them promising materials for wound healing and/or tissue scaffolding applications at beneficial levels (Peng et al. 2013; Shi et al. 2015). In summary, GO heterostructures have a wide range of applications in drug delivery and biomedical fields due to their diverse functions, including controlling surface properties, interacting with biological systems, and enhancing efficacy. These features are important for their use as GO scaffolds in the development of advanced therapeutic technologies.

Heterostructures of 0D graphene are also being explored for targeted drug delivery. Drugs can be loaded into nanoparticles or quantum dots and then released in response to specific stimuli, such as a change in pH within the body. GQD-drug conjugates can be designed to release their payload in the acidic tumor microenvironment, ensuring effective targeting and reduced side effects.

It is crucial to ensure the biocompatibility of these 0D graphene heterostructures to guarantee safe application in biomedical devices. Surface modification of these materials can overcome solubility, stability, or toxicity issues. They can be polymeric coatings, such as PEG, to improve biocompatibility, allowing them to circulate in the body without being immunogenic, or they could use peptide modifications. This is crucial in drug delivery applications, where nanoparticles are used to deliver therapeutic agents to specific locations within the body (Wang et al. 2019).

Despite this, graphene remains the top choice among 0D materials for bionanomaterials. The QD's toxicity is an issue that cannot be ignored (Wen et al. 2015). Therefore, QDs, typically carbon-based or other low-toxicity materials that degrade in the body after drug delivery, are being investigated for this purpose. Moreover, the flatness and surface chemistry of 0D materials play a pivotal role in establishing large-area contact with biological systems. Since these nanoparticles are small, they can be easily excreted from the body rather than accumulating and causing long-term effects.

3.2 1D Materials

One of the single-layered or few-layered structures, such as carbon nanotubes (CNTs), nanowires, and nanoribbons (see Fig. 1), is characterized by a long length and a high aspect ratio, which renders it unexpected mechanical, electrical, and thermal properties (Yoon et al. 2021). When mixed with these materials, graphene forms new graphene-based heterostructures (2D/1D) that are medically important in tissue engineering (Zhang et al. 2024) and biosensing (Prescher et al. 2007).

Graphene, being a 2D material, provides more surface area for functionalization, while CNTs, as one-dimensional materials (Ranasinghe et al. 2022), introduce additional electrical and mechanical properties. This combination results in heterostructures 2D/1D with improved electrical conductivity, mechanical strength, and surface area, is crucial for biomedical applications (Moses et al. 2007). Another application is their utility as nerve guides for tissue engineering, which has captured the attention of several research groups (Lee et al. 2019).

Therefore, understanding the biocompatibility of these heterostructures is crucial for their safe application in various biomedical environments. Functionalization, such as coating with biocompatible polymers like PEG, can mitigate the toxicity of mesoporous silica (Jianping Shi 2015). These modifications allow the materials to safely interact with biological systems, enhancing their potential in bioimaging, biosensing, and drug delivery.

The relatively high surface area of 2D/1D graphene-based heterostructures enables the incorporation of drug molecules into a drug delivery system, allowing for targeted release. For example, when ligands such as antibodies or peptides are attached to the heterostructure drug delivery system, this ensures that drugs are released only at the targeted site, minimizing side effects and enhancing treatment efficacy (Kim et al. 2020). Incorporating magnetic particles into 2D/1D heterostructures could help direct the heterostructure to the problem site and facilitate subsequent recovery. In Fig. 1a, a scheme illustrating one-dimensional structures is shown, with graphene

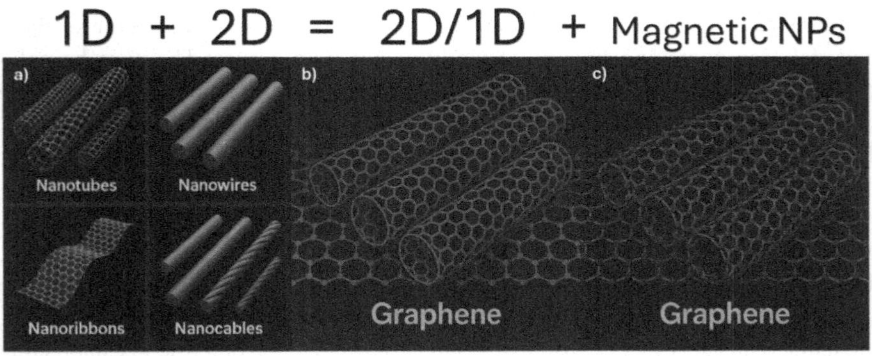

Fig. 1 **a** Examples of 1 Dimensional nanostructure, **b** 2D/1D heterostructure with graphene as the substrate, **c** 2D/1D heterostructure with magnetic nanoparticles at the surface

serving as the substrate, and the possible 2D/1D heterostructure featuring CNTs as 1D nanostructures (Fig. 1b). Subsequently, the incorporation of magnetic nanoparticles is depicted (Fig. 1c), which can serve as a recovery system. In the experimental field, researchers have explored rGO-quantum dot nanocomposites that combine photothermal therapy (PTT) with fluorescence imaging for targeting tumor cells. On the other hand, GO functionalized with porphyrin is a promising platform for PTT in brain cancer, demonstrating enhanced stability and improved "in vitro" depletion of cancer cells. However, PTT alone may not fully eradicate tumors due to uneven heat distribution, often requiring combination therapies for greater efficacy.

3.3 2D Materials

Genetically modified graphene heterostructures for bionanomaterials (Ghosal et al. 2019) have been widely applied in biosensing (Shankar et al. 2023), drug delivery (Tadyszak et al. 2018a), and bioimaging (Tadyszak et al. 2018b), due to their excellent electronic, optical, and mechanical properties. When 2D materials like molybdenum disulfide (MoS_2) are combined with graphene, they form van der Waals heterostructures or 2D/2D (Yang et al. 2013). These structures are largely unbound due to weak interlayer forces, allowing each layer to retain its unique properties while interacting synergistically. Biosensing applications benefit from this cooperation, where the optical and electrical properties of the materials are used to enhance the detection of biological molecules (Yang et al. 2013).

The large surface area of 2D materials also facilitates the decoration with biomolecules such as antibodies, proteins, or nucleic acids, enabling the development of biosensors and drug delivery systems with high sensitivity and specificity. Surface modifications further improve the biocompatibility of 2D heterostructures. The 2D graphene heterostructure is widely used in biosensing due to its high sensitivity. In drug delivery, graphene-based 2D materials can be functionalized with drugs for targeted release within the body. These structures have demonstrated excellent performance in biological viability and antioxidant applications, as evidenced by the concentration-dependent free-radical scavenging of the V_2O_5/GO nanocomposite, suggesting their potential for biological applications (Yang et al. 2012). Additionally, the high surface area and biocompatibility of 2D materials make them ideal for bioimaging applications, where they can be used as contrast agents for high-resolution imaging.

3.4 3D Materials

Due to their unique properties, graphene-based novel 3D materials, such as graphene foam, aerogels, and hydrogels, have demonstrated improved quality for tissue engineering (Kong et al. 2013), drug delivery (Novoselov et al. 2004), and biosensing

(Novoselov et al. 2005). The interconnected porous structure of these materials mimics the extracellular matrix (ECM) found in biological tissues, making them ideal for biomedical applications (Tang et al. 2023).

The high porosity of 3D graphene-based materials enables efficient transport of nutrients and waste, thereby facilitating cell adhesion and proliferation. This makes them particularly suitable for use as scaffolds in tissue engineering, where they support cell growth and differentiation. The large volume of 3D graphene materials enhances the biomolecules, such as growth factors, accelerating tissue restoration (Yue et al. 2017).

The electroactivity of 3D graphene materials also supports the debate on the need for scaffolds in electrically active tissues, such as neural and cardiac tissues. Researchers have demonstrated that electrical stimulation of 3D graphene foams enhances cell differentiation and proliferation, making them promising candidates for regenerative medicine (Meng et al. 2016). In addition to tissue engineering, 3D graphene-based materials are also utilized in drug delivery systems, where their porous structure enables efficient loading and release of therapeutic agents. These materials have also been applied in biosensing, where their properties enable the development of more sensitive and selective sensors for biomolecule detection.

3.5 Synthesis Techniques

Several simple and combined techniques have been developed for preparing these graphene-based heterostructures (Fig. 2). The details of these techniques are given below.

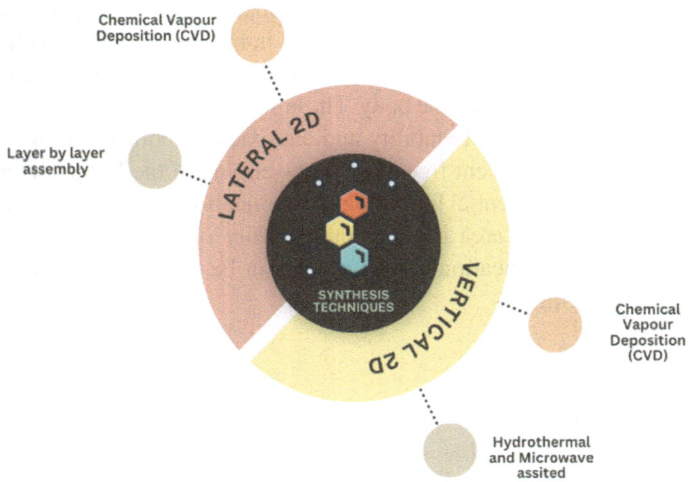

Fig. 2 Methods to synthesize heterostructures: vertical 2D assembly and lateral 2D assembly

4 Synthesis of Lateral 2D Heterostructures

4.1 *Chemical Vapor Deposition*

Lateral structures are typically fabricated using a chemical vapor deposition (CVD) process, which must be modulated to prevent alloy formation, as this process involves interfacial compositions. This ensures sharp interfaces, which are essential for achieving superior properties (Geiser et al. 2010).

By tuning the sublimation points of the precursors, controlling the temperature is very important in regulating the nucleation of 2D materials. This can be achieved by using higher temperatures, which increase domain size due to faster reaction rates; however, excessively high temperatures may lead to smaller domains resulting from higher nucleation density. The duration of growth also plays a significant role, as does temperature, in regulating the nucleation of 2D materials, which can be influenced by tuning the sublimation points of the precursors. Higher temperatures can enhance reaction rates and increase domain size; however, excessively high temperatures may lead to smaller domains due to an increased nucleation density. The duration of the growth process also plays a significant role. Extended growth times with low precursor supply can lead to the formation of nanovoids on the surface of the 2D material, rather than achieving the desired final structure.

The CVD processes can be classified into various types. One-step CVD methods prevent the presence of multiple vapor precursors but often do not allow complete separation of these vapors, and alloy formation occurs at the interface. Additionally, the size and orientation of the resultant heterostructures are hard to control. To get this, multi-step CVD processes are required. For example, Y. Gong and others employed a two-step CVD strategy to create WSe_2/MoS_2 lateral heterostructures (Legesse et al. 2020). The most noticeable advantage of this technique is that it can be beneficial, especially in 2D/2D heterostructures for tissue engineering (Mahmoudpour et al. 2021) and biosensors (Silva et al. 2021).

4.2 *Layer-By-Layer Structure*

Among the various techniques for assembling multilayer films, layer-by-layer (LbL) assembly is a simple and cost-effective method for preparing highly ordered 2D/2D heterostructures of various materials, with immense applications in biological systems. The multilayered assemblage of graphene sheets is very promising for emerging applications due to their concurrent electrical, optical, and thermal properties. Recent advancements in LbL assembly have enabled the development of graphene-based heterostructures with various other nanomaterials, including carbon-based materials, polymers, and inorganic nanoparticles. These graphene heterostructures exhibit enhanced physical and chemical properties, outperforming their individual constituents, and display synergistic effects within these nanocomposites, suggesting significant potential, particularly in medical applications.

5 Synthesis of Vertical 2D Heterostructures

5.1 Chemical Vapor Deposition

Vertical heterostructures, particularly those based on graphene, have remarkable electronic, biocompatibility, and mechanical properties (Silva et al. 2017). Using two approaches, vertical 2D structures with many layers can be constructed. These structures are constructed by stacking different layers to enhance the material's properties, rather than using individual layers. In top-down techniques, materials with large areas are exfoliated in a lower-dimensional form and then layered to build 2D heterostructures. On the other hand, bottom-up methods typically employ chemical vapor deposition to grow these structures by precisely monitoring these growth parameters. For instance, Zhang and colleagues synthesized monolayer MoS_2 via low-pressure CVD and monolayer graphene via atmospheric-pressure CVD. They then transferred and stacked the graphene on the MoS_2 to create vertical structures. Cross-sectional profiles revealed that the graphene and MoS_2 layers were well-stacked perfectly (Sup Choi 2013).

Another approach involves direct chemical vapor deposition growth of vertical structures by controlling the growth conditions to avoid contamination from manual processes. Another researcher, Ting Kang, has observed recent progress in the controlled growth of 2D materials using the CVD method. Then, they tried different methods for device fabrication (Maqsood Ahmed 2012). As the structure of these materials continues to evolve, their integration holds significant promise in the biomedical field. The synthesis of vertical 2D heterostructures for biomedical applications, such as biosensing, drug delivery, or tissue engineering, requires precise control over both material interfaces and functional properties to ensure their efficacy in biological environments (Guimarães et al. 2014).

5.2 Hydrothermal and Microwave-Assisted Technique

The preparation of such structures is a current trend due to their various applications and possibilities, primarily in the field of bionanomaterials. Among the methods used to synthesize these structures, hydrothermal and microwave-assisted techniques have proven effective, environmentally friendly, and scalable (Molaei et al. 2021; Das et al. 2011). These methods offer several advantages, including better control over reaction conditions, enhanced energy efficiency, and the formation of high-quality products, making them suitable for advanced materials in promising applications such as biosensing, drug delivery, and nanotechnology.

Hydrothermal synthesis is an established method that utilizes the pressure and temperature of water or other solvents to synthesize nanomaterials (Fuhrer et al. 2010). This technique, when used on heterostructures based on graphene, permits the incorporation of many elements (for example, metal oxides or organic compounds) with crystallinity for use on the substrate of graphene. This controlled environment enables simultaneous nucleation and growth during the hydrothermal process, resulting in homogeneously dispersed nanocomposites. One significant benefit of this approach is that it can yield very high-quality, mesostructured films with excellent electronic and mechanical properties. Furthermore, the materials obtained from hydrothermal synthesis usually have fewer defects, which is significant in some applications such as biosensors and drug delivery systems. Here, even small impurities can significantly alter the asset.

Therefore, a faster, lower-energy-demanding route to obtain these structures is microwave-assisted synthesis (Xia et al. 2019). They achieved this by developing a microwave-irradiation technique that heats their reactants more uniformly and faster than traditional methods. Microwave energy can directly interact with reactant molecules, rapidly creating these features within minutes. The lower reaction temperature and reaction time result in fewer side reactions and better control over the morphology and size of nanoscale structures. Additionally, this microwave-assisted approach can be applied to numerous precursor systems, enabling the production of tunable graphene heterostructures with distinct functionalities relevant to bionanomaterials applications.

With both synthesis methods, high tunability is reached, so you learn how to play the game by changing temperature, reaction time, and pressure with precursor concentrations and use this knowledge to achieve the desired structural/functional properties. That versatility comes in handy if you want to tailor your structures further for biological applications, whether to optimize biocompatibility, increase surface area, or achieve the ideal electrical properties. For instance, the metal oxide and graphene structure derived by these methods exhibits good electron transfer properties. It can be used for further functionalization purposes, thereby demonstrating impressive performance in biosensors. In summary, hydrothermal and microwave-irradiation synthesis strategies are widely used to produce bionanomaterial structures with significant potential, as demonstrated by earlier studies. It is beneficial for researchers to develop nanocomposites for biomedical devices, biosensing applications, and controlled release systems, as this enables the manufacture of defect-free, high-quality materials under specific environmental conditions.

5.3 Properties and Behavior of Graphene-Based Heterostructures

The properties and behavior of graphene-based heterostructures, which have garnered significant attention from an increasing number of researchers over the past several years in response to the need for integration with various components, have brought the field of bionanomaterials to the forefront. By blending graphene with various nanostructures, researchers can selectively enhance and harness its intrinsic properties for different biomedical applications. Due to their electrical, mechanical, and chemical properties, especially those of the structures fabricated with graphene, they have demonstrated significant potential. In this section, we provide a perspective on how such structures can be tailored to exhibit unique performance modifications (primarily in electrical conductivity, mechanical properties, and chemical reactivity), enabling their application in biosensors, tissue scaffolds, and therapeutic delivery systems.

6 Electrical Conductivity

Graphene shows a special electrical property (Dubey et al. 2015), which can be either enhanced or modulated depending on the materials combined with it in multilayered structures. These resultant structures could be used as biosensors in bionanomaterial applications due to their excellent electrical conductivity. One strategy to enhance the biocompatibility of graphene-based heterostructures is to introduce defects into the graphene lattice, such as nitrogen doping. Nitrogen-doped graphene alters its electronic properties by introducing localized states, which can enhance its chemical reactivity, making it suitable for "in vivo" applications. Here, nitrogen atoms are incorporated in place of carbon atoms into the graphene lattice during chemical synthesis to increase defects and change the surface energy for enhanced biological molecular interaction that can be useful for cell adhesive interactions as well as proliferation and differentiation. These changes also make pristine graphene more hydrophilic, thus improving its biocompatibility. Nitrogen-doped graphene is therefore better suited for applications such as drug delivery (Dubey et al. 2015), tissue engineering (Fatima et al. 2021), and biosensors (Li et al. 2019), where interactions with biological systems are necessary. Moreover, incorporating nitrogen atoms further enhances conductivity and improves bioelectronic interactivity when signal transduction between biological tissues and electronic devices is required.

Doping graphene with other materials, such as metals or semiconductors, can be used to adjust its conductivity, thereby increasing sensitivity and signal propagation in biosensors. The novelty of these changes lies in the detection of biomolecules at concentrations as low as a few hundred millimoles, making them well-suited for early-stage disease diagnosis and monitoring. This flexibility to adjust the material's electronic properties after structuring opens opportunities for biosensors with greater precision and design freedom.

7 Mechanical Properties

In addition to their optical response, these structures are also seen to enhance the mechanical properties. Graphene is known for its incredible strength, even in its pure form; however, when combined with other materials, it can significantly enhance their flexibility and toughness (Panwar et al. 2016). This helps to make graphene heterostructures ideal for the "Death Valley" of the mechanical properties map, which is typically relevant in biomedical engineering applications and tissue scaffold developments. The biomaterial's greater flexibility enables it to withstand mechanical stress within a biological matrix while retaining its structure. In addition, these two new properties, improved strength and flexibility, make it more suitable for replicating the mechanical nature of different tissues, thereby promoting cell growth and tissue regeneration (Rohaizad et al. 2021). Therefore, the advantages in mechanics through hosting graphene structures are highly desirable for tissue fabrication.

8 Chemical Reactivity

Another key aspect is chemical reactivity, which can be significantly enhanced by forming heterostructures. The interaction between two-dimensional materials and other nanomaterials of different dimensionality introduces new active sites and modifies the electronic environment, thereby promoting strong chemical activity. For instance, graphene-based heterostructures can be synthesized by integrating additional nanomaterials to create porous architectures with high surface areas, which improve their ability to interact with other molecules. This feature makes them particularly attractive for drug delivery systems, where the increased surface area allows efficient drug loading, and enhanced reactivity enables controlled release of therapeutic agents at specific rates and concentrations (Erol et al. 2018). Such tunable behavior makes these 2D heterostructures ideal candidates for precision and targeted medicine.

Finally, doping of the layers in graphene-based heterostructures leads to significant modifications in their chemistry, and these changes can strongly correlate with the final behavior of these nanostructures. These architectures, synthesized with graphene, can significantly modify and enhance the properties of functionalized molecules, potentially surpassing those of the parent molecules to uniquely suit them for biomedical applications. Such structures are thus built to suit different applications across biomedical fields, such as biosensors, tissue scaffolds, targeted drug delivery systems, and biocompatible bionanomaterials, by leveraging the compact synthesis and integration of these intrinsic properties. Such synergistic integration of doping and graphene-based synthesis enables the fine-tuning of properties, furthering these heterostructures closer to diverse biotechnological applicability.

9 Functionalization Techniques for Graphene-Based Heterostructures

Functionalization is critical for the modification and application of G-BFNs (Graphene-based functionalized nanostructures) across various biological and therapeutic applications. Surface modification of graphene opens new perspectives for applications, such as tissue engineering (Ajayan et al. 2016), regenerative medicine, drug delivery systems (Bellet et al. 2021), and biosensors (Blake et al. 2015), as well as the formation of new heterostructures using functionalization as an anchor to join other 0D, 1D, or 2D nanostructures. This section aims to review the prevalent functionalization techniques, engage with both their positive and negative aspects, and explore what the future holds for the use of graphene heterostructures.

10 Covalent Functionalization

Covalent modification involves attaching chemical groups to the basal plane of graphene, forming strong, rigid structures. This method is very effective in increasing stability in a biological medium. Graphene will also be resistant to degradation when certain functional groups are covalently attached to it, thereby retaining its properties for an extended period, even in a complex cellular environment. This type of functionalization is advantageous in clinical applications, such as drug targeting or tissue scaffolding, where materials are exposed to diverse biological environments (Choudhary et al. 2019).

There are several advantages of the covalent bond, including the following: one of the principal advantages of covalent modification is the ability to respond to external stimuli when the material is created. Dynamic covalent bonds, which can be adjusted or broken down by factors such as light, temperature, or pH, enable researchers to design materials that adapt to changing conditions. For example, techniques such as copper(I)-catalyzed azide-alkyne cycloaddition (CuAAC) and Diels–Alder reactions are used to attach bioactive molecules to graphene surfaces, thereby enabling the creation of multifunctional biomaterials (Kumar et al. 2019; Paras et al. 2023).

However, this functionalization has limitations too (Huang et al. 2013). These reactions may be complex, consisting of several steps, which can make the bond formation process intricate and potentially slow down large-scale production. However, it remains powerful for creating scalable graphene-based materials.

11 Non-covalent Functionalization

Non-covalent functionalization involves attaching molecules to graphene through weaker interactions, such as van der Waals forces or hydrogen bonding. This method is straightforward and rarely compromises the material's original electronic properties, making it suitable for electronic or biosensor applications where conductivity preservation is necessary (Guo et al. 2021).

One notable advantage of non-covalent modification is its relative simplicity. In contrast to covalent methods, this approach typically does not involve laborious chemical processes or purification steps, making it more feasible for bulk applications. However, the weaker bonds also mean there may be issues retaining such non-covalently modified graphene within biological matrices. To utilize these materials for medical or other implantable applications, significant improvements will be necessary to determine their behavior over extended periods in the body.

12 Green Chemistry Approaches

With the rise of environmental concerns, there is a need for sustainable and environmentally friendly methods. Functionalizing through green chemistry entails utilizing non-toxic and energy-efficient methods, resulting in reduced waste production and the avoidance of harmful chemicals (Kumar et al. 2023). For example, photoinduced thiol-ene reactions are such methods that allow molecules to be attached onto surfaces using light, thereby reducing the use of hazardous solvents and reagents.

Again, in this area, nature-based techniques also have a significant role. Its biocompatibility and environmental safety have made it popular in biomedical research (Sakthivel et al. 2023a). These researchers aim to develop high-performing yet eco-friendly functionalized materials by employing sustainable methods.

13 Hybrid Functionalization with Inorganic Materials

Graphene can be combined with other materials, such as black phosphorus (BP) or molybdenum disulfide (MoS_2) (Sakthivel et al. 2023b), to further enhance its properties (MoS_2) (Hauke et al. 2018), thereby forming 2D/2D heterostructures. In bioelectronics, biosensing, especially with these heterostructures, exhibits properties that combine optical, electronic, and mechanical properties, leading to improved device performance.

Incorporating inorganic materials allows for the development of highly sensitive biosensors and advanced tissue scaffolds that can interface more effectively with biological systems. However, integrating these materials while preserving their properties remains a challenge. Further research is needed to better understand how these heterostructures interact with biological tissues and to minimize any potential toxicity.

14 Application of Bionanomaterials

Graphene-based heterostructures are widely attractive in biomedical fields. Among these system approaches, the nanoconjugate based on acrylic has gained increasing interest for improving the effects of cancer therapeutics in polymeric and protein-based nanotechnologies. Jakus et al. were the first to investigate the use of smart implants comprising medical sensors in combination with 3D-engineered scaffolds. They developed a method to replace damaged bone tissue.

The vast array of medical applications for these heterostructures in device development promises to revolutionize the healthcare sector. Graphene in the core not only keeps the final structure light but also enables functionalization with pH-sensitive polymers. They comprise polymers such as poly (N,N-dialkyl aminoethyl methacrylate), polyacrylic acid, and polymethacrylic acid, which have been used in drug delivery systems (García-González et al. 2021), hydrogels for stimulus-responsive applications, and even dental restorative materials. For the past thirty years, improvements in resin-based filler composites have been made to achieve better clinical results (Bai et al. 2018). In dentistry, for example, amalgam compounds created through this mechanism have enabled their extensive use in various multifunctional medical applications (Gorbachev et al. 2018).

The excellent properties of graphene have made it an ideal candidate for biomedical applications, including bioimaging, medical sensors, drug delivery, tissue engineering, and antitumoral agents (Fig. 3). These innovations in formulation techniques have been utilized in research aimed at developing graphene-based heterostructures, leveraging the unique structures and properties of graphene and its two-dimensional forms to create a new generation of cutting-edge biomedical instruments, thereby enhancing healthcare. The following paragraphs will provide a more detailed description of these advances.

15 Bioimaging

Currently, research is focusing on graphene's two-dimensional properties to develop cutting-edge medical tools and devices that improve healthcare. Bioimaging enables the observation and study of biological systems at different levels, playing a vital role in medicine. Graphene-based heterostructures have demonstrated potential in various imaging techniques, including ultrasonography, photoacoustic imaging, magnetic resonance imaging, computed tomography, fluorescence/confocal imaging, surface-enhanced Raman scattering, coherent anti-Stokes Raman scattering, and electron paramagnetic resonance imaging. These technologies enable real-time monitoring

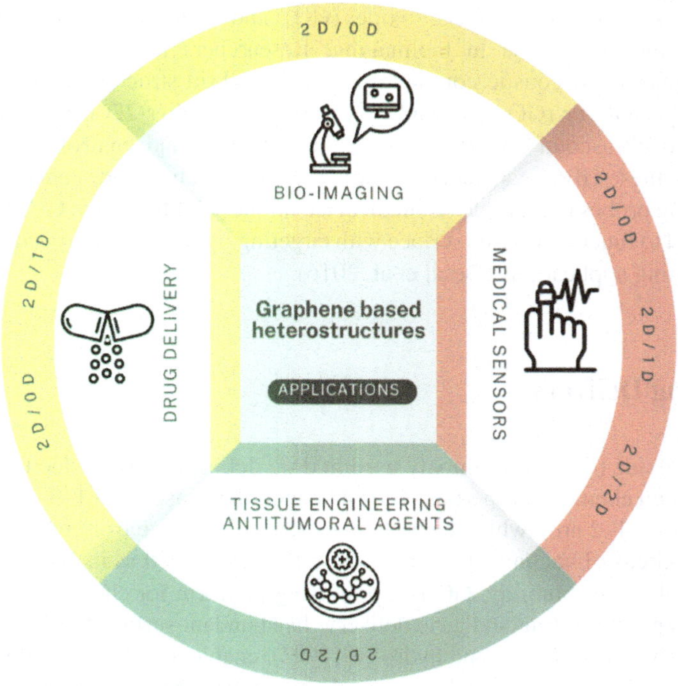

Fig. 3 Possible applications for graphene-based heterostructures

of biological processes, aiding in the detection of abnormalities such as cancer and necrosis (Bellet et al. 2021; Bai et al. 2018).

Sun et al. (2013) reported that the photoluminescent properties of nano-graphene oxide (nGO) with poly ethyl glycol are used for near-infrared (NIR) cell imaging. Both GO and nGO exhibited fluorescence across the visible to infrared range. Gonzalez et al. (Goenka et al. 2014) demonstrated the first use of a GBC contrast agent for "in vivo" magnetic resonance imaging (MRI) in tumor-bearing mice. Additionally, nGO–PEG has been adapted for in vivo positron emission tomography (PET) imaging, facilitating targeted tumor detection (Choudhary et al. 2019). Graphene quantum dots (GQDs), due to their ultra-small size, exhibit high photostability and low cytotoxicity, further enhancing their suitability for bioimaging (Priyadarsini et al. 2018).

Multimodal imaging, using multiple methods simultaneously, can provide more accurate diagnostics (Sengupta et al. 2023). This platform also allowed real-time monitoring of photothermal therapy, demonstrating potential for complete tumor ablation after treatment. Chen et al. (2016) presented another imaging agent, combining nano rGO-PEG with indocyanine green (ICG), creating a dual-modality system for fluorescence and photoacoustic imaging. Yue et al. (2017) further demonstrated the biocompatibility. Overall, multimodal imaging using graphene-based composites holds great promise for cancer diagnosis and therapy.

2D/2D systems of graphene oxide (GO) and reduced GO (rGO) demonstrate significant promise in bioimaging. Researchers have demonstrated high photothermal/photoacoustic contrast using these hybrid structures based on mono or multilayer GO or rGO, achieved by layering with other 2D nanomaterials, for optical and ultrasound imaging. Due to their stability and controlled fluorescent properties, these GBCs can act as carriers, contrast agents, fluorescence quenchers, or wrapping probes in multiple biomedical techniques. Additionally, GO/rGO can be engineered to functionalize its surface with targeting ligands for improved specificity in bioimaging applications (Desai et al. 2016).

16 Drug Delivery

Graphene oxide (GO) is commonly used in drug delivery systems due to its unique structural and chemical properties. The GO material consists of $\sim$ 1–3 layers (with a thickness of $\sim$1–2 nm), while the particulate size could range from several nanometers to hundreds of nanometers. Due to these factors, as well as its biocompatibility and physiological solubility, GO is a promising platform for chemical conjugation or physisorption for drug and gene delivery. Its abundant surface functional groups, such as carboxyl (–COOH) and hydroxyl (–OH), enable a wide array of biomedical applications. The biocompatibility of graphene can be enhanced (Haigh et al. 2014), and the toxicity can be reduced by incorporating graphene into hydrophilic biopolymers (Mousavi et al. 2020). For example, gelatin has been used as a functional component in doxorubicin (DOX)-loaded graphene nanosheets, as it can significantly enhance drug loading efficiency due to its high surface area and predominant stacking interactions. The studies mentioned above have shown that the combination of gelatin-graphene-DOX systems has selective toxicity on MCF-7 cells; therefore, it could be used as a promising intelligent drug delivery system (Laraba et al. 2022).

A different strategy involves using polyN-isopropylacrylamide (PNIPAM)-functionalized graphene sheets (GS) as a carrier system for camptothecin (CPT), a poorly water-soluble anticancer drug. The critical temperature for the hydrophilic-to-hydrophobic transition of PNIPAM-GS is 32.6 °C, slightly less than the transition degree temperature for PNIPAM alone (37.8 °C). This temperature sensitivity results in the controlled release of camptothecin (CPT), with a loading efficiency of 18.5%, primarily due to hydrophobic interactions and π-π stacking between the graphene sheets. PNIPAM-GS demonstrated excellent biocompatibility and significantly promoted CPT activity compared to the free drug (Shin et al. 2016).

Researchers synthesized a novel GO-based nanocomposite (GO-CSK) containing both chitosan (CHI) and hyaluronic acid (HA), which not only enhanced biocompatibility but also targeted tumor cells through the CD44 receptor. The GO-CHI-HA complex also demonstrated improved drug delivery capability of the anticancer agent SNX-2112. There was a significant increase in drug loading and cytotoxicity against cancer cells (A549), with minimal side effects, including hemolysis and coagulation (Shin et al. 2016). These findings suggest that GO-CHI-HA may be helpful in anticancer therapies.

Moreover, several functionalized graphene derivatives, such as Gr-Lys (lysine-treated graphene), GO-Rh2 (Ginsenoside Rh2-treated GO), and Gr-Arg (arginine-treated graphene), have been investigated for their superior anticancer effects. Amino acid functionalization, such as lysine and arginine, significantly reduces the toxicity of non-functionalized graphene, offering an improved biocompatible alternative for drug delivery applications. These outcomes illustrate that graphene-based composites (GBCs) hold great potential for use in drug delivery systems for cancer treatment (Shin et al. 2016). However, in real-world applications, practical considerations such as ease of administration, biocompatibility, reproducibility, and safety must be thoroughly addressed to ensure the clinical success of GBCs (Kang et al. 2022).

17 Tissue Engineering

Recently, the convergence of medical, biological, and engineering technologies has accelerated the rapid development of biomimetic tissues for repairing or regenerating organs in various devices. Tissue engineering is, by nature, an interdisciplinary field that involves cellular function, regulating cellular differentiation, and manipulating cell–cell interactions (Zhang et al. 2024). Various tissues exhibit distinct mechanical, electrical, and physical properties that differ significantly from one another. Graphene is a biocompatible material that supports cell attachment and growth, making it a valuable resource in tissue engineering and regenerative medicine due to its exceptional mechanical and electrical properties. The extraordinary properties of graphene can be harnessed to create tailored materials by incorporating a broad spectrum of bioactive components onto its surface.

The interesting atomic structure of graphene and its high adsorption power make graphene a good vehicle for gene and drug delivery. The facile preparation of graphene and its derivatives is a novel method for enhancing the mechanical strength and modifying the surface characteristics of biomaterials (Li et al. 2004). In addition, with its excellent electrical conductivity, graphene is expected to promote the growth and function of cardiac myocytes and neurons and improve the signal recording of individual cell changes triggered by electronic bipolarities. In addition, the researchers and their team developed a new approach inspired by 3D printing methodologies to create more intricate structures with tunable surface chemistry and machinable features (Gorbachev et al. 2018).

Research by Solanki et al. (2013) shows that neurobiologically relevant cellular matrices can be represented by hybrid nanostructures, such as monolayers of nanoparticles (NPs) overlaid with graphene oxide sheets, highlighting the potential of a type of hybrid nanostructure consisting of lipid NPs coated and functionalized with reduced graphene oxide. Silicon nanoparticles with positive charges were hybridized with GO by forming covalent bonds between graphene oxide and the groups on the silicon nanoparticle surface.

Graphene and its derivatives can be functionalized with other materials to develop multifunctional innovative materials that possess wettability, flexibility, or stimulus responsiveness. For example, carbon nanotube-based composites engineered to possess a range of functionalities, from shape-memory properties to self-folding capabilities, could significantly enhance their biological applications. By mixing graphene oxide (GO) with phase-changing materials, thermoresponsive drug delivery systems enhance both drug loading capacity and photothermal efficiency in photodynamic therapies. Self-folding 3D printing of graphene-based materials will catalyze advances in tissue engineering and usher in next-generation printing processes.

Despite the exciting biosensing applications of graphene and its derivatives, several issues should be considered. Although the cytotoxic and genotoxic effects of graphene have been well-studied, there is no standardized approach for using graphene in biological systems. Further studies are necessary to enhance graphene-based models for in vitro cellular behavior (Tandabany Dinadayalane 2022).

18 Fatal Cancer Agent Delivery

Graphene-based materials have the potential to carry a variety of diverse biological molecules, including polymers, proteins, carbohydrates, and anticancer agents. Graphene derivatives are frequently chemically modified to tune their hydrophobicity and hydrophilicity in biological environments, but such modifications can affect nanomaterials' biocompatibility. Graphene is also being developed to detect cancer (Ezike et al. 2023). This study, however, has demonstrated the growth-inhibiting properties of GO against tumors and cell lines. The greater toxicity of GO for cancer cells versus normal fibroblast cells has also been documented. In this context, it is hypothesized that GO activates toll-like receptors to stimulate autophagy, resulting in anticancer effects in malignant cells (Dasari Shareena 2018). Another example is a polyethylene glycol-graphene oxide conjugate (PEG–GO), which efficiently reduces tumor volume in xenograft models, suggesting potential applications in cancer therapy. The phototherapeutic effects of nGO likely result from oxidative stress, mitochondrial depolarization, and caspase activation, which may ultimately lead to autophagy and apoptosis (Vasilios Georgakilas 2016).

Although the application of graphene to cancer treatment is still in its infancy, significant hurdles must be overcome. A key area of study involves investigating how graphene interacts with various cells within the body. Understanding these biological properties and the toxicity of graphene will help enhance its potential for anticancer activity. Therefore, the toxicological effects and toxicity morphologies of graphene, depending on "in vitro" models, should be distinguished from those of "in vivo".

19 Antibacterial Activities

Numerous research studies have highlighted the potential of graphene-based composites (GBCs) for antibacterial applications (Vasilios Georgakilas 2016). Xia et al.'s work (Wang et al. 2021) identifies the primary microbial targets for GBCs, including Escherichia coli, Staphylococcus aureus, Pseudomonas aeruginosa, Streptococcus mutans, Porphyromonas gingivalis, Klebsiella pneumoniae, Salmonella typhimurium, and Candida albicans. Most importantly, the physicochemical properties of graphene, such as surface properties, dimensions, morphology, dispersibility, functionalization, and electronic structure, play a significant role in its antibacterial activity as a GBC.

Research further discussed the factors affecting the antimicrobial performance of graphene in GBCs. GBCs are more efficient in targeting Gram-negative bacteria than Gram-positive ones. Small graphene sheets exhibit a more pronounced antimicrobial activity due to their structural defects and increased contact area; however, they are also more cytotoxic. Single-layer graphene sheets display stronger interactions with bacteria than multilayered ones, and the greater their concentration, the more pronounced the antibacterial effect. Proper dispersibility and the functionalization of graphene with polymers further enhance its antimicrobial properties, as stable graphene-polymer mixtures integrate well into polymeric lattices, thereby improving overall activity.

20 3D-Printed Scaffolds

Graphene-based composites (GBCs) with various properties are showing significant promise for next-generation materials. Recent studies focus on developing cost-effective and straightforward methods for GBC preparation using 3D additive manufacturing. Printable graphene inkjet approaches demonstrate low-cost, scalable methods for integrating GBCs into modern technologies. (Wei et al. 2023) developed a graphene ink based on 3D printing that can be incorporated into other structures containing up to 60% graphene, combined with polylactide-co-glycolide (PLG), a biodegradable polymer. The resulting 3D-printed GBCs are not only electrically conductive but also mechanically robust and flexible.

Our in vivo experiments confirmed that the 3D-printed GBCs are biocompatible and could assist in various fine surgical operations. Furthermore, in vitro studies have shown that these GBCs can sustain the expansion of human mesenchymal stem cells, making them a promising material for nerve tissue engineering. It can be concluded that bioinks containing graphene can be formulated to enhance the printability of scaffolds with high graphene content, potentially for tissue regeneration applications.

21 Prospects

Graphene and its derivatives are of great interest as materials for biomedical research. Owing to their outstanding properties and pronounced progress observed so far, graphene-based nanomaterials have shown great potential and hold tremendous promise for various applications; however, they are still in the early stages of development. Standardized research direction is needed to upscale this field into a marketplace for biomedical solutions. One of the key aims in implementing the growing therapeutic potential of graphene and its derivatives is to better explore their toxicity profiles in both in vitro and in vivo studies. Therapeutic applications of these nanomaterials, which have been shown to have toxicological effects, are also relatively well-documented. From this research, the authors aim to modulate the bioactivities of potential graphene-based nanomaterials that are toxic by identifying the specific properties that cause toxicity. This will enable these nanomaterials to perform various functions, such as in antibiotic or anticancer therapy, in the future. Combinatorial therapies, especially when combined with conventional drug therapies such as photothermal therapy (PTT), photodynamic therapy (PDT), photoacoustic and photocatalytic techniques, and radiofrequency (RF) ablation, may also have a promising future when synergized with graphene-based agents. Not only would such combinatorial approaches make therapies more effective, but they could also address current chemotherapeutic issues, such as multidrug resistance, reducing drug dosages, and thus the risk of toxic side effects (Begum et al. 2020). Another aspect of graphene that is especially promising is its use in gene transfection. While in vitro studies using biofunctionalized graphene as gene delivery vectors have been successful, in vivo applications have been relatively underexplored. Progress in optimizing the surface chemistry of graphene could enable efficient and safe gene delivery to address genetic defects.

Thus, although graphene research in biomedicine is increasing rapidly, there are still few methods that can be applied on a large scale to produce stable nanoparticle dispersions. It is also necessary to develop new techniques for biofunctionalizing these materials to prevent agglomeration during biomedical applications. Further research will be necessary to investigate the fundamental properties and processes that govern the behavior of graphene in these environments. Graphene quantum dots (GQDs) have demonstrated effective bioimaging capabilities with low "in vivo" toxicity, showing great promise in various biological fields. Nevertheless, researchers should also pay attention to the poor production yield of GQDs and to a new issue that requires high quantum efficiency. Applying sensors to biosensing applications would require investigating how each chemical structure leads to its corresponding sensor function. This includes not only determining the most critical physical and chemical parameters that affect the operational performance of graphene-based biosensors but also enhancing their commercial viability. One of the most innovative applications of graphene-based materials in medicine is their ability to function simultaneously as both biomedical diagnostics and therapeutics. A real-time biosensing and imaging strategy integrated with targeted drug delivery offers a potential approach for simultaneous diagnosis and treatment. A recent advance has shown that graphene heterostructure films, i.e., incorporating graphene with other nanomaterials or metal nanoparticles, exhibit higher laser desorption/ionization (LDI) efficiency. Given the excellent performance of ND films, LD-MS with these biocompatible matrices is well-suited for phospholipase profiling, as well as for small-molecule and even brain-tissue analysis, making it a powerful tool in metabolomics and imaging. These parameters are also likely to influence the antibacterial properties of different graphene materials when applied in antimicrobial applications. Therefore, further studies should focus on how time, concentration, size, density, purity, and even the surface structure of these materials affect their sentinel-killing activity. Understanding the molecular level of these combinatorial features could help us design more effective nanomaterial-based antibiotics.

Graphene's potential also shows in the field of tissue engineering. Advancing its bio-applications from the laboratory to clinical practice requires strong interdisciplinary collaboration among physics, chemistry, biology, materials science and engineering. Despite the promising properties and numerous potential applications of graphene-based materials, many fundamental questions remain unresolved, and addressing these challenges will require coordinated and sustained efforts. This collaboration is expected to yield increased mechanistic insight into the function of graphene-based nanomaterials, thereby supporting their development as more widely accepted tools in biomedical applications.

22 Graphene and Selenium Nanoparticles: Antimicrobial Activity and Mechanisms

1. Graphene Nanoparticles: Properties and Synthesis

Graphene is a two-dimensional material composed of carbon atoms arranged in a hexagonal lattice. Its antimicrobial potential stems from high surface area, biocompatibility, and the ability to act as a mechanical barrier. The surface functionalization of graphene nanoparticles enables them to interact with microbial membranes, making them particularly effective for medical applications.

2. Antimicrobial Mechanisms of Graphene and Selenium Nanoparticles

Selenium nanoparticles (SeNPs) exhibit excellent biological compatibility and are essential micronutrients for human health. They possess significant antioxidant properties that contribute to their antimicrobial effects by disrupting bacterial cell walls and generating ROS. Additionally, selenium NPs can be functionalized to enhance selectivity against pathogens. SeNPs induce ROS, disrupting cellular components and compromising microbial viability (Liu et al. 2018; Ma et al. 2012). Selenium ions interact with thiol groups in microbial proteins, impairing their function and leading to cellular dysfunction (Sun et al. 2008). SeNPs can integrate into microbial membranes, altering permeability and causing leakage of cellular contents.

Graphene nanoparticles exhibit antimicrobial activity through various mechanisms, including physical disruption. The sharp edges of graphene sheets can physically damage microbial cell membranes. Graphene oxide induces ROS production, damaging cellular components such as proteins, lipids, and DNA (Wang et al. 2014). Due to the charge on functionalized graphene sheets, they can attach to negatively charged bacterial surfaces, thereby disrupting cell integrity (Xia et al. 2023).

3. **Comparative Analysis of Graphene and Selenium Nanoparticles**

Studies have shown that graphene nanoparticles are effective against Gram-positive and Gram-negative bacteria due to their mechanical strength and ROS production capabilities. For example, *E. coli* and *S. aureus* are notably susceptible to graphene nanoparticle treatment, with a significant reduction in colony formation observed (Xia et al. 2023).

Similarly, selenium nanoparticles have demonstrated inhibitory effects on bacteria such as *P. aeruginosa* and *L. monocytogenes.* Their biocompatibility and ROS-generating properties make them effective even at low concentrations, limiting bacterial growth without harming human cells. Graphene-based materials show promise against clinically relevant fungal pathogens, where ROS production damages fungal cell walls, inhibiting growth. Selenium nanoparticles have been tested against Candida species, demonstrating inhibition of fungal biofilms, which are often resistant to conventional antifungal agents (Vasilios Georgakilas 2016).

4. **Biomedical Applications and Potential Clinical Impact**

Graphene and selenium nanoparticles are increasingly being integrated into medical devices, such as surgical instruments and implant coatings, to prevent infections. Antimicrobial properties help reduce biofilm formation on medical devices, a common cause of hospital-acquired infections, as well as in dental surgical procedures such as endodontics (Fig. 4). In addition to their applications in medical devices, selenium nanoparticles are being investigated as potential supplements due to their antioxidant properties. Graphene nanoparticles are also being explored as drug-delivery vehicles, with the potential to co-deliver antimicrobial agents to enhance therapeutic outcomes (Gong et al. 2015).

5. **Safety and Toxicity Considerations**

While both graphene and selenium nanoparticles exhibit potent antimicrobial effects, their biocompatibility and potential cytotoxicity must be carefully considered. Research indicates that selenium nanoparticles are safe and beneficial to human cells at specific doses. In contrast, graphene nanoparticles may require more controlled applications due to the potential for oxidative damage to mammalian cells (Kang et al. 2021). Ensuring safe dosages and understanding body biodistribution are critical for clinical applications.

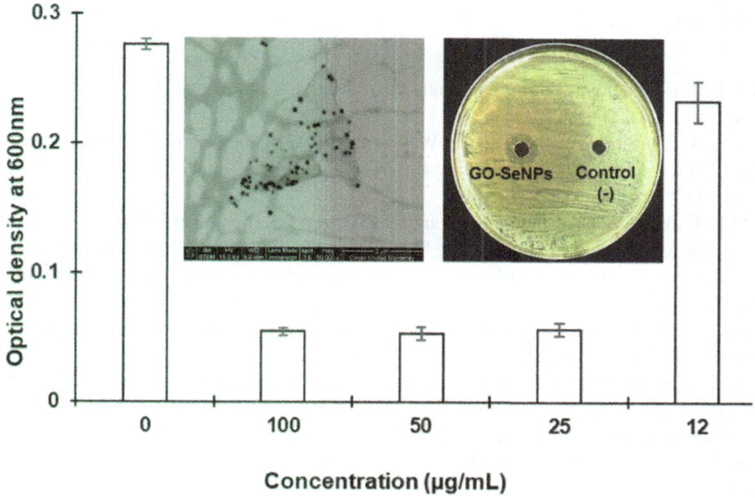

Fig. 4 Antimicrobial activity of GO-Se NPs on *E. faecalis* growth

6. **Conclusion and Future Prospects**

The antimicrobial capabilities of graphene and selenium nanoparticles present an innovative frontier in combating microbial resistance. While both types of nanoparticles are effective against a range of pathogens, their mechanisms of action and biocompatibility differ, providing unique advantages depending on the application. Future research should focus on optimizing synthesis, understanding long-term impacts, and expanding the scope of antimicrobial applications for these nanomaterials in clinical settings.

23 Challenges

Although graphene-based structures have been exploited in numerous applications, understanding their bio-interactions remains challenging in most cases. Most of the toxicological studies on these structures are experimental, with "in vitro" research as the primary focus, while "in vivo" animal models have received less emphasis. Human safety should be given top priority in the application of biomedicine, and additional studies are needed to evaluate chronic toxic effects due to the prolonged biosafety challenges that exist. In this regard, there is a shortage of comprehensive descriptions of the various synthesis and characterization methods in the literature, which should be carefully reviewed before initiating toxicological assessments. Future advances in this field will require considerable efforts to elucidate both the adsorption, scattering, and toxicity profiles.

References

M. Ahmed et al., Nanostructured materials for cardiovascular tissue engineering. J. Nanosci. Nanotechnol. (2012)

P. Ajayan et al., Two-dimensional van der Waals materials. Mater. Today. (2016)

C. Allard, *Advanced 1D Heterostructures Based on Nanotube Templates and Molecules* (Royal Society of Chemistry, 2024)

S. Bai et al., Enhancement of mechanical and electrical properties of graphene/cement composite due to improved dispersion of graphene by addition of silica fume. Constr. Build. Mater. (2018)

R.G. Bai et al., Graphene: a versatile platform for nanotheranostics and tissue engineering. Progr. Mater. Sci. (2018)

S. Begum et al., 2D and heterostructure nanomaterial based strategies for combating drug-resistant bacteria. ACS Omega. (2020)

P. Bellet et al., Graphene-based scaffolds for regenerative medicine. Nanomaterials. (2021)

P. Blake et al., Quality heterostructures from two-dimensional crystals unstable in air by their assembly in inert atmosphere. Nanoletters. (2015)

C.J. Bullock, C. Bussy, Biocompatibility considerations in the design of graphene. Mater. Interf. (2019)

F. Cadamuro et al., 3D printed tissue models: from hydrogels to biomedical applications. J. Controlled Release. (2023)

C. Castiello et al., GreenMedChem: the challenge in the next decade. Green Chem. (2023)

J. Chen et al., Indocyanine green loaded reduced graphene oxide for in vivo photoacoustic/ fluorescence dual-modality tumor imaging. Nanosc. Res. Lett. (2016)

H.L. Chia et al., Doping and decorating 2D materials for biosensing: benefits and drawbacks. Funct. Mater. (2021)

P. Choudhary et al., Bio-reduced graphene oxide as a nanoscale antimicrobial coating for medical devices. ACS Omega. (2019)

C.M. Corbet et al., van der Waals heterostructures with high accuracy rotational alignment. Nanoletters (2016)

M.R. Das et al., Synthesis of silver nanoparticles in an aqueous suspension of graphene oxide sheets and its antimicrobial activity. Colloids Surf. B: Biointerf. (2011)

T.P. Dasari Shareena et al., A review on graphene-based nanomaterials in biomedical applications and risks in environment and health. Nano-micro Lett. (2018)

A.F. de Faria et al., Anti-adhesion and antibacterial activity of silver nanoparticles supported on graphene oxide sheets. Colloids Surf. B: Biointerf. (2014)

C.R. Dean et al., Boron nitride substrates for high-quality graphene electronics. Nat. Nanotechnol. (2010)

S.B. Desai et al., Gold-mediated exfoliation of ultralarge optoelectronically-perfect monolayers. Adv. Mater. (2016)

T. Dinadayalane et al., Structures, properties, and applications of nitrogen-doped graphene. Theor. Comput. Chem. (2022)

N. Dubey et al., Graphene: a versatile carbon-based material for bone tissue engineering. Stem Cells Int. (2015)

O. Erol et al., Recent advances in bioactive 1D and 2D carbon nanomaterials for biomedical applications. Nanomed. Nanotechnol. Biol. Med. (2018)

T.C. Ezike et al., Advances in drug delivery systems, challenges and future directions. Heliyon. (2023)

N. Fatima et al., Recent developments for antimicrobial applications of graphene-based polymeric composites: a review. J. Ind. Eng. Chem. (2021)

M.S. Fuhrer et al., Graphene: materially better carbon. MRS Bull. (2010)

Y.X. Gan et al., Hydrothermal Synthesis of Nanomaterials. J. Nanomater. (2020)

C.A. García-González, Aerogels in drug delivery: From design to application. J. Control. Release. (2021)

A.K. Geim et al., Van der Waals heterostructures. Nature (2013)
A.K. Geim et al., The rise of graphene. Nat. Mater. (2007)
M. Geiser et al., Deposition and biokinetics of inhaled nanoparticles. Part. Fibre Toxicol. (2010)
V. Georgakilas et al., Noncovalent functionalization of graphene and graphene oxide for energy materials, biosensing, catalytic, and biomedical applications. ACS Publications. (2016)
K. Ghosal et al., Biomedical applications of graphene nanomaterials and beyond. ACS Biomater. Sci. Eng. (2019)
S. Goenka et al., Graphene-based nanomaterials for drug delivery and tissue engineering. J. Controlled Release. (2014)
Y. Gong et al., Two-step growth of two-dimensional WSe2/MoSe2 heterostructures. Nano Lett. (2015)
R.V. Gorbachev et al., Recent progress in the assembly of nanodevices and van der Waals heterostructures by deterministic placement of 2D materials. Chem. Soc. (2018)
M.H.D. Guimarães et al., Fast pick up technique for high quality heterostructures of bilayer graphene and hexagonal boron nitride. Appl. Phys. (2014)
R. Guo et al., Biomimetic 3D bacterial cellulose-graphene foam hybrid scaffold regulates neural stem cell proliferation and differentiation. Colloids Surf. B: Biointerf. (2021)
S.J. Haigh et al., Electronic properties of graphene encapsulated with different two-dimensional atomic crystals. Nanoletters. (2014)
H. Hashemzadeh et al., Understanding loading, diffusion and releasing of Doxorubicin and Paclitaxel dual delivery in graphene and graphene oxide carriers as highly efficient drug delivery systems. Appl. Surf. Sci. (2020)
A.H. Hauke et al., Post graphene 2D chemistry: the emerging field of molybdenum. Angewandte Chemie International Edition. (2018)
J. Heo et al., Controlling physicochemical properties of graphene oxide for efficient cellular delivery. J. Ind. Eng. (2022)
J. Hu et al., Chemistry and physics in one dimension: synthesis and properties of nanowires and nanotubes. Acc. Chem. Res. (1999)
P.Y. Huang et al., One-dimensional electrical contact to a two-dimensional material. Science (2013)
D. Iannazzo et al., Graphene quantum dots for cancer targeted drug delivery. Int. J. Pharmaceut. (2017)
A.E. Jakus et al., Three-dimensional printing of high-content graphene scaffolds for electronic and biomedical applications. ACS Nano (2015)
Y. Kang et al., Understanding the interactions between inorganic-based nanomaterials and biological membranes. Adv. Drug Deliv. Rev. (2021)
T. Kang et al., Strategies for controlled growth of transition metal dichalcogenides by chemical vapor deposition for integrated electronics. ACS Mater. (2022)
J.W. Kim et al., Effects of graphene oxide-gold nanoparticles nanocomposite on highly sensitive foot-and-mouth disease virus detection. Nanomaterials. (2020)
H. Kong, Hybrids of carbon nanotubes and graphene/graphene oxide. Curr. Opin. Solid State Mater. Sci. (2013)
R. Kumar et al., Graphene-based materials for biotechnological and biomedical applications: drug delivery, bioimaging and biosensing. Mater. Today Chem. (2023)
P. Kumar et al., Antibacterial properties of graphene-based nanomaterials. Nanomaterials. (2019)
S.R. Laraba et al., Graphene-based composites for biomedical applications. Green Chem. Lett. Rev. (2022)
J.H. Lee et al., Electrical property of graphene and its application to electrochemical biosensing. Nanomaterials. (2019)
M. Legesse et al., Tunable high workfunction contacts: doped graphene. Appl. Surf. Sci. (2020)
B.L. Li et al., Emerging 0D transition-metal dichalcogenides for sensors, biomedicine, and clean energy. Nano Micro Small. (2017)
J. Li et al., Promising graphene-based nanomaterials and their biomedical applications and potential risks: A comprehensive review. ACS Biomater. Sci. Eng. (2021)

N. Li et al., Electronic and photocatalytic properties of modified MoS2/graphene quantum dots heterostructures: a computational study. Appl. Surf. Sci. (2019)
J. Lin et al., Graphene-Based Nanomaterials for Bioimaging. Nanomaterials. (2018)
Y. Liu et al., Highly efficient gate-tunable photocurrent generation in vertical heterostructures of layered materials. Nanotechnology (2016)
T. Li et al., Ultrathin epitaxial graphite: 2D electron gas properties and a route toward graphene-based nanoelectronics. J. Phys. Chem. B. (2004)
T. Liu et al., 2D MoS2 Nanostructures for Biomedical Applications. Adv. Healthc. Mater. (2018)
Y. Liu et al., Van der Waals heterostructures and devices. Nat. Rev. Mater. (2016)
X. Liu et al., Targeted delivery of SNX-2112 by polysaccharide-modified graphene oxide nanocomposites for treatment of lung cancer. Carbohydr. Polym. (2018)
G. Liu et al., 0D to 2D carbon-based materials in flexible strain sensors: recent advances and perspectives. 2D Mater. (2023)
X. Ma et al., A functionalized graphene oxide-iron oxide nanocomposite for magnetically targeted drug delivery, photothermal therapy, and magnetic resonance imaging. Nano Res. (2012)
M. Mahmoudpour et al., Carbon-based aerogels for biomedical sensing: advances toward designing the ideal sensor. Adv. Colloid Interf. Sci. (2021)
Y. Mao et al., Environmentally friendly methodologies of nanostructure synthesis. Green Nanochem. (2007)
L. Maestro et al., CdSe quantum dots for two-photon fluorescence thermal imaging. Nano Lett. (2010)
L.Y. Meng et al., The progress of microwave-assisted hydrothermal method in the synthesis of functional nanomaterials. Mat. Today Chem. (2016)
A. Mirtaghavi et al., Recent advances in porous 3D cellulose aerogels for tissue engineering applications: a review. J. Compos. Sci. (2020)
M. Molaei, Two-dimensional (2D) materials beyond graphene in cancer drug delivery, photothermal and photodynamic therapy, recent advances and challenges ahead: a review. J. Drug Deliv. Sci. Technol. (2021)
J.E. Moses et al., The growing applications of click chemistry. Chem. Soc. Rev. (2007)
S.M. Mousavi et al., Development of graphene based nanocomposites towards medical and biological applications. Artif. Cells Nanomed. Biotechnol. (2020)
D. Mudusu et al., Multifunctional Metal-oxide Integrated Monolayer Graphene Heterostructures for Planar, Flexible, and Skin-mountable Device Applications. Nano Energy. (2021)
B.O. Murjani et al., Carbon nanotubes in biomedical applications: current status, promises, and challenges. Carb. Lett. (2022)
K.S. Novoselov et al., Electric field effect in atomically thin carbon films. Science. (2004)
K.S. Novoselov et al., Two-dimensional atomic crystals. Natl Acad. Sci. (2005)
N. Panwar et al., Nanocarbons for biology and medicine: sensing, imaging, and drug delivery. Chem. Rev. (2016)
K.-T.-R. Paras, A review on low-dimensional nanomaterials: nanofabrication, characterization and applications. Nanomaterials (2023)
J. Park et al., Covalent functionalization of graphene with reactive intermediates. Acc. Chem. Res. (2013)
J. Peng et al., Fabrication of graphene quantum dots and hexagonal boron nitride nanocomposites for fluorescent cell imaging. J. Biomed. Technol. (2013)
J.A. Prescher et al., Copper-free click chemistry for dynamic in vivo imaging. Proc. National Acad. Sci. (2007)
S. Priyadarsini et al., Graphene and graphene oxide as nanomaterials for medicine and biology application. J. Nanostruct. Chem. (2018)
Y. Qu et al., Advances on graphene-based nanomaterials for biomedical applications. Mater. Sci. Eng. C (2018)
B. Radisavljevic et al., Single-layer MoS2 transistors. Nat. Nanotechnol. (2011)

J.C. Ranasinghe et al., Engineered 2D materials for optical bioimaging and path toward therapy and tissue engineering. J. Mater. (2022)

G. Reina et al., Promises, facts and challenges for graphene in biomedical applications. Chem. Soc. Rev. (2017)

N. Rohaizad et al., Two-dimensional materials in biomedical, biosensing and sensing applications. Chem. Soc. (2021)

D. Roy et al., *0D, 1D, 2D & 3D Nano Materials: Synthesis and Applications* (Springer, India, 2024)

R. Sakthivel et al., Heterostructures of 2D materials and their applications in biosensing. Progr. Mater. Sci. (2023)

S. Sengupta et al., A review on synthesis, toxicity profile and biomedical applications of graphene quantum dots (GQDs). Inorganica Chimica Acta. (2023)

K. Shankar et al., A review on antimicrobial mechanism and applications of graphene-based materials. Biomaterials. (2023)

A. Sharma et al., Methods of preparation of metal-doped and hybrid tungsten oxide nanoparticles for anticancer, antibacterial, and biosensing applications. Surf. Interf. (2022)

J. Shi et al., Nanoparticle based fluorescence resonance energy transfer (FRET) for biosensing applications. J. Mater. Chem. B. (2015)

J. Shi et al., All chemical vapor deposition synthesis and intrinsic bandgap observation of MoS2/graphene heterostructures. Adv. Mater. (2015)

S.R. Shin et al., Graphene-based materials for tissue engineering. Adv. Drug Deliv. Rev. (2016)

C. Shuai et al., Additive manufacturing of promising heterostructure for biomedical applications. Int. J. Extr. Manuf. (2023)

M. Silva et al., 3D printing of graphene-based polymeric nanocomposites for biomedical applications. Funct. Compos. Mater. (2021)

M. Silva et al., Graphene-polymer nanocomposites for biomedical applications. Polym. Adv. Technol. (2017)

A. Solanki et al., Axonal alignment and enhanced neuronal differentiation of neural stem cells on graphene-nanoparticle hybrid structures. Adv. Mater. (2013)

S. Stankovich et al., Stable aqueous dispersions of graphitic nanoplatelets via the reduction of exfoliated graphite oxide in the presence of poly (sodium 4-styrenesulfonate). J. Mater. Chem. (2006)

H. Sun et al., Recent advances in graphene quantum dots for sensing. Mater. Today. (2013)

X. Sun et al., Nano-graphene oxide for cellular imaging and drug delivery. Nano Res. (2008)

M. Sup Choi et al., Controlled charge trapping by molybdenum disulphide and graphene in ultrathin heterostructured memory devices. Nat. Commun. (2013)

K. Tadyszak et al., Biomedical applications of graphene-based structures. Nanomaterials. (2018)

K. Tadyszak et al., Biomedical applications of graphene-based structures. Nanomaterials (2018)

A. Taghizadeh et al., Mussel-inspired biomaterials: from chemistry to clinic. Bioeng. Trans. Med. (2022)

Z. Tan et al., Control of cell growth on 3D-printed cell culture platforms for tissue engineering. J. Biomed. Mater. Res. (2017)

L. Tang et al., Recent advances in cardiovascular disease biosensors and monitoring technologies. ACS J. (2023)

A. Torres-Pinto et al., The effect of precursor selection on the microwave-assisted synthesis of graphitic carbon nitride. Catalysis Today (2023)

S. Villar-Rodil et al., Preparation, characterization and fundamental studies on graphenes by liquid-phase processing of graphite. J. Alloys Compounds. (2012)

W. Wang et al., Investigations of graphene and nitrogen-doped graphene enhanced polycaprolactone 3D scaffolds for bone tissue engineering. Nanomaterials. (2021)

J. Wang et al., Two-dimensional nanomaterials in cancer theranostics. Theranostic Bionanomat. (2019)

Z. Wang et al., Application of zero-dimensional nanomaterials in biosensing. Front. Chem. (2020)

X. Wang et al., Multifunctional graphene quantum dots for simultaneous targeted cellular imaging and drug delivery. Colloids Surf. B. (2014)

Y. Wang et al., Nitrogen-doped graphene and its application in electrochemical biosensing. ACS Nano. (2010)

W. Wei et al., Extraordinary physical properties of functionalized graphene. Micro Nano Small (2023)

J. Wen et al., Recent applications of carbon nanomaterials in fluorescence biosensing and bioimaging. Chem. Commun. (2015)

L. Xia, 0D/2D Schottky junction synergies with 2D/2D S-scheme heterojunction strategy to achieve uniform separation of carriers in 0D/2D/2D quasi CNQDs/TCN/ZnIn2S4 towards photocatalytic remediating petroleum hydrocarbons polluted marine. Appl. Catal. B: Environ. (2023)

M.Y. Xia et al., Graphene-based nanomaterials: the promising active agents for antibiotics-independent antibacterial applications. J. Control. Release. (2019)

Y. Xu et al., Graphene: two decades of revolutionizing material science. Innov. Mater. (2024)

H. Xu et al., Properties of graphene-metal contacts probed by Raman spectroscopy. Carbon. (2018)

K. Yang et al., Nano-graphene in biomedicine: theranostic applications. Chem. Soc. Rev. (2013)

K. Yang et al., Multimodal imaging guided photothermal therapy using functionalized graphene nanosheets anchored with magnetic nanoparticles. Adv. Mater. (2012)

J.V. Ye, Tailored carbon nanotubes for tissue engineering applications. Biotechnol. Progr. (2009)

J. Yoon et al., Graphene/MoS2 Nanohybrid for Biosensors. Materials. (2021)

L. Yue et al., pH-responsive, self-sacrificial nanotheranostic agent for potential in vivo and in vitro dual modal MRI/CT imaging, real-time, and in situ monitoring of cancer therapy. Bioconj. Chem. (2017)

Y.J. Yun et al., Highly elastic graphene-based electronics toward electronic skin. Adv. Funct. Mater. (2017)

Y.I. Zhang et al., Review of chemical vapor deposition of graphene and related applications. Account. Chem. Res. (2013)

Y. Zhang et al., Recent progress in CVD growth of 2D transition metal dichalcogenides and related heterostructures. Adv. Mater. (2019)

H. Zhang et al., Graphene-enabled wearable sensors for healthcare monitoring. Biosens. Bioelectron. (2022)

J. Zhang et al., Vertical graphene nanoarray decorated with Ag nanoparticles exhibits enhanced antibacterial effects. J. Colloid Interf. Sci. (2024)

F. Zhang et al., 3D graphene-based gel photocatalysts for environmental pollutants degradation. Environ. Pollut. (2019)

A. Zuchowska, M. Chudy, A. Dybko, Z.G. Brzozka, Graphene as a new material in anticancer therapy-in vitro studies. Sens. Actuat. B: Chem. (2017)

Eumelanin as a Key Material in Bioelectronic Interfaces and Eco-Friendly Technologies

Natan Luis Nozella, João Vitor Paulin, João Victor Morais Lima, and Carlos Frederico de Oliveira Graeff

Abstract Eumelanin (EuM), a natural pigment found in many organisms, is a versatile material with remarkable structural, optical, protective and electrical properties. In this book chapter, we present a comprehensive overview of EuM, highlighting its structural and multifunctional characteristics. We discuss its applications in photoconversion, pH sensors, transistor plataforms, energy storage and memory devices. We also adress current challenges and future prospects. These insights aim to guide the development of the next generation of sustainable bioelectronics materials and advanced healthcare solutions.

Keywords Bioelectronics · Eumelanin · Mixed ionic-electronic conductivity

1 Introduction

Melanin nanostructured systems have emerged as versatile materials that bridge the fields of electronics, biomedicine, and environmental science. Their unique attributes, including biocompatibility, tunable optical-electronic properties, and environmental stability, position them as promising candidates for next-generation energy storage systems, as well as for bioelectronic and sustainable devices.

Melanin, a naturally occurring biopolymer, is a remarkable material with diverse biological and functional properties. Found in organisms across all domains of life (Prota 1992; d'Ischia et al. 2015), it acts as both a pigment and a protective shield against environmental stressors, including ultraviolet radiation, oxidative damage, and, in some cases, microbial attacks (Corani et al. 2014; Mazur et al. 2023).

N. L. Nozella (✉) · J. V. M. Lima · C. F. de Oliveira Graeff
POSMAT—Graduate Program in Materials Science and Technology, School of Sciences, São Paulo State University (UNESP), Bauru, Brazil
e-mail: n.nozella@unesp.br

J. V. Paulin · C. F. de Oliveira Graeff
Department of Physics and Meteorology, School of Sciences, São Paulo State University (UNESP), Bauru, Brazil

R. Narayan (ed.), *Nanostructured Biomaterials and Their Applications*,
https://doi.org/10.1007/978-3-032-16316-5_13

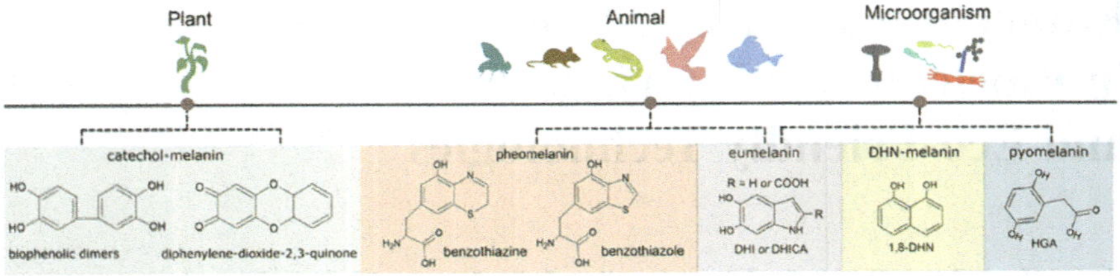

Fig. 1 Fundamental basic structure of various melanin types and their biological sources. Reprinted with permission from Xie et al. (2024) Copyright © 2024, American Chemical Society

It can be classified into four distinct groups based on its structure, composition, and biological roles: eumelanin (EuM), pheomelanin (PhM), neuromelanin (NeM), and allomelanin (AlM). Among these, EuM is the most abundant and widely studied type, responsible for the brown-to-black coloration (d'Ischia et al. 2015). This black-to-brown insoluble subgroup is primarily formed through the oxidative polymerization of 3,4-dihydroxyphenyl-L-alanine (L-dopa), involving polyindolequinone intermediates such as 5,6-dihydroxyindole (DHI) and 5,6-dihydroxyindole-2-carboxilic acid (DHICA) (Fig. 1). EuM is particularly effective at photoprotection and oxidant scavenger (Ito et al. 2018).

PhM imparts reddish to yellow hues, as seen in red-haired (d'Ischia et al. 2015). The yellow-to-reddish brown and alkali-soluble subgroup is derived from the oxidation of L-dopa and the cysteine amino acid, utilizing intermediates such as benzothiazine and benzothiazole (Fig. 1). Unlike EuM, PhM is less efficient in UV protection and can contribute to oxidative stress under prolonged UV exposure (Ito et al. 2018).

NeM is a specialized form of melanin found in certain areas of the brain, such as the substantia nigra and locus coeruleus (Bush et al. 2006; Zucca et al. 2014). This dark pigment is produced within neurons through the oxidation of dopamine or L-dopa, along with other catecholamine precursors. NeM is thought to have a neuroprotective function by sequestering toxic metals and mitigating oxidative stress. However, its dysfunction has been linked to neurodegenerative disorders such as Parkinson's disease (Zecca et al. 2006). Lastly, AlM is a diverse range of dark pigments predominantly found in bacteria, fungi, and plants (Solano 2014). It differs structurally from the other melanin types as it is formed through the oxidation and polymerization of phenolic precursors such as catechol (catechol-melanin), 1,8-dihydroxynaphthalene (DHN-melanin), and homogentisic acid (pyomelanin) (Fig. 1). Like the other groups in mammals, AlM plays various roles related to pigmentation, wound healing, camouflage, and defense mechanisms against pathogens, heavy metals, high salt concentrations, UV radiation, and extreme environmental conditions (Li et al. 2023).

Given the significant role played by the EuM group, this chapter will focus primarily on this specific type. It begins by examining its structural characteristics, followed by an in-depth discussion of its remarkable properties, including optical, protective, and electrical attributes, which underpin the foundation of its biological and functional significance. This chapter then examines the wide-ranging applications of EuM, from its role in photoprotection and medical therapies to its emerging potential in advanced technologies such as pH sensors, organic transistors, energy storage, and memory devices. By delving into these topics, this chapter aims to provide a comprehensive overview of EuM's multifaceted nature and relevance across diverse scientific and technological domains.

2 Eumelanin Properties

2.1 *Structure*

EuM is a complex and heterogeneous structure. Its primary components are polymerized derivatives of two key precursors: DHI and DHICA, both of which are products of the amino acid tyrosine via the eumelanogenesis pathway (d'Ischia et al. 2015). These monomers contain indole aromatic rings with hydroxyl, carbonyl groups, and carboxyl with different redox states: Fully reduced *o*-Hydroquinone (H_2Q), partially reduced/oxidized *o*-Semiquinone (SQ), fully oxidized *o*-Indole quinone (IQ), and tautomer form *o*-quinone imine (Fig. 2a) that contribute to EuM's ability to chelate metals and conduct charges due to the comproportionation redox equilibrium reaction (Fig. 2b) (Mostert et al. 2012).

These monomers couple to form oligomers through covalent bonds, primarily involving carbon-carbon linkages. The resulting oligomers are highly irregular, lacking a single-defined repeating unit, which contributes to EuM's amorphous and heterogeneous physical nature. The oligomers aggregate non-covalently into higher-order structures via π-π stacking and hydrogen bonding (Watt et al. 2009; d'Ischia et al. 2009). These aggregates form planar or twisted disordered layers, resulting in EuM characteristic amorphous and granular morphology.

The combination of carboxylate and non-carboxylate structures is an important characteristic of EuM, as different proportions of DHI and DHICA monomers can directly influence the final structure of the macromolecule (Panzella et al. 2013).

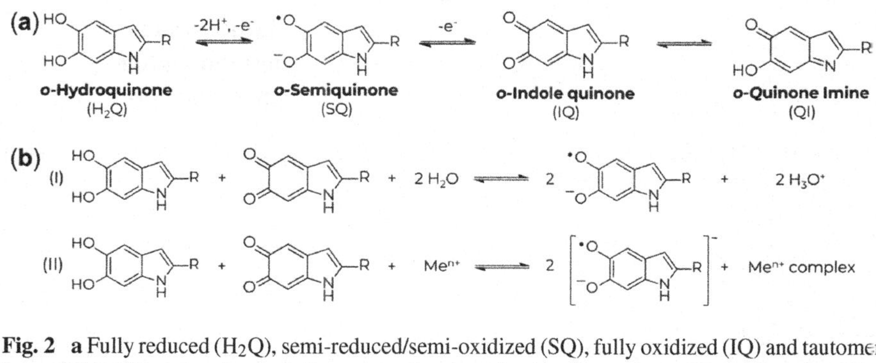

Fig. 2 **a** Fully reduced (H_2Q), semi-reduced/semi-oxidized (SQ), fully oxidized (IQ) and tautomer form (QI) EuM indole subunits. **b** Comproportional mechanism (I—water and II—cations metallics influence) responsible for EuM protonic conduction (R = H or COOH)

DHICA-rich EuMs are composed of smaller, elongated aggregates with limited inter-unit π-conjugation, while DHI-rich EuMs have larger structures with a globular tendency and efficient inter-unit π-conjugation (Fig. 3). This difference is related to the number and topology of cross-linking positions between the monomers. While DHICA predominantly polymerizes through positions C-4 and C-7, DHI can form adducts through positions C-2, C-3, C-4, and C-7.

The structure of EuM allows it to chelate metal ions (Fe^{2+}, Cu^{2+}, and Zn^{2+}, to mention a few), which can influence its electronic and optical properties (Hong and Simon 2006; d'Ischia et al. 2009). EuM's porous structure and hydrophilic functional groups allow it to retain water, which is critical for its ionic conductivity and environmental responsiveness (Mostert et al. 2010; Clulow et al. 2017). The combination of irregular supramolecular aggregation and functional group diversity makes EuM a highly versatile biomaterial. Its structural complexity underlies its multifaceted roles in photoprotection, free-radical scavenging, and potential applications in bioelectronics.

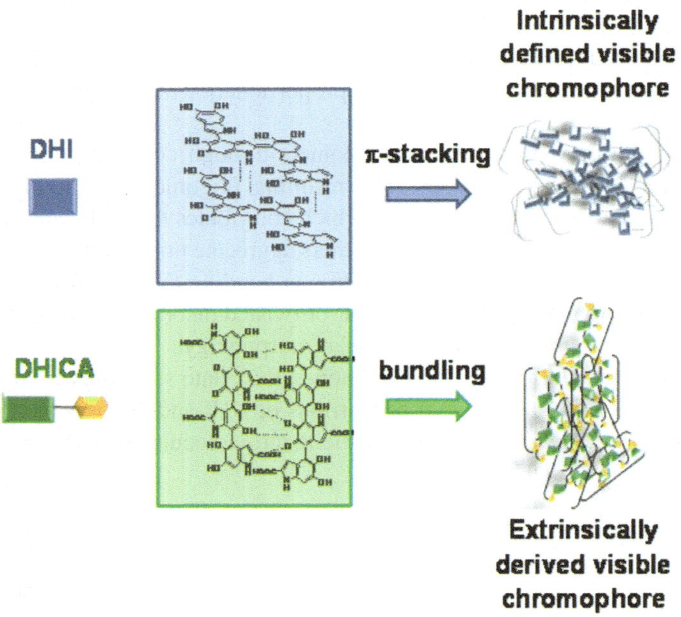

Fig. 3 DHI- and DHICA-based EuM structure. Reprint with permission from Micillo et al. (2017) Copyright © 2017, Springer Nature

2.2 Optical and Protective Properties

EuM exhibits a broad absorption spectrum that decreases monotonically with increasing wavelength (Tran et al. 2006). Additionally, it converts over 99% of the absorbed radiation into heat (Meredith and Riesz 2004), making it highly efficient at dissipating potentially harmful energy. These properties are attributed to the structural heterogeneity of EuM (Sect. 2), arising from variations in the oxidation states of its DHI and DHICA building blocks, diverse aggregation patterns, and differing degrees of π-electron delocalization (Tran et al. 2006; Pezzella et al. 2009; Chen et al. 2014; Grieco et al. 2020). This unique optical behavior allows EuM to absorb harmful UV radiation, minimizing its penetration into biological tissues and shielding them from UV-induced damage, maintaining cellular integrity (Corani et al. 2014; Mazur et al. 2023). Notably, its photoprotective efficacy is particularly pronounced in individuals with higher EuM content, as these individuals exhibit a lower incidence of skin cancers compared to those with albinism or high levels of PhM (Wright and Norval 2023; Mazur et al. 2023).

EuM is also a potent antioxidant. It neutralizes reactive oxygen species (ROS) generated during oxidative stress or UV exposure by participating in various redox reactions (Corani et al. 2014). This allows EuM to scavenge harmful free radicals, such as superoxide anions and hydroxyl radicals, reducing oxidative damage to cellular components. For instance, EuM's interaction with ROS protects photoreceptor cells in the retinal pigment epithelium from light-induced oxidative damage, preserving visual function (Ito et al. 2013).

2.3 Electrical Properties

EuM exhibits unique electrical properties that distinguish it from traditional organic and inorganic materials, such hydration-dependent and mixed ionic-electronic conductivity (Mostert et al. 2013; Wünsche et al. 2015; Bedran et al. 2021; Paulin et al. 2023a). The conductivity of EuM increases significantly in the presence of water, as hydration enhances proton generation, through the ionization of catechol and carboxyl groups. This dual effect makes EuM highly responsive to changes in environmental humidity (Mostert et al. 2013; Reali et al. 2020; Paulin et al. 2021a; Ambrico et al. 2024). For instance, the electronic conductivity values of EuM range from 10^{-13} to 10^{-2} S/cm depending on the hydration state (Reali et al. 2020).

The enhanced conductivity in EuM to hydration resulted from an increased concentration of protons. Consequently, the charge carriers in EuM consist of both protonic and electronic contributions, Wünsche et al. (2015) which arise from electrochemical doping induced by water (Bernardus Mostert et al. 2012; Mostert et al. 2012). This process generates positive ions (H^+) and electrons through the comproportionation equilibrium reaction (Fig. 2b). Based on this model, EuM can be classified as a mixed ionic-electronic conductor.

Other models have been proposed to explain the nature of charge transport in EuM. McGinness et al. (1974) demonstrated a reversible resistive switching behavior in wet EuM pellets, attributing this phenomenon to the amorphous semiconductor nature of EuM. The semiconducting behavior of melanin was also proposed by Santato's group (Reali et al. 2021). In their model, EuM exhibits both types of charge carriers (ionic and electronic), but the dominant conduction mechanism shifts from predominantly electronic to predominantly ionic/protonic, depending on the degree of hydration. Lastly, Paulin et al. (2023b) proposed a different mechanism in which ions migrate under an electric field and accumulate at the EuM/electrode interfaces. This accumulation generates strong fields that modify the energy levels of EuM, enabling electronic injections balanced by ionic compensation, a hallmark of electrochemical doping (Brizuela Guerra et al. 2024b). Beyond the electrical hydration dependence, EuM's conductivity is influenced by pH, as the ionization of functional groups affects charge transport (Mostert et al. 2013; Sheliakina et al. 2018b; Bedran et al. 2021).

Despite its intriguing properties, the low conductivity of EuM compared to traditional conductors limits its standalone applications in electronics. However, it can be combined with other materials or used in environments where its hybrid conductivity and environmental sensitivity are advantageous (Gargiulo et al. 2015; Migliaccio et al. 2017; Mostert et al. 2020; Pan et al. 2023).

3 Eumelanin Applications

3.1 Photoconversion

EuM's ability to absorb UV and visible light has inspired the development of advanced materials for photoprotection in both personal care and industrial contexts. In skin care, EuM reduces oxidative stress and inflammation in skin cells, making it an effective natural material for sunscreens (Menichetti et al. 2024). Additionally, incorporating EuM into polymers and other materials enhances their UV-shielding properties. For instance, adding EuM to polyvinyl alcohol significantly improves UV resistance, making it suitable for protective coatings, UV filters, and packaging (Wang et al. 2016; Albano et al. 2019). Outdoor eyewear incorporating EuM to block high-energy UV and blue light is also commercially available (TrueBlue).

Beyond its sunscreen role, EuM shows promise in photothermal therapy (Kim et al. 2017) by efficiently converting light, including near-infrared, into heat. This capability enables targeted tumor cell apoptosis with minimal harm to healthy tissues. This light-thermal conversion has also motivated research on thermoelectric devices. The combination of EuM with halide perovskites demonstrates high light absorption from UV to near-infrared, achieving a photothermal quantum yield of 99.56% and a conversion efficiency of 81% (Wang et al. 2019), surpassing materials like graphene. When applied on the hot side of a thermoelectric device, this composite coating significantly enhances power output under light, with increases of up to 7000% (Wang et al. 2019).

3.2 pH Sensors

As mentioned before, EuM's complex structure contains functional groups capable of donating or accepting protons depending on the surrounding environment, which directly influences its conductivity and electrochemical behavior (Wünsche et al. 2015; Paulin et al. 2023b). This property makes EuM a promising candidate for pH sensors, as variations in protonation and deprotonation result in measurable changes in its electrochemical response.

Studies have demonstrated the effectiveness of EuM-based sensors in detecting pH levels across various conditions (Piacenti da Silva et al. 2014; Paulin et al. 2022). For instance, Guerra et al. investigated the redox behavior of EuM electrodes in buffered aqueous solutions, showing that pH fluctuations significantly impact their electrochemical characteristics (Brizuela Guerra et al. 2024a). These findings highlighted the potential of EuM as a reliable material for applications where pH monitoring is essential, particularly in biological systems (Paulin et al. 2022).

Moreover, combining EuM with other materials can enhance its sensing performance (Tehrani et al. 2020; Whelan et al. 2022; Al-Shamery et al. 2023). For example, integrations such as EuM–graphene hybrids have been shown to improve sensitivity and response time, making the sensors more efficient (Tehrani et al. 2020; Whelan et al. 2022). These hybrid systems harness the strengths of both components, offering a versatile approach to developing advanced pH sensors.

3.3 Eumelanin in Transistors Platforms

In general, a transistor is composed of three terminals; the gate electrode is separated by an electrolyte or insulator from the semiconductor channel, which separates the source and drain electrodes. Studies have demonstrated the versatility of EuM to be used in various of these transistor components.

The first study reported a thin film of EuM as an active layer in an extended-gated field-effect transistor (EGFET) for pH sensing (Piacenti da Silva et al. 2014). The EGFETs demonstrated good sensitivity, from 31.3 mV/pH to 48.9 mV/pH in indium tin oxide and gold substrates, respectively. The detection of pH was linked to specific binding sites within its structure, as mentioned before.

Another study uses EuM as a solid electrolyte on a poly(3,4-ethylenedioxythiophene)-poly(styrenesulfonate) (PEDOT:PSS)-based organic electrochemical transistors (OECTs) with a 100 mm channel length, resulting in the development of an all-solid-state device (Sheliakina et al. 2018a). The devices demonstrated reliable modulation of channel conductance under low-voltage operation, achieving ON/OFF ratio exceeding 10^4. The gating mechanism was identified as volumetric, and the device exhibits exceptionally high channel capacitances, surpassing 200 F/cm^3, underscoring its potential for advanced bioelectronics and low-power applications.

The proton donation capacity and conductivity of EuM can be associated with its ion-chelating properties, in which the incorporation of Cu(II) into EuM solid electrolyte modulates the proton density within the layer. The effect of adding controlled amounts of Cu(II) ions into EuM solid electrolyte was studied by Mostert et al. (2020). The Cu-EuM-based OECTs demonstrated enhanced performance compared to neat EuM devices, with a higher transconductance peak (300 ± 60 vs. 150 ± 20 μA/V) and a shift to lower voltage operation (0.38 ± 0.05 vs. 0.52 ± 0.03 V). These results suggest a higher proton concentration and improved charge mobility in Cu-EuM. Overall, the findings strongly support the role of Cu in enhancing proton availability and device performance.

These interesting ionic properties of EuM make it well-suited for incorporation into the channel of the OECTs. Nozella et al. (2023) demonstrated an increase in the volumetric capacitance of PEDOT:PSS with the addition of EuM. They proposed that incorporating EuM into PEDOT:PSS increases the ionic-electronic coupling between the Na^+ ions from the electrolyte with the negative charges of PEDOT:PSS, which can improve OECTs responses, leading to higher transconductance, faster ion injection, and reduced ion removal in transient measurements.

The use of EuM as a new organic semiconductor reopens the enthusiasm of organic transistors for sustainable electronic, bio-interfacing technologies, and eco-friendly technologies.

3.4 Energy Storage

EuM can store electrical charge due to its redox-active functional groups. This property is attributed to reversible oxidation and reduction processes involving quinone, hydroquinone, and semiquinone species within its structure (Fig. 2a), as well as the capability of several of their functionalities to reversible bind cations (Fig. 2b). EuM has been explored for applications in organic batteries and supercapacitors.

Studies have demonstrated that EuM-inspired nanostructures can be applied to various battery components. For instance, Kim et al. (2013) reported sodium-ion batteries utilizing natural and synthetic EuM as anodes. The study revealed that the capacity of natural EuM (30.4 mAh g^{-1}) is 50% higher than its synthetic version due to the presence of pendant groups, like carboxylic and carboxylates, and a larger surface area.

The application of EuM in supercapacitors has gained increasing attention, particularly due to its pseudocapacitive properties. Although this device type has been less studied compared to batteries (Pan et al. 2023), recent research has shown significant progress in employing EuM as electrodes for supercapacitors. For instance, Kumar et al. (2016) developed EuM-coated carbon cloth electrodes. In a three-electrode system, the material exhibited a specific capacitance of 167 F g^{-1} (specific capacity of 24 mAh g^{-1}) in an aqueous electrolyte. The authors subsequently fabricated a flexible micro-supercapacitor on a plastic substrate. The results, combined with EuM's biocompatibility, biodegradability, and ambient-temperature processing capabilities, highlight its potential as an electrode material for supercapacitors.

Paulin et al. (2021b) observed photo-pseudocapacitive properties in symmetric EuM-based supercapacitors. Under illumination, the devices achieved a capacitance of 57.7 mF g^{-1}, which decreased by 53% in the absence of light. Furthermore, by utilizing different types of EuM, it was suggested that the quantity of carboxylic groups may directly influence the amount of charge stored in the device. Al-Shamery et al. (2024) developed a hybrid zinc-ion capacitor using natural EuM extracted from Black Soldier Fly. The system exhibited pseudocapacitive behavior, a wide electrochemical potential window, excellent thermal stability, and superior charge storage capacity (91.8 mAh g^{-1}) compared to synthetic EuM (17.3 mAh g^{-1}), underscoring the material's potential for this application.

In conclusion, EuM and its derivatives have demonstrated significant potential for energy storage applications. These materials have proven to be efficient in various components of such devices, including electrodes, electrolytes, and separators. Moreover, their inherent biocompatibility and biodegradability present significant opportunities for advancing the development of sustainable and environmentally friendly batteries and supercapacitors.

3.5 Memory

EuM has been used in metal-insulator-metal (MIM) (Ambrico et al. 2010, 2011, 2012) and metal-insulator-semiconductor (MIS) (Gurme et al. 2018) structures for memory applications. In MIM configurations, current-voltage (I–V) hysteresis demonstrates charge trapping and storage under applied bias or illumination (Ambrico et al. 2010, 2011). Additionally, this charge trapping enables transitions between high-resistance (HRS) and low-resistance (LRS) states essential for nonvolatile memory (Ambrico et al. 2012).

MIS device exhibits a pinched I–V hysteresis loop, characteristic of memristive behavior. Symmetric SET and RESET voltages ($\pm$ 0.6 V) facilitate abrupt transitions between resistance states, supporting precise memory operations (Gurme et al. 2018). Bipolar resistive switching, driven by ion and electron movement, occurs without electroforming, thanks to abundant mobile charge carriers (Gurme et al. 2018). This allows low-voltage switching (~ 0.6 V), reducing power consumption and enhancing reliability. These devices exhibit stable resistance states over 20,000 cycles and a memory window with a tenfold HRS/LRS ratio.

4 Prospective and Challenges

EuM's unique properties open exciting avenues for future applications in various scientific and technological fields. EuM's natural photoprotective properties could inspire the creation of advanced sunscreens, UV-blocking films, and materials for optoelectronic devices that require light sensitivity. In environmental applications, EuM's ability to bind metals and neutralize reactive oxygen species suggests potential use in water purification, heavy metal sequestration, and environmental remediation. The pigment's stability and ability to withstand harsh conditions could also make it valuable for protective coatings.

EuM's biocompatibility further enhances its suitability for medical implants, neural interfaces, and wearable devices designed to monitor or interact with biological systems. In bioelectronics, its mixed ionic-electronic conductivity and environmental stability position it as a key material for the development bio-interfacing sensors, OECTs, and energy storage solutions for implantable applications. In addition, the EuM materials have proven to be efficient in various components of such devices, including electrodes for sensing or electrolytes, and separators in supercapacitor and transistors.

However, significant challenges remain before EuM's full potential can be realized. A major obstacle is the variability in EuM's composition and properties, which depends on its source and extraction method, making standardization for industrial use difficult. Furthermore, the scalability of EuM production in a cost-effective and environmentally sustainable manner poses a critical challenge. Research is also needed to improve the understanding of its electronic and ionic transport mechanisms to optimize its performance in devices. Addressing these challenges will require interdisciplinary collaboration across materials scientist, physicist, chemists, microbiologists, and device engineers.

Despite these hurdles, the growing interest in EuM's multifunctional nature highlights its promise as a cornerstone for next-generation technologies that bridge biology and electronics. By overcoming these challenges, EuM-based innovations could significantly impact diverse areas, from sustainable electronic materials to advanced healthcare solutions.

Acknowledgements This study was financed, in part, by the São Paulo Research Foundation (FAPESP), Brazil. Process numbers #2013/07296-2, #2020/12356-8, #2021/03379-7, #2022/00410-3, , #2024/19323-9, #2025/00301-8, #2026/00697-1. C.F.O.G. is thankful for the support of CNPq under the Instituto Nacional de Ciência e Tecnologia de Nanomateriais para a Vida (INCT-NanoVIDA) n°406079/2022-6.

References

L.G.S. Albano, J.V. Paulin, L.D. Trino, et al., Ultraviolet-protective thin film based on PVA–melanin/rod-coated silver nanowires and its application as a transparent capacitor. J. Appl. Polym. Sci. **136**, 47805 (2019). https://doi.org/10.1002/app.47805

N. Al-Shamery, T. Benselfelt, P.S. Lee, Melanin and polypyrrole-coated nanocellulose hydrogel networks for environmental sensing and energy storage. Appl. Mater. Interfaces **15**, 25966–25979 (2023). https://doi.org/10.1021/acsami.3c03337

N. Al-Shamery, X. Gong, C. Dosche, et al., Sustainable organic electrodes using black soldier fly-derived melanin for zinc-ion hybrid capacitors. Commun. Mater. **5**, 156 (2024). https://doi.org/10.1038/s43246-024-00602-4

M. Ambrico, A. Cardone, T. Ligonzo, et al., Hysteresis-type current–voltage characteristics in Au/eumelanin/ITO/glass structure: towards melanin based memory devices. Org. Electron. **11**, 1809–1814 (2010). https://doi.org/10.1016/j.orgel.2010.08.001

M. Ambrico, P.F. Ambrico, A. Cardone, et al., Melanin layer on silicon: an attractive structure for a possible exploitation in bio-polymer based metal–insulator–silicon devices. Adv. Mater. **23**, 3332–3336 (2011). https://doi.org/10.1002/adma.201101358

M. Ambrico, P.F. Ambrico, T. Ligonzo, et al., Memory-like behavior as a feature of electrical signal transmission in melanin-like bio-polymers. Appl. Phys. Lett. **100** (2012). https://doi.org/10.1063/1.4729754

M. Ambrico, A.B. Mostert, P.F. Ambrico, et al., Exploring ion mobility mechanisms in poly indole-quinone polymers: a case study on black soldier fly melanin. J. Phys. D Appl. Phys. **57**, 265303 (2024). https://doi.org/10.1088/1361-6463/ad3765

Z.V. Bedran, S.S. Zhukov, P.A. Abramov, et al., Water-activated semiquinone formation and carboxylic acid dissociation in melanin revealed by infrared spectroscopy. Polymers (Basel) **13**, 4403 (2021). https://doi.org/10.3390/polym13244403

A. Bernardus Mostert, B.J. Powell, I.R. Gentle, P. Meredith, On the origin of electrical conductivity in the bio-electronic material melanin. Appl. Phys. Lett. **100** (2012). https://doi.org/10.1063/1.3688491

N. Brizuela Guerra, J.V.M. Lima, J.V. Paulin, et al., Electrochemical behavior of non-functionalized and sulfonated melanins at different pH values. Polym. Int. **73**, 992–1000 (2024a). https://doi.org/10.1002/pi.6678

N. Brizuela Guerra, J.V. Morais Lima, N.L. Nozella, et al., Electrochemical doping effect on the conductivity of melanin-inspired materials. ACS Appl. Bio Mater. **7**, 2186–2196 (2024b). https://doi.org/10.1021/acsabm.3c01166

W.D. Bush, J. Garguilo, F.A. Zucca, et al., The surface oxidation potential of human neuromelanin reveals a spherical architecture with a pheomelanin core and a eumelanin surface. Proc. Natl. Acad. Sci. **103**, 14785–14789 (2006). https://doi.org/10.1073/pnas.0604010103

C.-T. Chen, C. Chuang, J. Cao, et al., Excitonic effects from geometric order and disorder explain broadband optical absorption in eumelanin. Nat. Commun. **5**, 3859 (2014). https://doi.org/10.1038/ncomms4859

A.J. Clulow, A.B. Mostert, M. Sheliakina, et al., The structural impact of water sorption on device-quality melanin thin films. Soft Matter **13**, 3954–3965 (2017). https://doi.org/10.1039/C6SM02420C

A. Corani, A. Huijser, T. Gustavsson, et al., Superior photoprotective motifs and mechanisms in eumelanins uncovered. J. Am. Chem. Soc. **136**, 11626–11635 (2014). https://doi.org/10.1021/ja501499q

M. d'Ischia, A. Napolitano, A. Pezzella, et al., Chemical and structural diversity in eumelanins: unexplored bio-optoelectronic materials. Angew. Chem. Int. Ed. **48**, 3914–3921 (2009). https://doi.org/10.1002/anie.200803786

M. d'Ischia, K. Wakamatsu, F. Cicoira, et al., Melanins and melanogenesis: from pigment cells to human health and technological applications. Pigment Cell Melanoma Res. **28**, 520–544 (2015). https://doi.org/10.1111/pcmr.12393

V. Gargiulo, M. Alfè, R. Di Capua, et al., Supplementing π-systems: eumelanin and graphene-like integration towards highly conductive materials for the mammalian cell culture bio-interface. J. Mater. Chem. B **3**, 5070–5079 (2015). https://doi.org/10.1039/C5TB00343A

C. Grieco, F.R. Kohl, A.T. Hanes, B. Kohler, Probing the heterogeneous structure of eumelanin using ultrafast vibrational fingerprinting. Nat. Commun. **11**, 4569 (2020). https://doi.org/10.1038/s41467-020-18393-w

S.T. Gurme, T.D. Dongale, S.N. Surwase, et al., An organic bipolar resistive switching memory device based on natural melanin synthesized from *Aeromonas* sp. SNS. phys. status solidi (a) **215** (2018). https://doi.org/10.1002/pssa.201800550

L. Hong, J.D. Simon, Insight into the binding of divalent cations to sepia eumelanin from IR absorption spectroscopy. Photochem. Photobiol. **82**, 1265–1269 (2006). https://doi.org/10.1562/2006-02-23-RA-809

S. Ito, A. Pilat, W. Gerwat, et al., Photoaging of human retinal pigment epithelium is accompanied by oxidative modifications of its eumelanin. Pigment Cell Melanoma Res. **26**, 357–366 (2013). https://doi.org/10.1111/pcmr.12078

S. Ito, K. Wakamatsu, T. Sarna, Photodegradation of eumelanin and pheomelanin and its pathophysiological implications. Photochem. Photobiol. **94**, 409–420 (2018). https://doi.org/10.1111/php.12837

Y.J. Kim, W. Wu, S.-E. Chun, et al., Biologically derived melanin electrodes in aqueous sodium-ion energy storage devices. Proc. Natl. Acad. Sci. **110**, 20912–20917 (2013). https://doi.org/10.1073/pnas.1314345110

M. Kim, H.S. Kim, M.A. Kim, et al., Thermohydrogel containing melanin for photothermal cancer therapy. Macromol. Biosci. **17**, 1600371 (2017). https://doi.org/10.1002/mabi.201600371

P. Kumar, E. Di Mauro, S. Zhang, et al., Melanin-based flexible supercapacitors. J. Mater. Chem. C Mater. **4**, 9516–9525 (2016). https://doi.org/10.1039/C6TC03739A

Q. Li, Y. Guo, M. Wu, et al., Fluorinated polyimide/allomelanin nanocomposites for UV-shielding applications. Molecules **28**, 5523 (2023). https://doi.org/10.3390/molecules28145523

E. Mazur, D. Kwiatkowska, A. Reich, Photodynamic therapy in pigmented basal cell carcinoma—a review. Biomedicine **11**, 3099 (2023). https://doi.org/10.3390/biomedicines11113099

J. McGinness, P. Corry, P. Proctor, Amorphous semiconductor switching in melanins. Science **183**, 853–855 (1974). https://doi.org/10.1126/science.183.4127.853

A. Menichetti, D. Mordini, S. Vicenzi, M. Montalti, Melanin for photoprotection and hair coloration in the emerging era of nanocosmetics. Int. J. Mol. Sci. **25**, 5862 (2024). https://doi.org/10.3390/ijms25115862

P. Meredith, J. Riesz, Radiative relaxation quantum yields for synthetic eumelanin. Photochem. Photobiol. **79**, 211–216 (2004). https://doi.org/10.1111/j.1751-1097.2004.tb00012.x

R. Micillo, L. Panzella, M. Iacomino, et al., Eumelanin broadband absorption develops from aggregation-modulated chromophore interactions under structural and redox control. Sci. Rep. **7**, 41532 (2017). https://doi.org/10.1038/srep41532

L. Migliaccio, S. Aprano, L. Iannuzzi, et al., Eumelanin–PEDOT:PSS complementing en route to mammalian-pigment-based electrodes: design and fabrication of an ITO-free organic light-emitting device. Adv. Electron. Mater. **3** (2017). https://doi.org/10.1002/aelm.201600342

A.B. Mostert, K.J.P. Davy, J.L. Ruggles, et al., Gaseous adsorption in melanins: hydrophilic biomacromolecules with high electrical conductivities. Langmuir **26**, 412–416 (2010). https://doi.org/10.1021/la901290f

A.B. Mostert, B.J. Powell, F.L. Pratt, et al., Role of semiconductivity and ion transport in the electrical conduction of melanin. Proc. Natl. Acad. Sci. **109**, 8943–8947 (2012). https://doi.org/10.1073/pnas.1119948109

A.B. Mostert, G.R. Hanson, T. Sarna, et al., Hydration-controlled X-band EPR spectroscopy: a tool for unravelling the complexities of the solid-state free radical in eumelanin. J. Phys. Chem. B **117**, 4965–4972 (2013). https://doi.org/10.1021/jp401615e

A.B. Mostert, S.B. Rienecker, M. Sheliakina, et al., Engineering proton conductivity in melanin using metal doping. J. Mater. Chem. B **8**, 8050–8060 (2020). https://doi.org/10.1039/D0TB01390K

N.L. Nozella, J.V.M. Lima, R.F. de Oliveira, G. CFDO, Melanin/PEDOT:PSS blend as organic mixed ionic electronic conductor (OMIEC) for sustainable electronics. Mater. Adv. **4**, 4732–4743 (2023). https://doi.org/10.1039/D3MA00573A

J. Pan, Z. Xia, N. Deng, et al., Eumelanin-inspired nanomaterials in electrochemical energy storage devices: a review. Chem. Eng. J. **452**, 138607 (2023). https://doi.org/10.1016/j.cej.2022.138607

L. Panzella, G. Gentile, G. D'Errico, et al., Atypical structural and π-electron features of a melanin polymer that lead to superior free-radical-scavenging properties. Angew. Chem. Int. Ed. **52**, 12684–12687 (2013). https://doi.org/10.1002/anie.201305747

J.V. Paulin, A.P. Coleone, A. Batagin-Neto, et al., Melanin thin-films: a perspective on optical and electrical properties. J. Mater. Chem. C Mater. **9**, 8345–8358 (2021a). https://doi.org/10.1039/D1TC01440D

J.V. Paulin, S.L. Fernandes, C.F.O. Graeff, Solid-state electrochemical energy storage based on soluble melanin. Electrochem **2**, 264–273 (2021b). https://doi.org/10.3390/electrochem2020019

J.V. Paulin, L.G.S. Albano, D.H.S. Camargo, et al., Eumelanin-based multisensory platform: a case of study for photolithographic patterning. Appl. Mater. Today **28**, 101525 (2022). https://doi.org/10.1016/j.apmt.2022.101525

J.V. Paulin, S. Bayram, C.F.O. Graeff, C.C.B. Bufon, Exploring the charge transport of a natural eumelanin for sustainable technologies. ACS Appl. Bio Mater. **6**, 3633–3637 (2023a). https://doi.org/10.1021/acsabm.3c00469

J.V. Paulin, M.P. Pereira, B.A. Bregadiolli, et al., Controlling ions and electrons in aqueous solution: an alternative point of view of the charge-transport behavior of eumelanin-inspired material. J. Mater. Chem. C Mater. **11**, 6107–6118 (2023b). https://doi.org/10.1039/D3TC00490B

A. Pezzella, A. Iadonisi, S. Valerio, et al., Disentangling eumelanin "black chromophore": visible absorption changes as signatures of oxidation state- and aggregation-dependent dynamic interactions in a model water-soluble 5,6-dihydroxyindole polymer. J. Am. Chem. Soc. **131**, 15270–15275 (2009). https://doi.org/10.1021/ja905162s

M. Piacenti da Silva, J.C. Fernandes, N.B. de Figueiredo, et al., Melanin as an active layer in biosensors. AIP Adv. **4** (2014). https://doi.org/10.1063/1.4869638

G. Prota, *Melanins and Melanogenesis* (Elsevier, 1992)

M. Reali, A. Gouda, J. Bellemare, et al., Electronic transport in the biopigment sepia melanin. ACS Appl. Bio Mater. **3**, 5244–5252 (2020). https://doi.org/10.1021/acsabm.0c00373

M. Reali, P. Saini, C. Santato, Electronic and protonic transport in bio-sourced materials: a new perspective on semiconductivity. Mater. Adv. **2**, 15–31 (2021). https://doi.org/10.1039/D0MA00579G

M. Sheliakina, A.B. Mostert, P. Meredith, An all-solid-state biocompatible ion-to-electron transducer for bioelectronics. Mater. Horiz. **5**, 256–263 (2018a). https://doi.org/10.1039/C7MH00831G

M. Sheliakina, A.B. Mostert, P. Meredith, Decoupling ionic and electronic currents in melanin. Adv. Funct. Mater. **28** (2018b). https://doi.org/10.1002/adfm.201805514

F. Solano, Melanins: skin pigments and much more—types, structural models, biological functions, and formation routes. New J. Sci. **2014**, 1–28 (2014). https://doi.org/10.1155/2014/498276

Z. Tehrani, S.P. Whelan, B. Mostert, et al., Printable and flexible graphene pH sensors utilising thin film melanin for physiological applications. 2D Mater. **7**, 024008 (2020). https://doi.org/10.1088/2053-1583/ab72d5

M.L. Tran, B.J. Powell, P. Meredith, Chemical and structural disorder in eumelanins: a possible explanation for broadband absorbance. Biophys. J. **90**, 743–752 (2006). https://doi.org/10.1529/biophysj.105.069096

TrueBlue, *TrueBlue Vision: Your Best Eye Protection Against Harmful Blue Light*. https://www.truebluevision.com/. Accessed 4 Jan 2025

Y. Wang, T. Li, P. Ma, et al., Simultaneous enhancements of UV-shielding properties and photostability of poly(vinyl alcohol) via incorporation of sepia eumelanin. ACS Sustain. Chem. Eng. **4**, 2252–2258 (2016). https://doi.org/10.1021/acssuschemeng.5b01734

K. Wang, Y. Hou, B. Poudel, et al., Melanin–perovskite composites for photothermal conversion. Adv. Energy Mater. **9**, 1–11 (2019). https://doi.org/10.1002/aenm.201901753

A.A.R. Watt, J.P. Bothma, P. Meredith, The supramolecular structure of melanin. Soft Matter **5**, 3754 (2009). https://doi.org/10.1039/b902507c

S.P. Whelan, Z. Tehrani, M. Peacock, et al., Investigation into the suitability of screen printed graphene-melanin pH sensors for use in bacterial culturing applications. J. Electroanal. Chem. **904**, 115868 (2022). https://doi.org/10.1016/j.jelechem.2021.115868

C.Y. Wright, M. Norval, Solar ultraviolet radiation, skin cancer and photoprotective strategies in South Africa. Photochem. Photobiol. **99**, 509–518 (2023). https://doi.org/10.1111/php.13676

J. Wünsche, Y. Deng, P. Kumar, et al., Protonic and electronic transport in hydrated thin films of the pigment eumelanin. Chem. Mater. **27**, 436–442 (2015). https://doi.org/10.1021/cm502939r

W. Xie, A. Dhinojwala, N.C. Gianneschi, M.D. Shawkey, Interactions of melanin with electromagnetic radiation: from fundamentals to applications. Chem. Rev. **124**, 7165–7213 (2024). https://doi.org/10.1021/acs.chemrev.3c00858

L. Zecca, F.A. Zucca, A. Albertini, et al., A proposed dual role of neuromelanin in the pathogenesis of Parkinson's disease. Neurology **67** (2006). https://doi.org/10.1212/WNL.67.7_suppl_2.S8

F.A. Zucca, E. Basso, F.A. Cupaioli, et al., Neuromelanin of the human substantia nigra: an update. Neurotox. Res. **25**, 13–23 (2014). https://doi.org/10.1007/s12640-013-9435-y

Light Modulation of Biological/Semiconductor Interfaces for Affecting Cell Growth and for Advancing Artificial Retina Development

Manuela Ciocca, Luisa Petti, Paolo Lugli, Antonella Camaioni, and Thomas M. Brown

Contents

Abstract This chapter presents the concept of employing light as a tool to modulate the behavior of biological systems. In Sect. 1, a brief historical and scientific overview of light modulation of living systems, starting from the eighteenth century and reaching current days with the most recent progress in the field of bioelectronics is given. Then exogenous light stimulation approaches and the employment of bio-hybrid interfaces based on semiconducting polymers are described. In Sect. 2, the main features of widely used semiconducting polymers are detailed. Moreover, two

M. Ciocca (✉) · L. Petti · P. Lugli
Faculty of Engineering, Free University of Bozen-Bolzano, Bolzano, Italy
e-mail: manuela.ciocca@unibz.it

L. Petti
e-mail: luisa.petti@unibz.it

P. Lugli
e-mail: paolo.lugli@unibz.it

A. Camaioni
Department of Biomedicine and Prevention, University of Rome Tor Vergata, Rome, Italy
e-mail: camaioni@uniroma2.it

T. M. Brown
Department of Electronic Engineering, University of Rome Tor Vergata, Rome, Italy
e-mail: thomas.brown@uniroma2.it

R. Narayan (ed.), *Nanostructured Biomaterials and Their Applications*,
https://doi.org/10.1007/978-3-032-16316-5_14

key examples illustrating how light-sensitive bio-hybrid interfaces can be used for the control of cell proliferation as well as for the realization of an artificial retina model are exhaustively presented in Sects. 3 and 4. By the end of the chapter, the main elements and principles of light modulation of biological/semiconductor interfaces are explained. Finally, a discussion on the key concepts is included to show the relevant achievements and the thrilling future perspectives.

Keywords Semiconducting polymers. · Light stimulation of biological systems. · Optoelectrical stimulation. · Photosensitive bio-hybrid interfaces. · Bioelectronics.

1 Light Modulation of Living Systems

The possibility to modulate biological functions, in isolated cells as well as in tissues, has always been a fascinating perspective that has been historically addressed through electrode-mediated techniques.

Back in eighteenth century at the University of Bologna Luigi Galvani predicted for the first time the concept of integrating electric signals with biological systems. He induced muscular activity in the detached leg of a dead frog. Galvani's work, "De Viribus Electricitatis in Motu Musculari Commentarius" (Commentary on the Effect of Electricity on Muscular Motion) published in 1791 (Galvani 1792), pioneered the use of bioelectric forces to study tissues of living organisms (Berggren and Richter-Dahlfors 2007). Galvani coined the term "animal electricity" to describe these phenomena, indicating a form of energy generated by the tissues themselves in response to electrical stimuli, similar but in a way different from what was known as standard electricity. This was the first foray into the study of bioelectricity, a field that still studies the electrical patterns and signals from biological tissues and cells. Since the pioneering experiments of Galvani on frog's legs (1791) until nowadays, electrical stimulation of living systems (cells as well as tissues or organisms) has been intensively improved thanks to technological breakthroughs in electronics and their application in bioengineering and medicine.

Technological advancements such as lasers (Hu et al. 2020), optical tweezers (Corsetti and Dholakia 2021), and Raman spectroscopy (Pezzotti 2021) have paved the way to new noninvasive and nondestructive techniques for cell manipulation, based on the use of light. Indeed, the use of light as a mean of modulation of cellular properties dates back to 1891 when Jacques-Arséne d'Arsonval demonstrated that muscular tissues could be excited by light (Reif-Acherman 2017). Following this demonstration, Arvanitaki and Chalazonitis (Arvanitaki and Chalazonitis 1968) showed light-induced excitation and inhibition of ganglion cells of Aplysia californica. In 1960s, Fork reported a futuristic experiment about the selective stimulation of neurons via 488 nm laser radiation (Fork 1971).

The strong interest toward the use of light for the modulation of biological systems is due to the fact that it provides interesting solutions to overcome the limitations of traditional electrical approaches (Meng et al. 2021), such as the rigidity of metal-based electrodes (not conformable with the human body, tissues, and in general with biological systems), the erosion of electrodes due to the presence of culture medium or intra/extracellular fluids, as well as the cytotoxicity, and low biocompatibility of electrodes in general. Moreover, since no physical contact is required, light stimulation reduces the possibility of biological sample contamination, mechanical stress, and damage. Further advantages resulting from the ability to focus and shape the light beam are the high spatial (<1 μm) and temporal (<1 ms) resolution (Antognazza et al. 2015), and certainly the less invasive and wireless offered options.

This is why various techniques for exploiting the interaction of light with biological systems have been developed in recent years, indicating an increasing interest in optical approaches to stimulate living matter. These optical approaches include the development of light-sensitive proteins as well as photoactive molecules, materials, 2D surfaces, 3D scaffolds, and devices.

All these optical techniques rely on the property of light to propagate (to a certain extent and depending on the wavelength) through various biological tissues and to penetrate through biological membranes. However, light does not specifically interact with biological systems, unless some notable exception, like the mammalian retina and photosynthetic organisms. Therefore, light-sensitive transducers are commonly employed to optically modulate cellular or tissues activity. These materials can guarantee the required optoelectrical transduction mechanism, converting light into electrical signals suitable for cell and tissue stimulation. Hence, besides the standard electrical stimulation, optoelectrical manipulation of biological system, especially biophotovoltaics and photobiomodulation, have recently gained attention especially for cell and tissue engineering (Joseph et al. 2024; Yang et al. 2017).

Optoelectrical methods for light modulation of biological systems are usually classified in two main categories (Antognazza et al. 2019; Joseph et al. 2024): the endogenous and exogenous techniques (Fig. 1). The former focuses on exploiting photoactive mediators present in and expressed by living systems. The latter investigate photoactive materials (light-transducers) and their effect when interfaced with cells or tissues. In this case, the light-transducing materials can convert light excitation in electrical, chemical, or thermal stimuli.

In the following subsections of this chapter, both the stimulation approaches are described, starting with the endogenous one.

1.1 Endogenous Light Stimulation Approaches

Endogenous light stimulation method (Fig. 1, left) relies on photoactive/sensitive materials typical of biological systems and present in the extracellular environment, enclosed inside the cells or anchored on the cellular plasma membrane. Possible endogenous methods are:

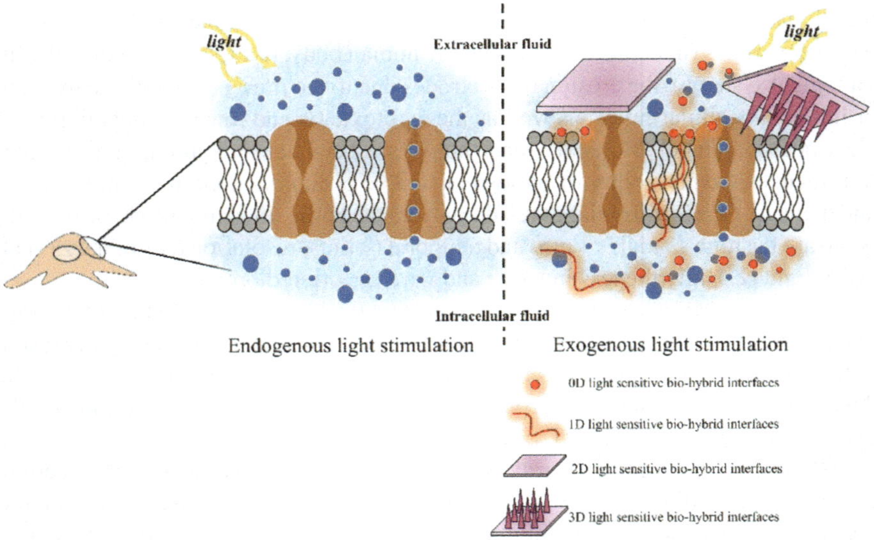

Fig. 1 Schematic representation of endogenous and exogenous methods for the light stimulation of living cells. Endogenous stimulation (left) comprises the use of direct light stimulation. Exogenous stimulation (right) techniques include the use of photosensitive 0D (nanoparticles), 1D (nanowires), 2D (thin film), or 3D (micropillars) bio-hybrid interfaces able to stimulate cells.

(i) *Direct Stimulation*: Ultrafast near infrared (NIR, 750 nm < λ < 2500 nm, from the femtosecond to the nanosecond range) and ultraviolet (UV, 100 nm < λ < 400 nm) light pulses have been used for different type of cell excitation (Iwanaga et al. 2005; Park et al. 2021; Smith et al. 2006). This method is relatively easy, but its limit is due to mechanical or biochemical stress activation of the biological system. Nevertheless, the infrared neural stimulation (INS), based on the employment of infrared light for cellular stimulation below the threshold (few mJ/mm^2) in case of tissue damage, gained interesting results linked to a transient cell depolarization due to the thermal effect (Airaghi Leccardi et al. 2020; Shapiro et al. 2012). The operating principle of INS is based on the absorption of IR light by water present in the intra- and extracellular environment, which generates local heating of cells and activates temperature-sensitive ion channels in the cell membrane.

(ii) *Light-Sensitive Bioactive Molecules*: One recent example of light-sensitive bioactive molecules is the acrylamide–azobenzene-quaternary ammonium (AAQ). This small molecule is a photoisomerizable compound (or photoswitch) that has been exploited as artificial photoreceptor (Tochitsky et al. 2014). Upon UV radiation, AAQ takes *cis*-form able to decease neural excitability, while the AAQ *trans*-form binds to the cell membrane ion channels and induces the opposite effect on cells. Photoisomerizable molecules can then be introduced inside or nearby the region of interest, with the advantage to light-stimulate the cells locally. However, photolysis and limited UV light penetration in tissues are the main drawbacks of this approach.

(iii) *Optogenetics:* Optogenetics is certainly one of the most powerful techniques to induce light sensitivity in a living system. This approach is based on the introduction of a photosensitive channel, which is a transmembrane photoswitchable protein encoded by an opsin gene introduced inside a cell through a molecular biology procedure, usually a viral transfection (Deisseroth 2015). Despite important results within the light interaction with the nervous systems and numerous applications, the major challenges are ethical concerns and safety issues regarding the use of viruses for gene transfection and expression.

1.2 Exogenous Light Stimulation Approaches

Exogenous light stimulation methods (Fig. 1, right) relies on light-sensitive bio-hybrid interfaces based on the combination of photoactive materials (light-transducers) and biological systems. The working principle of this approach is the light-transduction process actuated by the light-transducers in which the optical excitation is converted into an adequate stimulation affecting the behavior of cells or tissues under test. Possible exogenous methods include:

(i) *0D light-sensitive bio-hybrid interfaces*, based on light-transducer nanoparticles. 0D light-transducer nanoparticles can be made of organic or inorganic materials as well as a combination of both. Quantum dots are one of the most popular nanoparticles used in the field. QDs are semiconductor nanocrystals, typically with size in the range from 1.5 to 10 nm, which exhibit unique size and composition-dependent optoelectronic properties (Yadav and Raizaday 2016). When exposed to UV light, QDs can transport electrons and emit light of various colors. Therefore, QDs gained a lot of interest in biomedical applications and have been used for both *in vitro* and *in vivo* imaging analysis (Walling et al. 2009). Core or core/shell QDs such as cadmium selenide (CdSe), indium phosphide (InP), and aluminum antimonide (AlSb) were profitably used as bio-hybrid interfaces for optoelectrical stimulation of neurons employing external light excitation sources in the visible range (Bahmani Jalali et al. 2019; Han et al. 2021; Karatum et al. 2021). Organic nanoparticles based on conjugated polymers are also widely used for biophotonic applications, bio-sensing/stimulation (Allarà et al. 2025).

(ii) *1D light-sensitive bio-hybrid interfaces*, based on light-transducing nanorods and nanowires. One-dimensional (1D) structured materials are nanoscaled in two dimensions. Examples include nanotubes, nanowires, and nanorods. Silicon nanowires have been successfully used for photoelectric stimulation of myofibroblasts with subcellular resolution (Rotenberg et al. 2020). In this case, the 1D bio-hybrid nanowire–myofibroblast interface was profitably electrically coupled with cardiomyocytes, leading to increase in the spontaneous activation rate of cardiomyocytes by nanowires photostimulation.

(iii) *2D light-sensitive bio-hybrid interfaces*, based on light-transducer surfaces. Light-sensitive bio-hybrid surfaces, based on semiconducting polymers, were successfully used for light control of biotic and bioelectrical activity of different type of cells such as rat hippocampal neurons (Ghezzi et al. 2011), rat neocortical astrocytes (Benfenati et al. 2014), neuroblastoma cells (Ciocca et al. 2023), and endothelial colony forming cells (Negri et al. 2022). In these investigations, cells were cultured on top of the light-sensitive thin film. Upon light stimulation, in presence of the 2D bio-hybrid interface, it was possible to control the behavior of the cell network in terms of cell conductance, action potential, cell proliferation, ion fluxes through the cell membrane, cell angiogenesis.

(iv) *3D light-sensitive bio-hybrid interfaces*, based on light-transducing 3D scaffolds. 3D light-sensitive bio-hybrid interfaces consisting of semiconducting polymer micropillars were used for optical modulation of neuronal growth and orientation (Milos et al. 2021). Recently the design and fabrication of a 3D photosensitive bioprinted cell scaffold for biophotonic application was also demonstrated (Ciocca et al. 2025a, 2022), via mixing hydrogel-based ink with poly(3-hexylthiophene) nanoparticles (P3HT-NPs) suspended in water and also P3HT blended with [6, 6] phenyl-C61-butyric acid methyl ester (PCBM) nanoparticles mixed into polyethylene oxide (PEO) hydrogels to develop a bioelectronic interface for biophotonic applications (Ciocca et al. 2025b).

The following sections of this chapter focus on semiconducting polymers employed as 2D light-sensitive bio-hybrid interfaces since they are widely used for optoelectrical stimulation of living cells and other bio-interfaces. Firstly, some CPs examples and features are described (Sect. 2). Then, two examples of exogenous methods for the light modulation of living cells (Sect. 3) and for the mimicking of photoreceptors cells (Sect. 4) will be described together with the biophysical processes describing how these light-transducer interfaces can be used for affecting cell growth and for developing an artificial retina respectively.

2 Conjugated Polymers for Light Modulation of Living Cells

Conjugated polymers (CPs, also referred as semiconducting polymers) are organic semiconductors attracting increasing interest in the field of bioelectronics especially for light modulation and control of living cells (Gentile et al. 2025; Joseph et al. 2024). Semiconducting polymers have started to emerge in life science in the last decades as a new class of soft materials well suited for the design of light-sensitive bio-hybrid interfaces because of their remarkable properties:

- CPs are biocompatible photosensitive materials with adequate biological compatibility that can be tailored to achieve the desired electrical outputs for living systems stimulation.

- CPs show high efficiency of light absorption, thus employing CPs as light-transducers guarantees efficient light stimulation providing less invasiveness and avoiding electrode penetration inside cells or tissues.
- Photosensitive bio-hybrid interfaces based on CPs, within which living systems are interfaced or integrated, can be engineered, and controlled in order to be most suitable for the project needs, via specific fabrication steps and techniques, thanks to their tunable optical and electronic properties and easy processability.

Most importantly, these organic polymers show low production of heat, tailored interactions with photons thanks to the easy tuning of their optoelectronic properties, and good interactions with electrolytes due to the ionic nature of their electrical signals. Some CPs important features are described in Sect. 2.1.

2.1 Conjugated Polymers

Semiconducting organic polymers are a special class of polymers whose distinctive chemical property is conjugation: alternating double and single bonds in their structure (Moliton and Hiorns 2004). This conjugated system structure confers the semiconductive property to the polymer. Due to their favorable charge-transfer properties, CPs are largely used in organic photovoltaics, optoelectronics, and biological sensing application (Xie et al. 2016). The most widely used CPs are polyaniline, polypyrrole, polycarbazole, polythiophene, and their derivatives (Fig. 2, a). Thereby, as CPs present a carbon-based chemical structure resembling that of a basic compound of living matter, they bear an intrinsic affinity to biological systems and adequate biocompatibility. Furthermore, since they are soft materials, they match the mechanical properties of biological tissues better than inorganic materials.

CP's most important feature is light-sensitivity and the ability to transduce light into electrical energy. Since their chemical structure is based on conjugated carbon molecules, they have π-electrons delocalized along their backbone that induce strong coupling with light in the visible region. CP's optical bandgap can be properly engineered and tuned by chemical tailoring from the NIR to the UV. CPs work as light absorber, electron donor, acceptor, and/or hole transporting material (Peng et al. 2017). The phototransduction process and the consequent energy production involve the photovoltaic process with exciton generation, charge separation at heterostructure interfaces and transport of charge carriers. For a deep understanding of molecular orbits and photovoltaic processes, we recommend the readers to refer to the widely disseminated theoretical explanation and descriptions found in (Brédas et al. 2002; Hagberg et al. 2007; Mincuzzi et al. 2016; Vesce et al. 2019). For the aim of this chapter, the main steps of the photovoltaic process are briefly described and schematically represented in Fig. 2, b. The photovoltaic process starts with photoexcitation of an electron from the highest occupied molecular orbital (HOMO) to the lowest unoccupied molecular orbital (LUMO) and with the generation of an exciton (charged couple hole–electron bonded by Coulombian force) upon the absorption of light

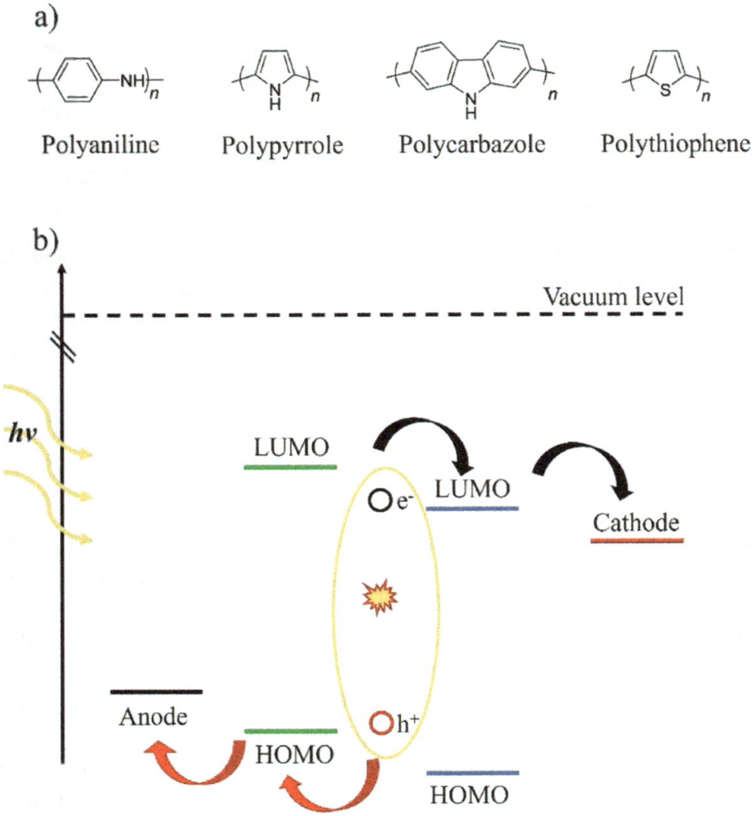

Fig. 2 **a** Structure of the most widely used conjugated polymers (CPs): polyaniline, polypyrrole, polycarbazole, polythiophene. **b** Representative schematic of the photovoltaic process occurring within the CP active materials upon light energy (*hv*) absorption with generation of an exciton, charge separation and subsequently collection of electrons (e^-) and holes (h^+) at the anode and cathode electrodes

energy (*hv*). In CPs, HOMO, and LUMO are separated by an energy gap typically in the range of 1.5–3 eV. The hole-electron pairs can dissociate into free carriers (electrons and holes) at the interface between two semiconductors with energy levels that differ by at least the binding energy of the exciton (donor and acceptor semiconductors). Subsequently, the free electrons and holes are collected at the anode and cathode electrodes (Fig. 2, b).

Considering all their excellent properties, CPs are well suited for the design of a bio-hybrid interface that interacts with light. Suitable CPs for bio-hybrid light-sensitive interfaces development, with biological and biomedical application, should offer a good trade-off between order and presence of amorphous structures, to guarantee good conduction across the molecules as well as surfaces that can ensure flexibility and adaptability to the various possible biological systems anatomy.

3 Bio-Photoelectrolytic Platform, Based on Conjugated Polymers, for Light Control of Cell Bioelectrical Activity

As an example of a planar (2D) light-sensitive bio-hybrid interface based on CPs and living cells, we present the work on a bio-hybrid photoelectrolytic platform (Fig. 3, a) described in reference (Ciocca et al. 2023). The platform was successfully employed for light control of SH-SY5Y neuroblastoma cells and to elicit and record cellular bioelectrical activity. It consists of two transparent and parallel electrodes separated by a thermoplastic encapsulant (Surlyn) chamber where an electrolyte solution, either culture medium or a buffer saline solution, is confined. The photosensitive electrode consists of an optically absorbing poly-3-hexylthiophene (P3HT) semiconductor thin film (100 nm thickness) spin-coated on a transparent conducting oxide (fluorine tin oxide [FTO]) glass substrate (UV–vis absorption spectra of P3HT-photoelectrode with a peak at 520 nm is shown in Fig. 3, b). The counter-electrode is an FTO-coated substrate with a platinum (Pt) overlayer deposited by screen-printing. The platform can be used in two different architectures: (1) the open-top Surlyn chamber with the photosensing substrate electrode (Glass|FTO|P3HT) that allows light stimulation of adhered cells during culture in a defined medium (Fig. 3, a—left); and (2) the sandwich-closed layout for bioelectrical signal measurements (Fig. 3, a—right). In the latter, the used electrolyte is a phosphate-buffered saline (PBS) solution that mimics extracellular fluids exhibiting pH, osmolality, and ion concentrations close to that of the human body fluids (Ciocca et al. 2023).

SH-SY5Y neuroblastoma cells were cultured in an incubator (at 37 °C, 5% CO_2) on Glass|FTO or Glass|FTO|P3HT -photosensitive surface up to 3 days (from T0 = 16 hours after cell seeding, to T3 or T4 = three or four days of culture) and kept in dark (not light-stimulated, NLS) or subjected to a light stimulation protocol (LS) via a white LED (1.26 mW/cm^2, light spectrum in Fig. 3, c), consisting in 1 s light and 1 s dark, sustained for 30 min twice a day, for 3 days. Firstly, biocompatibility and photocytotoxicity were investigated. Thus, viable and dead cells present in culture on Glass|FTO (CTRL) and Glass|FTO|P3HT (P3HT) samples at T0 and T3 for both NLS and LS protocols were counted by using in situ Cell Viability Imaging Kit (Fig. 4, a). The 2D bio-hybrid platform shows adequate biosafety with less than 2% of cell death on the total cells cultured on polymer thin films up to 3 days, for both LS and NLS conditions (Fig. 4, b). About biosafety concerns, the microenvironment temperature variation upon LS was measured by using a thermocouple near the polymer thin film placed in the same condition as during cell culture under LS (i.e., Glass|FTO|P3HT immersed in cell culture medium, inside incubator at 37 °C, 5% CO_2). Over the 30 minutes of LS, a temperature change of $\Delta T = 0.52 \pm 0.30$ °C (Fig. 4, c) was recorded. While during the 1 s light stimulus, the measured temperature variation was $\Delta T = 0.0006 \pm 0.0008$ °C (Fig. 4, d). This temperature variation can be considered negligible as it does not have any influence on the cellular microenvironment and/or it does not induce photothermal effects (Ciocca et al. 2023).

Afterward, the effect of polymer-mediated light stimulation on cells behavior was investigated. SH-SY5Y neuroblastoma cells were cultured on Glass|FTO (CTRL) or

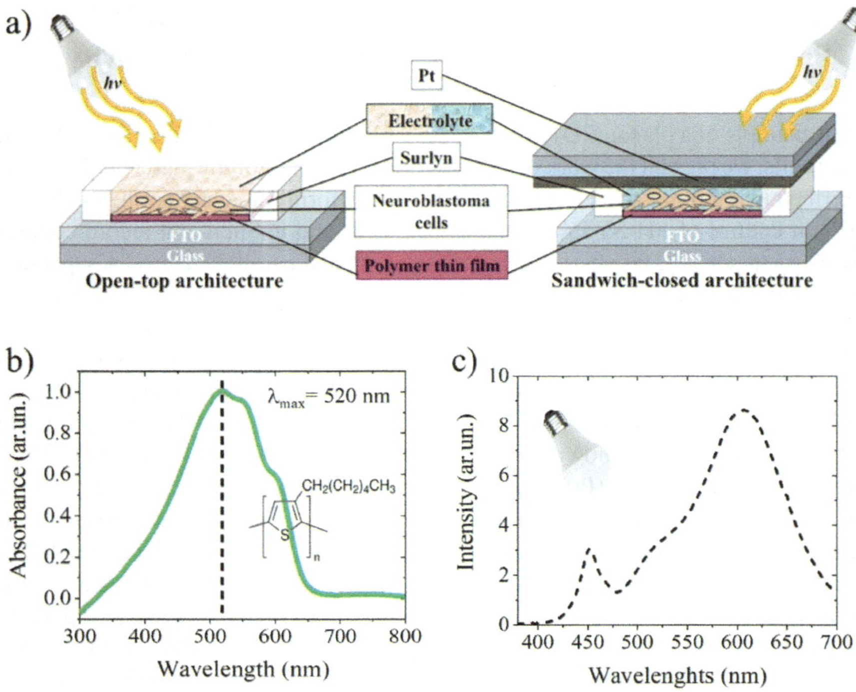

Fig. 3 **a** Schematic of the bio-photo electrolytic platform with the open-top (left) and sandwich-closed (right) architectures. Inside the chamber confined by Surlyn, neuroblastoma cells are cultured on the polymer thin film, immersed in culture medium, and subjected to a pulsed light stimulation (LS) protocol (left) while the closed configuration of the device, containing a buffer electrolyte solution confined in the Surlyn chamber, allows bioelectrical signal measurements (right). **b** UV-vis absorption spectra of P3HT thin film (maximum absorption peak at 520 nm). P3HT chemical structure is shown. **c** Standard warm white LED light spectrum. LED used for the light stimulation protocol (LS) of cells cultured on the bio-photo-electrolytic platform P3HT-photoelectrode. Light power was 1.26 mW/cm^2. Figure adapted with permission from (Ciocca et al. 2023)

Glass|FTO|P3HT (P3HT) up to 3 days in NLS or LS conditions. Cells proliferation was investigated via Click-iT EdU proliferation assay (Fig. 5, a). Data indicated that at T0 the cells cultured on Glass|FTO (CTRL) and Glass|FTO|P3HT (P3HT) substrates were proliferating with no significant differences between groups (CTRL-NLS = 45.96 ± 1.85%; P3HT-NLS = 43.92 ± 10.06%). However, growth of neuroblastoma cells on P3HT bio-hybrid surface in LS condition showed a 50% reduced proliferation activity when examined at T3. Only ~20% of total cells were actively synthesizing DNA when cultured on P3HT subjected to the LS protocol (P3HT-LS: 22.87 ± 1.18%), while all other groups showed ~40% of proliferating cells (CTRL-NLS: 41.92 ± 1.57%; P3HT-NLS: 44.3 ± 2.21%; CTRL-LS: 42.2 ± 1.16%) as quantified and shown in Fig. 5, b. This result indicates that the polymer-mediated LS protocol significantly affects cell proliferation by reducing to roughly one-half the percentage of cell that are actively synthesizing their DNA

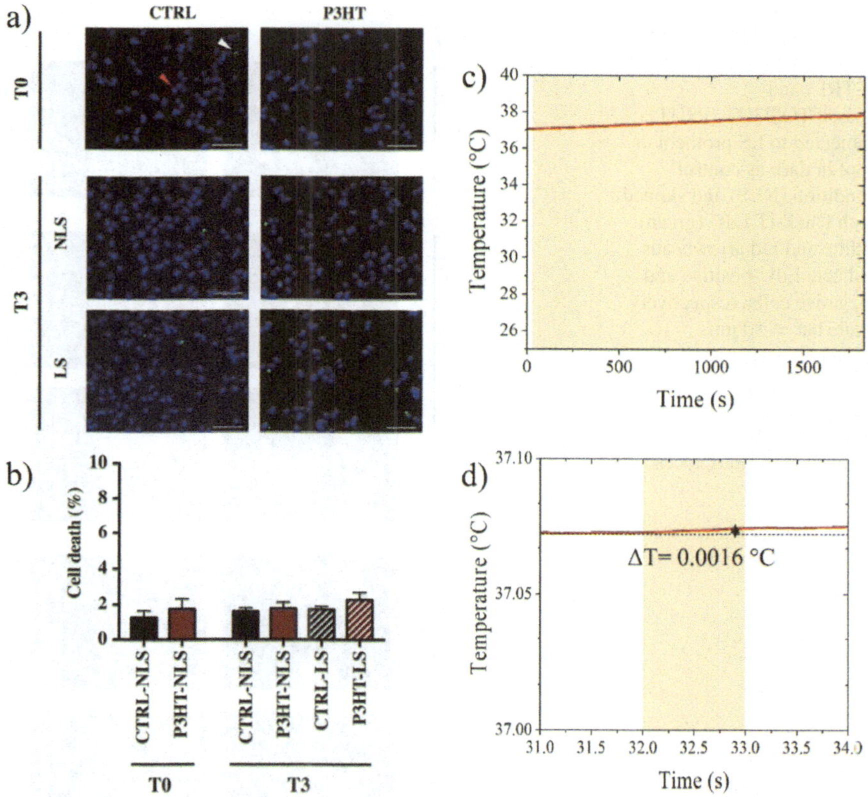

Fig. 4 **a** Evaluation of cell viability by in situ cell viability imaging assay. Representative fluorescence micrographs at T0 and T3 of SH-SY5Y cells cultured on Glass|FTO (CTRL) and Glass|FTO|P3HT (P3HT) subjected to the LS protocol or kept in dark as control (NLS). White and red arrowheads indicate dead (green emission) and live (blue emission) cells, respectively. Scale bar = 50 µm. **b** Quantitative analysis of cell death expressed as percentage of positive cells on total cells at the beginning (T0) and at the end (T3) of the culture. **c** Temperature variation (ΔT = 0.52 °C) of the extracellular bath upon light stimulation protocol over 30 min, 1 s on and 1 s off, as a function of time. **d** Temperature variation over 1 s of photoexcitation. Figure reproduced with permission from (Ciocca et al. 2023)

with respect to cells cultured in dark. More interestingly, after the supplementary day of culture in dark (T4), proliferation of LS cells cultured on P3HT resumed to the level displayed by all the other culture conditions (CTRL-NLS: 40.27 ± 1.34%; P3HT-NLS: 41.86 ± 1.01%; CTRL-LS: 40.55 ± 1.18%; P3HT-LS: 45.08 ± 1.42%) (Fig. 5, b). These results indicate that it is possible to control cell proliferation using a defined LS protocol during the culture in the presence of a polymer photosensitive 2D bio-hybrid interface, offering the possibility to light-regulate neuroblastoma cell proliferation in a reversible way. This effect can be mainly attributed to the P3HT-mediated optical excitation effect on SH-SY5Y cells.

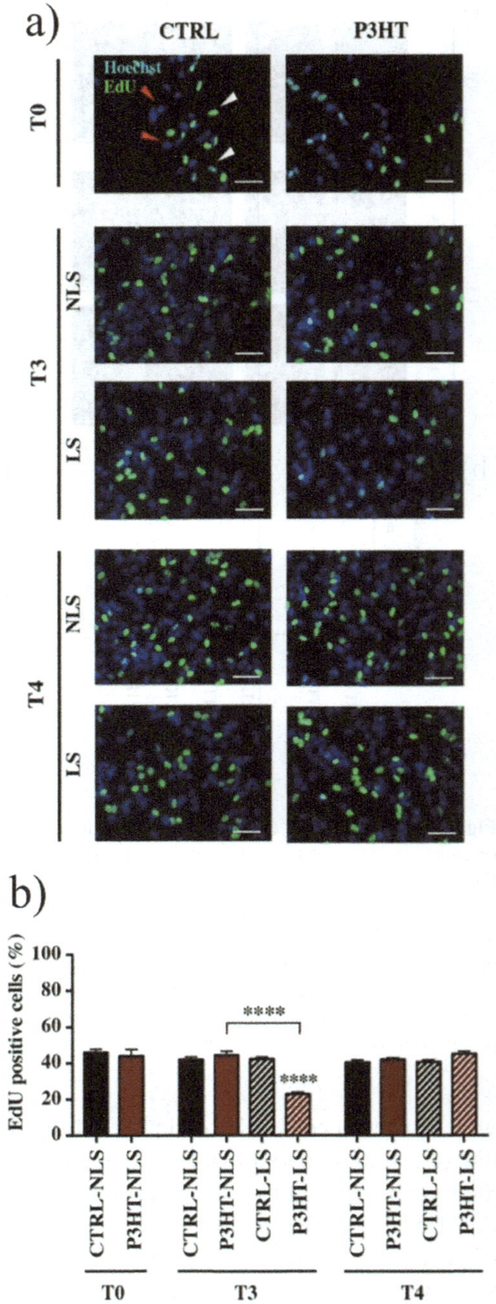

Fig. 5 **a** Representative micrographs of SH-SY5Y cells cultured on Glass|FTO (CTRL) and Glass|FTO|P3HT (P3HT) subjected to LS protocol or kept in dark as control condition (NLS) and stained with Click-iT EdU (green). White and red arrowheads indicate EdU-positive and -negative cells, respectively. Scale bar = 50 μm. **b** Quantification of Click-iT EdU-positive proliferating cells as percentage of total cells. Figure reproduced with permission from (Ciocca et al. 2023)

Intracellular Calcium (Ca^{2+}) evaluation was also conducted via FLUO-4 AM. SH-SY5Y cells cultured on Glass|FTO (CTRL) and on Glass|FTO|P3HT (P3HT) were loaded with the fluorescent dye FLUO-4 AM both at T0 and T3 in NLS and LS condition and then photostimulated for 30 min (white LED, 1.26 mW/cm^2, 1 s light and 1 s dark). The cellular fluorescence before (i.e., basal concentration of intracellular Ca^{2+}) and after photostimulation (i.e., induced concentration of intracellular Ca^{2+} after light stimuli) are shown in Fig. 6. Analysis performed at T0 and T3 in NLS condition on Glass|FTO (CTRL) and on Glass|FTO|P3HT (P3HT) showed a significant increase of fluorescence intensity induced in cells cultured on P3HT with respect to the basal fluorescence level, while no significant differences were observed before and after light stimuli in Glass|FTO (CTRL) groups (Fig. 7). Interestingly, when cells were cultured on P3HT and subjected to the LS protocol for 3 days (P3HT-LS/basal), a considerable increase in basal fluorescence was observed with respect to all the other conditions (CTRL-NLS/basal, CTRL-LS/basal, and P3HT-NLS/basal) as shown in Fig. 7. These levels remained unchanged also after photostimulation (P3HT-LS/induced). To investigate whether the observed Ca^{2+} increase arises from the extracellular milieu (through the opening of Ca^{2+}-permeable channels expressed on the cell membrane) or from intracellular storages (i.e., endoplasmic reticulum or mitochondria), EGTA, a Ca^{2+} chelator, was used. Pretreatment with EGTA significantly reduces intracellular Ca^{2+} elevation induced by LS protocol, although it did not restore basal levels (P3HT–EGTA/basal: 3907 $\pm$ 194 CTCF; P3HT + EGTA/basal: 4563 $\pm$ 238 CTCF; P3HT + EGTA/induced: 8963 $\pm$ 430 CTCF; P3HT + EGTA/induced: 6183 $\pm$ 320 CTCF) as depicted in Fig. 7.

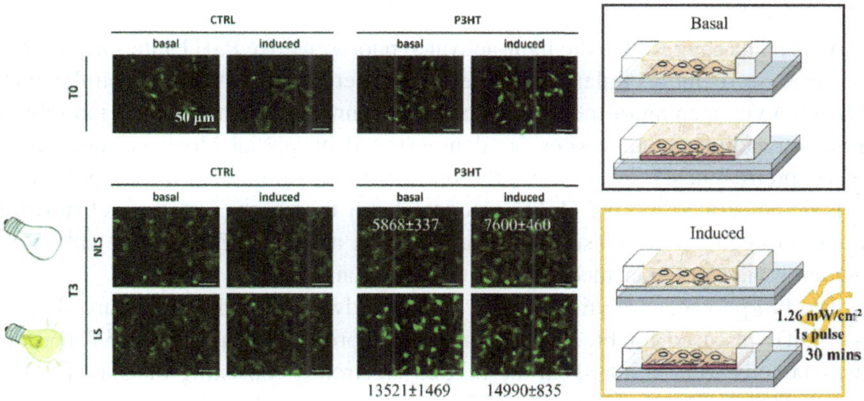

Fig. 6 Representative images of randomly selected fields of cells cultured on Glass|FTO (CTRL) and Glass|FTO|P3HT (P3HT) subjected to the LS protocol or kept in dark (NLS) analyzed at T0 (TOP) or T3 (BOTTOM). Images are acquired before (basal) and after (induced) 30 min of photostimulation (schematic on the right). Scale bar = 50 µm. Figure adapted with permission from (Ciocca et al. 2023)

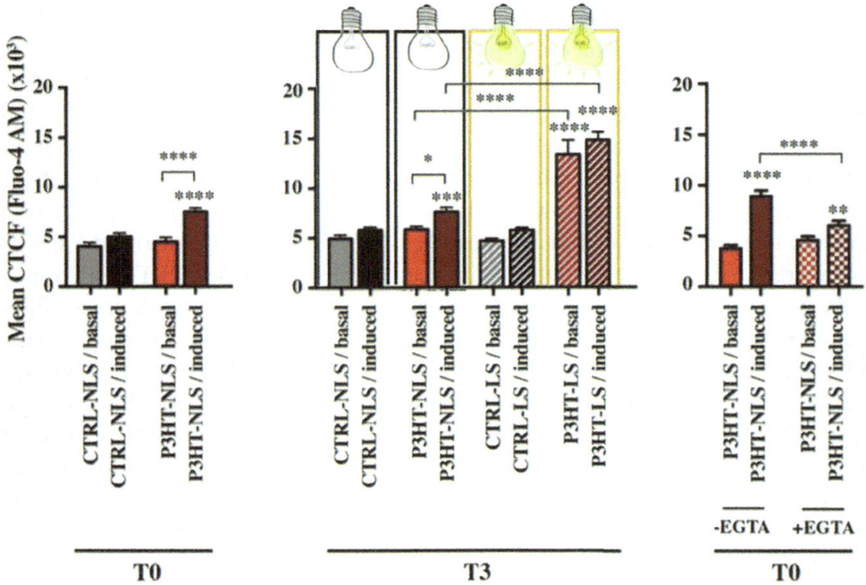

Fig. 7 The graphs report the quantification of FLUO-4 AM fluorescence in cultured cells at T0 or T3. Data are shown as mean correlated total cell fluorescence (CTCF) ± SEM. The bar chart on the right reports the quantification of FLUO-4 AM fluorescence in cells cultured on Glass|FTO|P3HT (P3HT) analyzed at T0 and pretreated without (−EGTA) and with (+EGTA) 100 μM EGTA. Data are shown as mean CTCF ± SEM of three experiments. Figure adapted with permission from (Ciocca et al. 2023)

These data suggest that the light-activated photosensitive P3HT interface induces the increase of intracellular Ca^{2+} levels (i.e., increased Fluo-4 AM cellular fluorescence) via opening of membrane calcium channels, and partially via ion release from intracellular storage sites (as demonstrated by partial blockade induced by EGTA pretreatment). In this case, the optoelectrical stimulation of neuroblastoma cells demonstrated the possibility to control cell membrane ion channel function modifying cellular response (proliferation) with a period of reversible cell cycle alteration via a polymer-mediated light stimulation of cells.

The bio-photoelectrolytic platform in its sandwich-closed architecture (Fig. 3, a—right) was used for bioelectrical signals recordings. Thus, SH-SY5Y neuroblastoma cells were cultured on the bottom electrodes consisting of Glass|FTO or Glass|FTO|P3HT and either subjected to LS protocol or kept in dark (NLS) for 3 days. At the end of culture time (T3), the open-top samples were taken from the incubator and assembled in the sandwich-closed architecture by applying the transparent platinized counter-electrode over the top. The closed-sandwich architecture was finally used to measure photogenerated voltage signals upon white light (standard cool white spectrum) pulses (300 ms) at fixed power density (15 mW/cm^2) in open-circuit condition ($I_{\text{applied}} = 0$ μA). Measurements were performed on Glass|FTO|SH-SY5Y (CTRL) samples without observing any signals. For P3HT only samples

(Glass|FTO|P3HT), the typical monotonical increase in the photo-voltage signal (V_{ph} in absolute value) upon light irradiation was observed (Fig. 8, left). Instead, recordings from P3HT/cells samples (Glass|FTO|P3HT|SH-SY5Y) showed two additional features when light was switched ON and OFF (Fig. 8, left), with a new peak arising a few ms from the time of the light being switched. The two new peaks, for P3HT/cells LS samples of $\approx$ 2 mV magnitude (Fig. 8, left), show that the impedance of the devices with cells was changed and this is a likely tell-tale signal of the depolarization–repolarization (light ON) and hyperpolarization recovery (light OFF) of the resting membrane potential in the cells. To prove that the recorded bioelectrical photo-voltage signals (obtained by using the bio-photoelectrolytic platform in its sandwich-closed architecture) are from the cells, and therefore to endorse the possibility to use the sandwich-closed bio-photoelectrolytic platform in its sandwich-closed architecture for an initial recording of bioelectrical signals, the variation of SH-SY5Y cell membrane potential was also investigated via patch-clamp recordings. Thus, whole-cell patch-clamp measurements in current clamp mode were performed (Fig. 8, right). While no variation of the cell membrane potential was observed for cells cultured on glass control (CTRL) in response to the photoexcitation, in the case of cells grown on the P3HT thin film (P3HT/cells) the illumination rapidly led to a variation in the membrane potential value in synchrony with the light stimulation pattern. Thus, an initial depolarization signal ($V_{ph,max} = 0.21 \pm 0.04$ mV) followed by a hyperpolarization peak ($V_{ph,min} = -0.99 \pm 0.05$ mV) was observed. Representative cellular responses recorded for Glass|FTO|SH-SY5Y (CTRL) samples and for Glass|FTO|P3HT|SH-SY5Y (P3HT/cells) are reported in Fig. 8, right.

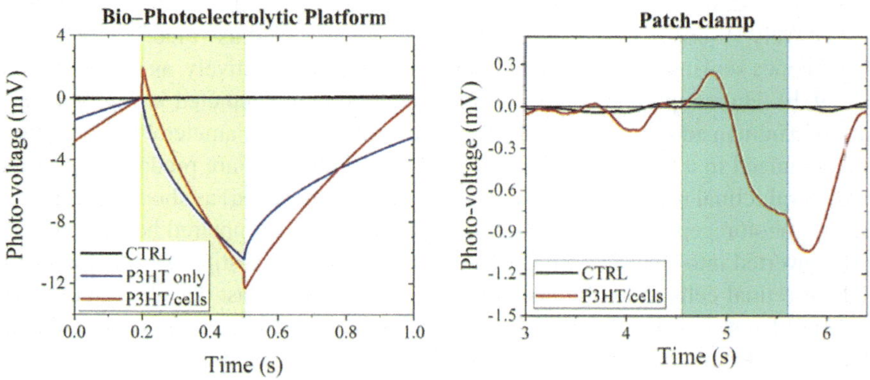

Fig. 8 Photo-voltage generated upon light irradiation at 15.0 mW/cm^2, recorded at the end of the culture period (T3) from samples (n = 3) subjected to the LS protocol via using the bio-photoelectrolytic platform (left) or the standard patch-clamp electrophysiology set-up in current clamp mode (right). The shaded areas represent the duration of the light stimulus: 300 ms and 1 s, respectively. For the patch-clamp setup, the light stimulus ($\lambda = 530$ nm) was provided by an epifluorescence system equipped with a 75 W Xenon lamp and a monochromator. Figure reproduced with permission from (Ciocca et al. 2023)

The bioelectrical photo-voltage signals recorded from P3HT/cells via the bio-photoelectrolytic platform can be described to the effect of the LS protocol on cells cultured on Glass|P3HT, which led to a significant increase of intracellular calcium level that can be due to the activation of voltage-gated calcium channels.

4 Three-Polymer Artificial Retinal Model

Another interesting example of light-sensitive (2D) bio-hybrid interface based on three different CPs and a biological medium is that of an artificial retina model described in reference (Ciocca et al. 2020). Differently from the first example in Sect. 3 where only one type of organic polymer (P3HT) is used as thin film for the bio-hybrid interface, the artificial retina model is composed of an array of 42,100 pixels made of three different CPs deposited on a transparent substrate (FTO|Glass) via inkjet printing with 110 pixels/mm^2 packing density (Ciocca et al. 2020). The three CPs pixels, disposed in a concentric annuli architecture, were conceived, and designed to mimic the spectral and spatial resolution of photoreceptors of mammalians retinas. A schematic of the retina, photoreceptors, and retina architecture is shown in Fig. 9, a and b. Photoreceptors are light-sensitive specialized neurons of the retina, the nervous tissue covering the inside-back of the eyeball. Being light-sensitive, photoreceptors convert light into electrical signals that are transmitted, traveling through the optical nerve, to the brain where they are processed, and where the vision is perceived. Human retina contains two kinds of photoreceptors, rods and cones, responsible for scotopic monochromatic and photopic trichromatic vision, respectively (S-cones, M-cones and L-cones, often labeled as "blue," "green," and "red" cones sensing short, mid and long wavelengths respectively, as represented in Fig. 9, b). Human photoreceptors absorbance spectra are depicted in Fig. 9, c. The size of a human adult retina is typically around 22.0 mm in diameter. Photoreceptors are organized in a well-defined mosaic where rod densities are predominant in the peripheral retinal region while cones in the central part (fovea) as shown in Fig. 9, d. In case photoreceptors do not function properly, vision is impaired because light is not converted into electrical triggers needed to change the resting membrane potentials of retinal cells to let the visual process begin. In the last decades, an exciting avenue of research has focused on interfacing degenerated retinas with semiconducting polymers, *in vitro* as well as *in vivo*, to elicit a response in the former upon photoexcitation of the latter through transduction of signals. In this scenario, P3HT has been the most employed CP. However, by considering the spectral responsivity of an individual CP, is not possible to provide a color sensitive artificial retinal model resembling the mammalians chromatic vision. Ciocca and co-authors proposed a color-sensitive inkjet-printed pixelated artificial retina model based on three different CPs for a spectrally sensitive retina depending locally on the absorption spectra of deposited polymer pixel (Ciocca et al. 2020). The proposed CPs were: regio-regular P3HT polymer and a blend of P3HT with [6,6]-Phenyl C61 butyric acid methyl ester (PC61BM) (P3HT:PCBM), mimicking well the green cone and rods respectively and Poly(9,9-di-n-octylfuorenyl-2,7-diyl) (PFO) to mimic S-cones. A comparison between the absorbance spectra of the chosen CPs and retinal photoreceptors is shown in Fig. 9, c. This achievement represents an important step toward a color-sensitive artificial retina realized via photosensitive bio-hybrid interfaces.

The artificial retina model is based on a bio-hybrid device architecture, as presented in Sect. 3, Fig. 3, a - right, sandwich close architecture. Thus, the developed device consists of two transparent and parallel electrodes separated by a 60 μm thick thermoplastic encapsulant (Surlyn). For the artificial retina model, spectral and spatial responsivity of the device composed of three different CPs was investigated together with the study of its biocompatibility.

Firstly, to verify the optoelectrical properties of the structure, the used working electrode (photosensitive electrode) was a 100 nm-thick P3HT thin film, spin-coated on Glass|FTO substrate. The photosensitive P3HT thin film planar electrode was interfaced with an electrolyte mediator, specifically a buffered isotonic solution (phosphate-buffered saline solution, PBS). PBS is commonly employed in biological contexts to reproduce a physiological extracellular fluid (Kaewsichan et al. 2011; Lim

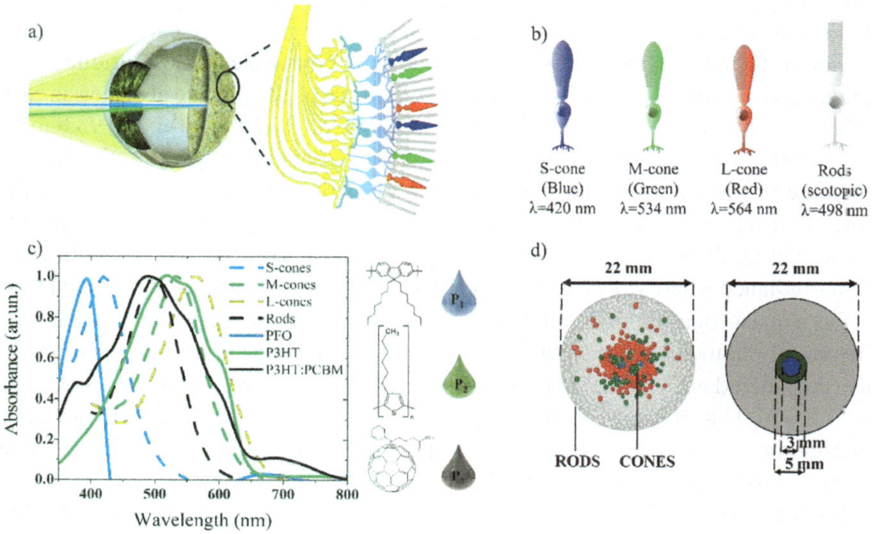

Fig. 9 **a** Representative schematics of the retina. The retina is the nervous tissues covering the inside-back of the eyeball. Retina is composed of different cells layers: photoreceptors (blue, green, and red), bipolar cells (purple), amacrine cells (turquoise) and ganglion cells (yellow). **b** Representative schematics of retinal photoreceptors, rods and cones. The human retina contains three different cones: S-cones, M-cones, and L-cones, often labeled as "blue," "green," and "red" cones sensing short, mid and long wavelengths, respectively. The maximum wavelength of the absorbance spectra for each type of photoreceptor is shown. **c** Comparison between the absorbance spectra of human photoreceptors and of the three different CPs. Chosen CPs are PFO, P3HT, and PCBM, represented as blue, green and gray drops, respectively. The chemical structure is also shown. **d** Representative schematics of the distribution of photoreceptors on a real retina and on the artificial retina design. Figure adapted with permission from (Ciocca et al. 2020)

and Sultana 2014); here it is used for mimicking eye microenvironment conditions. The top-electrode is the platinum (Pt) layer screen printed on Glass|FTO substrate and treated accordingly to guarantee high transparency (resulting transmittance of up to 79% between 400 and 700 nm) and a facile exchange of electrons/ions at the electrode/PBS interface. To gauge the effectiveness of the bio-hybrid device concept, 300 ms white light (17.8 mW/cm^2, standard cool white light spectrum) stimulus was applied to three different device architectures containing: (i) PBS, (ii) polymer, and (iii) polymer+PBS. No signals were recorded from the architectures containing only the PBS or only the polymer layer. While transient current density and voltage signals were generated upon photoexcitation for the complete device (Fig. 10, a and b). Current spikes occurring when light is turned ON or OFF are the result of a capacitive process due to electrostatic perturbation of accumulated carriers and ions with strong Coulomb interactions localized close to the polymer/PBS and PBS/Pt interfaces (e.g., Helmholtz layers). On the other hand, the steady state photocurrent after an initial spike is evidence of a Faradaic process at the electrode/PBS interface (Ciocca et al. 2020). Capacitive coupling is one of the most biologically safe mechanism used for cells and tissues electrical stimulation (Ghezzi et al. 2011). In this bio-hybrid device, the PBS solution maintains the physiological environment of biological cells and enables the movement and transport of charge carriers along the section of the device between photoelectrode and counter-electrode. Current densities at short circuit (J_{ph}) and photo-voltage at open circuit (V_{ph}) were also measured at different light power levels ranging from 17.8 mW/cm^2 ($\sim$10 $\times$ 10^3 lx) to 93.8 mW/cm^2 ($\sim$60 $\times$ 10^3 lx) representing the intensity range typically experienced in human photopic vision outdoors (Zwinkels et al. 2010) (from 10 to 100 $\times$ 10^3 lx) and the range of irradiance levels generally used for *in vitro* retinal stimulation experiments (Ciocca et al. 2020). Currents, $J_{ph,max}$ (J_{ph} first peaks, Fig. 10, c) increase linearly with irradiance whereas $V_{ph,max}$ (measured after 300 ms from the light switched ON) shows a quasi-logarithmic trend (Fig. 10, d). The total charge (calculated as the time integral of photocurrent) generated by the bio-hybrid device upon illumination was also considered and calculated to be 106.4 $\pm$ 23.7 nC/cm^2 and 331.9 $\pm$ 42.8 nC/cm^2 at 17.8 and 93.8 mW/cm^2 respectively (Fig. 10, e). Thus, the bio-hybrid device is appropriate to be used for neural stimulation since usually employed devices generate a charge level in the range of few nC/cm^2.

After the bio-hybrid device opto-electronic characterization, the biocompatibility of the identified CPs was assessed. Thus, human neuroblastoma cells SH-SY5Y were seeded on a P3HT, P3HT:PCBM and PFO layers and grown for up to 3 days. Cell death percentage analyzed at T0 (16 hours after cell seeding on the polymer thin films) and T3 (after 3 days of culture at 37 °C, 5% CO_2 in 95% humidified incubator) by the *in situ* Cell Viability Imaging assay was very low. No differences were found between the control (CTRL, cells grown on tissue culture tested polystyrene dishes) and P3HT, P3HT:PCBM and PFO. These results indicated no toxicity of all the polymers utilized (Fig. 11).

Once the biocompatibility of the identified CPs was assessed, a simplified model of the pixelated artificial retina system based on the resulting anatomical map of the

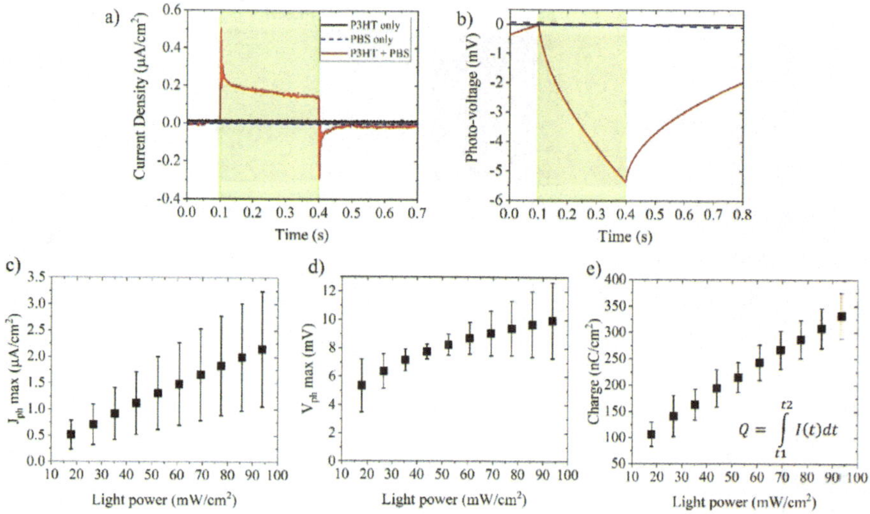

Fig. 10 Transient current density **a** and transient photo-voltage **b** signals recorded from the bio-hybrid device under 300 ms white light (17.8 mW/cm^2) stimulus. The shaded yellow areas represent the duration of the light stimulus (300 ms). **c** Current capacitive peaks (J_{ph} max referred to the J_{ph} first peaks) show a linear dependence with the light power intensity. J_{ph} values are the mean on samples $n = 3$. Y-error bar is also shown. **d** Photo-voltage as function of increasing light intensities. V_{ph} max values (in absolute value) are referred to the value reached after 300 ms from the light switched ON. Radiant intensities used for J_{ph} and V_{ph}: 17.8, 26.6, 35.3, 43.9, 52.4, 60.9, 69.3, 77.4, 85.7, and 93.8 mW/cm^2. **e** Photo-generated charge calculated from the time integral of the photocurrent response curves as a function of increasing light power for 300 ms light pulse duration. Samples $n = 3$. Y-error bar referred to the standard deviation (SD) are shown. Figure reproduced with permission from (Ciocca et al. 2020)

photoreceptors mosaic was designed (Fig. 9, d). The model consists in a concentric ring design where each annulus represents a different retinal photoreceptor region. Thus, different polymer semiconductors with specific absorbance spectra were displaced in concentric annuli via inkjet printing, on Glass|FTO substrates. Therefore, a pixelated retina system based on M-cones (P3HT), S-cones (PFO) and rods (P3HT:PCBM) was printed, providing a dichromatic inkjet-printed artificial retina model. The three-polymer bio-hybrid printed device mimics the dichromatic vision of most mammalian retinas, including rodents, and often used in biomedical studies (Ciocca et al. 2020). The outermost annulus of 360.5 mm^2 corresponds to rods (P3HT:PCBM), while the two central annuli correspond to the M-cones (P3HT) of 12.6 mm^2 and the S-cones (PFO) of 7.1 mm^2 areas, respectively. Total diameter was 22.0 mm. PFO, P3HT and P3HT:PCBM inks were obtained via a specific formulation mixing chlorobenzene (CB) and tetrahydronaphthalene (THN) (1:1) solvents. CB was used to achieve homogeneous film formation, owing to excellent solubility of the chosen polymers in CB. THN was used to prevent nozzle clogging and to provide reliable jetting over time. Inkjet parameters (pulse voltages, cartridge temperature, substrate temperature, drop spacing, waveform) were carefully adjusted in order to

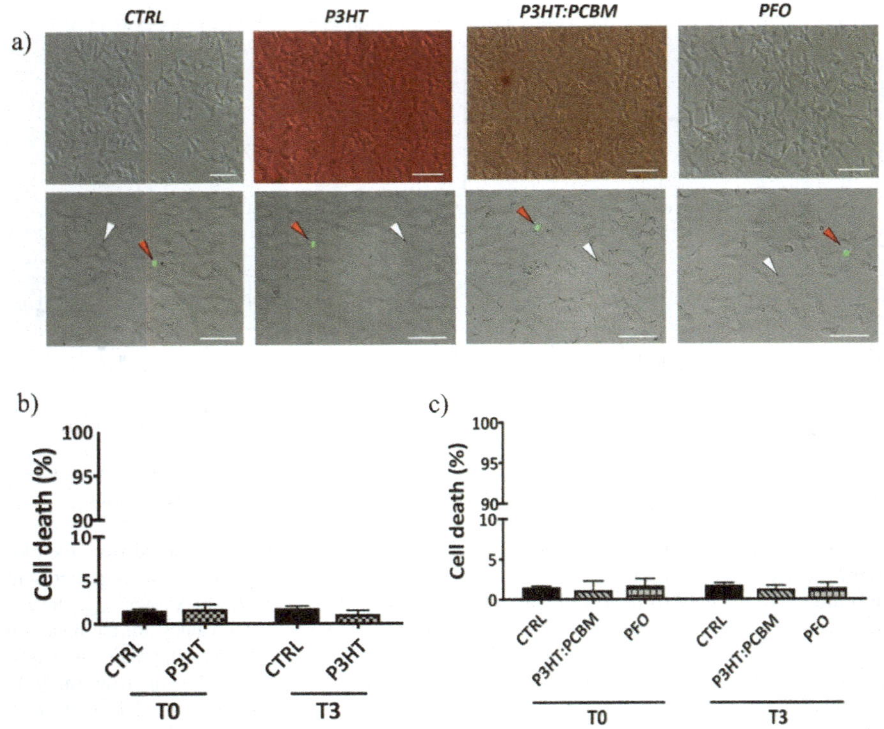

Fig. 11 **a** Representative phase contrast micrographs (top) and phase contrast/fluorescent micrographs (bottom) of SH-SY5Y cells cultured on standard polystyrene dish (CTRL), Glass|FTO|P3HT substrate (P3HT), Glass|FTO|P3HT:PCBM substrate (P3HT:PCBM), and Glass|FTO|PFO substrate (PFO) for 3 days. In the bottom panels, samples were analyzed via the in situ Cell Viability Imaging assay at the end of the culture time (T3). White and red arrowheads indicate live and dead (green) cells, respectively. Scale bar = 50 μm. **b, c** Bar plots representing the quantification of cell death measured by in situ Cell Viability Imaging assay, expressed as percentage of dead (green) cells on the total number of cells analyzed at the beginning (T0) and at the end (T3) of culture (Image J software 1.49 V was used) for P3HT, and for P3HT:PCBM and PFO, respectively. Figure adapted with permission from (Ciocca et al. 2020)

obtain stable droplet formation and to achieve rounded-pixels layout. The inkjet-printed device consisted of ~42,100 pixels over the total area of 380.1 mm^2. Optical microscope images showing the concentric layout of arrays of small round polymer pixels with an average diameter size of 95 ± 5 μm and of 50 to 60 nm thickness as measured by atomic force microscopy (AFM) and a packing density of ~110 pixels/mm^2 are shown in Fig. 12.

At this point, the spatial resolution of the photo-responses of the inkjet-printed artificial retina was investigated. The measured photocurrent (I_{ph}) as a function of wavelength of the light source is shown in Fig. 13 with the same measurements carried out on each of the single polymer (or blend) annulus of the printed artificial retina. Customized shadow masks were used to exclusively illuminate the polymer

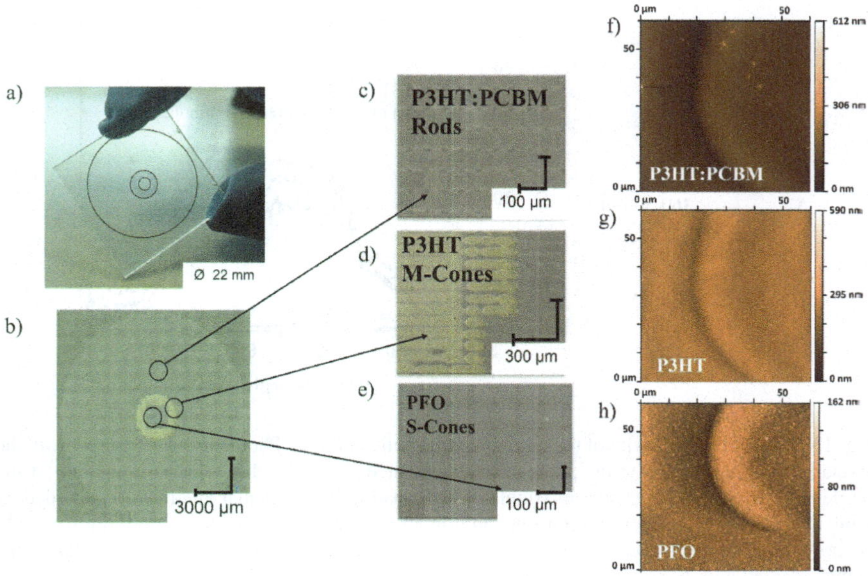

Fig. 12 Inkjet-printed artificial retina device prototype and related optical microscopy analysis. **a** Device picture and **b** optical microscopy image of polymer inkjet-printed artificial retina showing, **c–e** different regions of the concentrically organized polymer pixels. **f–h** AFM images of photosensitive round polymer pixels. AFM analysis allowed thickness and roughness measurements of the pixels. Figure reproduced with permission from (Ciocca et al. 2020)

annulus of interest. Notwithstanding the geometrical domination of the P3HT:PCBM component (PFO 2.0%, P3HT 3.3%, P3HT:PCBM 94.7% of total inkjet-printed artificial retina area), each pixelated polymer annulus contributes to the overall I_{ph} signal.

5 Conclusions

Light control and modulation of biological system is arising as a promising tool for bioelectronics. Among the possible options, exogenous light stimulation approaches are very promising. Thus, via employing photosensitive bio-hybrid interfaces, 0D, 1D, 2D, or 3D, it is possible to successfully stimulate cells and tissues with light, as well as to specifically control the cellular biotic and bioelectrical activity. Moreover, light stimulation of interfaces between photosensitive components (mainly semiconducting polymers) and biological systems allows avoiding or reducing harmful invasiveness of alternatives probes or stimuli.

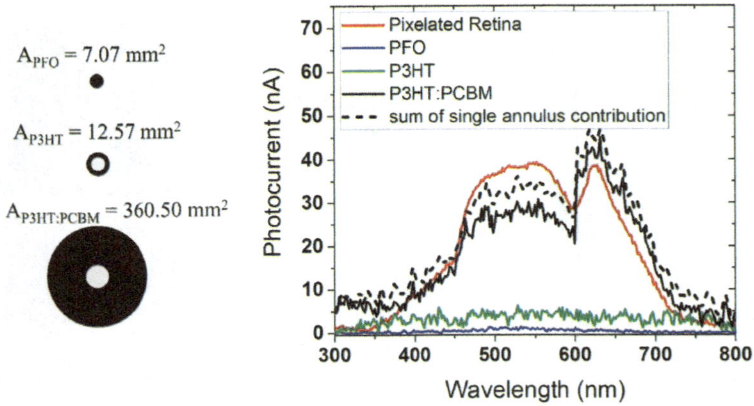

Fig. 13 Spectral responsivity of the inkjet-printed artificial retina. Photocurrent measured from the pixelated retina compared to the photocurrent calculated as the weighted linear summation of the single polymer-annuli contributions (right). I_{ph} originating from singular annuli were recorded by using a monochromator/lock-in set up and additional customized shadow masks to illuminate only the polymer annulus of interest (left) by covering the remaining part of the printed artificial retina. Figure adapted with permission from (Ciocca et al. 2020)

In this chapter, an overview about the possibility to use light as a tool for living cells control is given. Two different examples, based on the optoelectrical and biocompatible features of semiconducting polymers taken from recent advancements in the field, are described in detail.

A photosensitive bio-hybrid interface was used as building block for the realization of a bio-photoelectrolytic platform for light control of cell growth and for bioelectrical recordings (Ciocca et al. 2023). Proliferation of neuroblastoma cells cultured on P3HT and subjected to a specific light stimulation protocol was inhibited by roughly 50% compared with the cells cultured in dark. Interestingly, cell proliferation normally resumed 24 hours after the light protocol was suspended, indicating that the light protocol had resulted in a reversible alteration of the cell cycle. Moreover, cells cultured on P3HT and subjected to the light stimulation protocol showed a significant increase in the intracellular Ca^{2+} concentration both at the beginning (after 30 min illumination) and, more consistently, at the end of the 3-day culture period. Based on these results, the plausible hypothesis is that the bio-photoelectrolytic platform and the light stimulation protocol altered the electric/ionic microenvironment of neuroblastoma cells cultured on P3HT, due to the optoelectrical properties of the semiconducting polymer. This alteration was able to affect the functionality of the voltage-gated ion channels present on the surface of SH-SY5Y in contact with the polymer film by inducing the opening of cell membrane ion channels. The bio-photoelectrolytic platform in its sandwich-closed architecture allowed the optoelectrical recordings of these cell membrane potential alterations due to ionic channels opening. In fact, bioelectrical signals recorded from P3HT/cell samples showed transient membrane potential peaks at the light ON and OFF lasting few milliseconds, very similar to photo-responses obtained via standard patch-clamp recordings. As future perspectives, the platform can be considered as a tool for studies on *in vitro* photomanipulation of cell processes, retinal cells, and neural circuit. Furthermore, since through the optoelectrical stimulation of neuroblastoma cells by using the bio-photoelectrolytic platform was possible to inhibit cell proliferation in a cancer cell line, this approach paves the way for new tools in tumor progression control, possibly improving cancer therapy approaches such as photodynamic therapy.

The second example presented focused on the realization of a conjugated polymer-based bio-hybrid artificial retina model aiming to mimic the color response of mammalian cones and rods (Ciocca et al. 2020). The bio-hybrid artificial retina device optoelectrical and biocompatible features were demonstrated. Finally, the artificial retina was fabricated via inkjet printing technique. The inkjet-printed color-sensitive artificial retina consists of three different types of semiconducting round polymer pixels, with distinct absorption spectra, mimicking the chromatic sensitivity of photoreceptors. The number of pixels was 42.100, the density of the artificial photoreceptors was $\sim$11,000 pixels/cm^2 and the corresponding spatial resolution was 267 dpi (dots per inch), with pixel diameters of 95 $\pm$ 5 μm. The realization of such a bio-hybrid device represents an important step toward the construction of a desirable color-sensitive artificial retina to be used for alleviating the symptoms of patients with photoreceptors degenerative diseases.

Acknowledgments We acknowledge Lazio Region through the SIROH project "Sight Restoration via Organic and Hybrid thin films" (Progetto di Gruppo di Ricerca finanziato ai sensi della L.R. Lazio 13/08 n. 85-2017-15373), Air Force Office of Scientific Research's Biophysics program through award number FA9550-20-1-0157 for funding. We also thank the co-authors of references (Ciocca et al. 2023) and (Ciocca et al. 2020) from which contents and figures have been used in this chapter for Sects. 3 and 4, respectively, i,e., Serena Marcozzi, Paolo Mariani, Valentina Lacconi, Aldo Di Carlo, Lucio Cinà, Marcelo D. Rosato-Siri, Alessandra Zanon, Giada Cattelan, Enrico Avancini, Shashank Priya, Pavlos Giannakou, Mehmet O.Tas, Hiroki Asari, Maxim Shkunov.

References

M.J.I. Airaghi Leccardi, N.A.L. Chenais, L. Ferlauto, M. Kawecki, E.G. Zollinger, D. Ghezzi, Photovoltaic organic interface for neuronal stimulation in the near-infrared. Commun. Mater. **1**, 21 (2020)

C. Allarà, A. Orlando, G. Ciccone, S. Krik, M. Pompilio, A. Pedrielli, A. Gaiardo, P. Lugli, L. Petti, F. Cacialli, M. Ciocca, Conjugated polymer nanoparticles for biophotonic applications: preparation, characterization, and simulation in biohybrid interfaces. Adv. Electron. Mater. (2025)

M.R. Antognazza, I. Abdel Aziz, F. Lodola, Use of exogenous and endogenous Photomediators as efficient ROS modulation tools: results and perspectives for therapeutic purposes. Oxidative Med. Cell. Longev. **2019**, 1–14 (2019)

M.R. Antognazza, N. Martino, D. Ghezzi, P. Feyen, E. Colombo, D. Endeman, F. Benfenati, G. Lanzani, Shedding light on living cells. Adv. Mater. **27**, 7662–7669 (2015)

A. Arvanitaki, N. Chalazonitis, Electrical properties and temporal organization in oscillatory neurons, in *Neurobiology of Invertebrates*, (Springer US, Boston, MA, 1968), pp. 169–199

H. Bahmani Jalali, O. Karatum, R. Melikov, U.M. Dikbas, S. Sadeghi, E. Yildiz, I.B. Dogru, G. Ozgun Eren, C. Ergun, A. Sahin, I.H. Kavakli, S. Nizamoglu, Biocompatible quantum funnels for neural Photostimulation. Nano Lett. **19**, 5975–5981 (2019)

V. Benfenati, N. Martino, M.R. Antognazza, A. Pistone, S. Toffanin, S. Ferroni, G. Lanzani, M. Muccini, Photostimulation of whole-cell conductance in primary rat neocortical astrocytes mediated by organic semiconducting thin films. Adv. Healthc. Mater. **3**, 392–399 (2014)

M. Berggren, A. Richter-Dahlfors, Organic bioelectronics. Adv. Mater. **19**, 3201–3213 (2007)

J.L. Brédas, J.P. Calbert, D.A. da Silva Filho, J. Cornil, Organic semiconductors: a theoretical characterization of the basic parameters governing charge transport. Proc. Natl. Acad. Sci. **99**, 5804–5809 (2002)

M. Ciocca, C. Febo, G. Gentile, A. Orlando, F. Massoumi, A. Altana, G. Cantarella, A. Zanon, A. Gaiardo, P. Lugli, L. Petti, 3D-bioprinted light-sensitive cell scaffold based on alginate-conjugated polymer nanoparticles for biophotonics applications. BioNanoScience **15**, 251 (2025a)

Ciocca, M., Febo, C., Massoumi, F., Altana, A., Cantarella, G., Lugli, P., Petti, L., 2022. 3D bio-printed light-sensitive cell scaffolds based on polymer nanoparticles for bio-photonics applications, in *2022 IEEE International Flexible Electronics Technology Conference (IFETC)*. IEEE, pp. 1–2

M. Ciocca, P. Giannakou, P. Mariani, L. Cinà, A. Di Carlo, M.O. Tas, H. Asari, S. Marcozzi, A. Camaioni, M. Shkunov, T.M. Brown, Colour-sensitive conjugated polymer inkjet-printed pixelated artificial retina model studied via a bio-hybrid photovoltaic device. Sci. Rep. **10** (2020)

M. Ciocca, S. Krik, M. Pompilio, J.S. Gharehbagh, L. Petti, F. Cacialli, Conjugated polymer nanoparticles for multifunctional bioelectronics and sensing P3ht:Pcbm-Nps embedded in Peo hydrogel, in *2025 IEEE International Conference on Flexible and Printable Sensors and Systems (FLEPS). IEEE*, (2025b), pp. 1–4

M. Ciocca, S. Marcozzi, P. Mariani, V. Lacconi, A. Di Carlo, L. Cinà, M.D. Rosato-Siri, A. Zanon, G. Cattelan, E. Avancini, P. Lugli, S. Priya, A. Camaioni, T.M. Brown, A polymer bio–photo-electrolytic platform for electrical signal measurement and for light modulation of ion fluxes and proliferation in a neuroblastoma cell line. Adv. Nanobiomed. Res., 3 (2023)

S. Corsetti, K. Dholakia, Optical manipulation: advances for biophotonics in the 21st century. J. Biomed. Opt. **26** (2021)

K. Deisseroth, Optogenetics: 10 years of microbial opsins in neuroscience. Nat. Neurosci. **18**, 1213–1225 (2015)

R.L. Fork, Laser stimulation of nerve cells in *Aplysia*. Science **1979**(171), 907–908 (1971)

L. Galvani, De Viribus Electricitatis In Motu Musculari Commentarius. Apud Societatem typographicam (1792)

G. Gentile, M. Ravandeh, L. Petti, F. D'Elia, F. Santoro, *Multimodal platforms for light-mediated organic bioelectronics* (Adv. Mater. Interfaces, 2025)

D. Ghezzi, M.R. Antognazza, M. Dal Maschio, E. Lanzarini, F. Benfenati, G. Lanzani, A hybrid bioorganic interface for neuronal photoactivation. Nat. Commun. **2**, 166 (2011)

D.P. Hagberg, T. Marinado, K.M. Karlsson, K. Nonomura, P. Qin, G. Boschloo, T. Brinck, A. Hagfeldt, L. Sun, Tuning the HOMO and LUMO energy levels of organic chromophores for dye sensitized solar cells. J. Org. Chem. **72**, 9550–9556 (2007)

M. Han, H. Bahmani Jalali, E. Yildiz, M.H. Qureshi, A. Şahin, S. Nizamoglu, Photovoltaic neurointerface based on aluminum antimonide nanocrystals. Commun. Mater. **2**, 19 (2021)

W. Hu, Y. Zhang, B. Li, Q. Li, K. Ma, C. Zhang, X. Fu, Manipulation of living cells with 450 nm laser photobiomodulation. J. Photochem. Photobiol. B **209**, 111896 (2020)

S. Iwanaga, N. Smith, K. Fujita, S. Kawata, O. Nakamura, Single-pulse cell stimulation with a near-infrared picosecond laser. Appl. Phys. Lett. **87**, 243901 (2005)

E. Joseph, M. Ciocca, H. Wu, S. Marcozzi, M.A. Ucci, K. Keremane, L. Zheng, B. Poudel, C. Wu, A. Camaioni, K. Wang, S. Priya, T.M. Brown, Photovoltaic bioelectronics merging biology with new generation semiconductors and light in biophotovoltaics photobiomodulation and biosensing. npj Biosensing **1**, 15 (2024)

L. Kaewsichan, D. Riyapan, P. Prommajan, J. Kaewsrichan. ScienceAsia **37**, 240 (2011)

O. Karatum, M.M. Aria, G.O. Eren, E. Yildiz, R. Melikov, S.B. Srivastava, S. Surme, I.B. Dogru, H. Bahmani Jalali, B. Ulgut, A. Sahin, I.H. Kavakli, S. Nizamoglu, Nanoengineering InP quantum dot-based photoactive biointerfaces for optical control of neurons. Front. Neurosci. **15** (2021)

M.M. Lim, N. Sultana, Drug loading, drug release and in vitro degradation of poly(caprolactone) electrospun fibers, in *2014 IEEE Conference on Biomedical Engineering and Sciences (IECBES). IEEE*, (2014), pp. 356–359

S. Meng, M. Rouabhia, Z. Zhang, Electrical stimulation and cellular behaviors in electric field in biomedical research. Materials **15**, 165 (2021)

F. Milos, G. Tullii, F. Gobbo, F. Lodola, F. Galeotti, C. Verpelli, D. Mayer, V. Maybeck, A. Offenhäusser, M.R. Antognazza, High aspect ratio and light-sensitive micropillars based on a semiconducting polymer optically regulate neuronal growth. ACS Appl. Mater. Interfaces **13**, 23438–23451 (2021)

G. Mincuzzi, A.L. Palma, A. Di Carlo, T.M. Brown, Laser processing in the manufacture of dye-sensitized and perovskite solar cell technologies. ChemElectroChem **3**, 9–30 (2016)

A. Moliton, R.C. Hiorns, Review of electronic and optical properties of semiconductingπ-conjugated polymers: applications in optoelectronics. Polym. Int. **53**, 1397–1412 (2004)

S. Negri, P. Faris, G. Tullii, M. Vismara, A.F. Pellegata, F. Lodola, G. Guidetti, V. Rosti, M.R. Antognazza, F. Moccia, Conjugated polymers mediate intracellular Ca2+ signals in circulating endothelial colony forming cells through the reactive oxygen species-dependent activation of transient receptor potential Vanilloid 1 (TRPV1). Cell Calcium **101**, 102502 (2022)

Y. Park, S.-Y. Park, K. Eom, Current review of optical neural interfaces for clinical applications. Micromachines (Basel) **12**, 925 (2021)

H. Peng, X. Sun, W. Weng, X. Fang, Energy harvesting based on polymer, in *Polymer Materials for Energy and Electronic Applications*, (Elsevier, 2017), pp. 151–196

G. Pezzotti, Raman spectroscopy in cell biology and microbiology. J. Raman Spectrosc. **52**, 2348–2443 (2021)

S. Reif-Acherman, Jacques arsene d'arsonval: His life and contributions to electrical instrumentation in physics and medicine. Part ii: communications equipment and electrical measuring instruments [scanning our past]. Proc. IEEE **105**, 167–175 (2017)

M.Y. Rotenberg, B. Elbaz, V. Nair, E.N. Schaumann, N. Yamamoto, N. Sarma, L. Matino, F. Santoro, B. Tian, Silicon nanowires for intracellular optical interrogation with subcellular resolution. Nano Lett. **20**, 1226–1232 (2020)

M.G. Shapiro, K. Homma, S. Villarreal, C.-P. Richter, F. Bezanilla, Infrared light excites cells by changing their electrical capacitance. Nat. Commun. **3**, 736 (2012)

N.I. Smith, S. Iwanaga, T. Beppu, K. Fujita, O. Nakamura, S. Kawata, Photostimulation of two types of ca^{2+} waves in rat pheochromocytoma PC12 cells by ultrashort pulsed near-infrared laser irradiation. Laser Phys. Lett. **3**, 154–161 (2006)

I. Tochitsky, A. Polosukhina, V.E. Degtyar, N. Gallerani, C.M. Smith, A. Friedman, R.N. Van Gelder, D. Trauner, D. Kaufer, R.H. Kramer, Restoring visual function to blind mice with a Photoswitch that exploits electrophysiological remodeling of retinal ganglion cells. Neuron **81**, 800–813 (2014)

L. Vesce, A. Guidobaldi, P. Mariani, A. DI Carlo, M.L. Parisi, S. Maranghi, R. Basosi, *Scaling-Up of Dye Sensitized Solar Modules* (2019), pp. 423–485

M. Walling, J. Novak, J.R.E. Shepard, Quantum dots for live cell and in vivo imaging. Int. J. Mol. Sci. **10**, 441–491 (2009)

J. Xie, C. Zhao, Z. Lin, P. Gu, Q. Zhang, Nanostructured conjugated polymers for energy-related applications beyond solar cells. Chem. Asian J. **11**, 1489–1511 (2016)

H.K.S. Yadav, A. Raizaday, Inorganic nanobiomaterials for medical imaging, in *Nanobiomaterials in Medical Imaging*, (Elsevier, 2016), pp. 365–401

K. Yang, J.Y. Oh, J.S. Lee, Y. Jin, G.-E. Chang, S.S. Chae, E. Cheong, H.K. Baik, S.-W. Cho, Photoactive poly(3-hexylthiophene) Nanoweb for Optoelectrical stimulation to enhance neurogenesis of human stem cells. Theranostics **7**, 4591–4604 (2017)

J.C. Zwinkels, E. Ikonen, N.P. Fox, G. Ulm, M.L. Rastello, Photometry, radiometry and 'the candela': evolution in the classical and quantum world. Metrologia **47**, R15–R32 (2010)

Nanocarriers Immobilized Enzymes and Their Potential Industrial Applications

Madan L. Verma, Irfan Ahmad, John Jeslin, Sarita Devi, and Asim K. Jana

Abstract The impact of nanotechnology is evident in modern everyday life, ranging from biomedical applications to the agriculture sector. Nanotechnology involves the manufacturing of nanomaterials through various routes, including physico-chemical and biological methods. However, biological routes, also known as green routes, for nanomaterial synthesis offer a competitive edge over other contemporary physico-chemical routes due to their non-hazardous, environmentally benign, cost-effective, and safe biogenic process. The interaction between nanotechnology and living systems, specifically in the form of nanomaterial-immobilized enzymes, is discussed herein, emphasizing potential uses in industrial settings. Among the various applications of nanocarrier-bound enzymes, this chapter delves into the different kinds of nanomaterials and their characteristics employed for bioenergy production, particularly in the stabilization of bioenergy-producing enzymes involved in cellulose hydrolysis, such as cellulases, cellobiases, or β-1,4-glucosidases. Each nanomaterial-immobilized enzyme preparation is critically evaluated in terms of its biocatalytic potential. A comparison of nanomaterial-immobilized enzymes with their original form is made to assess their application in industries. Recent progress in the co-immobilization of cellulose-degrading biocatalytic proteins using nanocarriers are also discussed.

M. L. Verma (✉)
Department of Biotechnology, School of Basic Sciences, Indian Institute of Information Technology Una, Una, Himachal Pradesh, India
e-mail: madanverma@gmail.com; madanverma@iiitu.ac.in

I. Ahmad
Department of Plant Sciences, Akhibhagya PG College Ranapar, Gorakhpur, India

J. Jeslin
Department of Biotechnology, St. Joseph College of Engineering, Sholinganallur, Chennai, India

S. Devi
Biotechnology Division, CSIR-Institute of Himalayan Bioresource Technology, Palampur, Himachal Pradesh, India

A. K. Jana
Department of Biotechnology, Dr B R Ambedkar National Institute of Technology, Jalandhar, India

R. Narayan (ed.), *Nanostructured Biomaterials and Their Applications*,
https://doi.org/10.1007/978-3-032-16316-5_15

Keywords Biogenic · Nanoparticles · Enzymes · Immobilization · Cellulases · Biofuels

1 Introduction

In nanobiotechnology, nanomaterials are synthesized with dimensions ranging from 1–100 nm (Chandel et al. 2024; Verma et al. 2024). The applications of these nanomaterials are manifested in every sector, ranging from health to agriculture. Nanomaterials (NMs) are synthesized using various physico-chemical and biological methods (Verma et al. 2023a, b; Dhanya et al. 2020; Asmathunisha and Karthiresan, Asmathunisha and Kathiresan 2013). However, biological methods for nanomaterial synthesis offer competitive advantages over other contemporary methods due to their adherence to green chemistry principles (Paul et al. 2021). The biological method of nanomaterial production, known as green nanotechnology, involves various microorganisms, plants, and their parts or extracts (Fig. 1). Biological methods for the eco-friendly synthesis of nanomaterials hold tremendous potential, as they provide non-toxic, environmentally sustainable, economically viable, and safe biogenic methods. It is well known that conventional physico-chemical approaches to producing nanomaterials may require a significant amount of money, unproductive materials, and energy, potentially leading to the production of toxic chemicals. In contrast, bio-based techniques for producing nanomaterials involve the reduction/oxidation of metals, catalyzed by different enzymes provided by various organisms (Thakur et al. 2020; Verma et al. 2020a, 2020b; Das et al. 2012a, 2012b).

The distinctive properties of nanoparticles (NPs), combined with their biocompatibility, have led scientists to explore microbial-based approaches for nanoparticle production, utilizing organisms like bacteria, fungi, algae, and plants (Chandel et al. 2024; Dhanya et al. 2020; Elgorban et al. 2016; Ebrahiminezhad et al. 2016; Vago et al. 2015). Nanoparticles have distinct physico-chemical properties, such as well-defined dimensions, high surface area-to-volume ratio, enhanced chemical stability, and elevated reactivity, as well as a functionalized structure with desired biocompatibility (Arora et al. 2020; Kong et al. 2017; Neveen-Mohamed, Neveen-Mohamed 2014). Biogenic nanoparticles have gained attention due to their simplicity, ease of surface modification, and numerous applications, including data storage, antimicrobial agents, sensing, sustainable agriculture, environmental remediation, and biotechnology, particularly as nanocarriers for enzyme immobilization and drug delivery (Dhanya et al. 2020; Golchin et al. 2018; Verma 2018; Verma et al. 2016; Dykman and Khlebtsov 2017; Verma 2017a; b; c; Verma and Barrow 2015; Kumar et al. 2014; Verma et al. 2013a; b; c; d; Verma et al. 2012). Biogenic nanoparticles have tremendous potential for effectively delivering of a range of bioactive molecules, such as pharmaceuticals, proteins, vaccines, or oligonucleotides, to their targeted locations.

Recently, biofuels have garnered considerable attention due to the escalating consumption of non-renewable fossil reserves. The rapid consumption of fossil fuels

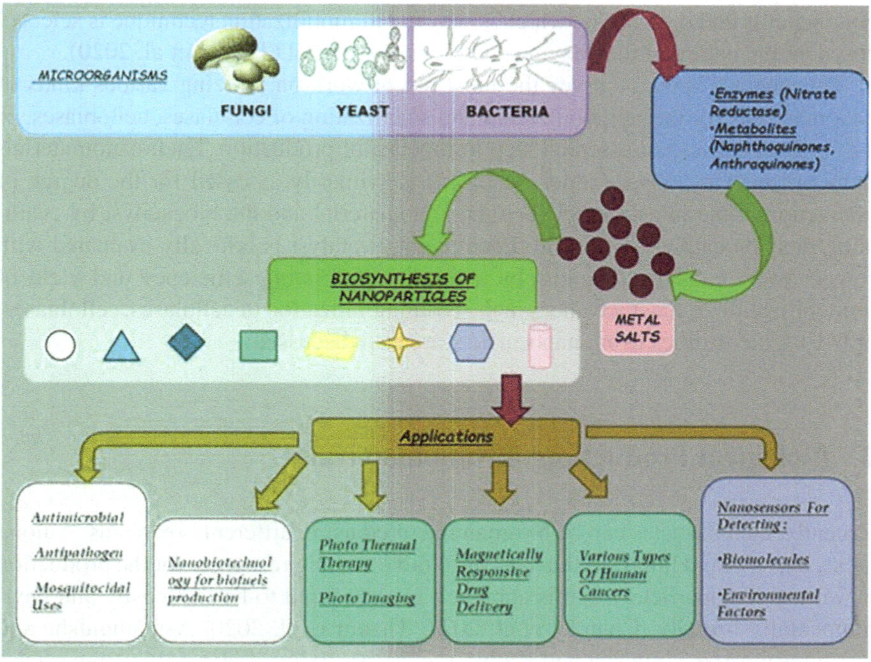

Fig. 1 Biogenic production of nanoparticles with potential biotechnological applications

has raised several concerns, including energy security, dwindling resources, escalating costs, and global warming (Thakur et al. 2020; Chandel et al. 2018; Abraham et al. 2014; Puri et al. 2013). Alternative renewable energy sources can serve as a renewable substitute for fossil fuels, as they rely on the accessibility of abundant cellulosic biomass and waste oils, making them a sustainable biofuel option. Among various enzymes, such as lipases and cellulases, cellulases play a crucial role in cellulosic biofuel production. Cellulase is a collection of hydrolytic enzymes that break down cellulosic materials into glucose through hydrolysis, specifically targeting β-1,4 bonds. Cellulose is present in the metabolic pathways of various microorganisms and can be converted into different products. The three primary enzymes responsible for catalyzing the biotransformation of cellulose to glucose are endoglucanases, exoglucanases/cellobiohydrolases, and β-glucosidase (Beguin and Aubert 1994). In nature, various types of cellulosic enzymes exhibit a wide distribution across species, acting on different celluloses (Kumar et al. 2021; Martinez et al. 2008).

The immobilization techniques play an important role in developing stable and recyclable nanobiosystems (Chandel et al. 2024; Arora et al. 2020; Verma et al. 2024; Puri et al. 2013; Verma et al. 2011; Kanwar et al. 2008; Verma et al. 2008; Kanwar et al. 2005). This is made possible by the distinctive features of enzyme-nanomaterial hybrids. The nano-immobilization technique can be achieved through physical absorption, covalent binding, or a combination of both. This technique has both benefits and drawbacks, which is why the immobilization technique is selected based on the nature of the enzyme and the nanomaterial (Thakur et al. 2020).

This chapter aims to survey the most recent work on utilizing various kinds of nanomaterials for the immobilization and stabilization of cellulases, cellobiases, or β-1,4-glucosidases, an essential step in bioethanol production. Each nanomaterial-immobilized biocatalyst (nanobiocatalyst) is primarily assessed for the degree of interaction at the interface between the nanomaterial and the biocatalyst by evaluating their biocatalytic potential. Each nanobiocatalyst is critically evaluated with respect to its catalytic potential by assessing the binding efficiency and yield of immobilization. Recent advances in the co-immobilization of cellulases, cellobiases, or β-1,4-glucosidases using nanocarriers are also discussed.

2 Biological Production of Nanomaterials

Recently, nanoparticles can be bio-manufactured using different organisms. Among these, bacteria and fungi are the most preferable starting resources for the production of various nanoparticles, as this approach is considered to be less costly and environmentally friendly (Chandel et al. 2024; Thakur et al. 2020; Asmathunisha and Karthiresan, Asmathunisha and Kathiresan 2013). Extracellular gold nanoparticles are produced through the reduction of Au^{3+} ions, which is facilitated by proteins present in the cell wall and cytoplasmic regions of fungi (Das et al. 2012a). The reduction of Au^{3+} to Au^0 is attributed to the electron-dense particles present in the intracellular and cell wall areas (Das et al. 2012b; Zhang et al., Zhang et al. 2011, Zhang et al. 2016). The two key starting materials used are $HAuCl_4$ and AuCl, which dissociate into Au^{3+} and Au + ions (Khan et al. 2013), respectively. However, it remains unclear whether Au^{3+} ions diffuse through the membrane via active biological uptake or passive adsorption. The toxicity of Au^{3+} ions may contribute to this diffusion by altering the membrane's permeability. Mukherjee et al. (2002) reported the involvement of NADPH-dependent reductases in the reduction process while working on the production of gold nanoparticles, using a soluble protein extract of the fungus *Fusarium Oxysporum.* Gupta and Bector (2013) reported that the reduction mechanism involving enzymes is the same for both intracellular and extracellular gold nanoparticles.

The fungus *Candida Albicans* produces chelatins, oligopeptide chains composed of cysteine, glycine, and glutathione, which are necessary for the production of gold nanoparticles (AuNPs). In pathogenic fungi, chelatins are synthesized via a transpeptidation reaction involving glutathione-derived dipeptides. Since small nanoparticles are unstable, extracellular enzymes can be utilized as capping agents by microorganisms to stabilize them and reduce aggregation. Zhang et al. (2011) reported that *Fusarium Oxysporum* has three capping agents: glyceraldehyde-3-phosphate dehydrogenase, 3-glucan binding protein, and ATPase. Microbes secrete various biomolecules that facilitate the homogeneous preparation of nanoparticles. Amino acids, such as L-histidine, can be utilized for nanoparticle synthesis. Maruyama and co-workers (Maruyama et al. 2015) employed L-histidine to reduce $AuCl_4$ to AuNPs. They further reported that particle size and aggregate size of nanoparticles were affected by the concentration of L-histidine. Additionally, the presence of amino and carboxylate groups in amino acids facilitates $AuCl_4$ reduction and nanoparticle surface functionalization. Polysaccharides can also be utilized as surface stabilizers in production of nanoparticles, using water as a solvent (Duan et al. 2015; Akhlaghi et al. 2013). For example, dextran has been used for coating many metal nanoparticles, as demonstrated by Virkutyte and Varma (2011), due to its hydrophilic, biocompatible, and non-toxic nature. Honey, which contains fructose and proteins, can also be used for nanoparticle synthesis. Fructose acts as a reductant, while proteins provide stability to the nanoparticles (Philip 2009). Another polysaccharide, aminocellulose, acts as a reducing agent and helps in the production of silver nanoparticles. Aminocellulose also maintains the dispersion of aqueous colloids of nanoparticles and exhibits considerable antimicrobial effective against most bacterial strains (Chandel et al. 2024; Cheng and Chang 2013).

In light of these findings, it is clear that green routes of nanoparticle production, ease of scale-up, and stabilization of homogeneous suspensions at an industrial setting have opened up new avenues for potential applications in various biotechnological sectors.

3 Advantages of Nanomaterial as Biomacromolecules Support

Adsorption or covalent methods can be utilized for the immobilization of enzymes on the exterior of cutting-edge nanomaterials (Chandel et al. 2024; Thakur et al. 2020; Dharela et al. 2013; Raj et al. 2011; Cao 2005). Immobilization techniques make bioprocesses cost-effective by facilitating quick separation and multiple reuses of enzymes (Verma et al. 2024; Arora et al. 2020; Verma et al. 2016; Abraham et al. 2014; Ansari and Hussain, Ansari and Husain 2012; Verma et al. 2008). Regulating the alignment of enzymes on nanoparticles or magnetic nanoparticles is advantageous. Moreover, compact nanoparticles do not have any dispersion issues (Xu et al. 2014).

Immobilization of enzymes can improve stability, whether the enzyme is denatured by high temperature or due to lysis. Improved and reusable enzymes may have a better price (Chandel et al. 2024; Thakur et al. 2020; Puri et al. 2013; Sheldon and van Pelt 2013). Immobilized enzymes must be usable for longer durations in industries, requiring derivatives with suitable functional properties, such as activity and selectivity, for a given reaction (Singh et al. 2013). Immobilization of enzymes, based on careful planning and optimization, can enhance the enzymatic catalytic performance. Chen et al. (2017) also highlighted that the association of nanomaterials with enzymes makes the enzymes stable and sensitive. Immobilization of enzymes is an attractive option that can improve efficacy and operational stability, while also lowering costs in industrial processes. Enzymes immobilized on nanomaterials can be reused, handled easily, and provide stability against denaturation in harsh chemical environments (Chauhan 2014). Moreover, repeated use of immobilized enzymes lowers operational costs, enhancing the economic feasibility of enzyme-catalyzed reactions. The advantages of immobilized biocatalysts, such as enhanced stability, and selectivity, can be maximized by choosing the optimal immobilization technique (Thakur et al. 2020; Kumar et al. 2016; Moteo et al. 2007).

The surface area of nanoparticles is quite large, and this surface area is readily modifiable to immobilize enzymes. Nanoparticles can immobilize enzymes in huge amounts, and with the assistance of nanoparticles, there is minimal risk of steric hindrance experienced by enzymes (Arora et al. 2020; Ansari et al. 2011; Khan et al. 2011). Similarly, magnetic nanoparticles recover with ease from the heterogeneous media using an external magnet after the completion of the reaction (Asmat et al. 2017). Magnetic nanoparticle (MNP)-based supports can immobilize diverse kinds of cellululases (Khan et al. 2016; Ansari and Hussain, Ansari and Husain 2012). Due to the advent of nanobiotechnology, nanocarriers with large and modifiable surface areas, high enzyme binding efficiency, and resistance to mass transfer can be utilized as an important nano-framework for enzyme immobilization (Verma et al. 2024; Arora et al. 2020; Verma 2018; Asmat et al. 2017; Verma 2017a, b, c; Hussain 2017; Verma et al. 2016; Abraham et al. 2014; Verma et al. 2013a, Verma et al. 2013b, Verma et al. 2013c, Verma et al. 2013d; Puri et al. 2013; Ansari and Hussain, Ansari and Husain 2012; Verma et al. 2012). Moreover, enzymes immobilized on MNPs exhibit excellent activity as well as the reusability properties (Zhou et al. 2013). Certain magnetic particles, such as magnetite (Fe_3O_4) and maghemite (Fe_2O_3), are utilized due to their minimal toxicity and biocompatible nature (Xu et al. 2014). Currently, nanomaterials have made various substances cheaper hosts to immobilize enzyme for enhanced stability (Chandel et al. 2024; Singh et al. 2013).

It is evident from the above-mentioned findings that nanomaterials offer unique advantages to biomacromolecules compared to bulk materials due to their small size, modifiable surface, and rapid separation.

4 Applications of the Nanocarrier in the Stabilization of Cellulase Enzyme, an Essential Step for Bioethanol Production

Enzymes are costly and prone to inactivation, whereas immobilized enzyme technology offers a cost-effective approach to bioprocess development, compared to using free enzymes. Various enzymes contributing to bioenergy production, as listed in Table 1, play a vital role in biofuel bioprocess. This discussion focuses on the significance of nanotechnology in biofuel production, specifically regarding the immobilization and stabilization of cellulase enzymes.

Table 1 Nanomaterials employed for immobilizing the bioenergy-producing enzymes

Type of enzymes	Types of nanocarriers	Types of immobilization methods	Improved properties of biocatalysts	References
Cellulase	Magnetic nanoparticle	Covalent bonding	Improved glucose production	Park and Johnson 2024
Cellulase	Nanocomposit e	Covalent bonding	Improved glucose production	John et al. 2023
Cellulase	Magnetic nanoparticle	Covalent bonding	Improved pH and temperature stabilities	Han et al. 2018
Cellulase	Magnetic nanocomposite	Covalent bonding	Improved operational stability	Poorakbar et al. 2018
Cellulase	Magnetic nanocomposite	Covalent bonding	Improved solvent tolerance, stability and reusability	Grewal et al. 2017
Cellulase	Magnetic nanocomposite	Cross linking	Improved the biomass saccharificatio n and bio separation process	Velmurugan and Incharoensakdi 2017
Cellulase	Polymeric nanoparticle	Covalent bonding	Improved pH stability	Wang et al. 2017
Cellulase	Poly(acrylic acid) nanogel	Adsorption	Improved acidic pH stability and thermal stability	Ahmed et al. 2017
Cellulase	Magnetic nanoparticles	Cross linking	Improved pH and temperature stability	Ladole et al. 2017
Cellulase	Magnetic nanoparticles	Cross linking	Improved higher pH stability	Selvam et al. 2016
Cellulase	Silica nanoparticles	Covalent bonding	Improved stability and reusability	Harmoko et al. 2016
Cellulase	Magnetic nanoparticles	Cross linking	Improved activity and stability	Zhang et al. 2016
Cellulase	Zinc oxide nanoparticles	Covalent bonding	Improved thermal and pH stability	Srivastava et al. 2016
Cellulase	Graphene oxide nanosheet	Cross linking	Improved self-life	Dutta et al. 2016

(continued)

Table 1 (continued)

Type of enzymes	Types of nanocarriers	Types of immobilization methods	Improved properties of biocatalysts	References
Cellulase	Magnetic nanoparticles	Adsorption and covalent bonding methods	Improved bioprocess	Kumar et al. 2016
Cellulase	Magnetic Nanocomposit e	Adsorption	Improved stability and nano emulsion	Roth et al. 2016
Cellulase	Chitosan functionalised magnetic nanoparticles	Covalent bonding	Improved operational stability	Sanchez-Ramırez et al. 2017
Cellulase	Cobalt ferrite nanoparticles	Covalent bonding	Improved operational	Bohara et al. 2016
Cellulase and glucosidase	Enzymogel nanoparticles	Adsorption	Improved biocatalyst performance at 50 °C	Samaratunga et al. 2015
Cellulase	Graphene oxide nanosheets	Covalent bonding	Improved operational stability	Xu et al. 2016
Cellulase	Silver and gold nanoparticles	Physical adsorption	Improved stability and reusability	Mishra and Sardar 2015
Cellulase	Manganese oxide nanoparticles	Covalent binding	Improved stability and reusability	Cherian et al. 2015
Cellulase	Magnetic nanocomposite	Covalent binding	Improved stability and reusability	Li et al. 2015
Cellulase	Magnetic nanocomposite	Cross linked	Improved stability and reusability	Khorshidi et al. 2014
Cellulase	Graphene nanosheet	Covalent bonding	Improved the bio-receptivity	Gokhale et al. 2013
Lipase	Magnetic cellulose nanocrystals	Precipitation-cross-linking	Improved stability and solvent tolerance	Cao 2005
Lipase	Magnetic nanocomposite	Covalent bonding	Improved stability, and reusability	Khoobi et al. 2016

(continued)

Table 1 (continued)

Type of enzymes	Types of nanocarriers	Types of immobilization methods	Improved properties of biocatalysts	References
Lipase	Carbon nanotube	Covalent bonding	Improved stability and selectivity	Verma et al. 2013b
ß-glucosidase	Magnetic nanoparticle	Covalent bonding	Improved thermal stability	Park et al. 2018
Endoglucanase and β-glucosidase	Magnetic nanoparticle	Reversibly immobilized on superparamagnetic polymeric membrane	Improved stability	Gebreyohannes et al. 2018
β-Glucosidase	Silica nanoparticles	Adsorption	Improved stability and reusability	Califano et al. 2018
β-Glucosidase	Magnetic nanocomposite	Covalent bonding	Improved catalytic activity and stability	Zhou et al. 2017
β-Glucosidase	Zinc oxide nanoparticle	Absorption	Improved thermostability	Kumar et al. 2017
β-Glucosidase	Chitosan-multiwalled carbon nanotubes	Covalent bonding	Improved operational stability	Çelik et al. 2016
β-Glucosidase	Polymeric nanomaterials	Entrapment	Improved stability and activity	Javed et al. 2016
β-Glucosidases	Silica nanoparticles	Covalent bonding	Improved stability	Agrawal et al. 2015
Endoglucanase and β-glucosidase	Magnetic nanoparticles	Magnetosome display system	Improved activity towards carboxymethyl cellulose	Honda et al. 2015
β-Glucosidase	Magnetic nanoparticles	Absorption	Improved biocatalytic performance	Chen et al. 2014
β-Glucosidase	Magnetic nanoparticle	Covalent binding	Improved operational stability	Verma et al. 2013c
Endoglucanase, cellobiohydrolase and β-glucosidase	Magnetic modified chitosan	Covalent bonding	Improved activity and stability	Yuan et al. 2016

(continued)

Table 1 (continued)

Type of enzymes	Types of nanocarriers	Types of immobilization methods	Improved properties of biocatalysts	References
β-Glucosidase and Cellobiohydrolase	Magnetic nanoparticles	Covalent bonding	Improved stability	Song et al. 2016

4.1 Cellulase

Cellulases are widely present in nature, produced by plants, parasites, microorganisms, protozoa, mollusks, and nematodes (Chandel et al. 2024; Arora et al. 2020; Dowe 2009; Bayer et al. 2007; Watanabe and Tokuda 2001). The application of cellulolytic enzymes has gained significant interest in cellulose-derived products across various industrial sectors. Recently, cellulases extracted from various origins, have been bound to diverse nanoparticles for various uses (Arora et al. 2020; Hussain 2017; Verma et al., 2020; Puri et al. 2013). To examine the influence of cellulase immobilization, Han et al. (2018) developed a four-arm polyethylene glycol dendrimer on the surface of Fe_3O_4 nanoparticles to design a novel polymer-based nanomaterial. The magnetic nanocomposite was employed for cellulase immobilization. Cellulase immobilized system displayed excellent thermostability, pH resistance, and best practical and storage capabilities, making it more appealing for various applications.

Another nano-framework was developed by Poorakbar et al. (2018) to facilitate cellulase immobilization. A nanocomposite comprising magnetic gold mesoporous silica nanoparticle core shells was composed to immobilize cellulase through covalent bonding. Whatman filter paper was used to estimate enzymatic activity at various pH and temperatures using the filter paper activity assay. This setup improved thermal dependability and enhanced storage capacity for a long period. Additionally, the nanomaterial bound enzymes can withstand a broad temperature and pH spectrum, and the enzyme can be easily separated using the insoluble support (Arora et al. 2020).

Thakur et al. (2018) utilized the nanocomposite bound immobilized cellulase for effective cellulose hydrolysis. The immobilized cellulase demonstrated superior heat stability and excellent activity across a range of reaction variables such as pH, temperature, and storage conditions. In repeated hydrolysis processes, the immobilized cellulase showed a high state of activity even after multiple reusability studies.

Grewal et al. (2017) first immobilized cellulase from *Trichoderma Reesei* onto magnetic nanoparticles and silica nanoparticles. These nanoconjugates were effectively reused for five repeated cycles and were found to be stabilized in the green solvent used for breaking down complex carbohydrates into simple sugars. The method of immobilizing enzymes showed higher catalytic effectiveness, enhanced thermal reliability, reusability, and improved resilience to ionic liquids. The authors inferred that magnetic nanoparticle-immobilized cellulase can be easily applied to break down carbohydrates present in wheat straw and sugarcane bagasse into simple sugars when treated with ionic liquid, resulting in three times higher yields.

Velmurugan and Incharoensakdi (2017) developed a unique compound by mixing cellulase enzyme with MgO, which can activate the substrate and stabilize the enzyme. Subsequently, cellulose sourced from *Chlorella* sp. CYB2 was incubated with this unique compound via xylan aldehyde linking molecules, which enhanced the binding of enzymes onto metal nanoparticles. To fasten cellulose hydrolysis, magnesium oxide was mixed with magnetic nanoparticles, resulting in improved immobilization yield, restoration of enzymatic activity, and enhanced cellulose hydrolysis. Under these conditions, the glucose yield was found to be 91%. Moreover, the hydrolysis process was improved due to the degradation of complex carbohydrates by the enhanced activity of metal oxides.

Wang et al. (2017) developed a straightforward procedure to immobilize cellulase. Cellulase was bound to copolymer-based nanoparticles through covalent bonding under normal conditions. The immobilized biocatalyst showed greater thermostability and higher activity at alkaline pH compared to free cellulase. Additionally, it demonstrated better reusability during the hydrolysis of carboxymethylcellulose.

Ahmed et al. (2017) synthesized polyacrylic nanogel to immobilize cellulase, enhancing its viability, strength, and reusability. The adsorption of cellulase onto the nanogel was pH-dependent. Nanomaterial bound cellulase showed good thermostability and hydrolytic activity, particularly at high temperatures (i.e., 80 °C). The enzyme bound immobilization system enables effortless recovery and reuse, rendering them ideal for repeated industrial processes.

Cellulase activity was found to increase when using non-invasive, low-power ultrasonic stimulation compared to the control (Subhedar and Gogate 2014). Ladole et al. (2017) evaluated the low-frequency, low-intensity ultrasound effects on magnetic nanoparticle-immobilized cellulase and reported improvements in catalytic potential and pH-thermal stability. Additionally, they observed conformational modification of free enzyme and nanomaterial bound cellulase when sonicated, which showed improved activity after ultrasonication.

Selvam et al. (2016) observed an upgrade in thermostability and activity when cellulase was immobilized onto Fe_3O_4 magnetic nanoparticles (prepared through a chemical coordination method) using a suitable glutaraldehyde cross-linker. The immobilization was optimized based on several critical parameters, including pH levels, temperature ranges, reusability potential, and storage durability.

Two cubic mesostructures of silica materials, with sizes of 8 μm and 300 nm, were prepared using F127 surfactant. Harmoko et al. (2016) developed cellulase-immobilized silica nanomaterials modified with vinyl. The vinyl-modified nanoparticles showed better biocatalytic potential compared to micron-sized particles. They concluded that the vinyl-modified cellulase enzymes exhibited better activity.

Magnetic nanoparticles were synthesized by immobilizing cellulase onto Fe_3O_4 nanoparticles and made functionalized with silane coupling agent (Zhang et al. 2016). Under ideal conditions (pH 6.0, 40 °C, and 4 h), the activity of the nanomaterial bound enzyme was found to be 99% than to the free enzyme, and after 15 cycles, the activity of the immobilized enzyme reduced to 91%. The immobilized enzyme was used to degrade corncobs, with a disintegration rate of 62%. Srivastava et al. (2016) optimized the bioprocessing of cellulosic biomass using thermostable cellulase obtained from *Aspergillus Fumigatus* and immobilized onto ZnO nanoparticles prepared using the sol-gel technique. The immobilized enzyme showed thermal stability at 65 °C and pH stability at pH 10.5 for up to 10 h. It can be concluded that these methods can be employed for biofuel production.

Dutta et al. (2016) synthesized a nanohybrid of magnesium nanoparticles with graphene oxide. This nanohybrid was utilized for cellulase immobilization using a multifunctional cross-linker. This setup demonstrated a threefold increase in enzymatic activity at low temperatures. Even at high temperatures (i.e., 90 °C), a nearly fourfold increase in activity was reported. The activity of GO-MgN-cellulase ceased after 12 repeated cycles and was optimally stored at 4 °C for over 120 days, indicating its storage capability.

Kumar et al. (2016) demonstrated the application of holocellulolytic immobilized enzymes for the breakdown of complex carbohydrates in paddy straw into simple sugars, yielding better results in terms of sugar yield. The enzyme holocellulase was extracted from Aspergillus niger and immobilized onto nanoparticles using adsorption and covalent coupling techniques. Among the five immobilized biocatalyst systems, magnetic enzyme-nanoparticle complexes (MENC) demonstrated better results in terms of sugar yield from alkali-treated paddy straw compared to free enzymes. MENC also showed efficiency in immobilizing enzymes.

Roth et al. (2016) immobilized cellulase onto magnetic nanoparticles modified by silica through electrostatic means, which showed better colloidal stability. This enzyme complex exhibited better enzymatic activity, i.e., 76%, compared to the free enzyme. The stability of the cellulase enzyme also increased, indicating its potential use for industrial applications.

Sanchez-Ramírez et al. (2017) used chitosan-modified magnetic nanoparticles to covalently immobilize cellulase using glutaraldehyde as a cross-linker. Nanomaterial bound enzyme retained around 37% of its original activity, indicating the excellent thermal and storage capabilities than to the free enzyme. Bound enzyme could easily hydrolyze the lignocellulose present in the leaves of *Agave Atrovirens* and could be reused up to 4 repeated cycles with maximum activity of 50%. This demonstrates that bioethanol can be produced using less enzyme complex during the saccharification of lignocellulose.

Bohara et al. (2016) reported that cellulase, when immobilized covalently onto amine-treated magnetic nanoparticles through covalent coupling using carbodiimide coupling, showed higher stability, reusability, and thermal capability than free cellulase. TEM micrographs and FTIR spectroscopy demonstrated no change in the size of MNPs and enzyme coating on the surface of MNPs after combining with cellulase.

Xu et al. (2016) employed ionic liquid (IL) resilience of nanomaterial bound cellulase for biorefinery applications. A nanocomposite was prepared through the chemical binding of polymeric-nanocomposite for cellulase immobilization. A significant improvement of over 30 times in IL stability was observed. This arrangement was utilized for the hydrolysis of rice straw treated with 1-butyl-3-methylimidazolium chloride and diluted to 15% (w/v), which gave a high hydrolysis rate of 87%. It also showed great reusability when pretreated with IL.

Samaratunga et al. (2015) immobilized cellulase and β-glucosidase onto silica nanoparticles modified with enzyme-gel nanoparticles having grafted polymer brushes stacked with cellulases. This complex exhibited remarkable stability as compared to the native form. Subsequently, Cherian et al. (2015) also immobilized cellulase onto manganese oxide nanoparticles. This immobilized enzyme proved to be stable in terms of activity, pH, temperature, thermal capability, and reusability.

This indicated the potential use of this enzyme complex for hydrolyzing cellulosic substances over a wide range of reaction conditions.

Due to the availability of carboxyl functional groups on its large surface, water solubility, graphene oxide, a precursor of graphene, can be utilized for enzyme immobilization. Utilizing the unique properties of graphene oxide, Li et al. (2015) prepared $Fe_3O_4@SiO_2$-graphene oxide nanosupport for the covalent binding of cellulase. High immobilization yields and proficiency (90%) were achieved. The properties of this immobilized enzyme, such as thermal stability and reusability, can be utilized in industrial applications.

Khorshidi et al. (2014) developed a setup consisting of cellulase cross-linked enzyme crystals and magnetic nanoparticles combined covalently through 3-aminopropyltriethoxysilane. The hydrolytic activity was found to be increased due to the activity of this setup, indicating the production of a biocatalyst that can withstand extreme conditions. Gokhale et al. (2013) prepared nanoparticles by combining polyelectrolytes and maghemite-magnetite nanoparticles on graphene nanosheets, which were utilized for the immobilization of cellulase when covalently bound. The activity of the immobilized enzyme, i.e., 55%, was maintained after four repeated cycles of reuse. The swelling level of the polyelectrolyte can be altered by managing pH and temperature, indicating that this setup can control the activity of immobilized enzymes.

In summary, it is evident from the above-discussed recent studies that cellulases were effectively stabilized on unique nanocarriers using efficient immobilization strategies. Immobilized cellulases demonstrated increased stability and recyclability in various operating modes of industrial reactors. The immobilized cellulases showed broad affinities for synthetic substrates as well as natural substrates.

4.2 *β-Glucosidase*

β-glucosidase is widely present in organisms and has numerous industrial applications. However, it has certain limitations due to its structural instability, which makes enzyme recovery after repeated cycles expensive (Chandel et al. 2024). With the introduction of enzyme immobilization methods, it has become easier to reuse enzymes without losing their activity, and they can also be recovered after repeated cycles (Zhou et al. 2013). Before industrial use, β-glucosidases are immobilized on solid supports, as enzyme immobilization provides easy separation from reactants after reaction completion, reusability, and thermostability (Misson et al. 2015). β-glucosidases is further stabilized via immobilization route using various supports, such as silica gel (Jung et al. 2012), magnetic chitosan microspheres (Chang et al. 2013), Eupergit C (Khan et al. 2012), gold nanoparticles (Cho et al. 2012), magnetic nanoparticles (Verma et al. 2013a), and silicone polymeric thin films (Javed et al. 2016). Recently, β-glucosidases from different sources immobilized on diverse nanocarriers have been comprehensively reviewed (Arora et al. 2020; Hussain 2017;

Verma et al., 2020; Puri et al. 2013). Park et al. (2018) developed a method to bind β-glucosidase with magnetic nanoparticles through a glutaraldehyde cross-linker with various polyethylene glycol space-linkers, which improved the thermostability of the immobilized enzyme under conditions where the free enzyme gets inactivated. The immobilized enzyme showed reusing capability even after ten rounds when p-nitrophenyl β-d-glucoside was hydrolyzed by it. Based on their findings, it can be concluded that cellulose hydrolysis can be achieved with a smaller amount of enzyme consumption, making ethanol production more cost-effective.

Superparamagnetic enzymes prepared by immobilizing endoglucanase and β-glucosidase on superparamagnetic nanoparticles were utilized for membrane cleaning to remove clogging caused by the hydrolysis of cellulosic materials (Gebreyohannes et al. 2018). They reported reusability, clogging removability, and a higher loading rate of enzymes under the influence of a biocatalytic membrane. Based on their findings, they concluded that immobilization of various enzymes can be utilized for the conversion of cellulose to glucose via cellobiose in a single reactor.

Wrinkled silica nanoparticles (WSN) with a central radial pore were manufactured, showing improved characteristics such as smaller size, allowing for simple dispersion and reduced diffusion. Recently, Califano et al. (2018) immobilized β-glucosidase onto WSNs by physical adsorption and executed cellobiose hydrolysis, assessed by kinetic studies. Immobilization improved enzyme activity by preserving auxiliary structures. Additionally, enzyme-substrate affinity was increased, as shown by the lower KM value. Cellobiose was hydrolyzed four times, indicating the stability of the biocatalyst. β-glucosidase was restricted to the nickel doped surface of nanoparticles by covalent binding with imidazolyl and nickel groups (Zhou et al. 2017). This showed better activity, stability, reusability, and purification of chemicals. Bacterial derived β-glucosidase was surface-bound on zinc oxide nanoparticles using an absorption method (Kumar et al. 2017) remained reusable up to ten times without losing its activity and showed better thermostability.

Javed et al. (2016) extracted fungal β-glucosidase was immobilized on polymeric nanomaterials (polyurethane, latex, and silicone) using entrapment. This immobilization method improved the biocatalytic potential, resulting in improved cellulose hydrolysis. Nanomaterial immobilized biocatalyst preserved 70% of its original activity. Thus, this setup can be utilized for industrial biotechnology applications.

Agrawal et al. (2015) devised a plan to improve the properties of sugarcane juice by extracting β-glucosidase sourced from *Bacillus subtilis* and immobilizing it onto SiO_2 nanoparticles. As a result of sugarcane juice treatment with the immobilized β-glucosidase, it showed an increase in phenolic content, resulting in a 2.6-fold and 2.4-fold increase in p-hydroxybenzoic acid and gallic acid, respectively. Nanomaterial immobilized biocatalyst demonstrated the improved thermostability and reusability for a longer duration.

Honda et al. (2015) immobilized endoglucanase and β-glucosidase on magnetic nanoparticles for cellulose hydrolysis. This combination demonstrated improved hydrolytic activity and reported better outcomes.

Chen et al. (2014) first combined magnetic Fe_3O_4 nanoparticles (MNPs) with agarose (AMNPs) and then associated it with Span-80 surfactants through an alkaline medium in an organic solvent (AMNPs-ECH-IDA-Co^{2+}). Subsequently, β-glucosidase was immobilized onto this setup. This setup exhibited improvements in hydrolytic activity, thermostability, and functional stability, making it suitable for industrial applications.

Verma et al. (2013a) demonstrated the biochemical properties of the purified β-glucosidase (BGL) sourced from *Aspergillus Niger* and covalently immobilized it onto magnetic nanoparticles for cellobiose hydrolysis. Transmission electron microscopy, Fourier transform infrared spectroscopy, and enzyme assays confirmed the immobilization of BGL on the surface of magnetic nanoparticles. Due to this immobilization, conformational changes were observed, resulting in adjustments in pH and kinetic constants. This setup improved enzyme activity, thermostability, and reusability, making it suitable for biofuel production.

Based on the above-discussed studies, it is concluded that immobilizing β-glucosidase on various nanostructured forms improved the operational stability and reusability of the enzyme-nanoparticle complex.

Various enzymes such as cellulase, lipase, xylanase, β-glucosidases, and a combination of these enzymes has been immobilized using magnetic nanocarriers or in combination of other nanocarriers. Performance of enzymes improved with respect to broader pH and temperature, enhanced biocatalytic potential and operational stability.

4.3 Co-Immobilization of Cellulolytic Enzymes

Co-immobilization of different cellulase enzymes plays a crucial role in the decomposition of celluloses. Immobilizing just a single type of cellulase does not provide the synergistic function mandatory for cellulose saccharification to glucose (Arora et al. 2020; Song et al. 2016). Different nanosupports for co-immobilization of cellulolytic enzymes for effective industrial applications have been recently reviewed (Chandel et al. 2024; Arora et al. 2020; Hussain 2017; Verma et al. 2016; Puri et al. 2013). For the hydrolysis of cell walls of Nannochloropsis sp., cellulase and lysozyme were co-immobilized onto magnetic nanoparticles treated with an amino group using glutaraldehyde as a cross-linker (Chen et al. 2018). The immobilization of multiple enzymes improved the activity of both enzymes (cellulase: 79% and lysozyme: 70%). It also enhanced thermostability, half-life, reusability, and catalytic efficiency to hydrolyze cell walls. Even after six repeated cycles, the co-immobilized enzymes maintained their activity up to 60%. A magnetic nanobiocatalyst made by immobilizing a mixture of pectinase, xylanase, and cellulase onto magnetic nanoparticles exhibited better cellulase activity and can be utilized for juice clarification and bioethanol production (Perwez et al. 2017).

Yuan et al. (2016) developed a robust nanobiocatalytic system by immobilizing endoglucanase, cellobiohydrolase, and β-glucosidase onto magnetic nanoparticles coated with aminated starch to explore the effects of pH, temperature, reusability, and catalytic activity of co-immobilized enzymes. This catalytic system was also utilized to explore the reusability of anthocyanins present in biowaste. The blended immobilized cellulases were utilized for decomposition, whereas productivity was enhanced by β-glucosidase.

Song et al. (2016) covalently co-immobilized β-glucosidase A (BglA) and cellobiohydrolase D (CelD) on nanoparticles, which provided a better optimum temperature compared to the free enzyme, while BglA displayed better thermostability. The immobilization of multiple cellulases on nanoparticles can possibly significantly decrease enzyme utilization and benefit from the synergistic activity of cellulases during sugar production.

Cho et al. (2012) developed nanobiocatalyst system by co-immobilizing three forms of modified cellulases on gold nanoparticles as well as silica-modified gold nanoparticles. This nanobiocatalyst exhibited better stability, reusability, and activity compared to mixtures of free cellulases. Both immobilized forms showed higher hydrolytic degradation of cellulose.

It is concluded from the above discussion that co-immobilization could be an effective tool for cellulose hydrolysis.

5 Conclusion

The green route of nanoparticle production is the most sought-after technology. It offers ease of scale-up and stabilization of homogeneous nanosuspensions, opening up new avenues for potential applications in various biotechnological sectors. Nanoparticles-bound cellulolytic enzymes exhibited greater efficiency in terms of biocatalytic potential, thermostability, and recycability against different types of physico-chemical denaturants during the hydrolysis of cellulosic materials. Similarly, co-immobilized enzymes also proved to be a potent agent for hydrolyzing cellulose into glucose and other valuable compounds, thus providing a viable route for bioethanol production.

Acknowledgments One of the authors (Dr Madan L. Verma) thankfully acknowledge the support and encouragement received from the Director, Indian Institute of Information Technology Una, Himachal Pradesh for pursuing the present work.

References

R.E. Abraham, M.L. Verma, C.J. Barrow, M. Puri, Suitability of magnetic nanoparticle immobilised cellulases in enhancing enzymatic saccharification of pretreated hemp biomass. Biotechnol. Biofuels **7**, 90 (2014). https://doi.org/10.1186/1754-6834-7-90

R. Agrawal, A.K. Verma, A. Satlewal, Application of nanoparticle-immobilized thermostable β-glucosidase for improving the sugar cane juice properties. Innov. Food Sci. Emerg. Technol. **33**, 472–482 (2015). https://doi.org/10.1016/j.ifset.2015.11.024

I.N. Ahmed, R. Chang, W. Tsai, Poly(acrylic acid) nanogel as a substrate for cellulase immobilization for hydrolysis of cellulose. Colloids Surf. B Biointerfaces **152**, 339–343 (2017). https://doi.org/10.1016/j.colsurfb.2017.01.040

S.P. Akhlaghi, B. Peng, Z. Yao, K.C. Tam, Sustainable nano materials derived from polysaccharides and amphiphilic compounds. Soft Matter. **9**(33), 7905–7918 (2013). https://doi.org/10.1039/C3SM50358E

S.A. Ansari, Q. Husain, Potential applications of enzymes immobilized on/in nano materials: a review. Biotechnol. Adv. **30**, 512–523 (2012). https://doi.org/10.1016/j.biotechadv.2011.09.005

S.A. Ansari, Q. Husain, S. Qayyum, A. Azam, Designing and surface modification of zinc oxide nanoparticles for biomedical applications. Food Chem. Toxicol. **49**, 2107–2115 (2011). https://doi.org/10.1016/j.fct.2011.05.025

A. Arora, P. Nandal, J. Singh, M.L. Verma, Nanobiotechnological route for the biomass pretreatment. Mater. Sci. Energy. Technol. **3**, 308–318 (2020). https://doi.org/10.1016/j.mset.2019.12.003

S. Asmat, Q. Husain, A. Azam, Lipase immobilization on facile synthesized polyaniline-coated silver-functionalized graphene oxide nanocomposites as novel biocatalysts: stability and activity insights. RSC Adv. **7**, 5019–5029 (2017). https://doi.org/10.1039/C6RA27926K

N. Asmathunisha, K. Kathiresan, A review on biosynthesis of nanoparticles by marine organisms. Colloids Surf. B Biointerfaces **103**, 283–287 (2013). https://doi.org/10.1016/j.colsurfb.2012.10.030

E.A. Bayer, R. Lamed, M.E. Himmel, The potential of cellulases and cellulosomes for cellulosic waste management. Current Opin. Biotechnol. **18**, 237–245 (2007). https://doi.org/10.1016/j.copbio.2007.04.004

P. Beguin, J.P. Aubert, The biological degradation of cellulose. FEMS Microbiol. Rev. **13**, 25–58 (1994). https://doi.org/10.1111/j.1574-6976.1994.tb00033.x

R.A. Bohara, N.D. Thorat, S.H. Pawar, Immobilization of cellulase on functionalized cobalt ferrite nanoparticles. Korean J. Chem. Eng. **33**(1), 216–222 (2016). https://doi.org/10.1007/s11814-015-0120-0

V. Califano, F. Sannino, A. Costantini, J. Avossa, J. Cimino, A. Aronne, Wrinkled silica nanoparticles: efficient matrix for β-glucosidase immobilization. J. Phys. Chem. **122**(15), 8373–8379 (2018). https://doi.org/10.1021/acs.jpcc.8b00652

L. Cao, Immobilized enzymes: science or art? Curr. Chem. Biol. **9**(2), 217–226 (2005). https://doi.org/10.1016/j.cbpa.2005.02.014

A. Çelik, A. Dinçer, T. Aydemir, Characterization of β-glucosidase immobilized on chitosan-multiwalled carbon nanotubes (MWCNTS) and their application on tea extracts for aroma enhancement. Int. J. Biol. Macromol. **89**, 406–414 (2016). https://doi.org/10.1016/j.ijbiomac.2016.05.008

A.K. Chandel, V.K. Garlapati, A.K. Singh, F.A.F. Antunes, S.S. da Silva, The path forward for lignocellulose biorefineries: bottlenecks, solutions, and perspective on commercialization. Bioresour. Technol. (2018). https://doi.org/10.1016/j.biortech.2018.06.004

J. Chang, Y.S. Lee, S.J. Fang, D.J. Park, Y.L. Choi, Hydrolysis of isoflavone glycoside by immobilization of β-glucosidase on a chitosan-carbon in two-phase system. Int. J. Biol. Macromol. **61**, 465–470 (2013). https://doi.org/10.1016/j.ijbiomac.2013.08.014

G.S. Chauhan, Evaluation of nanogels as supports for enzyme immobilization. Polym. Int. **63**(11), 1889–1894 (2014). https://doi.org/10.1002/pi.4734

H. Chandel, P. Kumar, A. Chandel, M.L. Verma, Biotechnological advances in biomass pretreatment for bio-renewable production through nanotechnological intervention. Biomass Convers Biorefin. **14**, 2959–2981 (2024). https://doi.org/10.1007/s13399-022-02746-0

M. Chen, G. Zeng, P. Xu, C.L.L. Tang, How do enzyme 'meet' nanoparticles and nanomaterials? Trends Biochem. Sci. **42**(11), 914–930 (2017). https://doi.org/10.1016/j.tibs.2017.08.008

Q. Chen, D. Liu, C. Wu, K. Yao, Z. Li, N. Shi, F. Wen, I.D. Gates, Co-immobilization of cellulase and lysozyme on amino-functionalized magnetic nanoparticles: an activity-tunable biocatalyst for extraction of lipids from microalgae. Bioresour. Technol. **263**, 317–324 (2018). https://doi.org/10.1016/j.biortech.2018.04.071

T. Chen, W. Yang, Y. Guo, R. Yuan, L. Xu, Y. Yan, Enhancing catalytic performance of β-glucosidase via immobilization on metal ions chelated magnetic nanoparticles. Enzyme Microb. Technol. **63**, 50–57 (2014). https://doi.org/10.1016/j.enzmictec.2014.05.008

C. Cheng, K.C. Chang, Development of immobilized cellulase through functionalized gold nanoparticles for glucose production by continuous hydrolysis of waste bamboo chopsticks. Enzyme Microb. Technol. **53**, 444–451 (2013). https://doi.org/10.1016/j.enzmictec.2013.09.010

E. Cherian, M. Dharmendirakumar, G. Baskar, Immobilization of cellulase onto MnO2 nanoparticles for bioethanol production by enhanced hydrolysis of agricultural waste. Chinese J. Catal. **36**, 1223–1229 (2015). https://doi.org/10.1016/S1872-2067(15)60906-8

E.J. Cho, S. Jung, H.J. Kim, Y.G. Lee, K.C. Nam, H.J. Lee, H.J. Bae, Co-immobilization of three cellulases on Au-doped magnetic silica nanoparticles for the degradation of cellulose. Chem. Commun. **48**, 886–888 (2012). https://doi.org/10.1039/C2CC16661E

S.K. Das, C. Dickinson, F. Laffir, D.F. Brougham, E. Marsili, Synthesis, characterisation and catalytic activity of gold nanoparticles, biosynthesised with *Rhizopus oryzae* protein extract. Green Chem. **14**, 1322–1344 (2012a). https://doi.org/10.1039/C2GC16676C

S.K. Das, J. Liang, M. Schmidt, F. Laffir, E. Marsili, Biomineralization mechanism of gold by zygomycete fungi *Rhizopous oryzae*. ACS Nano. **6**, 6165–6173 (2012b). https://doi.org/10.1021/nn301502s

B.S. Dhanya, A. Mishra, A.K. Chandel, M.L. Verma, Development of sustainable approaches forconverting the organic waste to bioenergy. Sci. Total Environ. **723**, 138109 (2020). https://doi.org/10.1016/j.scitotenv.2020.138109

R. Dharela, G.S. Chauhan, J.H. Ahn, Immobilization of urease onto new nanogels. Curr. Catal. **2**(2), 122–129 (2013). https://doi.org/10.2174/2211544711302020006

N. Dowe, Assessing cellulase performance on pretreated lignocellulosic biomass using saccharification and fermentation-based protocols. Method. Mol. Biol. **581**, 233–245 (2009). https://doi.org/10.1007/978-1-60761-214-8_15

H. Duan, D. Wang, Y. Li, Green chemistry for nanoparticle synthesis. Chem. Soc. Rev. **44**(16), 5778–5792 (2015). https://doi.org/10.1039/C4CS00363B

N. Dutta, S. Biswas, M.K. Saha, Biophysical characterization and activity analysis of nano magnesium supplemented cellulase obtained from a psychrobacterium following graphene oxide immobilization. Enzyme Microb. Technol. **95**, 248–258 (2016). https://doi.org/10.1016/j.enzmictec.2016.04.012

L.A. Dykman, N.G. Khlebtsov, Immunological properties of gold nanoparticles. Chem. Sci. **8**, 1719–1735 (2017). https://doi.org/10.1039/C6SC03631G

A. Ebrahiminezhad, M. Bagheri, S.M. Taghizadeh, A. Berenjian, Y. Ghasemi, Biomimetic synthesis of silver nanoparticles using microalgal secretory carbohydrates as a novel anticancer and antimicrobial. Adv. Nat. Sci. Nanosci. Nanotechnol. **7**, 015018 (2016)

A.M. Elgorban, A.N. Al-Rahmah, S.R. Sayed, A. Hirad, A.A.F. Mostafa, A.H. Bahkali, Antimicrobial activity and green synthesis of silver nanoparticles using *Trichoderma viride*. Biotechnol. Biotechnol. Equip. **30**, 299–304 (2016). https://doi.org/10.1080/13102818.2015.1133255

A.Y. Gebreyohannes, M. Dharmjeet, T. Swusten, M. Mertens, J. Verspreet, T. Verbiest, C. Courtin, I.F.J. Vankeleco, Simultaneous glucose production from cellulose and fouling reduction using a magnetic responsive membrane reactor with superparamagnetic nanoparticles carrying cellulolytic enzymes. Bioresour. Technol. **263**, 532–540 (2018). https://doi.org/10.1016/j.biortech.2018.05.002

A.A. Gokhale, J. Lu, I. Lee, Immobilization of cellulase on magnetoresponsive graphene nanosupports. J. Mol. Catal. B Enzym. **90**, 76–86 (2013). https://doi.org/10.1016/j.molcatb.2013.01.025

K. Golchin, J. Golchin, S. Ghaderi, N. Alidadiani, S. Eslamkhah, M. Eslamkhah, S. Davaran, A. Akbarzadeh, Gold nanoparticles applications: from artificial enzyme till drug delivery. Artif. Cells Nanomed. Biotechnol. **46**(2), 250–254 (2018). https://doi.org/10.1080/21691401.2017.1305393

J. Grewal, R. Ahmad, S.K. Khare, Development of cellulase-nanoconjugates with enhanced ionic liquid and thermal stability for in situ lignocellulose saccharification. Bioresour. Technol. **242**, 236–243 (2017). https://doi.org/10.1016/j.biortech.2017.04.007

S. Gupta, S. Bector, Biosynthesis of extracellular and intracellular gold nanoparticles by *Aspergillus fumigatus* and *A. flavus*. Anton Leeuw **103**, 1113–1123 (2013). https://doi.org/10.1007/s10482-013-9892-6

J. Han, L. Wang, Y. Wang, J. Dong, X. Tang, L. Ni, L. Wang, Preparation and characterization of Fe_3O_4-NH_2@4-arm-PEG-NH_2, a novel magnetic four-arm polymer-nanoparticle composite for cellulose immobilization. Biochem. Eng. J. **130**, 90–98 (2018). https://doi.org/10.1016/j.bej.2017.11.008

C. Harmoko, K.I. Sucipto, E.S. Retnoningtyas, S.B. Hartono, Vinyl functionalized cubic mesoporous silica nanoparticles as supporting material to enhance cellulase enzyme stability. ARPN J. Eng. Appl. Sci. **11**(5), 2981–2992 (2016)

T. Honda, T. Tanaka, T. Yoshino, Stoichiometrically controlled immobilization of multiple enzymes on magnetic nanoparticles by the magnetosome display system for efficient cellulose hydrolysis. Biomacromolecules **16**(12), 3863–3868 (2015). https://doi.org/10.1021/acs.biomac.5b01174

Q. Hussain, Nanomaterials immobilized cellulolytic enzymes and their industrial applications: a literature review. JSM Biochem. Mol. Biol. **4**(3), 1029 (2017) https://www.jscimedcentral.com/Biochemistry/earlyonline.php

M.R. Javed, A. Buthe, M.H. Rashid, P. Wang, Cost efficient entrapment of β-glucosidase in nanoscale latex and silicone polymeric thin films for use as stable biocatalysts. Food Chem. **190**, 1078–1085 (2016). https://doi.org/10.1016/j.foodchem.2015.06.040

J.A. John, M.S. Samuel, E. Selvarajan, Immobilized cellulase on Fe3O4/GO/CS nanocomposite as a magnetically recyclable catalyst for biofuel application. Fuel **333**(1), 126364 (2023). https://doi.org/10.1016/j.fuel.2022.126364

Y.R. Jung, H.Y. Shin, Y.S. Song, S.B. Kim, S.W. Kim, Enhancement of immobilized enzyme activity by pretreatment of β-glucosidase with cellobiose and glucose. J. Ind. Eng. Chem. **18**, 702–706 (2012). https://doi.org/10.1016/j.jiec.2011.11.133

S.S. Kanwar, C. Sharma, M.L. Verma, S. Chauhan, S.S. Chimni, G.S. Chauhan, Short-chain ester synthesis by transesterification employing poly (MAc-co-DMA-cl-MBAm) hydrogel-bound lipase of *Bacillus coagulans* MTCC-6375. J. Appl. Polym. Sci. **109**, 1063–1071 (2008). https://doi.org/10.1002/app.25320

S.S. Kanwar, R.K. Kaushal, M.L. Verma, Y. Kumar, G.S. Chauhan, R. Gupta, S.S. Chimni, Synthesis of ethyl laurate by hydrogel immobilized lipase of *Bacillus coagulans* MTCC-6375. Ind. J. Microbiol. **45**, 187–193 (2005)

J.A. Khan, S. Qayyum, F. Alam, Q. Husain, Effect of tin oxide nanoparticle binding on the structure and activity of α-amylase from *Bacillus amyloliquefaciens*. Nanotechnology **22**, 455708 (2011). https://doi.org/10.1088/0957-4484/22/45/455708

M. Khan, Q. Husain, A.H. Naqvi, Graphene based magnetic nanocomposites as versatile carriers for high yield immobilization and stabilization of β-galactosidase. RSC Adv. **6**(53493–53), 503 (2016). https://doi.org/10.1039/C6RA06960F

M.M. Khan, S. Kalathil, T.H. Han, J. Lee, M.H. Cho, Positively charged gold nanoparticles synthesized by electrochemically active biofilm-a biogenic approach. Nanosci. Nanotechnol. **13**, 6079–6085 (2013). https://doi.org/10.1166/jnn.2013.76666079

S. Khan, C. Lindahl, C. Turner, E.N. Karlsson, Immobilization of thermostable β-glucosidase variants on acrylic supports for biocatalytic processes in hot water. J. Mol. Catal. B. Enzym. **80**, 28–38 (2012). https://doi.org/10.1016/j.molcatb.2012.01.004

M. Khoobi, M.K. Sedagheh, A. Ramazani, Z. Asadgol, H. Forootanfar, M.A. Faramarzi, Synthesis of polyethyleneimine (PEI) and βcyclodextrin grafted PEI nanocomposites with magnetic cores for lipase immobilization and esterification. J. Chem. Technol. Biotechnol. **91**, 375–384 (2016). https://doi.org/10.1002/jctb.4579

K.J. Khorshidi, H. Lenjannezhadian, M. Jamalan, M. Zeinali, Preparation and characterization of nanomagnetic cross-linked cellulase aggregates for cellulose bioconversion. J. Chem. Technol. Biotechnol. **91**(2), 539–546 (2014). https://doi.org/10.1002/jctb.4615

F.Y. Kong, J.W. Zhang, R.F. Li, Z.X. Wang, W.J. Wang, W. Wang, Unique roles of gold nanoparticles in drug delivery, targeting and imaging applications. Molecules **22**, 1445–1451 (2017). https://doi.org/10.3390/molecules22091445

A. Kumar, S. Singh, R. Tiwari, R. Goel, L. Nain, Immobilization of indigenous holocellulase on iron oxide (Fe2O3) nanoparticles enhanced hydrolysis of alkali pretreated paddy straw. Int. J. Biol. Macromol. **96**, 538–549 (2016). https://doi.org/10.1016/j.ijbiomac.2016.11.109

S. Kumar, R. Kushwaha, S. Kumar, M.L. Verma, Decongestion of lignocellulosics: a critical assessment of physicochemical approaches, in *Handbook of Biofuels*, (Elsevier, 2021). https://doi.org/10.1016/B978-0-12-822810-4.00009-9

P. Kumar, B. Ryan, G.T.M. Henehan, β-Glucosidase from *Streptomyces griseus*: nanoparticle immobilisation and alkyl glucoside synthesis. Protein Exp. Purif. **132**, 164170 (2017). https://doi.org/10.1016/j.pep.2017.01.011

S. Kumar, C. Malarkodi, K. Paulkumar, M. Vanaja, G. Gnanajobitha, G. Annadurai, Algae-mediated green fabrication of silver nanoparticles and examination of its antifungal activity against clinical pathogens. Int. J. Metals **2014**, 692643 (2014). https://doi.org/10.1155/2014/692643

M.R. Ladole, J.S. Mevada, A.B. Pandit, Ultrasonic hyperactivation of cellulase immobilized on magnetic nanoparticles. Bioresour. Technol. **239**, 117–126 (2017). https://doi.org/10.1016/j.biortech.2017.04.096

Y. Li, X.Y. Wang, X.P. Jiang, J.J. Ye, Y.W. Zhang, X.Y. Zhang, Fabrication of graphene oxide decorated with Fe_3O_4@SiO_2 for immobilization of cellulose. J. Nanopart Res. **17**, 8 (2015). https://doi.org/10.1007/s11051-014-2826-z

D. Martinez, R.M. Berka, B. Henrissat, M. Saloheimo, M. Arvas, S.E. Baker, J. Chapman, O. Chertkov, P.M. Coutinho, D. Cullen, et al., Genome sequencing and analysis of the biomass-degrading fungus *Trichoderma reesei* (syn. *Hypocrea jecorina*). Nat. Biotechnol. **26**, 553–560 (2008). https://doi.org/10.1038/nbt1403

T. Maruyama, Y. Fujimoto, T. Markawa, Synthesis of gold nanoparticles using various amino acids. J. Colloid Interf. Sci. **447**, 254–257 (2015). https://doi.org/10.1016/j.jcis.2014.12.046

A. Mishra, M. Sardar, Cellulase assisted synthesis of nano-silver and gold: Application as immobilization matrix for biocatalysis. Int. J. Biol. Macromol. **77**, 105–113 (2015). https://doi.org/10.1016/j.ijbiomac.2015.03.014

M. Misson, H. Zhang, B. Jin, Nanobiocatalyst advancements and bioprocessing applications. J. R. Soc. Interface **12**(102), 20140891 (2015). https://doi.org/10.1098/rsif.2014.0891

C. Moteo, J.M. Palomo, G. Fernandez-Lorente, J.M. Guison, R. Fernandez-Lafuante, Improvement of enzyme stability and selectivity via immobilization techniques. Enzyme Microb. Technol. **40**(16), 1451–1463 (2007). https://doi.org/10.1016/j.enzmictec.2007.01.018

P. Mukherjee, S. Senapati, D. Mandal, A. Ahmad, M.I. Khan, R. Kumar, M. Sastry, Extracellular synthesis of gold nanoparticles by the fungus *Fusarium oxysporum*. Chembiochem **3**, 461–463 (2002). https://doi.org/10.1002/1439-7633(20020503)3:5<461::AID-CBIC461>3.0

K. Neveen-Mohamed, Biogenic silver nanoparticles by *Aspergillus terreus* as a powerful nanoweapon against *Aspergillus fumigates*. Afr. J. Microbiol. Res. **7**, 5645–5651 (2014). https://doi.org/10.5897/AJMR2013.6429

H.J. Park, A.J. Driscoll, P.A. Johnson, The development and evaluation of β-glucosidase immobilized magnetic nanoparticles as recoverable biocatalysts. Biochem. Eng. J. **133**, 66–73 (2018). https://doi.org/10.1016/j.bej.2018.01.017

H. Park, P.A. Johnson, The development and evaluation of chitosan-coated enzyme magnetic nanoparticles for cellulose hydrolysis. Front. Chem. Eng. **6**, 2024 (2024). https://doi.org/10.3389/fceng.2024.1479798

D. Paul, A. Arora, M.L. Verma, Advances in Microbial Biofuel production. Front. Microbiol. **12**, 2768 (2021). https://doi.org/10.3389/fmicb.2021.746216

M. Perwez, R. Ahmad, M. Sardar, A reusable multipurpose magnetic nanobiocatalyst for industrial applications. Int. J. Biol. Macromol. **103**, 16–24 (2017). https://doi.org/10.1016/j.ijbiomac.2017.05.029

D. Philip, Biosynthesis of Au, Ag and Au-Ag nanoparticles using edible mushroom extract. Spectochim. Acta Part A Mol. Biomol. Spectrosc. **73**(2), 374–381 (2009). https://doi.org/10.1016/j.saa.2009.02.037

E. Poorakbar, A. Shafiee, A.A. Saboury, B.L. Rad, K. Khoshnevisan, L. Ma'mani, H. Derakhshankhah, M.R. Ganjali, M. Hosseini, Synthesis of magnetic gold mesoporous silica nanoparticles core shell for cellulase enzyme immobilization: improvement of enzymatic activity and thermal stability. Process Biochem. **71**, 92–100 (2018). https://doi.org/10.1016/j.procbio.2018.05.012

M. Puri, C.J. Barrow, M.L. Verma, Enzyme immobilization on nanomaterials for biofuel production. Trends Biotechnol. **31**(4), 215–216 (2013). https://doi.org/10.1016/j.tibtech.2013.01.002

L. Raj, G.S. Chauhan, W. Azmi, J.H. Ahn, J. Manuel, Kinetics study of invertase covalently linked to a new functional nanogel. Bioresour. Technol. **102**(3), 2177–2184 (2011). https://doi.org/10.1016/j.biortech.2010.11.062

H.C. Roth, S.P. Schwaminger, F. Peng, S. Berensmeier, Immobilization of cellulase on magnetic nanocarriers. Chemi. Open **5**, 183–187 (2016). https://doi.org/10.1002/open.201600028

A. Samaratunga, O. Kudina, N. Nahar, A. Zakharchenko, S. Minko, A. Voronov, S.W. Pryor, Modeling the effect of pH and temperature for cellulases immobilized on enzymogel nanoparticles. Appl. Biochem. Biotechnol. **176**(4), 1114–1130 (2015). https://doi.org/10.1007/s12010-015-1633-z

J. Sanchez-Ramırez, J.L. Martınez-Hernandez, P. Segura-Ceniceros, G. Lopez, H. Saade, M.A. Medina-Morales, R. Ramos-Gonzalez, C.N. Aguila, A. Ilyina, Cellulases immobilization on chitosan-coated magnetic nanoparticles: application for *Agave atrovirens* lignocellulosic biomass hydrolysis. Bioprocess Biosyst. Eng. **40**(1), 9–22 (2017). https://doi.org/10.1007/s00449-016-1670-1

K. Selvam, M. Govarthanan, D. Senbagam, S.K. Kamala Kannan, B. Senthilkumar, T. Selvankumar, Activity and stability of bacterial cellulase immobilized on magnetic nanoparticles. Chinese J. Catal. **37**, 1891–1898 (2016). https://doi.org/10.1016/S1872-2067(16)62487-7

R.A. Sheldon, S. van Pelt, Enzyme immobilisation in biocatalysis: why, what and how. Chem. Soc. Rev. **42**, 6223–6235 (2013). https://doi.org/10.1039/C3CS60075K

R.K. Singh, M.K. Tiwari, R. Singh, J.K. Lee, From protein engineering to immobilization: promising strategies for the upgrade of industrial enzymes. Int. J. Mol. Sci. **14**, 1232–1277 (2013). https://doi.org/10.3390/ijms14011232

Q. Song, Y. Mao, M. Wilkins, F. Segato, R. Prade, Cellulase immobilization on superparamagnetic nanoparticles for reuse in cellulosic biomass conversion. AIMS Bioeng. **3**(3), 264–276 (2016). https://doi.org/10.3934/bioeng.2016.3.264

N. Srivastava, M. Srivastava, P.K. Mishra, P.W. Ramteke, Application of ZnO nanoparticles for improving the thermal and pH stability of crude cellulase obtained from *Aspergillus fumigatus* AA001. Frontiers Microbiol. **7**, 1–9 (2016). https://doi.org/10.3389/fmicb.2016.00514

P.B. Subhedar, P.R. Gogate, Enhancing the activity of cellulase enzyme using ultrasonic irradiations. J. Mol. Catal. B Enzym. **101**, 108–114 (2014). https://doi.org/10.1016/j.molcatb.2014.01.002

N. Thakur, B.S. Dhanya, M.L. Verma, Nano-immobilized biocatalysts and their potential biotechnological applications in bioenergy sector. Mater. Sci. Energy Technol. **3**, 808–824 (2020). https://doi.org/10.1016/j.mset.2020.09.006

S.S. Thakur, A. Kumar, G.A. Chauhan, Cellulase immobilization on to zirconia-gelatin-based mesoporous hybrid matrix for efficient cellulose hydrolysis. Trends Carbohy. Res. **10**(1), 45–55 (2018)

A. Vago, G. Szakacs, G. Safran, R. Horvath, B. Pecz, I. Lagzi, One-step green synthesis of gold nanoparticles by mesophilic filamentous fungi. Chem. Phys. Lett. **645**, 1–4 (2015). https://doi.org/10.1016/j.cplett.2015.12.019

R. Velmurugan, A. Incharoensakdi, MgO-Fe_3O_4 linked cellulase enzyme complex improves the hydrolysis of cellulose from *Chlorella* sp. CYB2. Biochem. Eng. J. **122**, 22–30 (2017). https://doi.org/10.1016/j.bej.2017.02.012

M.L. Verma, B.S. Dhanya, B. Wang, M. Thakur, V. Rani, R. Kushwaha, Bio-nanoparticles mediated transesterification of algal biomass for biodiesel production. *Sustainability.* **16**(1), 295 (2024). https://doi.org/10.3390/su16010295

M.L. Verma, P. Kumar, H. Chandel, Nanobiotechnological Routes in Lignocellulosic Waste Pretreatment for Bio-renewables Production, in *Recent Advances in Bio-Energy Research. ICRABR-2022 2022. Springer Proceedings in Energy*, ed. by N. Gakkhar, S. Kumar, A.K. Sarma, N.T. Graham, (Springer, Singapore, 2023a). https://doi.org/10.1007/978-981-99-5758-3_3

M.L. Verma, P.J. Joseph, D. Sen Karaman, Microbial nanotechnology: a new frontier in microbiology. Front. Microbiol. **14** (2023b). https://doi.org/10.3389/fmicb.2023.1296573

M.L. Verma, B.S. Dhanya, T.M. Sukriti, J. Jeslin, R. Kushwaha, Carbohydrate and protein based biopolymeric nanoparticles: current status and biotechnological applications. Int J Biol Macromol **154**, 390–412 (2020a). https://doi.org/10.1016/j.ijbiomac.2020.03.105

M.L. Verma, S. Kumar, A. Das, J.S. Randhawa, M. Chamundeeswari, Chitin and chitosan-based support materials for enzyme immobilization and biotechnological applications. Environ Chem Lett **18**, 315–323 (2020b). https://doi.org/10.1007/s10311-019-00942-5

M.L. Verma, Critical evaluation of toxicity tests in context to engineered nanomaterials: an introductory overview, in *Nanotoxicology: Toxicity Evaluation, Risk Assessment and Management*, ed. by V. Kumar, N. Dasgupta, S. Ranjan, (CRC Press, Boca Raton, 2018), pp. 1–21

M.L. Verma, Fungus-mediated bioleaching of metallic nanoparticles from agro-industrial by-products, in *Fungal Nanotechnology. Fungal Biology*, ed. by R. Prasad, (Springer, Cham, 2017a), pp. 89–102. https://doi.org/10.1007/978-3-319-68424-6_5

M.L. Verma, Nanobiotechnology advances in enzymatic biosensors for the agri-food industry. Environ. Chem. Lett. **15**(4), 555–560 (2017b). https://doi.org/10.1007/s10311-017-0640-4

M.L. Verma, Enzymatic nanobiosensors in the agricultural and food industry, in *Nanoscience in Food and Agriculture 4, Sustainable Agriculture Reviews*, ed. by S. Ranjan, N. Dasgupta, L. E, vol. 24, (Springer, Cham, 2017c), pp. 229–245. https://doi.org/10.1007/978-3-319-53112-0_7. isbn:978-3-319-53111-3

M.L. Verma, M. Puri, C.J. Barrow, Recent trends in nanomaterials immobilised enzymes for biofuel production. Crit. Rev. Biotechnol. **36**(1), 108–119 (2016). https://doi.org/10.3109/07388551.2014.928811

M.L. Verma, C.J. Barrow, Recent advances in feedstocks and enzyme-immobilised technology for effective transesterification of lipids into biodiesel, in *Microbial Factories*, ed. by V. Kalia, (Springer, New Delhi, 2015), pp. 87–103. https://doi.org/10.1007/978-81-322-2598-0_6. isbn:978-81-322-2597-3

M.L. Verma, R. Rajkhowa, C.J. Barrow, X. Wang, M. Puri, Exploring novel ultrafine Eri silk bioscaffold for enzyme stabilisation in cellobiose hydrolysis. Bioresour. Technol. **145**, 302–306 (2013a). https://doi.org/10.1016/j.biortech.2013.01.065

M.L. Verma, M. Naebe, C.J. Barrow, M. Puri, Enzyme immobilisation on amino-functionalised multi-walled carbon nanotubes: structural and biocatalytic characterisation. PLOS One **8**(9), e73642 (2013b). https://doi.org/10.1371/journal.pone.0073642

M.L. Verma, R. Chaudhary, T. Tsuzuki, C.J. Barrow, M. Puri, Immobilization of β-glucosidase on a magnetic nanoparticle improves thermostability: application in cellobiose hydrolysis. Bioresour. Technol. **135**, 2–6 (2013c). https://doi.org/10.1016/j.biortech.2013.01.047

M.L. Verma, C.J. Barrow, M. Puri, Nanobiotechnology as a novel paradigm for enzyme immobilization and stabilisation with potential applications in biofuel production. Appl. Microbiol. Biotechnol. **97**, 23–39 (2013d). https://doi.org/10.1007/s00253-012-4535-9

M.L. Verma, C.J. Barrow, J.F. Kennedy, M. Puri, Immobilization of β-galactosidase from *Kluyveromyces Lactis* on functionalized silicon dioxide nanoparticles: characterization and lactose hydrolysis. Int. J. Biol. Macromol. **50**, 432–437 (2012). https://doi.org/10.1016/j.ijbiomac.2011.12.029

M.L. Verma, W. Azmi, S.S. Kanwar, Enzymatic synthesis of isopropyl acetate catalysed by immobilized Bacillus cereus lipase in organic medium. Enzym. Res., 919386 (2011). https://doi.org/10.4061/2011/919386

M.L. Verma, C.G.S. Chauhan, S.S. Kanwar, Enzymatic synthesis of isopropyl myristate using immobilized lipase from *Bacillus cereus* MTCC 8372. Acta Microbiol. Immunol. Hung. **55**(3), 327–342 (2008). https://doi.org/10.1556/AMicr.55.2008.3.4

M.L. Verma, R.E. Abraham, M. Puri, Nanobiocatalyst designing strategies and their applications in food industry, in *Biomass, Biofuels, Biochemicals Advances in Enzyme Catalysis and Technologies* ed. by S. P. Singh, A. Pandey, R. R.Singhania, C. Larroche, Z. Li (Elsevier, London UK, 2020), pp. 171–189. https://doi.org/10.1016/B978-0-12-819820-9.00010-7

J. Virkutyte, R.S. Varma, Green synthesis of metal nanoparticles: biodegradable polymers and enzymes in stabilization and surface functionalization. Them. Sci. **2**(5), 837–846 (2011). https://doi.org/10.1039/C0SC00338G

Y. Wang, D. Chen, G. Wang, C. Zhao, Y. Ma, W. Yang, Immobilization of cellulase on styrene/maleic anhydride copolymer nanoparticles with improved stability against pH changes. Chem. Eng. J. **336**, 152–159 (2017). https://doi.org/10.1016/j.cej.2017.11.030

H. Watanabe, G. Tokuda, Animal cellulases. Cell Mol. Life Sci. **58**, 1167–1178 (2001). https://doi.org/10.1007/PL00000931

J. Xu, Z. Sheng, X. Wang, X. Liu, J. Xia, P. Xiong, B. He, Enhancement in ionic liquid tolerance of cellulase immobilized on PEGylated graphene oxide nanosheets: Application in saccharification of lignocellulose. Bioresour. Technol. **200**, 1060–1064 (2016). https://doi.org/10.1016/j.biortech.2015.10.070

J. Xu, J. Sun, Y. Wang, J. Sheng, F. Wang, M. Sun, Application of iron magnetic nanoparticles in protein immobilization. Molecules **19**(11465–11), 486 (2014). https://doi.org/10.3390/molecules190811465

B. Yuan, X.Q. Yang, L.W. Xue, Y.N. Feng, J.H. Jiang, A novel recycling system for nano-magnetic molecular imprinting immobilised cellulases: Synergistic recovery of anthocyanin from fruit and vegetable waste. Bioresour. Technol. **222**, 14–23 (2016). https://doi.org/10.1016/j.biortech.2016.09.088

Q. Zhang, J. Kang, B. Yang, L. Zhao, Z. Hou, B. Tang, Immobilized cellulase on Fe_3O_4 nanoparticles as a magnetically recoverable biocatalyst for the decomposition of corncob. Chinese J. Catal. **37**, 389–397 (2016). https://doi.org/10.1016/S1872-2067(15)61028-2

X. Zhang, X. He, K. Wang, X. Yang, Different active biomolecules involved in biosynthesis of gold nanoparticles by three fungus species. J. Biomed. Nanotechnol. **7**, 245–254 (2011). https://doi.org/10.1166/jbn.2011.1285

Y. Zhou, S. Pan, X. Wei, L. Wang, Y. Liu, Immobilization of β-glucosidase onto magnetic nanoparticles and evaluation of the enzymatic properties. Bio Resour. **8**, 2605–2619 (2013). https://doi.org/10.15376/biores.8.2.2605-2619

Y. Zhou, S. Yuan, Q. Liu, D. Yan, Y. Wang, L. Gao, J. Han, H. Shi, Synchronized purification and immobilization of His-tagged β-glucosidase via Fe_3O_4/PMG core/shell magnetic nanoparticles. Sci. Rep. **7**, 41741 (2017). https://doi.org/10.1038/srep417411-11

Materials, Technologies, and Applications of 3D/4D Printing in Tissue Engineering

Shangsi Chen, Xiaodie Chen, Jie Huang, and Min Wang

Abstract This article gives an overview of 3D and 4D printing and bioprinting in tissue engineering and looks into 3D printing and bioprinting technologies, biomaterials, and applications in regenerative medicine. Generally, 3D and 4D printing and bioprinting are powerful manufacturing platforms and have unique advantages over other fabrication techniques. Each 3D printing or bioprinting technology has its advantages and limitations and the use of a particular printing technology in tissue engineering mainly depends on the structure and properties of the targeted tissue for regeneration and available biomaterial(s) for the printing ink/inks or bioink/bioinks. There have been successes in clinical applications or clinical trials for 3D/4D printed tissue engineering scaffolds and bioprinted living structures. But there are still many challenges for applying 3D/4D printing and bioprinting in the tissue engineering field. Concerted efforts need to be made to tackle these challenges successfully, which will lead to new and better tissue engineering products and consequently, desired clinical outcomes.

Keywords 3D printing · 4D printing · Bioprinting · Biomaterial · Ink · Bioink · Scaffold · Cell-scaffold construct · Tissue engineering · Regenerative medicine · Printability · Fidelity · Biocompatibility · Biodegradability · Performance

S. Chen · X. Chen · M. Wang (✉)
Department of Mechanical Engineering, The University of Hong Kong, Pokfulam, Hong Kong
e-mail: memwang@hku.hk

J. Huang
Department of Mechanical Engineering, University College London, London, UK

R. Narayan (ed.), *Nanostructured Biomaterials and Their Applications*,
https://doi.org/10.1007/978-3-032-16316-5_16

1 Introduction

1.1 Tissue Engineering

Tissue and organ dysfunction caused by aging, disease or injury has always been an unavoidable aspect of human lives, which impairs both physical and mental well-being of people and puts a huge pressure on the healthcare system of the society (Wang et al. 2024a; Villanueva-Flores et al. 2023). Tissue repair using autografts or allografts and organ transplantation have been the gold standard for treating failed tissues or organs in human bodies. However, problems of donor shortage, immunological rejection and possible disease transmission have severely limited use of autografts and allografts and particularly, organ transplantation. According to the latest data published on USA's Health Resources and Services Administration (HRSA) website (Resources and Administration 2023), 106,837 patients were on the transplant wait list while only 46,629 transplants were performed in 2024. Specifically, out of the total number of patients waiting for kidney transplantation, which was 89,792, only 27,332 received a transplant in 2024. Regrettably, an average of 17 individuals lost their lives each day while waiting for organ transplantation in the USA.

Over the past two decades, tissue engineering strategies have shown the promise of overcoming problems of donor shortage and organ transplantation issues by providing novel approaches for treating human tissue or organ dysfunction. The term "tissue engineering" first appeared in the late 1980s. In 1993, Langer and Vacanti provided the definition of tissue engineering as "an interdisciplinary field that applies the principles of engineering and life sciences toward the development of biological substitutes that restore, maintain, or improve (biological tissue) function or a whole organ" (Langer and Vacanti 1993). Tissue engineering strategies can be divided into cell-based, biomolecule-based, and scaffold-based tissue engineering, and the field is dominated by scaffold-based tissue engineering. In scaffold-based tissue engineering, there are three essential components: cells, biomolecules, and scaffolds. Therefore, most current tissue engineering strategies aim to construct three-dimensional (3D) structures to mimic the physiological structure and functions of the targeted tissue or organ through the combination of suitable biomaterials (natural or synthetic) and cells (mature cells or stem cells, particularly autologous stem cells in recent years) with the incorporation of appropriate biomolecules (for guiding cell growth and differentiation) (Pajooh et al. 2024; Rana and Siegler 2024). After implantation in the body, the 3D scaffolds or constructs perform to restore, maintain, or improve the functions of the targeted tissue or organ. There are sets of requirements for scaffolds targeting as specific tissues/organs. Generally, a tissue engineering scaffold should possess

(1) Biocompatibility: The scaffold [and hence the scaffold material(s)] should not elicit an unfavorable immune response after implantation, and the biodegradation product(s) must be non-toxic and should not affect normal cell behavior and new tissue formation.
(2) Biodegradability: The scaffold after implantation should degrade in the body environment so as to allow cells to produce their own extracellular matrix (ECM) to occupy the space in the porous scaffold, resulting in the formation of new tissue (i.e., tissue regeneration). It is ideal that the biodegradation rate of implanted scaffold matches the speed of tissue regeneration.
(3) Suitable porous structure: Interconnected pores and high (or, adequate) porosity are essential for oxygen and nutrient transportation and waste removal. Furthermore, the pore size and pore shape play a crucial role in affecting/guiding cell behavior, including cell attachment, migration, proliferation, and differentiation.
(4) Appropriate mechanical properties: The scaffold should have the strength and modulus appropriate for the implantation site and be sufficiently strong to provide mechanical support for the surrounding tissue. It must have adequate mechanical properties for handling during operation.

Today, tissue engineering is a thriving and rapidly evolving field. There are thousands of companies, large or small, involved in tissue engineering and the global tissue engineering market is projected to have a robust growth, with an anticipated increase from US$17.48 billion in 2025 to US$29.92 billion in 2029, reflecting a remarkable compound annual growth rate (CAGR) of 14.4% (Research and Markets 2025).

1.2 Developments of 3D/4D Printing

Many fabrication techniques, including solvent casting and particle leaching, freeze-drying, gas foaming, thermal-induced phasing separation (TIPS), and electrospinning, have been extensively investigated and used to construct 3D tissue engineering scaffolds. However, most of these techniques are unable to precisely control the microstructure (e.g., pore shape, pore size, porosity, and pore interconnectivity) of resulting 3D scaffolds. Therefore, 3D printing technologies and four-dimensional (4D) printing have flourished in the tissue engineering field as they can provide unprecedented capabilities for engineering customized, complex biomedical products accurately and show high reproducibility for manufactured products through layer-by-layer positioning of material(s), biomolecules, and in bioprinting, living cells in 3D structures according to the designs of these products that are achieved by computer-aided design (CAD). 3D/4D printing and bioprinting, which involves bioinks that contain living cells, are gaining popularity in the biomedical field.

The concept of 3D printing can be traced back to the early 1980s in Japan (Fig. 1). In 1981, Kodama attempted to develop a rapid prototyping system using the layer-by-layer approach for fabrication, employing an ultraviolet (UV) light to polymerize photosensitive resin. This was the predecessor of stereolithography (SLA). Unfortunately, Kodama was unable to file a patent for his technology. Hull of USA proposed stereolithography in 1984 and patented the first 3D printer for SLA in the US in 1986 (Hull 1984), opening the era of 3D printing. Also in 1986, Deckard developed another 3D printing technology, selective laser sintering (SLS), at University of Texas at Austin, USA, using a laser beam to sinter solid powders layer-by-layer to form 3D structures (Deckard 1989). Bioprinting was first demonstrated in 1988 when Klebe used a standard Hewlett-Packard (HP) inkjet printer to deposit cells for constructing synthetic tissues in 3D (Klebe 1988). In 1989, fused deposition modeling (FDM), which uses heat to soften filaments of a polymer and extrudes the filaments layer-by-layer to form 3D objects, was patented by Crump, co-founder of Stratasys Inc. (Crump 1992). Subsequently, binder jet 3D printing was developed at Massachusetts Institute of Technology (MIT), USA, and Sachs et al. patented this technology in 1993 (Sachs et al. 1993). 4D printing emerged in 2013 when Tibbits of MIT introduced the concept and term of "4D printing" in a TED talk. In addition to the physical three dimensions in 3D printing, time is the fourth dimension in 4D printing. 4D printed objects during their service time can change their shape and/or properties over time in response to suitable external/internal stimulus/stimuli (e.g., temperature, pH, humidity, and light), while objects fabricated via 3D printing stay static without shape or property changes. Generally, 4D printed structures having shape morphing and/or property-change capabilities are fabricated via 3D printing technologies but use the so-called smart materials that are sensitive to external stimulus/stimuli, i.e., stimulus-responsive materials.

Using 3D printing of a human ear model as an example, a typical 3D printing process for producing tissue engineering products is illustrated in Fig. 2. Generally, a 3D printing operation can be divided into two stages: the pre-printing stage and 3D printing stage. The pre-printing stage involves acquisition of image data from modern medical imaging techniques such as computed tomography (CT) and magnetic resonance imaging (MRI) and on computers, construction of 3D models from the image data for subsequent use in 3D printing (Lai et al. 2021a). In brief, images of a patient's tissue(s) and organ are obtained via CT, MRI, or ultrasound imaging. Then, the image data is used to construct 3D models on a computer using CAD software. The constructed 3D models are subsequently converted into the stereolithography

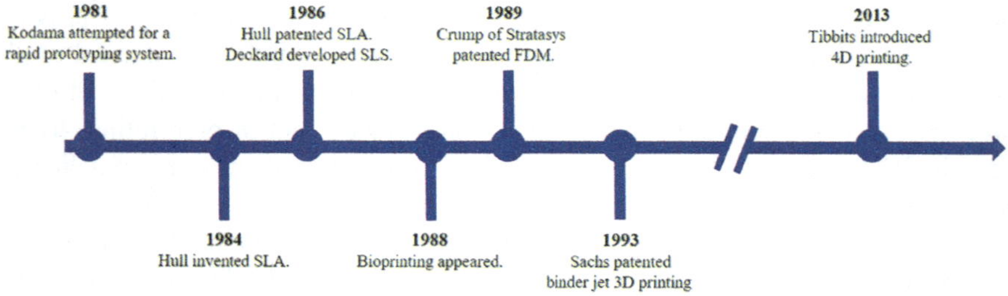

Fig. 1 Timeline for developments of 3D printing and 4D printing

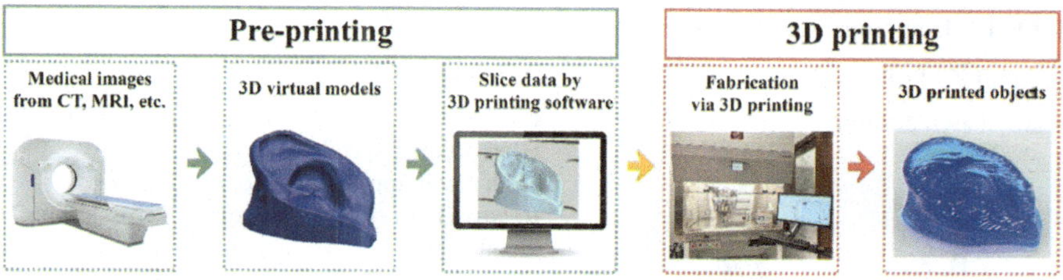

Fig. 2 Typical 3D printing process for fabricating tissue engineering products

(STL) file format, which is a commonly accepted file format for most 3D printers in the market. The 3D printing stage involves importing the STL file into a 3D printer and operating the 3D printer to perform 3D printing. After importing the STL file and during the printing operation, the 3D printer can recapitulate precisely computer-created 3D models by placing biomaterial(s), biomolecules, and in bioprinting, living cells in the 3D structure in a lay-by-layer manner, thereby fabricating the designed 3D structure.

2 3D/4D Printing Technologies

On the basis of their working principles, 3D printing technologies can be classified into three major categories: (1) inkjet-based printing, (2) laser-assisted printing, and (3) extrusion-based printing. Each 3D printing technique has its own particular advantages and limitations. Table 1 provides illustrations and also comparisons for 3D printing technologies in these three categories.

2.1 Inkjet-Based 3D Printing

An inkjet-based printer ejects inks or bioinks out of a nozzle, forming droplets and then depositing the droplets onto a substrate to fabricate 3D structures layer-by-layer. Inkjet-based printing can be sub-divided into two different systems: continuous inkjet printing and drop-on-demand inkjet printing. A continuous inkjet printer can eject continuously ink or bioink droplets under pressure. Although the movement of droplets can be tuned during printing, the printing process can be unstable and the manipulation cannot be precise. A drop-on-demand inkjet printer enables precise control and positioning of ejected droplets because it uses an actuator to generate pluses to eject droplets on-demand. Based on the types of actuators, a drop-on-demand inkjet printer can be a thermal or piezoelectrical system. In thermal drop-on-demand inkjet printing, when a voltage pulse is applied to the thermal actuator to locally heat the ink or bioink, a vapor bubble forms, expands and explodes and

Table 1 3D printing technologies and their comparisons

3D printing technology	Advantages	Shortcomings
Inkjet-based printing 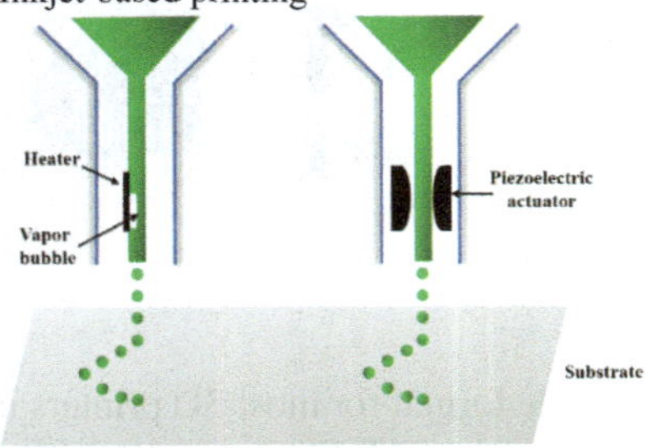 	Low cost High printing speed High resolution Relative high cell viability for bioprinting	Low viscosity of inks or bioinks Nozzle clogging Requiring crosslinking treatment Low cell density for bioprinting
Laser-assisted printing 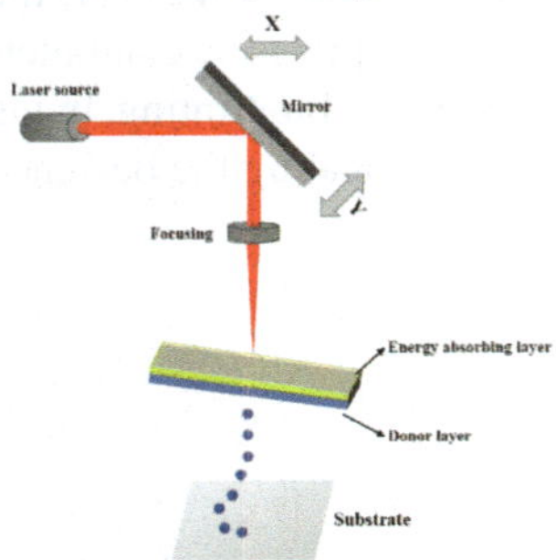 	Nozzle-free printing High resolution High cell viability for bioprinting	High cost Complexity of controlling laser pulse Risk of laser irradiation
Extrusion-based printing 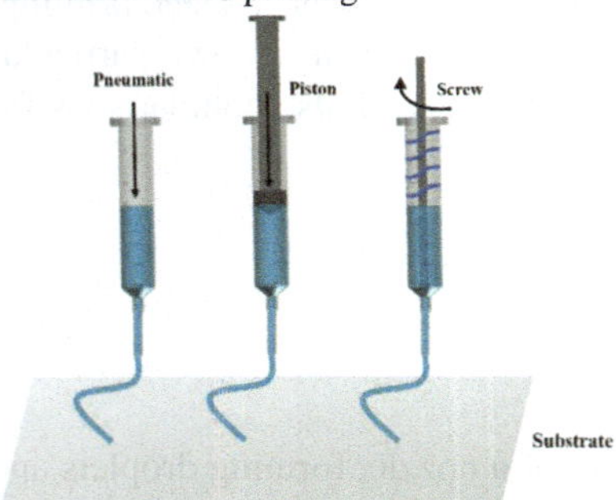 	Applicable for a wide range of biomaterials High viscosity Scalability	Low resolution Nozzle clogging Low cell viability for bioprinting

then the printer ejects droplets out of the nozzle. On the other hand, a piezoelectrical drop-on-demand inkjet printer uses a piezoelectrical actuator to generate expansion or contraction upon the application of voltage pulses. As a result, the expansion or contraction can cause the deformation of printing chamber and therefore generate pressure to eject droplets from the nozzle (Li et al. 2020).

Advantages of inkjet-based printing include

(1) Affordability: Due to the similar structure to commercial office printers, the cost of inkjet-based printers is low and they are affordable.

(2) High printing speed: Inkjet-based printers can eject ~ 10,000 droplets per second.
(3) High resolution: The resolution of printed structures can be 50–500 μm.
(4) Relative high cell viability for bioprinting: The cell viability for inkjet-based bioprinting is usually up to 80–90%.

On the other hand, inkjet-based printing has limitations, including

(1) Low viscosity of inks or bioinks: Only inks or bioinks with a low viscosity (3–12 mPa s) can be printed.
(2) Nozzle clogging: The nozzle can be easily blocked during printing.
(3) Crosslinking treatment: An additional crosslinking treatment is necessary for maintaining the printed structure and its good fidelity.
(4) Low cell density for bioprinting: The low viscosity of bioinks limits the concentration of cells ($< 1 \times 10^6$ cells/mL).

2.2 Laser-Assisted 3D Printing

Laser-assisted printing utilizes laser energy to pattern inks or bioinks in a 3D spatial arrangement layer-by-layer. A typical laser-assisted printing system consists of three main components: a laser source (either pulsed or continuous), a layer of printing inks or bioinks placed under the laser transparent print ribbon (with or without a laser energy absorbing layer), and a substrate to collect the deposited inks or bioinks (Vijayavenkataraman et al. 2018). During the printing process, a focused laser pulse is applied to the energy absorbing layer and then vaporize a small area of a donor layer, causing a high-pressure bubble at the interface of ink or bioink layer, thereby propelling the suspended inks or bioinks. The falling inks or bioinks are then received by the substrate and crosslinked to form a 3D structure. Laser-assisted printing has many advantages, such as nozzle-free printing (thus avoiding the nozzle clogging problem), high resolution, (~ 50 μm) and high cell viability (> 95%) for bioprinting. However, the high cost of laser systems, the complexity of controlling laser pulses, low viscosity of inks or bioinks (1–300 mPa s), and the risk of laser exposure to cause cell apoptosis are the challenges that still need to be addressed.

2.3 Extrusion-Based 3D Printing

Extrusion-based printing provides the most popular 3D printing technologies for fabricating 3D tissue engineering products. Unlike inkjet-based printing that ejects only inks or bioinks with a low viscosity (~ 10 mPa s), inks or bioinks with a high viscosity ($30–6 \times 10^7$ mPa s) can be pneumatically (via pressure) or mechanically (via a piston or rotating screw) printed in extrusion-based printing (Matai et al.

2020). Also, instead of droplets being ejected in inkjet-based printing, extrusion-based printing can print out continuously filaments to fabricate 3D structures layer-by-layer upon applying the pressure for extrusion. In extrusion-based printing, inks or bioinks are placed in a printing syringe. By optimizing printing parameters (e.g., pressure, printing speed, and temperature), continuous filaments are extruded from the nozzle of the printing head of the machine onto the substrate to form 3D structures. Subsequently, the polymer(s) in printed objects can be crosslinked by UV light, heat, ionic solution, or enzymes.

Extrusion-based printing has many advantages, including

(1) Suitable for a wide range of biomaterials: Almost all types of solutions or suspensions (from, e.g., polymer, ceramic or metal) with the shear thinning behavior can be printed for fabricating 3D objects.
(2) High viscosity: Compared to inkjet-based or laser-assisted printing, extrusion-based printing can process inks and bioinks with very high viscosity through modulating printing parameters such as pressure and printing speed.
(3) Scalability: Extrusion-based printing can fabricate large-size 3D structures, e.g., human-scale tissues or organs, after laboratory-scale, small-size printing investigations.

However, compared with inkjet-based or laser-based printing, extrusion-based printing shows the lowest printing resolution (~ 100 μm). Also, the nozzle clogging problem often occurs. Furthermore, due to the high (or, relatively high) shear stress generated in the nozzle of the printing head for 3D printing, which can cause cell death, extrusion-based printing usually exhibits a low cell viability for bioprinting.

3 Requirements for Printing Inks and 3D Printed Structures

Many biomaterials have been developed and used for printing inks or bioinks for fabricating 3D structures for tissue engineering applications. There are specific requirements for inks and bioinks and also printed structures, as shown in Fig. 3, in order to create desirable tissue engineering products via 3D printing and bioprinting. For 3D printing and bioprinting in tissue engineering, two important aspects must be considered:

(1) Printing inks or bioinks: Properties of the materials for the inks or bioinks and the inks or bioinks themselves should possess good (or, appropriate) printability, biocompatibility, and biodegradability.
(2) Printed objects: The fidelity of printed structures, when compared to their designs, must be high, or, at least acceptable, which will ensure proper properties and functions.

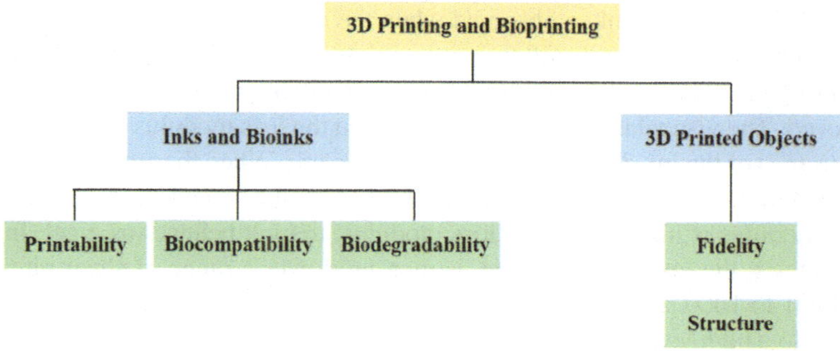

Fig. 3 Summary of requirements for 3D printing and bioprinting in tissue engineering

3.1 Printability

Printability is a crucial factor that characterizes the suitability of inks or bioinks for 3D printing or bioprinting. In general, printability refers to the ability of an ink or bioink to be printed continuously and consistently and to form and maintain a 3D structure in accordance with the design obtained through CAD prior to 3D printing. Inks of suitable printability determine the final structure of 3D printed objects, such as pore shape, pore size, and porosity, and, as a result, affect the mechanical properties and biological performance of the printed object. Many factors can affect the printability of an ink or bioink, including design features (e.g., scaffold external shape and dimensions, pore shape, pore curvature, pore size, and layer thickness), materials properties (e.g., viscosity, thixotropy, and mechanical properties), and printing parameters (e.g., printing pressure, nozzle inner diameter, and printing speed). Layer thickness is a structure design-related factor that significantly affects ink printability. Inks or bioinks having low printability can result in inconsistency of layer thickness, increase in filament diameter and decrease in both pore size and printing resolution. Viscosity is another crucial material-related parameter. For example, gelatin (Gel) is a popular biomaterial for 3D printing in tissue engineering. Gel solutions with low Gel concentrations and, hence, low viscosity exhibit poor printability in extrusion-based 3D printing. When added by other materials to increase the viscosity of Gel-based inks or bioinks, the printability could be improved (Ivone et al. 2021). Furthermore, in extrusion-based printing, the printing pressure determines the extrusion speed for inks or bioinks, while the extrusion speed equates to the printing speed. A high pressure can cause over-deposition of an ink or bioink, resulting in an increase in filament thickness, a decrease in pore size and distortion of the pore shape. A low pressure can result in inconsistency in ink or bioink extrusion.

The flow behavior of an ink or bioink significantly influences its printability for extrusion 3D printing and hence rheological properties of the ink or bioink are usually investigated prior to 3D printing. The rheological study of an inks or bioink is conducted typically using three types of tests: shear thinning tests, angular frequency sweep tests, and thixotropy tests (Lai et al. 2021b; Chen et al. 2024a). The shear thinning behavior of an ink is observed when the viscosity of its samples decreases with an increase in shear rate, allowing the ink to flow easily through the nozzle of the printing head during 3D printing and form stable filaments once the shear stress is removed. The viscoelastic relationship between the loss modulus (G'') and storage modulus (G') of the ink determines the state of the ink. When the storage modulus of the ink is lower than the loss modulus, it exhibits sol-like behavior; conversely, if the storage modulus is higher than the loss modulus, the ink behaves as a gel. In shear thinning tests, the viscosity of an ink is measured over a range of shear rates, e.g., from 0.001 to 1000 s^{-1}. In angular frequency sweep tests, the strain sweeps from a low level to a high level (e.g., from 0.1 to 100%) over a range of angular frequencies (e.g., 0.1–100 rad^{-1}) so as to locate the linear viscoelastic region (LVR). Thixotropy tests are performed in three steps to assess the recoverability of an ink in the gel state. In Step I, a low shear rate, e.g., 0.1 s^{-1}, is applied to the ink sample to observe the state of the ink without a shear force, simulating the situation prior to 3D printing. In Step II, the shear rate is instantaneously and substantially increased to a high level and held for a short period to observe the shear state of the ink, simulating the situation during 3D printing. In Step III, the shear rate is restored to the low level and held for a period to observe the recovery of viscosity of the ink, simulating the situation after printing. During the process of shearing, the polymer chains in the ink undergo alignment. However, once the shearing ceases, the polymer networks gradually return to their original state, thereby restoring their higher viscosity level. The ink structure change and recovery take a certain amount of time, which is the thixotropy of the ink. A quick return to a high viscosity after a high shear rate is removed means good thixotropy and hence good printability of the ink. Good thixotropy of an ink also suggests high fidelity of 3D printed structures from the ink (refer to Sect. 3.4).

Given its great importance for 3D printing, the printability of an ink under development should be measured accurately and assessed. Currently, many methods and formulae have been employed for this purpose (Naghieh and Chen 2021). Generally, indexes taking into account the overall geometry and inner structure of printed objects, such as external shape irregularity, pore printability, strand printability, and diffusion rate, are the major parameters for indicating/comparing printability. These parameters can be calculated using equations shown below. The irregularity (I) of a 3D printed object defines the overall accuracy of 3D printing by comparing the experimental length of the three dimensions (X, Y, and Z) with the design length in the three dimensions (Eq. 1). Pore printability (P) is now commonly used to determine the difference between the experimental pore shape and design pore shape (Eq. 2), which is also used to assess the fidelity of 3D printed structures (refer to Sect. 3.4). Strand printability (P_s) is calculated for the comparison between the experimental strand diameter and design strand diameter (Eq. 3). Diffusion rate (D) characterizes the decreasing tendency of the actual pore area in comparison with the design pore area (Eq. 4). The irregularity of a 3D printed object, I, is calculated by

$$I\ (\%) = \frac{L'x, y, z}{Lx, y, z} \times 100 \tag{1}$$

where $L'x, y, z$ is the experimental length of the three dimensions (X, Y, and Z) of the 3D printed object, and Lx, y, z is the design length of the three dimensions. The pore printability, P, is calculated by

$$P = \frac{L^2}{16A} \tag{2}$$

where L is the perimeter of the pore and A is the area of the pore. The strand printability, P_s, is calculated by

$$P_s = \frac{D'}{D_s} \tag{3}$$

where D' is the experimental strand diameter and D_s is the design strand diameter. The diffusion rate, D, is calculated by

$$D\,(\%) = \frac{A - A'}{A} \times 100 \tag{4}$$

where A is the area of design pore and A' is the area of actual pore.

3.2 *Biocompatibility*

Biocompatibility is the foremost criterion for inks or bioinks for 3D printing in tissue engineering application, which enables printed structures to support cell activities (i.e., adhesion, migration, proliferation, and differentiation) without eliciting unwanted immune reaction and severe inflammatory response. It should be noted that biocompatible materials are allowed to trigger appropriate inflammatory reaction after being implanted in the body. Many studies have shown that an inflammatory response is inevitable when biomaterials are implanted in vivo. Moreover, an appropriate inflammatory response is beneficial for tissue regeneration. The implanted materials, whether they are metals, ceramics, polymers, or composites, are surrounded by the host biological tissues, react with the adjacent environment (water, enzymes, pH, cells, etc.), and in most situations, become corroded or degraded, thereby releasing degradation and ionic products and debris. The degradation products or debris should be biocompatible and should not elicit severe unwanted host response. Ideally, the degradation products should be easily cleared up by the host. In many circumstances, while the material inks are biocompatible, but in order to maintain the structures after printing, printed scaffolds are crosslinked by some chemicals that show cytotoxicity. For example, Gel-based scaffolds have been commonly crosslinked by glutaraldehyde for improving their mechanical properties. Cytotoxic photoinitiators [e.g., 2-Hydroxy-4′-(2-hydroxyethoxy)-2-methylpropiophenone] are mixed in gelatin methacryloyl (GelMA)-based inks to enable chemical crosslinking upon exposure to a UV light. In this context, residual chemicals should be removed before scaffold implantation or the amount of these chemicals should be reduced below the safety limit. Overall, printing inks and bioinks and 3D printed products should be biocompatible.

There are national and international standards for biocompatibility testing to evaluate the materials intended for biomedical applications. These standards can be used for evaluating biomaterials for inks and bioinks, as well as 3D printed products. Generally, biological evaluations include in vitro and in vivo experiments related to the cytocompatibility, genotoxicity, sensitization, irritation, acute and chronic toxicity, hemocompatibility, reproductive and developmental toxicity, and carcinogenicity (Huzum et al. 2021).

3.3 Biodegradability

Biodegradability is another important property for 3D printed tissue engineering products. Biodegradability refers to the ability of a material to decompose or degrade in the biological environment. After a material is implanted in the body, its biodegradation occurs when it interacts with various biological molecules and species. Biodegradation is unavoidable for all types of materials. According to the definition provided by International Union of Pure and Applied Chemistry (IUPAC), biodegradation is material degradation caused by enzymatic process resulting from the action of cells. In Europe, the EU 13432 standard defines biodegradation as chemical breakdown of at least 90% of a material into CO_2, water, and minerals in six months by biological reactions. Vert et al. suggested that biodegradation is chemical breakdown of a material mediated by any component of the physiological environment (water, ions, proteins, cells, bacteria, etc.) into smaller constituents or low molecular weight products which are then processed, resorbed or cleared by the body (Vert et al. 2012). Even though tissue engineering materials are generally required to be biodegradable, a good number of well-established biomaterials that are non-biodegradable and can maintain their structure and properties in the biological environment for a period of time have also been used in investigations for 3D printing in tissue engineering. For example, Ti and Ti–6Al–4V alloy are known non-biodegradable orthopedic metals but they have been made into porous cages via selective laser melting (SLM) 3D printing for spinal fusion applications. Also, some non-biodegradable bioceramics (e.g., alumina and zirconia ceramics) have been mixed with bioactive hydroxyapatite (HAp) and made via digital light processing (DLP)-based 3D printing into dental devices. Nevertheless, in the conventional sense of tissue engineering, biomaterials used for tissue engineering should be biodegradable and consequently, it will be ideal that all materials that make up individual inks and bioinks should be biodegradable. With current status and availability of biodegradable materials, biodegradable polymers (natural or synthetic) dominate and therefore, currently, inks and bioinks are mainly based on polymers, polymer blends, and polymer-based composites, with some systems being based on biodegradable bioceramics, while reports appearing occasionally for 3D printing of biodegradable Mg-based alloys.

It is important that the biodegradation rate of a 3D printed tissue engineering product should be comparable with the speed of tissue regeneration in the body. The biodegradation rates of different biomaterials can vary greatly. There are different strategies that can be used to control the biodegradation rates of biomaterials and hence those of the 3D printed products of these materials. Natural polymers [e.g., collagen (Col), Gel and alginate (Alg)] degrade very fast in the biological environment. Ceramics such as β-tricalcium phosphate (β-TCP) and synthetic polymers, such as poly(lactic acid) (PLA), poly(ε-caprolactone) (PCL), and poly(lactic-co-glycolic acid) (PLGA), exhibit relatively slow biodegradation. Therefore, natural polymers can be mixed with synthetic polymers or ceramics to obtain polymer blends or composites for achieving the desired degradation rates. Also, many polymers, natural, or synthetic, can be physically or chemically crosslinked through different mechanisms so as to achieve desirable biodegradation rates, thereby controlling the structural integrity and properties of their 3D printed products during biodegradation processes. Furthermore, the structural characteristics (porous or non-porous, porosity, pore size, etc.) significantly affect the biodegradation rate of 3D printed products. Compared with non-porous structures, porous scaffolds of the same biomaterial can be degraded more quickly in the biological environment.

3.4 *Fidelity of 3D Printed Objects*

Fidelity is an important parameter that shows the structural closeness between the 3D printed object and its design made via computer software for 3D printing. It can also be defined as the ability to maintain the structure of a 3D printed object. Since fidelity is used to evaluate how similar the final printed structure is to the original design, the deformation of printed and laid-down filaments and also the whole printed structure can be employed for assessing fidelity. It needs to be point out that fidelity can determine the resolution of 3D printing. For a printed structure, poor fidelity can cause diffusion of printed filaments and hence an increase in filament diameter (i.e., width) and a decrease in filament height, thereby impairing 3D printing resolution. Furthermore, a printed object with poor fidelity is unable to maintain its spatial structure and may collapse, especially in the case of multilayered structures with a high number of layers. Fidelity significantly affects the pore shape and pore size of printed objects. In 3D tissue engineering scaffolds, pores are intended for the transport of oxygen and nutrients and removal of the waste. Printed objects with poor fidelity will have had their pore shape and pore size changed, which may compromise the transportation of oxygen and nutrients and removal of waste. For extrusion-based 3D printing, printability and fidelity are closely linked parameters. Equations 2, 3, and 4 shown in Sect. 3.1 can also be used for calculations for the fidelity of 3D printed structures, with Eq. 2 being very often used by many researchers.

Several factors can significantly affect the fidelity of 3D printed objects. They include:

(1) Rheological properties (particularly viscosity) of inks or bioinks: For extrusion-based 3D printing, inks or bioinks with high viscosity result in better fidelity (Schwab et al. 2020). For example, a polymer-based ink with a high polymer concentration has high viscosity and hence its 3D printed objects exhibit high fidelity.
(2) Printing parameters: Printing parameters, including pressure, printing speed, and nozzle shape and inner diameter, determine the shape and diameter of printed and laid-down filaments and hence the fidelity of 3D printed objects.
(3) Crosslinking of polymer(s): After (or, during) 3D printing, in many situations, the printed objects need to be crosslinked, physically, or chemically, in order to maintain the printed structure and avoid shape deformation. For example, to improve shape fidelity, Alg-based inks or bioinks can be printed in a Ca^{2+} water bath that will ionically crosslink the Alg polymer.

4 Biomaterials for 3D Printing

3D printing is a powerful manufacturing platform that has been increasingly used to fabricate porous scaffolds with complex structures and cell-scaffold constructs for body tissue regeneration. One challenge for 3D printing in tissue engineering is to find suitable materials or develop new materials that have desirable properties (biocompatibility, printability, biodegradability, fidelity, etc.) (Mathur et al. 2025; Kumar et al. 2025). Up until now, commonly used materials for 3D printing for tissue engineering are mainly biomedical polymers and their blends and composites while 3D printing of bioceramics and metallic biomaterials are also reported from time to time.

4.1 Biomedical Polymers

Due to their good biocompatibility and biodegradability and the ability to mimic the structure of ECM by natural polymers, a great variety of biomedical polymers, natural or synthetic, have been employed to construct tissue engineering scaffolds via 3D printing (Satchanska et al. 2024; Tao et al. 2025a).

4.1.1 Natural Polymers

Natural polymers are mainly derived from living organisms (animals, plants, microorganisms, etc.). They are biomacromolecules that usually consist of a single or several functional monomers. Because these polymer macromolecules can retain the biochemical cues and possess high similarity in structure to the ECM of native tissues which modulate cell activities, such as cell migration, attachment, proliferation, and differentiation, they have been extensively employed for fabricating tissue engineering scaffolds via 3D printing. Polysaccharides [e.g., Alg, hyaluronic acid (HA), chitosan (CS), and cellulose] and proteins [e.g., Col, silk, Gel, and fibrin] are two main compositions for natural polymers for 3D printing (Behrooznia et al. 2025; Kantaros et al. 2025). However, the intrinsic drawbacks, including batch-to-batch variation, possible immunological reaction, uncontrollable degradation rate, and poor mechanical strength, make it difficult for widely applying natural polymers in 3D printing for tissue engineering.

Collagen (Lee et al. 2021; Li et al. 2024) is the main component of ECM in human bodies and can provide specific cell binding sites to modulate cell behavior, such as offering RGD sequences (arginine, glycine, and aspartic acid) to promote cell adhesion. Consequently, 3D printed Col scaffolds have been widely seen for treating defects in various tissues, including bone, skin, blood vessel, and neural tissue (Debnath et al. 2025). For example, many studies have shown that 3D printed Col-based scaffolds are conducive to enhance osteogenesis in vitro and in vivo. Gel is a denatured protein that is obtained from the hydrolysis of Col. Different from Col, Gel preserves the RGD sequences and lacks immunogenicity. Because of its thermosensitive property (i.e., at room temperature, Gel molecules in a solution can be physically crosslinked and thus Gel changes from liquid to the solid state and when the temperature rises to the physiological temperature, Gel becomes liquid), Gel is a remarkable biomaterial and has been explored for 3D printing. In many investigations, Gel has been utilized to improve the printability of other materials. But Gel can be quickly degraded at the physiological temperature. To overcome this problem, GelMA (Van Hoorick et al. 2019; Chen et al. 2023), a modified Gel, is synthesized for 3D printing work in many recent investigations. GelMA retains the thermosensitive property and can be chemically crosslinked upon exposure to a UV light, which improves its properties (printing, mechanical, biodegradation, etc.), making it a focus in recent 3D printing and bioprinting research (Das et al. 2024). Many studies have used GelMA-based inks or bioinks to fabricate hydrogel scaffolds and cell-laden structures for tissue engineering applications.

Alginate is a natural polysaccharide derived from the cell wall of brown marine algae (seaweed) or bacteria (Rastogi and Kandasubramanian 2019). Alg is built up mainly from two primary monomers, 1,4-β-D-mannuronic acid (M) and 1,4-α-L-guluronic acid (G). It should be noted that Alg extracted from different sources possesses the configuration difference in the content of M and G units which can affect mechanical and physicochemical properties. Although Alg is biocompatible and biodegradable, the insufficient mechanical strength and biological performance (e.g., lacking RGD sequence for promoting cell attachment) is its weakness. To improve structure stability and mechanical strength, 3D printed Alg-based scaffolds can be crosslinked by several cation ions, such as Ca^{2+}, Mg^{2+}, Sr^{2+}, and Ba^{2+}. In addition, Alg can be oxidized to synthesize derivatives for providing more reactive sites in the polymer chains and thus improve biodegradability and biological performance.

Hyaluronic acid is a linear macromolecule composed of anionic non-sulfated glycosaminoglycans (GAGs) and is widely distributed in soft connective tissues (Ding et al. 2023; Yadav et al. 2025). Owing to its high molecule weight (1×10^5 to 1×10^7 Da) and extraordinary ability to absorb water, it can maintain structure integrity and viscoelasticity and helps lubrication of tissues. In addition to its excellent biocompatibility and biodegradability, HA plays important roles in modulating cell activities and inflammation and tissue regeneration by interacting with its transmembrane receptor CD44 to initiate intracellular signaling. HA can not only be used to construct 3D printed hydrogel scaffolds for tissue regeneration but also employed as cell-laden bioinks in 3D bioprinting for encapsulating and delivering cells.

4.1.2 Synthetic Polymers

Unlike natural polymers that are poor in controlling biodegradation, the structure, and physiochemical properties of synthetic polymers can be controlled/tailored by chemical reactions for specific tissue engineering applications. The biodegradation behavior and mechanical properties of synthetic polymers can be tuned by adjusting their chemical compositions, average molecular weight and crystallinity (if it is a semi-crystalline polymer). Generally, synthetic polymers are bioinert and exhibit higher mechanical strength and slower biodegradation as compared to natural polymers (Shanno et al. 2025). So far, the most commonly used synthetic polymers for fabricating 3D printed tissue engineering scaffolds include PCL, PLA, and PLGA. All of these synthetic polymers have been approved by the U.S. Food and Drug Administration (FDA) for tissue engineering applications.

Poly(ε-caprolactone) is a thermoplastic aliphatic polyester with a semi-crystallinity structure (Arif et al. 2022). It can be degraded by the hydrolysis of its ester bonds in the physiological environment. However, the biodegradation duration can be up to three to four years. The melting point of PCL is around 60 °C. Therefore, PCL is usually heated up over its melting points and then extruded from the nozzle for fabrication of 3D scaffolds via FDM. Alternatively, PCL can be dissolved in an organic solvent to form viscoelastic inks for 3D printing. Owing to excellent mechanical properties, 3D printed PCL scaffolds exhibit great potential for hard tissue regeneration including spine. On the other hand, due to the hydrophobic nature and lack of bioactive motifs that provide specific binding sites for cells, PCL should combine with other function biomaterials (e.g., natural polymers and bioceramics) to create 3D composite scaffolds for promoting biological performance.

Poly(lactic acid) is an industrially produced polyester via polymerization of lactic acid monomer and can be poly(L-lactic acid) (PLLA) or poly(D,L-lactic acid) (PDLLA) (Bhagia et al. 2021). As a commercial PLA, the structure and physicochemical properties of PDLLA vary significantly. The biodegradation rate and crystallinity of PDLLA can be tuned through controlling the ratio of stereoisomer distribution (the *L/D* ratio). When the content of poly(D-lactic acid) (PDLA) is over 20%, PDLLA can be an amorphous polymer. If the content of PLLA is more than 90%, PDLLA can have a high crystallinity. Additionally, by changing the *L/D* ratio, PDLLA can be completely biodegraded within 12 months. Since the hydrolysis of backbone ester groups in PDLLA can release LA monomer into the surrounding environment, the acidic degradation products can cause a local inflammation response in vivo, which needs to be avoided for tissue regeneration.

Poly(lactic-co-glycolic acid) is a biocompatible and biodegradable aliphatic amorphous polymer produced by the polymerization of two monomers, lactic acid and glycolic acid (Jin et al. 2021). Owing to the different LA:GA ratio in PLGA, the molecular weight of PLGA varies from several thousands of Daltons to hundreds of thousands of Daltons, which significantly affects properties of PLGA. For example, PLGA exhibits a glass transition temperature (T_g) at 40–60 °C. The increase in LA content and molecular weight of PLGA can cause the increase of T_g. On the other hand, the biodegradation of PLGA can be tuned from several weeks to several months by varying the LA:GA ratio. Generally, PLGA with the LA:GA ratio at 75:25 is the most commonly used PLGA because of its suitable biodegradation rate and mechanical strength. Similar to PLA, the acidic biodegradation product of PLGA can trigger inflammation response in vivo.

4.1.3 Polymer Blends

Although natural polymers are biodegradable and can provide biological cues for modulating cell activities, their poor mechanical strength and fast biodegradation have limited their applications (Guo et al. 2024; Gayathri et al. 2025). On the other hand, synthetics polymers have their advantages and disadvantages for biomedical applications as discussed in the previous section. Therefore, polymer blends, which are made by physically blending two polymers, are often created for targeted applications. Particularly, polymer blends combining natural polymers with synthetic polymers can have much improved strength while retaining the very useful biological properties. For example, Col is essential component in bone. Many studies have shown the effectiveness of employing Col for bone tissue reconstruction. However, 3D printed Col scaffolds are rarely made and used for treating load-bearing bone defects due to poor mechanical strength and rapid biodegradation. Therefore, Col is mixed with other biomaterials (e.g., PLA, PCL, Hap, or β-TCP) to fabricate bone tissue engineering scaffolds (Nguyen et al. 2022; Han et al. 2015). Both in vitro and in vivo studies have shown that 3D printed PLA/Col, PCL/Col, HAp/Col, and β-TCP/Col scaffolds all have good mechanical properties and suitable biodegradation rate, which are beneficial for bone tissue regeneration. On the other hand, synthetic polymers possess tunable biodegradation rate and good mechanical strength but usually lack bioactivity and appropriate surface cues for regulating cell behavior. Therefore, synthetic polymers are mixed with natural polymers to improve biological properties. In addition, a pure natural or synthetic polymer may exhibit low viscosity, which is not suitable for extrusion-based 3D printing. Using a polymer blend may solve this problem. Chen et al.'s investigation demonstrated that the incorporation of methylcellulose into methacrylated-modified CS significantly improved the rheological properties and thus improved the printability of inks for 3D printing of scaffolds (Chen et al. 2024a).

4.2 *Bioceramics*

Bioceramics, including alumina (Al_2O_3), zirconia (ZrO_2) ceramics, carbons, bioactive glass (BG, such as Bioglass®), HAp, β-TCP, and biphasic calcium phosphate (BCP), have been used to construct 3D printed structures for tissue substitution or tissue regeneration. According to their interaction with the host tissue after implantation, they are classified as bioinert or bioactive ceramics. Bioactive ceramics can be further divided into resorbable and non-resorbable ceramics, depending on whether they will be degradable or resorbable in the biological environment.

Bioinert bioceramics (e.g., alumina, zirconia and carbons) are inert biomaterials and cause foreign body response after implantation in vivo, thereby forming acellular Col capsule surrounding them (Zhou et al. 2023). Even so, bioinert bioceramics have been used in clinical applications, particularly as dental implant and porous bone scaffolds because of their moderate mechanical strength (i.e., sufficient compression, tensile, and bending resistance). Moreover, bioinert bioceramics have significant stability in the biological environment and hence maintain their structure and functions for a long time, making them good implants for repairing bone defects in load-bearing areas. Alumina crystals have robust ionic bond between Al^{3+} and O^{2-} ions, which has led to, for alumina, great mechanical strength, hardness, melting point, and chemical stability to resist the attack of body fluid in vivo. Similarly, zirconia is also an ionic ceramic that possesses great chemical stability, hardness, and melting point and an even better mechanical behavior than alumina. Carbons, particularly graphene and carbon nanotubes (CNTs), have gain interest for 3D printing for tissue engineering applications because of their excellent electrical properties and photothermal effect.

HAp (Chen et al. 2019) and BG (Rahaman et al. 2011) are two typical bioactive bioceramics and have received great attention for bone tissue engineering because they enable the formation, in vitro or in vivo, of a layer of so-called bone-like apatite on their surfaces to promote interfacial bond formation with the host bone tissue in vivo. Many studies have investigated the use of 3D printed porous HAp or BG scaffolds for repairing bone. HAp [$Ca_{10}(PO_4)_6(OH)_2$] has the thermodynamically stable hexagonal crystalline structure in the biological environment. Owing to acceptable mechanical strength, low solubility, excellent bioactivity, and possibility in modulating cell activities (e.g., cell migration, attachment, proliferation, and differentiation), 3D printed HAp scaffolds are often used in orthopedics and dentistry. BG comprises silicate-based glasses. Hench and his coworkers developed world's first bioactive glass (45S5 Bioglass®) in 1969 and found that it could bond chemically with rat bone in vivo. Due to the superior interfacial bioactivity, 3D printed BG scaffolds have been used for bone and articular cartilage regeneration.

β-TCP (Lai et al. 2019) and BCP (Wang et al. 2023) are the most commonly used biodegradable bioceramics for 3D printing for bone regeneration. Like HAp and BG, β-TCP and BCP possess good bioactivity. A layer of hydroxycarbonate apatite (HCA) or bone-like apatite will form on the surface of β-TCP and BCP when they are put in a simulated body fluid (SBF) or biological environment. Both β-TCP and BCP can decompose in the biological environment and their biodegradation rate can be controlled by modulating their structure, crystallinity and porosity. TCP [$Ca_3(PO_4)_2$] has three polycrystalline morphologies: α, β, and α′. β-TCP is a metastable state of TCP and shows stability at room temperature. Although α-TCP and β-TCP are of the same chemical composition, they have differences in crystal structure and thus possess different properties. Compared to α-TCP, β-TCP has a lower biodegradation rate. Physical mixing HAp particles with β-TCP particles and followed by sintering the greenbody makes non-porous BCP. BCP printing inks can be formulated for 3D printing of BCP scaffolds using technologies such as DLP. BCP combines excellent bioactivity of HAp and good biodegradability of β-TCP. The biodegradation rate, mechanical strength, and biological performance of BCP and hence its scaffolds can be tuned by controlling the HAp-to-β-TCP ratio.

4.3 Metallic Biomaterials

Metallic biomaterials, including pure metals and their alloys (e.g., 316 L stainless steel, Co-based alloys, Ti and Ti-based alloys, and Mg-based alloys), have been used for 3D printing for medical applications because of their reasonable biocompatibility and excellent mechanical strength (Bandyopadhyay et al. 2023). Metallic biomaterials are chosen for bone tissue engineering, mainly as load-bearing bone implants, mainly due to their mechanical properties. 316 L stainless steel and Co-based alloys (e.g., Co–Cr alloys) can form a thin layer of compact oxide on their surface and hence have high resistance to corrosion in the human body, thereby avoiding excessive heavy metal ion release and thus adverse effects. 3D printed 316 L stainless steel can be processed into personalized structures as orthopedic or dental implants at a low cost. Compared with 316 L stainless steel, Co–Cr alloys provide better wear resistance but have lower plasticity and workability. 3D printed Co–Cr alloys are mostly likely to be used as joint prostheses. However, it should be noted that the Young's modulus of 316 L stainless steel and Co–Cr alloys is much higher than that of human bone, which can cause stress shielding effect. Stress shielding can lead to bone tissue resorption, accompanying the reduction of bone density. Furthermore, these metallic biomaterials are bioinert and hence cannot form direct chemical bonding with the host tissue after implantation.

Owing to excellent biocompatibility and corrosion resistance properties, lower density (as compared to steel and Co-based alloys), high mechanical strength and fracture toughness, Ti and Ti-based alloys are increasingly used for biomedical applications (Guo et al. 2022), including 3D printing. Pure Ti has poor shear strength but Ti-based alloys have increased shear strength and corrosion resistance owing to alloying by Ta, Nb, Zr, Mo, etc. Moreover, Ti-based alloys containing these alloying elements have lower Young's modulus that is closer to that of natural bone, reducing the stress shielding effect. Ti–6Al–4V is a typical Ti-based alloy and has been popularly used for artificial joints, bone implants and spine fixators (bone screws, bone nails, etc.). 3D printed Ti–6Al–4V are used as cervical spine implants and dental frameworks. Another Ti-based metal attracting attention in the medical field is Ni–Ti shape memory alloy (SMA, with Nitinol being mainly used). Recently, 4D printing have been investigated for fabricating porous Nitinol structures.

In addition to their good biocompatibility and also relatively high mechanical strength (as compared to polymers), Mg-based alloys degrade in vivo owing to their low corrosion resistance and hence second surgical operations to remove implants after tissue reconstruction can be avoided. Pure Mg is light and has a low elastic modulus and can be quickly degraded in the physiological environment, resulting in the production of H_2 gas and OH^- ions, which are detrimental to the host tissue. To enhance mechanical strength and decrease the degradation rate, Mg can be alloyed with other elements (e.g., Zr and Zn) to form Mg-based alloys. Mg and Mg-based alloys can generate Mg^{2+} ions via corrosion in vivo. Mg^{2+} ions can activate intracellular signaling pathways and promote cells attachment, proliferation, and differentiation to support bone formation. Therefore, 3D printed Mg-based alloys are promising for bone tissue engineering (Zeng et al. 2022).

4.4 Biomedical Composites

Individual materials (i.e., polymers, metals, or ceramics) have respective limitations for tissue engineering applications. For example, polymers have poor mechanical strength, ceramics are brittle, and metallic biomaterials are bioinert. Therefore, biomedical composites that combine at least two types of biomaterials and can avoid shortcomings of the constituents biomaterials and provide synergistic effect are created for 3D printing of tissue engineering scaffolds. Using the main phase (i.e., the matrix) as a criterion, composites can be categorized as polymer matrix composites, ceramics matrix composites and metal matrix composites. In the biomedical field, composites can also be classified as bioinert composites, bioactive composites, and biodegradable composites. Polymer matrix composites have been discussed in Sect. 4.1.3.

Bioinert bioceramics (alumina, zirconia, and carbon) exhibit poor bioactivity (osteoinductivity and/or osteoconductivity). They can be mixed with other suitable biomaterial to form ceramic matrix composites to overcome these problems. On the other hand, 3D printed bioactive bioceramics (e.g., HAp, BG, and β-TCP) scaffolds are usually brittle and have insufficient mechanical strength. By combining with metals, bioactive ceramics matrix composites can have sufficient mechanical strength and exhibit osteoconductivity (Wang et al. 2020a). Metallic biomaterials possess show excellent mechanical performance but exhibit poor bioactivity. Metal matrix composites can possess suitable mechanical properties and good interfacial response by combining metallic biomaterials with appropriate bioactive bioceramics (Zhang et al. 2020a).

5 Biomaterials for 4D Printing

Compared with 3D printed objects, 4D printed structures can change their shapes, properties or functions when they are exposed to appropriate stimulus or stimuli (Liu et al. 2024; Wan et al. 2024). Stimuli can be categorized as physical stimuli (e.g., temperature, moisture, light, magnetic field, and electrical field), chemical stimuli (e.g., pH and ionic concentration) and biological stimuli (e.g., glucose and enzyme). Accordingly, materials for 4D printing can be defined as physical stimulus-responsive materials, chemical stimulus-responsive materials, and biological stimulus-responsive materials.

For physical stimulus-responsive materials, temperature-responsive materials are the most widely used for 4D printing, showing shape morphing phenomenon when triggered by a change in temperature. Due to their good biocompatibility, printability and processability, temperature-responsive polymers, including poly(*N*-isopropylacrylamide) (PNIPAM), poly(ethylene glycol) (PEG), Col, Gel, poly(ε-caprolactone)dimethacrylate (PCLDMA), and PLA, have been used for 4D printing for tissue engineering applications. Among them, PNIPAM is one of the most studied temperature-responsive polymer. Moisture-responsive materials enable changes in structure configurations or properties upon absorbing or losing moisture in a humid environment. For example, Zhang et al synthesized a moisture-responsive material by modifying cellulose with stearoyl moieties (Zhang et al. 2015). Consequently, 4D printed objects can perform quick reversible bending movements and continuous shape transition after being placed in water. Light-responsive materials are sensitive to light exposure. Generally, light-responsive materials are polymers containing stilbene, derivatives of nitrobenzene, azobenzene, fulgide or spiropyran. Magneto- and electro-responsive materials can use magnetic field or electrical field to control shape morphing of 3D printed structures. Magneto-sensitive materials [e.g., para- or ferro-magnetic nanoparticles (MNPs)] or electro-sensitive materials (e.g., CNT and graphene) usually function as additives in 4D printed structures.

pH-responsive materials typically contain functional groups such as pyridine, carboxyl, or sulfonic phosphate. These functional groups can deliver or gain protons when the environment pH changes, thereby causing the swelling or collapse of 4D printed structures. HA, Col, Gel, Alg, CS, poly(histidine) (PHIS), poly(acrylic acid) (PAA), poly(L-glutamic acid) (PGA), and poly(aspartic acid) (PASP) are the main pH-responsive biomaterials used for 4D printing. The ionic strength can also be a potential stimulus for 4D printing. 4D printed objects can exhibit shape morphing upon a change in salt concentration in the environment. For example, Kirillova et al demonstrated that 4D printed Alg-based hydrogel scaffolds could form tubes in response to calcium ions crosslinks (Kirillova et al. 2017). Glucose and enzyme are two primary biological stimuli for 4D printing. Glucose-responsive biomaterials can be used to print devices that monitor the glucose level in the human body.

6 Application of 3D/4D Printing in Tissue Engineering

Tissue engineering is an interdisciplinary subject and requires multidisciplinary efforts. IoT aims to construct biological substitutes to restore, maintain, and/or improve tissue and organ functions. 3D and 4D printing enable precise spatial-temporal control over the shape, structure and properties of tissue substitutes and hence can fabricate customized biological products for patients. 3D and 4D printing have been increasingly used to fabricate tissue engineering scaffolds and cell-laden structures for regenerating various human body tissues, including skin, blood vessel, bone, articular cartilage, neural tissue, and other tissues.

6.1 Skin

Skin is the largest organ of the human body and has a hierarchical structure comprising three layers from skin surface to the inner part: epidermis, dermis, and hypodermis. It provides a protection barrier between the internal human body and external environment against pathogens. After minor skin wounds or burns, skin can self-regenerate due to the presence of stem cells. However, in case of large skin damages (e.g., full-thickness skin wounds or extensive burns), which significantly compromise the function of skin, medical treatment is necessary (Tavakoli et al. 2024; Derman et al. 2025). Each year, more than 70,000 burn cases require surgical treatments and the costs of skin wound treatments are over $20 billion in the US. Like the treatments for bone defects, autograft, allograft, and xenograft are mainly used for severe skin injuries. However, limited donor sites and secondary surgical damages are major constraints for autografts and allografts. On the other hand, xenografts cause concerns on possible disease transmission and immune rejection.

Tissue engineering strategies have been explored for over two decades now and synthetic grafts fabricated via 3D or 4D printing are seen as potential substitutes for skin regeneration. Compared with autograft, allograft, and xenograft, 3D and 4D printing can produce with ease patient-tailored tissue engineering products for treating large skin wounds. Furthermore, 3D and 4D printing can construct substitutes that mimic the hierarchical structure of skin and may, therefore, achieve better skin regeneration outcomes. Zhou et al constructed a functional living skin (FLS) via DLP 3D printing using a biomimetic bioink comprising GelMA and *N*-(2-aminoethyl)-4-(4-(hydroxymethyl)-2-methoxy-5-nitrosophenoxy) butanamide (NB) linked hyaluronic acid (HA-NB) (Zhou et al. 2020). They precisely positioned human skin fibroblasts (HSFs) and human umbilical vein endothelial cells (HUVECs) in the different areas in FLS for mimicking the

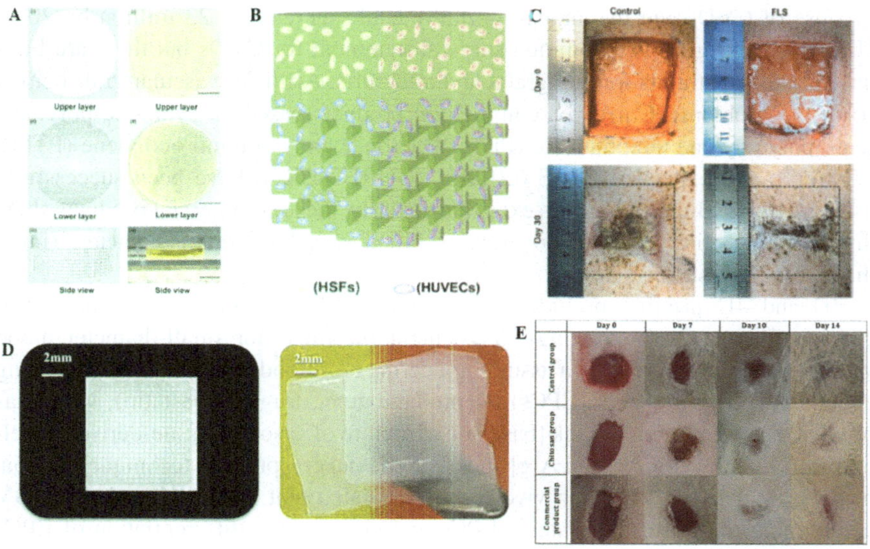

Fig. 4 **a** CAD designs and micro- and macrographs showing the structure of 3D printed functional living skin (FLS). **b** Schematic illustration showing cell distribution inside 3D printed FLS. **c** Appearance of a skin wound before and after wound healing through the use of 3D printed FLS (Zhou et al. 2020). **d** Photographs of 3D printed CS scaffolds without or with a film of CS at the base. **e** Appearance of skin wounds in treated and untreated groups of rats: each photo corresponds to an area of 1 cm^2 (Intini et al. 2018)

physiological structure of natural skin. After implantation in vivo, FLS had a superior performance in promoting skin regeneration (Fig. 4a–c). In another study, Intini et al 3D printed CS-based porous scaffolds for promoting skin regeneration (Intini et al. 2018). In vivo experiments on a rat model with diabetes showed that 3D printed CS scaffolds could promote wound healing with an improved skin functionality as compared to wounds treated with a commercial product, suggesting the usefulness of printed CS scaffolds for the treatment of chronic dermal wounds (Fig. 4d, e).

6.2 Blood Vessel

Vascular networks are vital for the regeneration of vascularized tissues due to their great ability to provide oxygen and nutrient transportation and the removal of wastes. Therefore, developing synthetic grafts for vascular tissue engineering is highly important. For example, cardiovascular diseases (CVDs) are one of the leading causes of mortality globally and are often related to blood vessel stenosis or occlusion. The narrowed or blocked coronary arteries can cause myocardial infarction and sudden death due to insufficient blood and oxygen supply to myocardium. According to American Heart Association, there were more than 19.1 million deaths in 2020 because of CVDs and the annual mortality could increase to 23 million by 2030. Using vascular graft is a common surgical treatment for CVDs but there are limitations and constraints for autografts and allografts. Artificial vascular graft help to solve the problems. Currently, commercial products based on synthetic polymers [e.g., polyethylene terephthalate (PET: "Dacron"), polytetrafluoroethylene (PTFE: "Teflon"), and expanded PTFE (ePTFE: "GORE-TEX")] have been successfully used in clinics. But problems do exist: particularly, these commercial products show disappointing clinical results for treating blood vessels of small diameters (inner diameters of less than 5 mm).

3D and 4D printing provides great ability and flexibility to fabricate artificial vascular grafts for treating CVDs, including those for small-diameter blood vessels. Gao et al constructed a tissue engineering bio-blood-vessel (BBV) containing endothelial progenitor cells (EPCs) and proangiogenic drug (atorvastatin), which was produced using a hybrid bioink [based on a mixture of vascular-tissue-derived decellularized ECM (VdECM) and Alg] and a 3D coaxial cell printing technique (Fig. 5a, b) (Gao et al. 2017). Their in vivo results indicated that the cell/drug-laden BBV could enhance the survival rate of EPCs and promote the differentiation of EPCs to endothelial cells and hence increase neovascularization. In another investigation, Jeong et al fabricated a small-diameter vessel (SDV) with a multilayered structure and controlled pore size based on a natural polymer bioink that contained HUVECs and human aorta smooth muscle cells (HAoSMCs) using a dragging 3D printing technique (Fig. 5c) (Jeong et al. 2024). Their in vitro experiments showed that the SDV could allow blood flow without any leakage and had sufficient flexibility, burst pressure, and suturing tension for transplantation.

Vascular stents, particularly biodegradable stents, have also gained great attention for CVD treatment and blood vessel repair. Compared to artificial vascular grafts which are used to replace the narrowed or blocked blood vessels, vascular stents are usually implanted in the disease sites to support the stenotic or occlusive vessels. Shen et al 3D printed PCL vascular stents and then modified the stents with heparin via covalent grafting (Fig. 5d) (Shen et al. 2022). In vitro experiments showed that the heparinized 3D printed PCL stents promoted adhesion, spreading and proliferation of HUVECs and inhibited the excessive proliferation of smooth muscle cells (SMCs). After implantation in the abdominal aorta of rabbits, the stents exhibited rapid endothelialization and prevention of neointimal restenosis (Fig. 5e, f).

6.3 Bone

Bone is a hierarchically organized connective tissue in the body to provide shape and mechanical support for the body and protection for internal organs (brain, spine cord, heart, etc.) (Fan et al. 2025; Nasiripour et al. 2025; Sabahi et al. 2025). Human bone consists of inorganic and organic substances. The organic substances are mainly collagen type I (Col I) fibril (10–20 wt%), collagen type III, collagen type IV, and other biomacromolecules, i.e., lipids, proteins, and polysaccharides. The inorganic

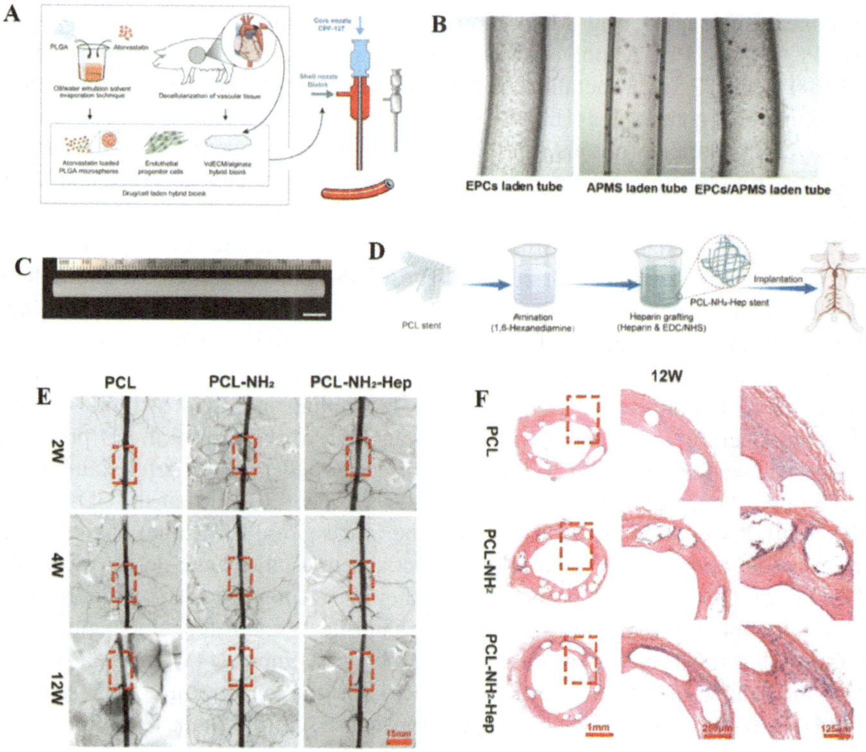

Fig. 5 **a** Schematic illustration for bio-blood-vessel (BBV) fabrication. **b** 3D printed EPC-, AMPS-, and EPC/AMPS-laden BBVs (scale bar: 500 μm) (Gao et al. 2017). **c** A photo showing an SDV fabricated by dragging 3D printing (inner diameter of 5 mm) (Jeong et al. 2024). **d** Schematic illustration showing fabrication of heparinized 3D printed PCL vascular stent. **e** Angiography images of PCL, $PCL-NH_2$ and $PCL-NH_2$-Hep stents after 2-week, 4-week, and 12-week implantation. **f** H&E staining images of PCL, $PCL-NH_2$, and $PCL-NH_2$-Hep stents after 12-weeks implantation (Shen et al. 2022)

part is bone apatite, which is similar to synthetic HAp but with calcium deficiency and heavy substitutions. Injuries, diseases, bone tumor-related resections, degenerative conditions, aging, and congenital disabilities are common causes for large bone defects (Yu et al. 2024; He et al. 2022; Liu et al. 2025). Considering the limited regeneration capacity of bone, the treatment of large bone defects is a major clinical challenge. Currently, more than 75 million people suffer from bone diseases and need to have bone implants in Europe, the United States, and Japan (Jaiswal and Wadetwar 2025).

Although autografts and allografts provide main treatments for bone defects, the inherent problems, such as limited donor sites, possible disease transmission and immune rejection, have put constraints on their applications (Li et al. 2025; Koushik et al. n.d.). Therefore, 3D and 4D printing that can fabricate customized porous scaffolds to match the physiological properties of human bone is increasingly using for bone tissue engineering. Many biomaterials, including polymers [CS, HA, Gel, Col, PLA, PCL, PLGA, polyether-ether-ketone (PEEK), etc.], bioceramics (HAp, BG, β-TCP, BCP, etc.), metallic biomaterials (Ti–6Al–4V, Mg-based alloys, etc.), and biomedical composites (HAp/PCL, β-TCP/PLLA, HAp/PEEK, etc.), have been employed to fabricate porous scaffolds with controlled structure and mechanical properties for bone tissue regeneration. For example, Zhang et al designed and fabricated via DLP 3D printing a Haversian bone-mimicking scaffold with integrated hierarchical Haversian bone structure using bioactive akermanite ceramic as the matrix (Fig. 6a) (Zhang et al. 2020b). The porosity and mechanical strength of this Haversian bone-mimicking scaffold could be well-controlled. Moreover, this Haversian bone-mimicking scaffold showed great potential in inducing osteogenic, angiogenic, and neurogenic differentiation of stem cells in vitro and could promote the repair of femoral defects in rabbits by facilitating ingrowth of blood vessels and consequently, new bone formation. In another work, Yan et al. 3D printed a biodegradable PCL scaffold to release in a controlled manner deferoxamine for accelerating bone regeneration (Yan et al. 2019). They found that the 3D printed PCL scaffolds with controlled deferoxamine release could facilitate angiogenesis and promote bone regeneration at the defect site in a large bone defect rat model (Fig. 6b, c). Our group 4D printed a photothermal-responsive shape memory bone scaffold by incorporating black phosphorus nanosheets and osteogenic peptide into β-TCP/poly(L-lactic acid-co-trimethylene carbonate) composite (Wang et al. 2020b). With the irradiation of a near-infrared (NIR) laser, the temperature of the scaffold could rise to 45 °C quickly and could therefore cause scaffold shape reconfiguration, which enabled easy scaffold implantation in the body and precise fitting in irregular bone defects (Fig. 6d).

6.4 *Articular Cartilage*

Articular cartilage is an avascular connective tissue comprising collagen type II (Col II) network and aggrecan that provides lubrication between joint surfaces (Tao et al. 2025b). The only cells in this hyaline cartilage tissue are chondrocytes. Because articular cartilage has a very limited regenerative capability, it is very important to employ tissue engineering scaffolds that combine with stem cells and appropriate biomolecules to treat articular cartilage defects (Culma et al. 2025). 3D scaffolds should provide mechanical and structural support for chondrocytes to attach and grow, leading to forming natural ECM. In addition, 3D scaffolds should have suitable microstructures (e.g., pore shape, pore size, and porosity) to allow chondrocyte ingrowth and maturation.

For articular cartilage regeneration, the scaffolds are usually made from biodegradable polymers. Polymeric biomaterials, especially natural polymers (e.g., HA, Col, Gel, Alg, and CS), have gained tremendous interests for cartilage regeneration because they can provide temporary ECM-like microenvironment, which is very conducive for cell attachment, proliferation and differentiation (Wang et al.

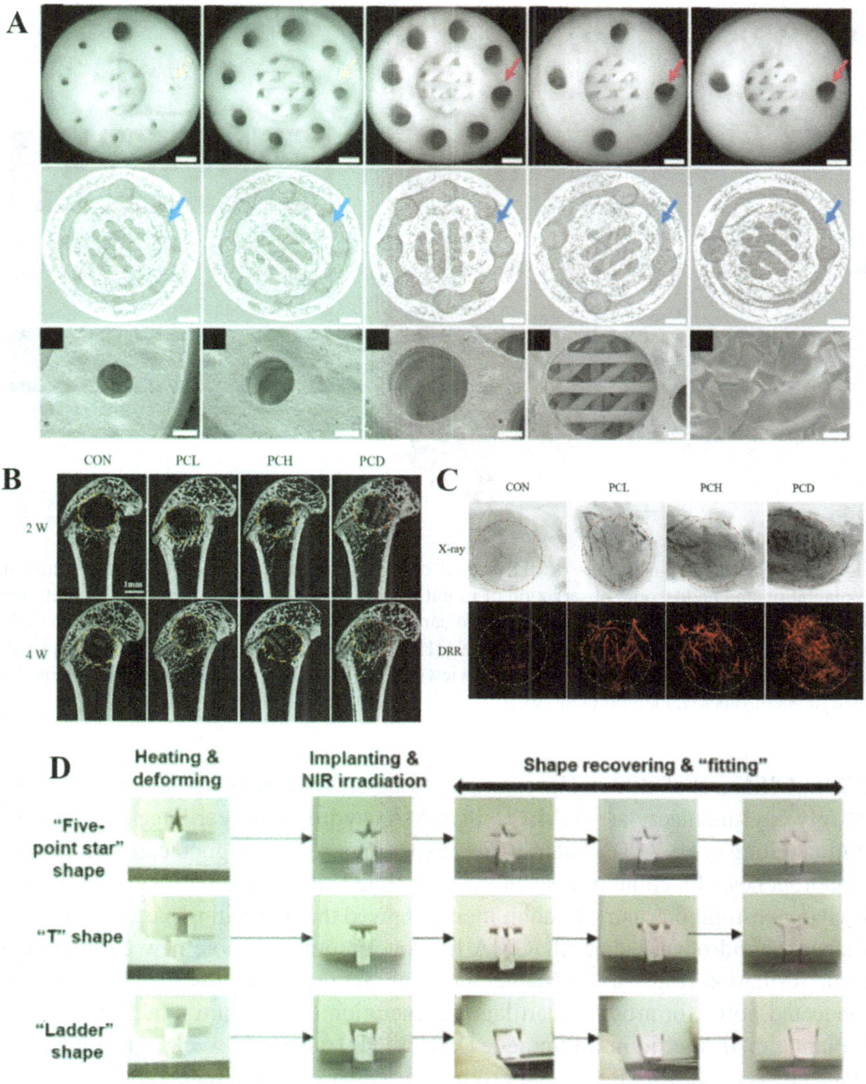

Fig. 6 **a** 3D printed Haversian bone-mimicking bioceramic scaffolds with cortical bone and cancellous bone structures (Zhang et al. 2020b). **b** Micro-CT images showing the effect of PCL-based scaffolds on bone tissue regeneration. **c** X-ray photographic images and digital reconstructed radiographs (DRR) after micro-CT scanning of the new vasculature formed inside the bone defect site 2 weeks after scaffolds insertion (Yan et al. 2019). **d** Shape morphing triggered by NIR laser irradiation of three types of bone tissue engineering scaffolds inserted in model bone defects (Wang et al. 2020b)

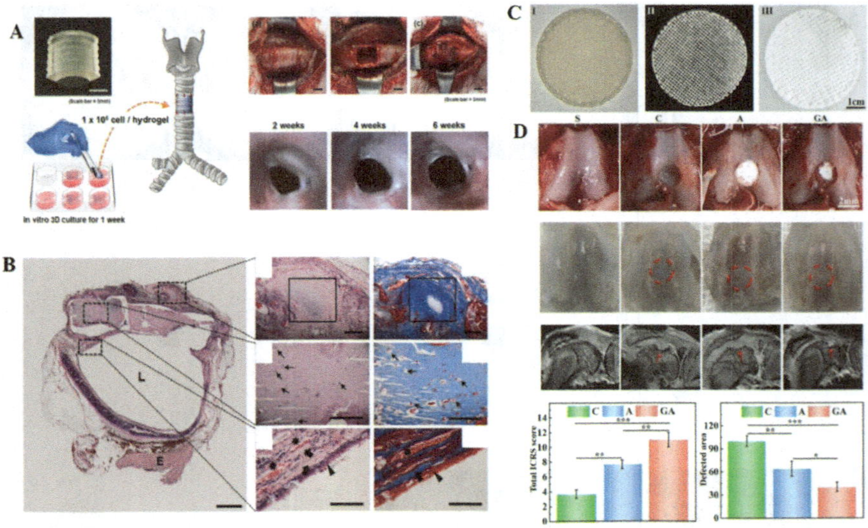

Fig. 7 **a** Schematic illustrations of 3D printed chondrocyte-laden silk/GMA hydrogels and its implantation and endoscopic observation of rabbit trachea after 6 weeks of hydrogel implantation. **b** Histological images showing development of cartilage tissue after 6 weeks of implantation of 3D printed chondrocyte-laden silk/GMA hydrogels (Hong et al. 2020). **c** General views of 3D printed Gel scaffolds. **d** General views, macroscopic views and MRI images of Gel scaffolds implanted in knee joints of rats (Maihemuti et al. 2023)

2024b; O'Shea et al. 2024). For example, Hong et al. 3D printed chondrocyte-laden silk/glycidyl-methacrylate (GMA) (silk/GMA) hydrogel for cartilage tissue regeneration (Hong et al. 2020). Their in vitro experiments showed good cell viability and chondrogenesis by chondrocytes in the 3D printed silk/GMA hydrogels. Moreover, in vivo investigations using a rabbit model showed that in treating partially defected trachea, chondrocyte-laden silk/GMA hydrogels could promote new cartilage-like tissue formation (Fig. 7a, b). Maihemuti et al. 3D printed Gel scaffolds with interconnected pores for articular cartilage regeneration (Maihemuti et al. 2023). After implantation in knee joints of Sprague Dawley (SD) rats for 12 weeks, 3D printed Gel scaffolds were shown effective to promote articular cartilage regeneration (Fig. 7c, d).

6.5 *Neutral Tissue*

The human nervous system comprising the central nervous system (CNS, including brain and spine cord) and peripheral nervous system (PNS, originating from CNS and including cranial and spinal nerves along with ganglia connecting CNS to various parts of the body) has the most complex and intricate biological structures and plays an essential role in the communication and interactions between body activities

(Tiong et al. 2025). Functions of the nervous system can be impaired due to trauma, diseases, and other factors. The impairment will cause disruptions in the connection between motor, sensory, and autonomic neurons within the neural circuit, resulting in paralysis, organ dysfunction, and potentially death. Owing to the low regeneration capability of the nervous system, transplantation of autologous or allogenic nerve grafts is usually performed for the treatment of sever nerve injuries. However, due to the inherent limitations of tissue or organ transplantation, i.e., limited source, possible disease transmission and immune rejection, nerve tissue engineering provides an promising option by fabricating and applying artificial grafts for neural regeneration. 3D printing of nerve tissue engineering scaffolds enables mimicking the complex structure and function of the nervous system.

Although PNS and CNS share many key anatomical and molecular features, the process of axon regeneration differs significantly. Neural regeneration for either PNS or CNS is not easy, and a much greater challenge exists for CNS owing to the complexity of the brain and spinal cord, as well as factors that inhibit repair. Nevertheless, many investigations have been conducted on applying 3D/4D printing and bioprinting in nerve tissue engineering, particularly for PNS. Ye et al. fabricated via DLP 3D printing nerve guidance conduits (NGCs) for treating large-gap nerve injuries (Ye et al. 2020). In this study, they printed multichannel NGCs with different inner diameters for peripheral nerve regeneration using GelMA for the printing ink (Fig. 8a). In vitro experiments using PC-12 cells and neural crest stem cells (NCSCs) revealed that the NGCs could support the migration and proliferation of PC-12 cells and the differentiation of NCSCs into neurons, suggesting the great potential of GelMA NGCs for peripheral nerve regeneration (Fig. 8b, c) In another study, Joung et al. constructed a bioengineered spine cord via 3D bioprinting (Joung et al. 2018). As shown in Fig. 8d, they precisely positioned clusters of induced pluripotent stem cell (iPSC)-derived spinal neuronal progenitor cells (sNPCs) and oligodendrocyte progenitor cells (OPCs) in 3D bioprinted scaffolds for mimicking the spatial distributions of cellular components in spinal cord. During in vitro culture, sNPCs differentiated into neurons projecting axons throughout the scaffold channels and OPCs differentiated into oligodendrocytes to myelinate the axons, thereby creating an effective relay across the injury site.

6.6 *Other Body Tissues*

3D and 4D printing and bioprinting have also been investigated to construct various tissue engineering scaffolds and cell-scaffold constructs for the regeneration of other body tissues and organs, such as heart, muscle and uterine. Currently, heart transplantation is practiced as the only treatment for end-stage heart failure. Using 3D printing to construct tissue engineering scaffolds that integrate biomaterials with stem cells and biomolecules provides an attractive route to regenerate heart tissues or even whole heart. As shown in Fig. 9a, a personalized cardiac patch could be 3D printed using personalized cell-laden hydrogel for cardiac tissue engineering (Noor et al. 2019).

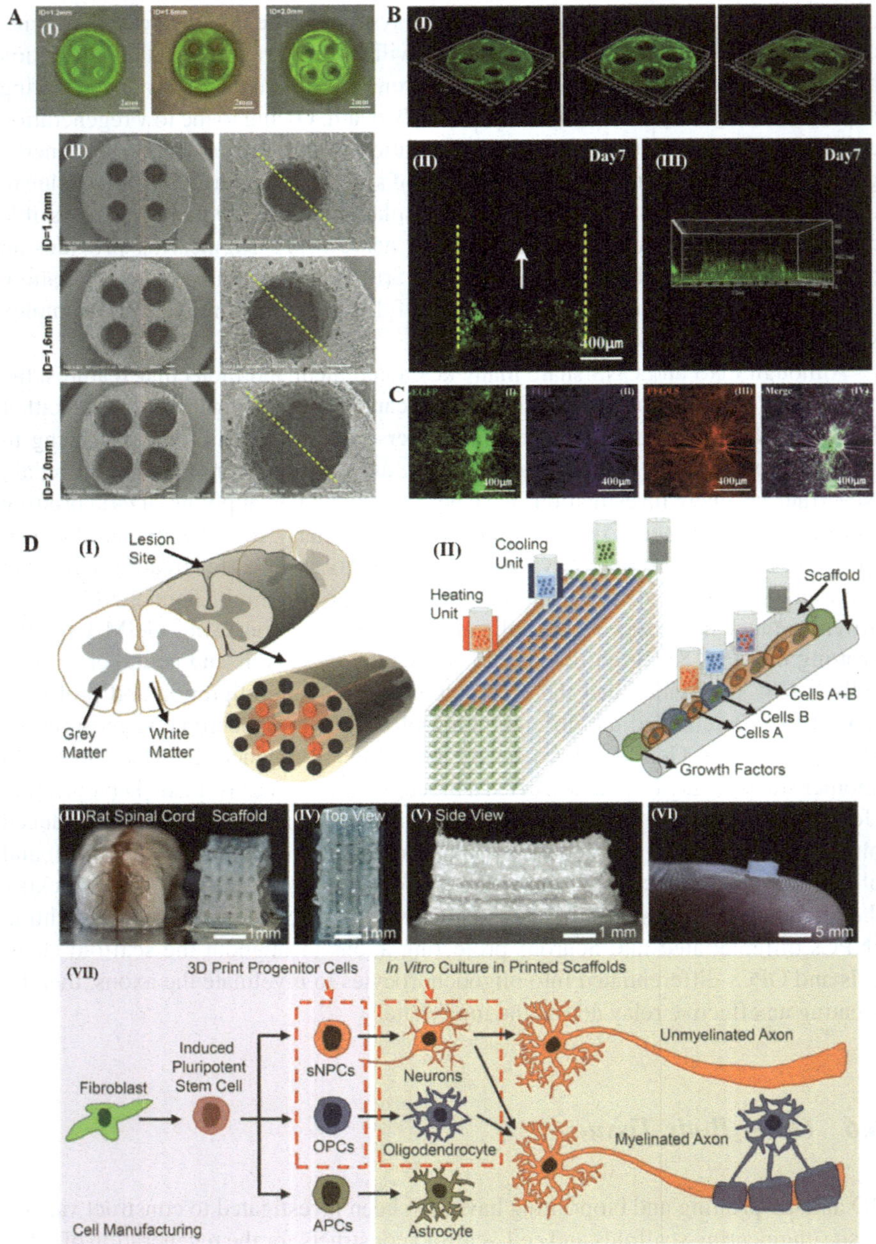
A
(I)
(II)
ID=1.2mm
ID=1.6mm
ID=2.0mm
B
(I)
(II)
Day7
400μm
(III)
Day7
C
Merge
D
(I)
Lesion Site
Grey Matter
White Matter
(II)
Cooling Unit
Heating Unit
Scaffold
Cells A+B
Cells B
Cells A
Growth Factors
(III)Rat Spinal Cord
Scaffold
1mm
(IV) Top View
1mm
(V) Side View
1 mm
(VI)
5 mm
(VII)
3D Print Progenitor Cells
In Vitro Culture in Printed Scaffolds
Fibroblast
Induced Pluripotent Stem Cell
sNPCs
OPCs
APCs
Neurons
Oligodendrocyte
Astrocyte
Unmyelinated Axon
Myelinated Axon
Cell Manufacturing

◂**Fig. 8** **a** 3D printed multichannel NGCs: (I) Photos of multichannel NGCs with different inner diameters. (II) SEM images showing cross-sectional morphology of multichannel NGCs with different inner diameters. **b** Cell survival and migration of PC-12 cells on 3D printed multichannel NGCs: (I) Confocal images of PC-12 cells after live/dead staining. (II) Confocal images of PC-12 cells in longitudinal channel at Day 7 of culture after live/dead staining. (III) 3D confocal image showing PC-12 cell migration on NGCs at Day 7 of culture. **c** Differentiation of NCSCs on NGCs: (I) Enhanced green fluorescent protein (EGFP, in green) fluorescence image showing neuronal differentiation of NCSCs cultured on NGCs. (II) Tuj1-positive neurons (in blue). (III) PGP9.5-positive neurons (in red). (IV) Merged image of EGFP/Tuj1/PGP9.5/DAPI (Ye et al. 2020). **d** 3D bioprinted bioengineered spine cord: (I) Schematic illustration of a spine cord with gray matter and white matter boundaries and a corresponding design for a spinal cord scaffold. (II) Schematic illustration of the 3D bioprinting process for the designed spinal cord scaffold. (III) to (VI) Photos for different views of 3D bioprinted spine cord scaffolds. (VII) Schematic illustration of iPSC reprogramming and differentiation into sNPCs or OPCs for spinal cord regeneration (Joung et al. 2018)

The 3D printed cardiac patch could be implanted on the heart of the patient to repair the dysfunctioning heart with no or low risk of rejection (Fig. 9b). Noor et al. were also able to produce via 3D printing a model of human heart of reduced size (Fig. 9c). Compared to heart, muscles exhibit better regeneration capability. However, when the muscle loss is greater than 20%, which is known as critical volumetric muscle loss (VML), the damage is irreversible and muscle tissue is unable to self-heal. In such circumstances, clinical intervention is necessary. Several studies have shown that 3D printed muscle grafts could perform well to promote de novo muscle regeneration and functional recovery. For example, as shown in Fig. 9d, Choi et al. fabricated via 3D printing a 3D muscle construct by using human skeletal muscle cell (hSMC)-laden decellularized ECM (dECM) bioinks (Choi et al. 2019). After implantation in a VML rat model, the 3D muscle grafts exhibited high cell survival rate of hSMCs and promoted de novo muscle formation, showing its great potential for muscle tissue engineering (Fig. 9e, f). The uterus in females is essential for biological functions in human reproduction. Damages of uterine tissues owing to disease or injury can result in dysfunction of the uterus and may cause infertility. Various tissue engineering scaffolds have been constructed to promote uterine tissue regeneration and recover uterus function. 3D bioprinting and 4D printing were used in a recent study to construct novel tissue engineering scaffolds mimicking the hierarchical structure of the uterine tissue (Chen et al. 2024b). As shown in Fig. 9g, h, biomimicking trilayer scaffolds having the shape morphing ability, possessing comparable mechanical properties with human uterine tissue, providing sustained release of estradiol (E2) and delivering in situ bone marrow-derived mesenchymal stem cells (BMSCs) were fabricated. These trilayer scaffolds exhibited great similarity to uterine tissues and showed high potential for uterine regeneration.

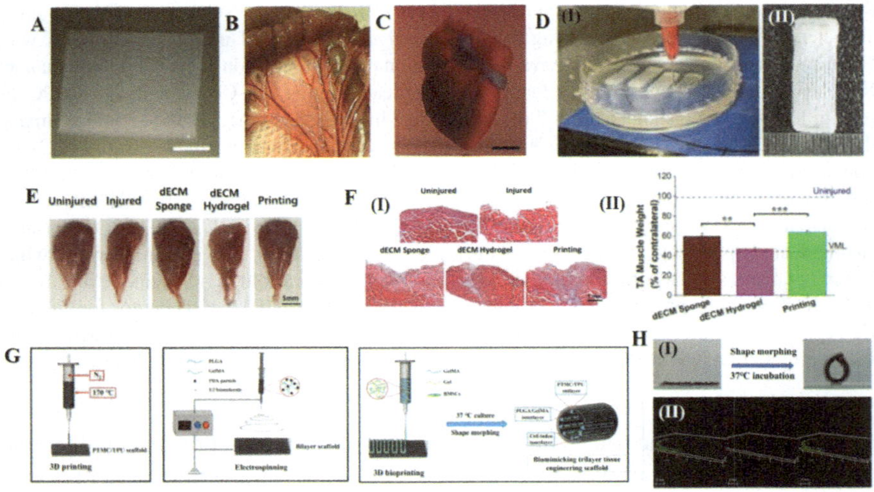

Fig. 9 **a** A 3D printed vascularized cardiac patch (scale bar: 1 cm). **b** Implantation of a 3D printed patch in between two layers of rat omentum (dashed, white line highlights the borders of the patch). **c** A 3D printed small-scale human heart model (scale bar: 0.5 cm) (Noor et al. 2019). **d** (I) 3D bioprinting of muscle constructs using hSMC-laden dECM bioinks. (II) A 3D bioprinted muscle construct. **e** Photos of tibialis anterior (TA) muscles after treatment in a VML rat model. **f** (I) Masson's trichrome staining of TA muscle tissue. (II) TA muscle mass (% of contralateral uninjured TA muscle) (the dashed blue line indicates the uninjured muscle and the dashed black line indicates the VML injured muscle) (Choi et al. 2019). **g** Schematic illustration of fabrication of biomimicking trilayer uterine tissue engineering scaffolds. **h** (I) Shape morphing of a trilayer uterine tissue engineering scaffold. (II) Confocal image showing cell distribution of BMSCs in the hydrogel layer of trilayer scaffolds (Chen et al. 2024b)

7 Concluding Remarks

This article has provided an introduction to 3D and 4D printing and bioprinting and a concise review of their technologies, materials, and applications in tissue engineering. According to their working principles, 3D and 4D printing technologies are generally categorized into three groups: inkjet-based, laser-assisted, and extrusion-based 3D printing. Many of these technologies can be employed for tissue engineering applications, and a large number of biomaterials (which are mostly biodegradable), including natural and synthetic biomedical polymers, bioceramics, metallic biomaterials, and biomedical composites, can be 3D or 4D printed into different types of tissue engineering scaffolds or medical implants for different body tissues or, when used in bioinks, be bioprinted into living structures for different medical applications including human body tissue regeneration. Each 3D printing technology has its advantages and limitations and the use of a particular 3D printing technology in tissue engineering mainly depends on the structure and properties of the targeted tissue for regeneration and available biomaterial(s) for the printing ink/inks or bioink/bioinks. Other factors, including resolution, precision, efficiency, scalability, and cost of 3D/4D printing and requirements for printing inks and hence biomaterials, are also important. Particularly, among the wide variety of biomaterials for 3D/4D printing and bioprinting, the selection of a suitable biomaterial (or, biomaterials) for constructing specific scaffolds or implants for a target tissue primarily relies on material properties (which decide on ink/bioink properties), including rheological properties, printability (of ink/bioink), biocompatibility, biodegradability and mechanical properties, and the fidelity of 3D/4D printed structures.

Due to the exceptional capability of fabricating customized patient-specific scaffolds and implants, 3D/4D printing has been increasingly used in tissue engineering for developing various biological substitutes for skin, blood vessel, bone, articular cartilage, nerve tissue, and other body tissues and organs. While the safety and efficacy of many of these biological grafts are now assessed at the preclinical stage, a good number of tissue engineering products have shown their benefits and potential on body tissue regeneration through clinical trials and successful commercialization. Over the past three to four decades, significant advances have been made for 3D printing technologies toward tissue engineering applications. Among new technological inventions and innovations, further improvements in printing resolution and scalability are needed, Even though there is already a good pool of biomaterials for 3D/4D printing and bioprinting in tissue engineering, new or better biomaterials still need to be developed for making better-performance products and/or achieving better clinical outcomes. Particularly, the material choices for 4D printing in the biomedical field are still very limited. Successfully addressing challenges in 3D printing technologies and also biomaterials for printing inks and consequently scaffolds and implants will enable the developments of high-performance tissue engineering products and new designs and products for regenerating complex body tissues and eventually human organs. There are these technical challenges, but the future of 3D/4D printing and bioprinting in tissue engineering looks bright. Millions of people, as well as the healthcare systems in different countries, will benefit hugely from the products that these technologies can and will provide.

Acknowledgements Min Wang's research in tissue engineering and additive manufacturing has been supported by Hong Kong's Research Grants Council (RGC) and China's National Natural Science Foundation (NSFC) through various research grants (including recent grants 17200519, 17202921, 17201622, N_HKU749/22, and 17201324) and also by The University of Hong Kong (HKU) with research grants from its Seed Fund for Basic Research Scheme. Shangsi Chen thanks HKU for awarding him with Ph.D. scholarships for conducting research on 3D printing and bioprinting at HKU. Assistance provided by members of Min Wang's research group at HKU and by technical staff in HKU's Department of Mechanical Engineering, Faculty of Medicine, Faculty of Dentistry and Electron Microscopy Unit is acknowledged. Min Wang thanks his collaborators in HKU's Faculty of Medicine and Faculty of Dentistry.

Data Availability The data that support the findings of our own research in 3D/4D printing and bioprinting in tissue engineering are available from the corresponding author (memwang@hku.hk) upon reasonable request. The data that support the findings in others' publications and presented in this article are available from the corresponding authors of publications cited in this article. Restrictions may apply to the availability of these data.

Statement of Usage of Artificial Intelligence No artificial intelligence tools were used for writing this article.

Author Contributions Shangsi Chen: research and drafting of the manuscript; Xiaodie Chen: research and drafting of the manuscript; Jie Huang: writing, reviewing, and editing; Min Wang: funding acquisition, design of the review, research supervision, writing, reviewing, and editing.

Conflict of Interest Statement There are no conflicts of interest to declare.

References

Z.U. Arif, M.Y. Khalid, R. Noroozi, A. Sadeghianmaryan, M. Jalalvand, M. Hossain, Recent advances in 3D-printed polylactide and polycaprolactone-based biomaterials for tissue engineering applications. Int. J. Biol. Macromol. **218**, 930–968 (2022)

A. Bandyopadhyay, I. Mitra, S.B. Goodman, M. Kumar, S. Bose, Improving biocompatibility for next generation of metallic implants. Prog. Mater. Sci. **133** (2023)

Z. Behrooznia, J. Nourmohammadi, Z. Mohammadi, F. Shabani, R. Mashhadi, Biological evaluation of 3D-printed chitosan-based scaffolds for tissue engineering. Carbohydr. Res. **551**, 109416 (2025)

S. Bhagia, K. Bornani, R. Agrawal, A. Satlewal, J. Ďurkovič, R. Lagaňa, M. Bhagia, C.G. Yoo, X. Zhao, V. Kunc, Y. Pu, S. Ozcan, A.J. Ragauskas, Critical review of FDM 3D printing of PLA biocomposites filled with biomass resources, characterization, biodegradability, upcycling and opportunities for biorefineries. Appl. Mater. Today **24**, 101078 (2021)

S. Chen, Y. Shi, X. Zhang, J. Ma, Biomimetic synthesis of Mg-substituted hydroxyapatite nanocomposites and three-dimensional printing of composite scaffolds for bone regeneration. J. Biomed. Mater. Res. A **107**(11), 2512–2521 (2019)

S. Chen, Y. Wang, J. Lai, S. Tan, M. Wang, Structure and properties of gelatin methacryloyl (GelMA) synthesized in different reaction systems. Biomacromolecules **24**(6), 2928–2941 (2023)

X.D. Chen, X.Y. Zhang, H.Q. Zhu, H.H. Lu, M. Wang, Three-dimensional printing of hydrogel blend tissue engineering scaffolds with in situ delivery of anticancer drug for treating melanoma resection-induced tissue defects. J. Funct. Biomater. **15**(12), 381 (2024a)

S. Chen, J. Li, L. Zheng, M. Wang, Biomimicking trilayer scaffolds with controlled estradiol release for uterine tissue regeneration. Exploration **4**(5), 20230141 (2024b)

Y.J. Choi, Y.J. Jun, D.Y. Kim, H.G. Yi, S.H. Chae, J. Kang, J. Lee, G. Gao, J.S. Kong, J. Jang, W.K. Chung, J.W. Rhie, D.W. Cho, A 3D cell printed muscle construct with tissue-derived bioink for the treatment of volumetric muscle loss. Biomaterials **206**, 160–169 (2019)

S.S. Crump, Apparatus and method for creating three-dimensional objects, U.S. Patents 5,121,329, 1992

J.J.S. Culma, J.M.G. Morales, Y.A.H. Uribe, D.A. Garzón-Alvarado, S. Leal-Marin, B. Glasmacher, J.J. Vaca-González, Effects of electric fields on the modulation of chondrocytes dynamics in gelatin scaffolds: a novel approach to optimize cartilage tissue engineering. J. Biomater. Sci. Polym. Ed. 1–20 (2025)

S. Das, J.T. Jegadeesan, B. Basu, Gelatin methacryloyl (GelMA)-based biomaterial inks: process science for 3D/4D printing and current status. Biomacromolecules **25**(4), 2156–2221 (2024)

S. Debnath, A. Agrawal, N. Jain, K. Chatterjee, D.J. Player, Collagen as a bio-ink for 3D printing: a critical review. J. Mater. Chem. B **13**(6), 1890–1919 (2025)

C.R. Deckard, Method and apparatus for producing parts by selective sintering, U.S. Patent 4,863,538, 1989

I.D. Derman, T. Rivera, L.G. Cerda, Y.P. Singh, S. Saini, H.E. Abaci, I.T. Ozbolat, Advancements in 3D skin bioprinting: processes, bioinks, applications and sensor integration. Int. J. Extreme Manuf. **7**(1), 012009 (2025)

Y.-W. Ding, X.-W. Zhang, C.-H. Mi, X.-Y. Qi, J. Zhou, D.-X. Wei, Recent advances in hyaluronic acid-based hydrogels for 3D bioprinting in tissue engineering applications. Smart Mater. Med. **4**, 59–68 (2023)

J.X. Fan, Z.C. Ding, Y.R. Cai, Y.H. Lai, C. Huang, B.Y. Jiang, Z.K. Zhou, Z.Y. Luo, Revolutionizing Bone regeneration: vascularized bone tissue engineering with advanced 3D printing technology. Aggregate **6**(4), e731 (2025)

G. Gao, J.H. Lee, J. Jang, D.H. Lee, J.S. Kong, B.S. Kim, Y.J. Choi, W.B. Jang, Y.J. Hong, S.M. Kwon, D.W. Cho, Tissue engineered bio-blood-vessels constructed using a tissue-specific bioink and 3D coaxial cell printing technique: a novel therapy for ischemic disease. Adv. Funct. Mater. **27**(33), 1700789 (2017)

V. Gayathri, T. Khan, M. Gowtham, R. Balan, T.A. Sebaey, Functionalized conductive polymer composites for tissue engineering and biomedical applications- a mini review. Front. Bioeng. Biotechnol. **13**, 1533944 (2025)

A.X.Y. Guo, L. Cheng, S. Zhan, S. Zhang, W. Xiong, Z. Wang, G. Wang, S.C. Cao, Biomedical applications of the powder-based 3D printed titanium alloys: a review. J. Mater. Sci. Technol. **125**, 252–264 (2022)

Y.B. Guo, D.L. Qiao, S.M. Zhao, P. Liu, F.W. Xie, B.J. Zhang, Biofunctional chitosan-biopolymer composites for biomedical applications. Mater. Sci. Eng. R Rep. **159**, 100775 (2024)

F. Han, F. Zhou, X. Yang, J. Zhao, Y. Zhao, X. Yuan, A pilot study of conically graded chitosan-gelatin hydrogel/PLGA scaffold with dual-delivery of TGF-beta1 and BMP-2 for regeneration of cartilage-bone interface. J. Biomed. Mater. Res. B Appl. Biomater. **103**(7), 1344–1353 (2015)

S. He, J. Fang, C.X. Zhong, F.Z. Ren, M. Wang, Controlled pVEGF delivery via a gene-activated matrix comprised of a peptide-modified non-viral vector and a nanofibrous scaffold for skin wound healing. Acta Biomater. **140**, 149–162 (2022)

Health Resources & Services Administration, Organ donation statistics (2023). https://www.organdonor.gov/learn/organ-donation-statistics. Accessed 3 Apr 2025

H. Hong, Y.B. Seo, D.Y. Kim, J.S. Lee, Y.J. Lee, H. Lee, O. Ajiteru, M.T. Sultan, O.J. Lee, S.H. Kim, C.H. Park, Digital light processing 3D printed silk fibroin hydrogel for cartilage tissue engineering. Biomaterials **232**, 119679 (2020)

C.W. Hull, Apparatus for production of three-dimensional objects by stereolithography, U.S. Patents 5,556,590A, 1984

B. Huzum, B. Puha, R.M. Necoara, S. Gheorghevici, G. Puha, A. Filip, P.D. Sirbu, O. Alexa, Biocompatibility assessment of biomaterials used in orthopedic devices: an overview (Review). Exp. Ther. Med. **22**(5), 1315 (2021)

C. Intini, L. Elviri, J. Cabral, S. Mros, C. Bergonzi, A. Bianchera, L. Flammini, P. Govoni, E. Barocelli, R. Bettini, M. McConnell, 3D-printed chitosan-based scaffolds: an in vitro study of human skin cell growth and an in-vivo wound healing evaluation in experimental diabetes in rats. Carbohydr. Polym. **199**, 593–602 (2018)

R. Ivone, Y. Yang, J. Shen, Recent advances in 3D printing for parenteral applications. AAPS J. **23**(4), 87 (2021)

R. Jaiswal, R. Wadetwar, Technique of 3D printing for scaffolding in tissue engineering of bones: opportunities and challenges. Mater. Today Commun. **42**, 111249 (2025)

H.J. Jeong, H. Nam, J.S. Kim, S. Cho, H.H. Park, Y.S. Cho, H. Jeon, J. Jang, S.J. Lee, Dragging 3D printing technique controls pore sizes of tissue engineered blood vessels to induce spontaneous cellular assembly. Bioact. Mater. **31**, 590–602 (2024)

S. Jin, X. Xia, J. Huang, C. Yuan, Y. Zuo, Y. Li, J. Li, Recent advances in PLGA-based biomaterials for bone tissue regeneration. Acta Biomater. **127**, 56–79 (2021)

D. Joung, V. Truong, C.C. Neitzke, S.Z. Guo, P.J. Walsh, J.R. Monat, F. Meng, S.H. Park, J.R. Dutton, A.M. Parr, M.C. McAlpine, 3D printed stem-cell derived neural progenitors generate spinal cord scaffolds. Adv. Funct. Mater. **28**(39), 1801850 (2018)

A. Kantaros, T. Ganetsos, F.I.T. Petrescu, E. Alysandratou, Bioprinting and intellectual property: challenges, opportunities, and the road ahead. Bioengineering-Basel **12**(1), 76 (2025)

A. Kirillova, R. Maxson, G. Stoychev, C.T. Gomillion, L. Ionov, 4D biofabrication using shape-morphing hydrogels. Adv. Mater. **29**(46), 1703443 (2017)

R.J. Klebe, Cytoscribing: a method for micropositioning cells and the construction of two-and three-dimensional synthetic tissues. Exp. Cell Res. **179**(2), 362–373 (1988)

T.M. Koushik, C.M. Miller, E. Antunes, Graded hydroxyapatite triply periodic minimal surface structures for bone tissue engineering applications. Adv. Healthc. Mater. **14**(25), 2402953 (2025)

M.S. Kumar, P. Varma, B. Kandasubramanian, From lab to life: advances in in-situ bioprinting and bioink technology. Biomed. Mater. **20**(1), 012004 (2025)

Y. Lai, Y. Li, H. Cao, J. Long, X. Wang, L. Li, C. Li, Q. Jia, B. Teng, T. Tang, J. Peng, D. Eglin, M. Alini, D.W. Grijpma, G. Richards, L. Qin, Osteogenic magnesium incorporated into PLGA/TCP porous scaffold by 3D printing for repairing challenging bone defect. Biomaterials **197**, 207–219 (2019)

J. Lai, C. Wang, M. Wang, 3D printing in biomedical engineering: processes, materials, and applications. Appl. Phys. Rev. **8**(2), 021322 (2021a)

J. Lai, X. Ye, J. Liu, C. Wang, J. Li, X. Wang, M. Ma, M. Wang, 4D printing of highly printable and shape morphing hydrogels composed of alginate and methylcellulose. Mater. Des. **205**, 109699 (2021b)

R. Langer, J.P. Vacant, Tissue engineering. Science **260**(5110), 920–926 (1993)

J.M. Lee, S.K.Q. Suen, W.L. Ng, W.C. Ma, W.Y. Yeong, Bioprinting of collagen: considerations, potentials, and applications. Macromol. Biosci. **21**(1), e2000280 (2021)

J. Li, C. Wu, P.K. Chu, M. Gelinsky, 3D printing of hydrogels: rational design strategies and emerging biomedical applications. Mater. Sci. Eng. R Rep. **140**, 100543 (2020)

S.S. Li, X.Y. Li, Y.D. Xu, C.R. Fan, Z.A. Li, L. Zheng, B.C. Luo, Z.P. Li, B.F. Lin, Z.G. Zha, H.T. Zhang, X.Y. Wang, Collagen fibril-like injectable hydrogels from self-assembled nanoparticles for promoting wound healing. Bioact. Mater. **32**, 149–163 (2024)

Y.B. Li, X.D. Li, L.W. Zhu, T.Y. Liu, L.F. Huang, Chitosan-based biomaterials for bone tissue engineering. Int. J. Biol. Macromol. **304**, 140923 (2025)

B. Liu, H. Li, F.Z. Meng, Z.Y. Xu, L.Z. Hao, Y. Yao, H. Zhu, C.M. Wang, J. Wu, S.Q. Bian, W.W. Lu, W.G. Liu, H.B. Pan, X.L. Zhao, 4D printed hydrogel scaffold with swelling-stiffening properties and programmable deformation for minimally invasive implantation. Nat. Commun. **15**(1), 1587 (2024)

Y. Liu, Y. Wan, C.J. Li, G.P. Guan, F.J. Wang, J. Gao, L. Wang, Gradient scaffolds in bone-soft tissue interface engineering: structural characteristics, fabrication techniques, and emerging trends. J. Orthop. Transl. **50**, 333–353 (2025)

A. Maihemuti, H. Zhang, X. Lin, Y. Wang, Z. Xu, D. Zhang, Q. Jiang, 3D-printed fish gelatin scaffolds for cartilage tissue engineering. Bioact. Mater. **26**, 77–87 (2023)

I. Matai, G. Kaur, A. Seyedsalehi, A. McClinton, C.T. Laurencin, Progress in 3D bioprinting technology for tissue/organ regenerative engineering. Biomaterials **226**, 119536 (2020)

V. Mathur, P. Agarwal, M. Kasturi, V. Srinivasan, R.N. Seetharam, K.S. Vasanthan, Innovative bioinks for 3D bioprinting: exploring technological potential and regulatory challenges. J. Tissue Eng. **16**, 20417314241308022 (2025)

S. Naghieh, X. Chen, Printability—a key issue in extrusion-based bioprinting. J Pharm Anal **11**(5), 564–579 (2021)

S. Nasiripour, F. Pishbin, S.A.S. Ebrahimi, 3D printing of a self-healing, bioactive, and dual-cross-linked polysaccharide-based composite hydrogel as a scaffold for bone tissue engineering. ACS Appl. Bio Mater. **8**(1), 582–599 (2025)

T.T. Nguyen, C.C. Hu, R. Sakthivel, S.C. Nabilla, Y.W. Huang, J. Yu, N.C. Cheng, Y.J. Kuo, R.J. Chung, Preparation of gamma poly-glutamic acid/hydroxyapatite/collagen composite as the 3D-printing scaffold for bone tissue engineering. Biomater. Res. **26**(1), 21 (2022)

N. Noor, A. Shapira, R. Edri, I. Gal, L. Wertheim, T. Dvir, 3D printing of personalized thick and perfusable cardiac patches and hearts. Adv. Sci. (Weinh) **6**(11), 1900344 (2019)

D.G. O'Shea, T. Hodgkinson, C.M. Curtin, F.J. O'Brien, An injectable and 3D printable pro-chondrogenic hyaluronic acid and collagen type II composite hydrogel for the repair of articular cartilage defects. Biofabrication **16**(1), 015007 (2024)

A.M.D. Pajooh, M. Tavakoli, M.H. Al-Musawi, A. Karimi, E. Salehi, S. Nasiri-Harchegani, F. Sharifianjazi, K. Tavamaishvili, M. Mehrjoo, A. Najafinezhad, J. Varshosaz, M. Mirhaj, Biomimetic VEGF-loaded bilayer scaffold fabricated by 3D printing and electrospinning techniques for skin regeneration. Mater. Des. **238**, 112714 (2024)

M.N. Rahaman, D.E. Day, B.S. Bal, Q. Fu, S.B. Jung, L.F. Bonewald, A.P. Tomsia, Bioactive glass in tissue engineering. Acta Biomater. **7**(6), 2355–2373 (2011)

M.M. Rana, H.D. Siegler, Evolution of hybrid hydrogels: next-generation biomaterials for drug delivery and tissue engineering. Gels **10**(4), 1–50 (2024)

P. Rastogi, B. Kandasubramanian, Review of alginate-based hydrogel bioprinting for application in tissue engineering. Biofabrication **11**(4), 042001 (2019)

Research and Markets, Tissue engineering global market report 2025 (2025). https://www.researchandmarkets.com/reports/5792890/tissue-engineering-global-market-report?gclid=CjwKCAjwyY6pBhA9EiwAMzmfwVa7n3SIBukJBolOntKq-ZyC8EtL_jUC4AQclCJHn5nQsa8f4W0pDhoCw9kQAvD_BwE. Accessed 3 Apr 2025

N. Sabahi, I. Roohani, C.H. Wang, X.P. Li, Material extrusion 3D printing of bioactive smart scaffolds for bone tissue engineering. Addit. Manuf. **98**, 104636 (2025)

E.M. Sachs, J.S. Haggerty, M.J. Cima, P.A. Williams, Three-dimensional printing techniques, U.S. Patents 5,204,055, 1993

G. Satchanska, S. Davidova, P.D. Petrov, Natural and synthetic polymers for biomedical and environmental applications. Polymers **16**(8), 1159 (2024)

A. Schwab, R. Levato, M. D'Este, S. Piluso, D. Eglin, J. Malda, Printability and shape fidelity of bioinks in 3D bioprinting. Chem. Rev. **120**(19), 11028–11055 (2020)

K. Shanno, P. Mangala, T.S. Shanmugarajan, B. Bhyan, M.G. Shinde, B.Y. Rane, S.S. Ali, M. Kumar, P. Kumar, 3D-printed polyurethane scaffolds for bone tissue engineering: techniques and emerging applications. Regen. Eng. Transl. Med. 1–23 (2025)

Y. Shen, C. Tang, B. Sun, Y. Zhang, X. Sun, M. El-Newehy, H. El-Hamshary, Y. Morsi, H. Gu, W. Wang, X. Mo, 3D printed personalized, heparinized and biodegradable coronary artery stents for rabbit abdominal aorta implantation. Chem. Eng. J. **450**, 138202 (2022)

H. Tao, X.Y. Zhang, X.M. Yuan, Z.Q. Lian, J. Xu, D.B. Shan, B. Guo, 3D bioprinting technology in tissue engineering printing method and material selection. BioNanoScience **15**(1), 1–19 (2025a)

H.C. Tao, M.L. Feng, H. Feng, H.C. Ren, Research advance of 3D printing for articular cartilage regeneration. Regen. Med. **20**(1), 45–55 (2025b)

M. Tavakoli, M.H. Al-Musawi, A. Kalali, A. Shekarchizadeh, Y. Kaviani, A. Mansouri, S. Nasiri-Harchegani, A.Z. Kharazi, F. Sharifianjazi, M. Sattar, J. Varshosaz, M. Mehrjoo, A. Najafinezhad, M. Mirhaj, Platelet rich fibrin and simvastatin-loaded pectin-based 3D printed-electrospun bilayer scaffold for skin tissue regeneration. Int. J. Biol. Macromol. **265**, 130954 (2024)

A.E. Tiong, X.Y. Zhang, C. Wang, Q.L. Zhao, M. Wang, 3D printing and bioprinting in neural tissue engineering. Nano Life **15**(06), 2541004 (2025)

J. Van Hoorick, L. Tytgat, A. Dobos, H. Ottevaere, J. Van Erps, H. Thienpont, A. Ovsianikov, P. Dubruel, S. Van Vlierberghe, (Photo-)crosslinkable gelatin derivatives for biofabrication applications. Acta Biomater. **97**, 46–73 (2019)

M. Vert, Y. Doi, K.H. Hellwich, M. Hess, P. Hodge, P. Kubisa, M. Rinaudo, F. Schué, Terminology for biorelated polymers and applications (IUPAC recommendations 2012). Pure Appl. Chem. **84**(2), 377–408 (2012)

S. Vijayavenkataraman, W.C. Yan, W.F. Lu, C.H. Wang, J.Y.H. Fuh, 3D bioprinting of tissues and organs for regenerative medicine. Adv. Drug Deliv. Rev. **132**, 296–332 (2018)

F. Villanueva-Flores, I. Garcia-Atutxa, A. Santos, J. Armendariz-Borunda, Toward a new generation of bio-scaffolds for neural tissue engineering: challenges and perspectives. Pharmaceutics **15**(6), 1750 (2023)

X. Wan, Z.M. Xiao, Y.J. Tian, M. Chen, F. Liu, D. Wang, Y. Liu, P.J.D. Bartolo, C.Z. Yan, Y.S. Shi, R.R. Zhao, H.J. Qi, K. Zhou, Recent advances in 4D printing of advanced materials and structures for functional applications. Adv. Mater. **36**(34), 2312263 (2024)

C. Wang, L. He, M. Wang, Nanocomposites for human body tissue repair, in *Composites in Biomedical Applications*, ed. by S.M. Sapuan, Y. Nukman, N.A. Abu Osman, R.A. Ilyas (CRC Press, 2020a), pp. 239–261

C. Wang, H. Yue, J. Liu, Q. Zhao, Z. He, K. Li, B. Lu, W. Huang, Y. Wei, Y. Tang, M. Wang, Advanced reconfigurable scaffolds fabricated by 4D printing for treating critical-size bone defects of irregular shapes. Biofabrication **12**(4), 045025 (2020b)

Y. Wang, S. Chen, H. Liang, J. Bai, M. Wang, Design and fabrication of biomimicking radially graded scaffolds via digital light processing 3D printing for bone regeneration. J. Mater. Chem. B **11**(41), 9961–9974 (2023)

W.Z. Wang, L. Wang, B.Q. Zhang, S.H. Shang, C.X. Zhao, W.C. Zhang, J. Chen, C.C. Zhou, H.X. Zhou, S.Q. Feng, 3D printing of personalized magnesium composite bone tissue engineering scaffold for bone and angiogenesis regeneration. Chem. Eng. J. **484**, 149444 (2024a)

M.K. Wang, Y. Wu, G.F. Li, Q.S. Lin, W.C. Zhang, H. Liu, J.C. Su, Articular cartilage repair biomaterials: strategies and applications. Mater. Today Bio. **24**, 100948 (2024b)

A. Yadav, D.S. Waghmare, A. Ahir, A. Srivastava, Comprehensive exploration on chemical functionalization and crosslinked injectable hyaluronic acid hydrogels for tissue engineering applications. Regen. Eng. Transl. Med. 1–28 (2025)

Y. Yan, H. Chen, H. Zhang, C. Guo, K. Yang, K. Chen, R. Cheng, N. Qian, N. Sandler, Y.S. Zhang, H. Shen, J. Qi, W. Cui, L. Deng, Vascularized 3D printed scaffolds for promoting bone regeneration. Biomaterials **190–191**, 97–110 (2019)

W. Ye, H. Li, K. Yu, C. Xie, P. Wang, Y. Zheng, P. Zhang, J. Xiu, Y. Yang, F. Zhang, Y. He, Q. Gao, 3D printing of gelatin methacrylate-based nerve guidance conduits with multiple channels. Mater. Des. **192**, 108757 (2020)

X.G. Yu, S.J. Jiang, D.J. Li, S.G.F. Shen, X.D. Wang, K.L. Lin, Osteoimmunomodulatory bioinks for 3D bioprinting achieve complete regeneration of critical-sized bone defects. Compos. Part B Eng. 273 (2024)

Z. Zeng, M. Salehi, A. Kopp, S. Xu, M. Esmaily, N. Birbilis, Recent progress and perspectives in additive manufacturing of magnesium alloys. J. Magnesium Alloys **10**(6), 1511–1541 (2022)

K. Zhang, A. Geissler, M. Standhardt, S. Mehlhase, M. Gallei, L. Chen, C. Marie Thiele, Moisture-responsive films of cellulose stearoyl esters showing reversible shape transitions. Sci. Rep. **5**, 11011 (2015)

G. Zhang, H. Lu, S. Mamidwar, M. Wang, Composites, in *Biomaterials Science: An Introduction to Materials in Medicine*, ed. by W. Wagner, S. Sakiyama-Elbert, G. Zhang, M. Yaszemski (Elsevier, The Netherlands, 2020a), pp. 415–429

M. Zhang, R.C. Lin, X. Wang, J.M. Xue, C.J. Deng, C. Feng, H. Zhuang, J.G. Ma, C. Qin, L. Wan, J. Chang, C.T. Wu, 3D printing of Haversian bone-mimicking scaffolds for multicellular delivery in bone regeneration. Sci. Adv. **6**(12), eaaz6725 (2020b)

F. Zhou, Y. Hong, R. Liang, X. Zhang, Y. Liao, D. Jiang, J. Zhang, Z. Sheng, C. Xie, Z. Peng, X. Zhuang, V. Bunpetch, Y. Zou, W. Huang, Q. Zhang, E.V. Alakpa, S. Zhang, H. Ouyang, Rapid printing of bio-inspired 3D tissue constructs for skin regeneration. Biomaterials **258**, 120287 (2020)

Q. Zhou, X. Su, J. Wu, X. Zhang, R. Su, L. Ma, Q. Sun, R. He, Additive manufacturing of bioceramic implants for restoration bone engineering: technologies, advances, and future perspectives. ACS Biomater. Sci. Eng. **9**(3), 1164–1189 (2023)

Nanoparticle Designs for Specific Targeting in Precision Theranostics

Zicheng Deng, Vladimir V. Kalinichenko, and Donglu Shi

Abstract There is a growing fascination with the progression of nanomaterials in the field of biomedical applications. Nanoparticles refer to particle materials that possess dimensions on a nanoscale. These types of nanomaterials offer numerous advantages due to their unique abilities, particularly in targeting specific cells, tissues, or organs. Currently, the greatest challenge in clinical therapy is to design a delivery system for delivery of therapeutics to the lesion sites with spatial and temporal precision without affecting the normal tissues. An effective delivery system can not only boost the therapeutic outcome at a lower dose, but also decrease the damage or toxicity to the normal tissues. Some superparamagnetic nanoparticles can serve as effective tumor therapeutics based on their intrinsic properties such as the photothermal effect and magnetic hyperthermia therapy. These therapeutic approaches require even more precise confinement of nanoparticles within the targeted area. Hence, the key to addressing critical issues in various biomedical fields lies in the design of nanoparticles with high selectivity for specific cells or tissues. This chapter introduces a range of nanoparticle designs that facilitate targeting specific cells, tissues, or organs. Nanoparticle targeting strategies are commonly categorized as passive targeting and active targeting. Passive targeting primarily relies on physicochemical properties, while active targeting involves the use of biomarkers on the nanoparticle surface to recognize specific molecules on the targeted cell. This chapter explores the latest advancements in nanoparticle design for efficient and specific targeting, aiming to facilitate the delivery of nanoparticles to their intended sites. Recently, charge-based targeting has garnered significant attention as a biomarkerless targeting strategy. Early studies revealed a unique metabolic characteristic in cancer cells

Z. Deng · V. V. Kalinichenko
Children's Research Institute, Department of Child Health, University of Arizona College of Medicine-Phoenix, Phoenix, USA

V. V. Kalinichenko
Division of Neonatology, Phoenix Children's Hospital, Phoenix, USA

D. Shi (✉)
The Materials Science and Engineering Program, Department of Mechanical and Materials Engineering, Department of Biomedical Engineering, College of Engineering and Applied Science, University of Cincinnati, Cincinnati, USA
e-mail: shid@ucmail.uc.edu

R. Narayan (ed.), *Nanostructured Biomaterials and Their Applications*,
https://doi.org/10.1007/978-3-032-16316-5_17

known as glycolysis, which results in a net negative surface charge that can be exploited for electrical-charge-mediated targeting. In addition to targeting cancer cells, our previous research also utilized charge-based targeting for the specific targeting of pulmonary endothelial cells. However, surface charge is not the sole physicochemical property that influences targeting efficiency; nanoparticle size also plays a crucial role in nanoparticle biodistribution and targeting. Another significant aspect of targeting strategy design involves the use of biomarkers such as antibodies, peptides, or other biomolecules to actively recognize or be recognized by specific cells. Active targeting is considered a flexible and effective strategy, leading to the development of various ligands that can be decorated on the nanoparticle surface to target different cells. Furthermore, for certain nanoparticles, external forces can be employed to drive them to specific sites. For example, a magnetic field can assist in the accumulation of superparamagnetic nanoparticles in a particular area. Additionally, to achieve maximum targeting efficiency, researchers have started combining different designs to synergistically integrate the effectiveness of multiple targeting strategies. This chapter will dedicate a significant section to summarize the most recent advancements in combined targeting design.

Keywords Nanoparticles · Nanomaterials · Biomedicine · Targeting strategies · Surface charge · Biomarker · Magnetic guide targeting · Combination targeting

1 Introduction

1.1 Opportunities and Challenges in Precision Theranostics

In modern medicine, there is a growing need for high-precision diagnosis and therapeutics at the cellular and genetic levels. As our understanding of disease mechanisms improves, innovative approaches are being developed to diagnose and combat the most critical diseases. For instance, in the field of cancer management, early detection of tumors is of utmost importance but often challenging. The discovery of Circulating Tumor Cells (CTCs) has brought new hope for tumor liquid biopsy (Sharma et al. 2018). CTCs refer to tumor cells that have detached from the primary tumor and entered the peripheral blood circulation system (Deng et al. 2022). Recently, the significance of CTCs in cancer biology research and precision medicine has been widely acknowledged (Deng et al. 2022). Compared to other biomarkers in tumor liquid biopsy, such as circulating tumor DNA (ctDNA) or exosomes, Circulating Tumor Cells (CTCs) represent a complete biological entity that can provide more dynamic information. Clinical studies have confirmed the association between cancer metastasis and CTC counts, demonstrating that changes in the number of CTCs in peripheral blood offer greater accuracy in predicting drug efficacy compared to conventional methods, especially in prostate cancer (Heller et al. 2018; Bidard et al. 2014; Goldkorn et al. 2014). Beyond CTC counts, the heterogeneity of CTCs holds immense value in bridging fundamental cancer biology with clinical theranostics (Lim et al. 2019; Sinkala et al. 2017). Recent research has shown that analyzing the phenotypic, morphological, and molecular characteristics of CTCs is a promising approach for predicting cancer migration, metastatic outgrowth, and proliferation (Liu et al. 2019a). Furthermore, the in vitro culture of CTCs collected from clinical samples can be utilized for further studies in cancer biology and precision diagnosis (Liu et al. 2021). However, the clinical applications of CTCs still face challenges in accurately detecting and isolating them from blood samples. Clinical blood samples contain millions of blood cells, while CTCs in the bloodstream are rare (1–100 CTCs in 1 mL of blood) (Shiriny and Bayareh 2021). Therefore, the most pressing task in tumor liquid biopsy is to develop a precise method that can efficiently and reliably isolate CTCs from blood samples with high efficiency and purity. In the field of cancer therapy, novel treatment opportunities are accompanied by significant challenges.

Recent studies have highlighted the strong association between the Forkhead box M1 (FOXM1) transcription factor and human solid cancers (Borhani and Gartel 2020). FOXM1 is a crucial transcription factor associated with proliferation and is frequently overexpressed in various human cancers (Liao et al. 2018). It is found to be overexpressed in multiple carcinoma types, including lung, prostate, breast, ovary, colon, pancreas, stomach, bladder, liver, and kidney (Pilarsky et al. 2004). High expression of FOXM1 in carcinomas, glioblastomas, and acute myeloid leukemia indicates the tumor cells' dependence on FOXM1 (Raychaudhuri and Park 2011; Teh et al. 2002; Liu et al. 2006; Nakamura et al. 2010). FOXM1 plays a critical role in regulating cell cycle progression by stimulating the expression of genes involved in G1-S and G2-M transitions, and its expression is primarily restricted to proliferative cells (Raychaudhuri and Park 2011). In tumorigenesis, abnormal activation of FOXM1 hampers cellular senescence and promotes cancer initiation by stimulating stem cell-like self-renewal (Koo et al. 2012).

Studies have also demonstrated that FOXM1 is involved in cancer progression, including cell proliferation, tissue homeostasis, tumor angiogenesis, migration, and invasion (Koo et al. 2012). Importantly, FOXM1 can modulate drug sensitivity and resistance in various tumor types, as it is associated with the control of DNA damage response and regulation of reactive oxygen species (ROS) (Raychaudhuri and Park 2011; Alvarez-Fernandez and Medema 2013). Due to its minimal-to-no expression in normal healthy tissue and its involvement in all stages of many cancer types, FOXM1 is considered an ideal molecular target for precise tumor growth inhibition without harming normal cells. In fact, FOXM1 was named the Molecule of the Year in 2010 (Liao et al. 2018). A small molecule compound called Robert Costa Memorial drug-1 (RCM-1) has recently been identified as a FOXM1 inhibitor (Sun et al. 2017a). Studies have confirmed that RCM-1 inhibits tumor growth by: (1) Preventing FOXM1 nuclear accumulation, leading to protein ubiquitination and proteasomal degradation; (2) Inhibiting cancer cell proliferation associated with FOXM1 by increasing the duration of mitotic/cell cycle phases; (3) Decreasing the protein interaction between FOXM1 and β-catenin, which reduces the levels and stability of β-catenin, a regulator associated with carcinogenesis (Shukla et al. 2019). Although RCM-1 holds promise as a candidate for cancer therapy, its application, like other FOXM1 inhibitors, is limited by the lack of an efficient delivery system to target cancer cells. The major challenge is the high hydrophobicity of RCM-1. Its poor solubility in aqueous solutions prevents intravenous administration and results in low RCM-1 concentrations in tumors, leading to insufficient anticancer effects. Therefore, there is a critical need to develop a delivery system capable of stabilizing hydrophobic compounds and efficiently delivering them to cancer cells.

Gene therapy provides another approach for regulating transcription factors by delivering specific genes to cells carrying mutations, thus correcting the abnormal activity of transcription factors. One example is the Forkhead Box (FOX) family member, FOXF1, which has been found to be involved in various pulmonary diseases (Clark et al. 1993). For instance, bronchopulmonary dysplasia (BPD), a complication of preterm birth, can lead to respiratory insufficiency and a high risk of pulmonary hypertension (Abman 2010). Previous studies have demonstrated that FOXF1 promotes vascular endothelial cell proliferation and angiogenesis. In a mouse model of BPD, delivery of the Foxf1 gene significantly improves lung angiogenesis (Bolte et al. 2020). The STAT3 signaling pathway has also been identified as important in pulmonary angiogenesis (Pradhan et al. 2019a). Depletion or mutations in the FOXF1 gene can disrupt the STAT3-FOXF1 protein–protein interactions, which are associated with Alveolar Capillary Dysplasia with Misalignment of Pulmonary Veins (ACDMPV), a fatal congenital disorder characterized by reduced capillary density and impaired lobular development (Pradhan et al. 2019a, b; Kim et al. 2005). ACDMPV has a mortality rate close to 100% due to respiratory insufficiency and impaired lung tissue development. Therefore, there is a critical need for new therapies to treat ACDMPV in infants with defective FOXF1. Our previous work has shown that increasing STAT3 gene and protein levels can activate endothelial cell proliferation and enhance angiogenesis, making gene therapy an ideal approach for ACDMPV treatment (Pradhan et al. 2019a). FOXF1 is also expressed in the adult lung, where it helps maintain the endothelial barrier and pulmonary homeostasis (Cai et al. 2016). Recent studies have demonstrated its role in lung tissue repair and regeneration after injury by providing angiocrine growth factors. Lack of Foxf1 in mouse models exacerbates pulmonary fibrosis caused by dysregulated tissue repair (Bian et al. 2023). Given the crucial roles of FOXF1 in embryonic development and organ repair and regeneration, it could be considered a potential therapeutic target for ACDMPV and lung fibrosis treatment. However, gene therapy faces major challenges. The therapeutic gene cannot be used directly in vivo due to various reasons: (1) Enzymes in the biological system, such as Deoxyribonuclease (DNase) and Ribonuclease (RNase), may degrade the therapeutic genes. (2) Nucleic acids lack cell selectivity, making it difficult for therapeutic genes to accumulate in specific tissues or cells spontaneously. (3) The cell membrane penetration efficiency of nucleic acids is insufficient, making it challenging for therapeutic genes to enter cells easily. Therefore, an ideal delivery system needs to be developed that can protect therapeutic genes from degradation and precisely and efficiently deliver them to the targeted cells.

1.2 *Advantages of Nanoparticles in Biomedical Applications*

The advancement of medical sciences has brought about new opportunities and possibilities for precision theranostics. However, a common challenge faced by these advancements is the lack of an effective targeting system. To address this issue, multidisciplinary scientific efforts have explored novel ideas in biomedicine, with nanoparticles emerging as one of the most promising candidates. Nanoparticles offer numerous benefits in biomedical applications due to their unique properties and capabilities (Fig. 1).

Firstly, nanoparticles possess a distinct size range typically ranging from 1 to hundreds of nanometers. Recent studies have demonstrated that the cellular uptake efficiency of therapeutics is greatly influenced by their sizes.

For small molecules with a molecular weight below 1 kDa, their cellular internalization primarily occurs through simple diffusion, and their penetration efficiency is largely influenced by the nature of the molecules (Mosquera et al. 2018). Small molecule drugs that are insoluble in the lipid bilayers of cell membranes often struggle to effectively enter cells (Yang and Hinner 2015). On the other hand, biological macromolecules with a molecular weight above 1 kDa, such as proteins and nucleic acids, cannot directly cross cell membranes through diffusion. Instead, they are primarily transported via active processes like endocytosis. However, they exhibit inefficient endocytic uptake due to factors such as their larger size range and the

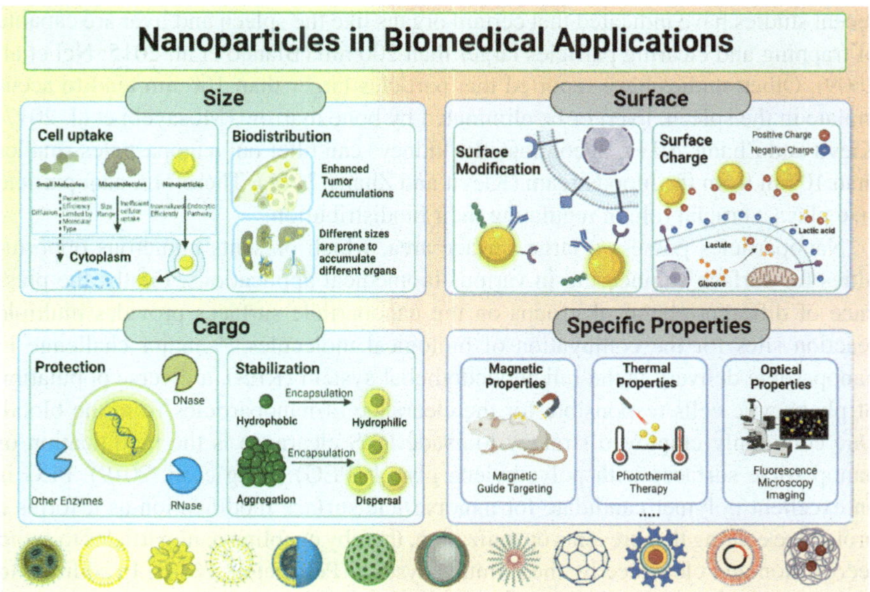

Fig. 1 Nanoparticles in biomedical applications (Created with Biorender.com)

absence of specific receptor interactions (Mosquera et al. 2018). Even if successfully endocytosed, macromolecules can become trapped in endosomes due to their limited escape capability (Torchilin 2008). In comparison to small molecules and biological macromolecules, nanoparticles with even larger sizes can be actively internalized into cells through endocytic pathways (Behzadi et al. 2017). Nanoparticles with a nanoscale size possess a high surface-to-volume ratio, which enhances their binding affinity to cell surfaces (Mosquera et al. 2018). Therefore, well-designed nanoparticles with suitable sizes can facilitate the more efficient cellular uptake of therapeutics.

Beyond the cellular level, the biodistribution of injected biomedical particles is highly influenced by their sizes. For example, the enhanced permeability and retention (EPR) effect in tumor vessels contributes to the improved accumulation of particles within a specific size range in tumors. In cancer therapies, nanoparticles with specific sizes can passively transport into tumors due to the EPR effect, resulting in the accumulation of drug-loaded nanoparticles within the tumor tissue (Goos et al. 2020). The EPR effect is a unique phenomenon where the gaps between endothelial cells in tumor blood vessels are larger than those in normal tissues (Wu 2021). These gaps provide higher permeability in tumor blood vessels for therapeutics within certain size ranges, and the solid tumor tissue has a higher retention rate for such particles (Fang et al. 2011). Studies have shown that nanoparticles with diameters of approximately 100–200 nm are considered optimal for exploiting the EPR effect and achieving tumor accumulation (Wu 2021). Apart from tumors, the biodistribution of nanoparticles in other organs is also highly dependent on their sizes. For instance, recent studies have indicated that certain organs like the spleen and liver are capable of trapping and clearing particles larger than 200 nm (Blanco et al. 2015; Nel et al. 2009). Other studies have reported that particles larger than 100 nm tend to accumulate in the spleen, liver, or be eliminated by bone marrow (Mosayebi et al. 2017; Kievit and Zhang 2011). In contrast, the kidneys can filter out nanoparticles smaller than 10 nm from the bloodstream (Kievit and Zhang 2011). Therefore, nanoparticle size plays a crucial role in regulating their biodistribution.

Nanoparticles possess a large surface area, which presents numerous opportunities for surface engineering in various biomedical applications. Firstly, the presence of different chemical groups on the nanoparticle surfaces provides multiple reaction sites for the conjugation of biological molecules. A major challenge in nanoparticle delivery is the reticuloendothelial system (RES), a diverse population of phagocytic cells responsible for the clearance of nanoparticles from the blood. One commonly employed strategy to evade RES clearance is the modification of nanoparticle surfaces with polyethylene glycol (PEG) (Tang et al. 2019). PEG is an excellent polymer candidate for nanoparticle surface modification as it forms a protective coating that prevents opsonization, thereby enabling nanoparticles to avoid recognition and clearance by the immune system (Perry et al. 2012). In addition to PEGylation, other polymers such as polyvinylpyrrolidone (PVP), polyphosphoesters (PPEs), and zwitterionic polymers have been used to protect nanoparticles from RES clearance (Izci et al. 2021).

For specific cell targeting, nanoparticles can be decorated with biomolecules or ligands. One example is the utilization of antibodies as targeting ligands on nanoparticle surfaces. The amine or thiol groups of antibodies can be coupled to nanoparticles using established chemical reactions. The high specificity of antibodies significantly enhances the interaction of nanoparticles with target cells or antigens (Richards et al. 2016). Since the expression levels of receptors vary among different cells and in specific physiological processes, other surface decoration strategies have been employed to improve nanoparticle targeting efficiency in addition to antibody conjugation. For instance, mannose-decorated nanoparticles have demonstrated enhanced targeting efficiency toward alveolar macrophages in the treatment of pulmonary tuberculosis, where the infected macrophages overexpress mannose receptors (Truzzi et al. 2020). Another advantage of the large surface area of nanoparticles is the ability to control surface charge. Previous studies have shown that different cells exhibit variations in surface metabolism, resulting in differences in surface charge. Cancer cells, for example, often possess a highly negatively charged surface due to the Warburg effect (Shi 2017). In contrast, normal cell lines typically maintain a neutral or slightly positive surface charge (Chen et al. 2016). Consequently, nanoparticles with positively charged surfaces can bind more efficiently to cancer cells through electrostatic interactions (Han et al. 2017). Similarly, surface charge has been utilized for targeting pulmonary endothelial cells, where positively charged nanoparticles exhibit higher efficiency in targeting pulmonary endothelium. This is attributed to the negatively charged surface of endothelial cells, which is covered by glycocalyx containing sialic acids with abundant carboxylates (Dunn et al. 2018; Fu et al. 2022).

Protecting cargos, particularly in gene delivery, is a crucial aspect when utilizing nanoparticle delivery systems. A significant challenge in gene delivery arises from the inherent instability of nucleic acids, which can be degraded by nucleases. Encapsulation of nucleic acids into polymeric nanoparticles, forming polyplexes, provides effective protection against nuclease-mediated degradation (Berg et al. 2020). Polyethylenimine (PEI) is a widely used polymer for nucleic acid delivery, as studies have demonstrated that PEI-based polymeric nanoparticles can efficiently condense DNA and offer excellent resistance against DNase degradation (Thapa and Narain 2016). In addition to nucleic acids, certain drugs, especially hydrophobic ones, cannot be directly employed in vivo due to their poor solubility in aqueous solutions. An example is Paclitaxel (PTX), a common chemotherapy drug for cancer treatment. However, PTX's limited clinical application is attributed to its instability and high cytotoxicity. To address this issue, nanoparticles have been designed as carriers to stabilize PTX. These nanocarriers typically consist of amphiphilic molecules such as lipids or amphiphilic polymers. This structure enables the creation of a hydrophobic core that accommodates the therapeutic agent while maintaining a hydrophilic surface, thereby ensuring nanoparticle stability (Massey et al. 2019). Furthermore, nanoparticles with mesoporous structures have the capability to deliver hydrophobic drugs by loading them into the nanoparticle pores, protecting them from aggregation (Sun et al. 2017b).

Nanoparticles are valuable for biomedical applications due to their specific properties. For instance, iron oxide nanoparticles, known as superparamagnetic nanoparticles, find utility in magnetic-guided targeting and MRI. Wang et al. synthesized a superparamagnetic nanoparticle coated with PEI and PEG using $Fe(acac)_3$ for MR imaging in mouse brains. This nanoparticle exhibited good water solubility and contrast effect, crucial for in vivo delivery and MR imaging (Wang et al. 2015a). Apart from magnetic properties, nanoparticles' thermal characteristics offer new possibilities in disease prevention and control, particularly in cancer. Nanoparticle-mediated hyperthermia is a well-known example in cancer therapy. Gold nanoparticles, with strong near-infrared (NIR) absorption, hold promise as therapeutic agents in cancer photothermal therapies (Yang et al. 2018). Recent studies on superparamagnetic iron oxide nanoparticles have demonstrated their potential in cancer hyperthermia therapy. These nanoparticles generate heat when subjected to an alternating magnetic field, leading to tumor cell death (Gavilán et al. 2021). Iron oxide nanoparticles also possess a photothermal effect that can be utilized in cancer photothermal therapy. Activation of iron oxide nanoparticles with a NIR laser increases the local temperature, effectively killing cancer cells through hyperthermia (Estelrich and M. 2018). Semiconductor nanoparticles, such as quantum dots, with unique optical properties at the nanoscale, have become popular tools in medical imaging. Unlike conventional fluorescent dyes, quantum dots have a relatively broad absorption spectra, enabling excitation with a wide range of excitation light. They also offer a narrower emission spectrum that can be tuned based on their formulation and size. Additionally, quantum dots interact closely with biological entities due to their specific size scale, making them attractive in biomedical applications (Jamieson et al. 2007; Wagner et al. 2019).

Overall, nanoparticles serve as excellent tools in biomedical applications. The key to nanoparticle design lies in employing appropriate targeting strategies to maximize their cell and tissue selectivity, as the therapeutic outcomes heavily rely on the nanoparticles' targeting efficiency. The following sections introduce the latest nanoparticle designs and targeting strategies, including active targeting, passive targeting, and strategies that utilize external forces to accumulate nanoparticles in specific regions. Moreover, the synergistic enhancement of targeting efficiency through the combination of different strategies is also discussed in this chapter.

2 Nanoparticle Design for Active Targeting

Active targeting, also known as receptor-mediated targeting, involves the conjugation of nanoparticles with specific ligands such as antibodies, peptides, and other molecules that can be recognized by the target cells (Rasal and Reddy 2021). By employing ligands that exhibit a high affinity for biomarkers that are only overexpressed on the target cells, the binding efficiency of the nanoparticles to the target cells can be significantly enhanced, while minimizing non-specific interactions with other cell types. The crucial aspect of designing active targeting nanoparticles lies

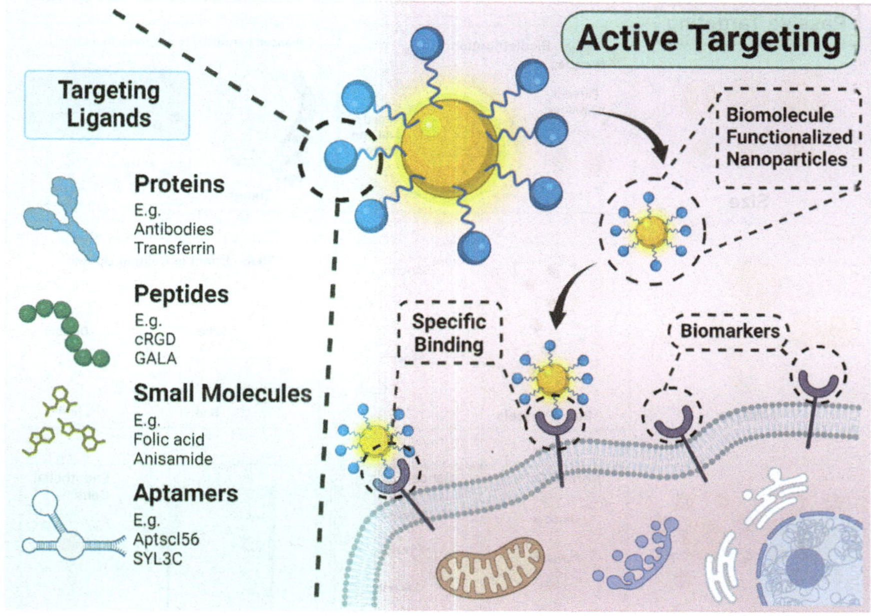

Fig. 2 Typical design of nanoparticles for active targeting. The nanoparticles are modified with targeting ligands that can be recognized by the specific biomarkers on the target cell surface. By using active targeting, the functionalized nanoparticle can have a strong specific binding to target cells. (Created with Biorender.com)

in the careful selection of highly specific ligands that can efficiently interact with the target cells. Proteins (including antibodies and non-antibody proteins), peptides, small molecules, and aptamers are among the most commonly used ligands in active targeting nanoparticle design. This section will discuss these ligands, along with the latest studies and typical designs (refer to Fig. 2).

2.1 Protein-Mediated Targeting

Antibodies are the most well-known proteins used for specific targeting in biological systems. Also known as immunoglobulins (Ig), antibodies are glycoproteins that play crucial roles in the immune system (Marques et al. 2020). They exhibit high affinity for specific receptors, making them ideal targeting agents (Goddard et al. 2020). There are five main antibody isotypes (IgG, IgA, IgM, IgD, and IgE), classified based on their heavy chain type. Among these, IgG antibodies are widely used for therapeutic purposes and nanoparticle functionalization (Marques et al. 2020). IgG antibodies have a Y-shaped structure consisting of a constant (Fc) region and a variable (Fab) region (Goddard et al. 2020). One strategy for conjugating antibodies to nanoparticle surfaces is through adsorption, which can be achieved via

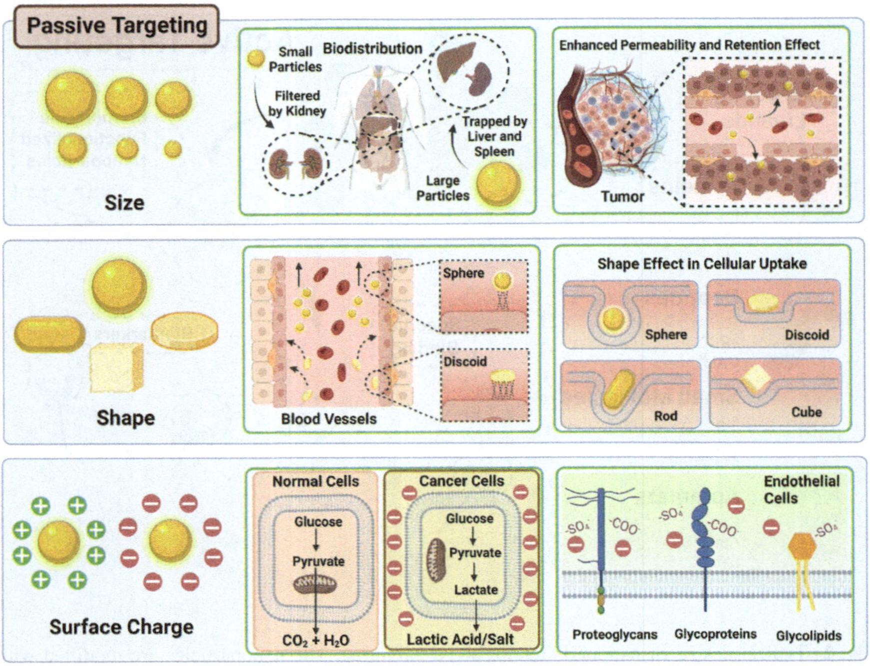

Fig. 3 Typical nanoparticle design for passive targeting. (1) Sizes: Nanoparticle sizes have a great impact on the biodistribution of the nanoparticles (large nanoparticles are prone to accumulate to liver or spleen, while small nanoparticles can be filtered by kidney), and the enlarged endothelial gap in tumor vasculature allows nanoparticles with specific size to leak and accumulate in tumor tissue. (2) Shapes: Different shapes may lead to different fate of the nanoparticle in circulation (discoidal nanoparticles have more tumbling and oscillatory effect which can increase the nanoparticle-vascular endothelial cell contact) and cellular uptake (different shape requires to overcome different membrane bending energy barrier). (3) Surface charge: Bioelectricity can mediate the nanoparticles to bind to the cells with opposite surface charge. The fundamental of the surface charge of the cells are from their unique metabolism (aerobic glycolysis in cancer cells) or contents on cell membranes (glycocalyx, including proteoglycans, glycoproteins, and glycolipids on endothelial cells). (Created with Biorender.com)

physical adsorption or ionic adsorption (Juan et al. 2020). Physical adsorption, such as hydrophobic interaction-based adsorption, often leads to significant conformational changes and random orientation of the antibodies on the nanoparticle surface, resulting in reduced biological activity (Marques et al. 2020). On the other hand, ionic adsorption depends on the density of charged groups on the antibody surface, allowing for oriented adsorption that avoids immobilizing the antigen recognition site and preserves antibody binding capacity (Marques et al. 2020). However, nonspecific ionic adsorption of serum proteins may lead to competitive displacement (Montenegro et al. 2013). Both physical and ionic adsorption strategies require a high concentration of antibodies for functionalization, which increases costs and

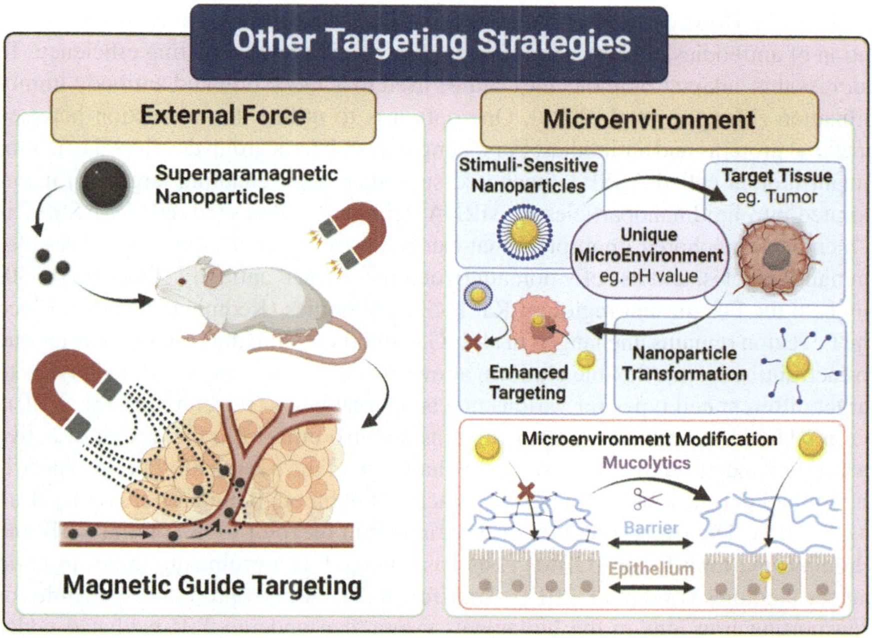

Fig. 4 Examples of other targeting strategies. (1) External magnetic field can be applied to help the superparamagnetic nanoparticles to accumulate to the target site. (2) Microenvironment plays an important role in nanoparticle targeting. First is using stimuli-sensitive nanoparticles that can be triggered by microenvironment. For example, nanoparticles covered with biologically inert polymer can avoid systemic clearance, once the nanoparticles enter the tumor tissue, the low pH value of tumor microenvironment can disassemble the polymer layer to enhance the tumor cell uptake and accumulation of the nanoparticles. Second is changing the microenvironment with specific agents, for example, mucus layer is the major barrier causes low epithelial targeting efficiency, by using mucolytics, the viscosity of the mucus layer can be decreased, and the epithelial targeting efficiency can be improved. (Created with Biorender.com)

limits the application of antibody-mediated targeting nanoparticles (Jazayeri et al. 2016).

Alternatively, covalent conjugation is another widely used strategy for antibody-nanoparticle conjugation. It involves simple chemical reactions based on the presence of amine (-NH2) groups in antibodies, which can easily conjugate to nanoparticles with carboxylic acid or activated succinimidyl ester on their surfaces (Goddard et al. 2020; Lim et al. 2014). For instance, Penon et al. reported the functionalization of porphyrin-gold nanoparticles with anti-erbB2 antibodies for cancer thermodynamic therapy (Penon et al. 2017). In this study, gold nanoparticles were functionalized with porphyrin and thiolated carboxyl-terminated PEG to enhance water solubility, and the antibodies were conjugated to the nanoparticles through EDC/NHS coupling between the amine groups on the antibodies and carboxyl groups on the PEG linker. The anti-erbB2 antibody-modified nanoparticles exhibited high targeting efficiency toward the erbB2 receptor overexpressed on SK-BR-3 breast cancer cells (Penon et al. 2017). However, a limitation of most covalent strategies is the random orientation of antibodies, which can reduce antibody activity and targeting efficiency. To address this, adapter biomolecules can be used to achieve oriented antibody immobilization (Marques et al. 2020). One option is to utilize the interaction between artificial proteins and antibodies. For example, Dan Peer's group developed a recombinant protein called ASSET (anchored secondary scFv enabling targeting) incorporated into lipid nanoparticles for siRNA delivery (Kedmi et al. 2018). ASSET is a membrane-anchored lipoprotein that can be easily inserted into the lipid vesicles on nanoparticles, and its scFv domain (from monoclonal antibody clone RG7/1.30) binds to the Fc constant region of Rat IgG2a antibodies (Kedmi et al. 2018). Since the Fc region remains unchanged in all IgG antibodies while the Fab region is unique to each antibody, this flexible platform allows for easy switching of antibody types to target different cell types for various precision treatments (Rosenblum et al. 2020).

In addition to antibodies, other proteins are also utilized in the design of active targeting nanoparticles. One significant challenge in the treatment of brain cancer is the limited permeability of therapeutics across the blood–brain barrier (BBB) (Luo et al. 2019). The overexpression of the transferrin receptor (TfR) on the BBB and glioblastoma multiforme (GBM) cells has emerged as a promising target in brain cancer therapies (Luo et al. 2019). Transferrin (Tf), a glycoprotein responsible for transporting iron ions in the biological system, can undergo TfR-mediated endocytosis. Tf molecules, composed of amino acids, can be conjugated to carboxyl-terminated silicon nanoparticles using EDC/NHS chemistry (Luo et al. 2019). Additionally, maleimide-thiol chemistry is widely employed for Tf-nanoparticle conjugation. Muntoni et al. developed a solid lipid nanoparticle delivery system modified with Tf and insulin to enhance the targeting efficiency for GBM treatments (Muntoni et al. 2019). In this study, proteins were thiolated using 2-iminothiolane, and the lipid nanoparticles were coated with Stearyl-PEG-Maleimide. Subsequently, the proteins were grafted onto the nanoparticle surface through simple mixing under acidic conditions (Muntoni et al. 2019).

Similar to antibodies, proteins like Tf can bind to specific biomolecules. For instance, the Tf-binding peptide (TBP) CGGGHKYLRW has shown high affinity for Tf and was employed as a linker to modify Tf onto nanoparticles for the delivery of the anticancer drug doxorubicin hydrochloride (Wei et al. 2020). Compared to non-functionalized nanoparticles, the Tf-binding peptide-functionalized nanoparticles exhibited approximately a 2.5-fold improvement in HCT-16 cancer cell uptake in vitro and over a twofold increase in tumor accumulation in vivo (Wei et al. 2020). These results confirm the feasibility and effectiveness of utilizing proteins to enhance the targeting capability of nanoparticles.

2.2 *Peptide-Mediated Targeting*

Peptides, which are short chains of amino acids with chemical groups similar to proteins, can be conjugated to nanoparticles using similar chemistry. Peptides have the advantage of being small and easy to synthesize, making them ideal candidates for nanoparticle functionalization (Ruoslahti 2012). One widely recognized peptide used for nanoparticle decoration is the Arg-Gly-Asp (RGD) peptide, which is an integrin binding motif (Sheikh et al. 2021; Yadav et al. 2023). Despite its small size, the RGD motif exhibits high specific affinity for integrin ($\alpha_v\beta_3$), which is highly overexpressed on cancer cells and tumor vascular endothelial cells (Yadav et al. 2023; Gong et al. 2021). In a recent study, linear RGD peptides were conjugated to carboxylated Pluronic F127 through a simple EDC/NHS reaction, resulting in the synthesis of RGD-Pluronic F127 (Yadav et al. 2023). Here, Pluronic F127 stabilized the hydrophobic core composed of Poly(D,L-lactic-co-glycolic acid) (PLGA) and anticancer drugs to form PLGA nanoparticles, while the RGD on the nanoparticle surface facilitated targeted delivery to lung cancer cells (Yadav et al. 2023). However, linear RGD peptides are prone to chemical degradation, whereas cyclic RGD (cRGD) peptides exhibit higher bioactivity and targeting efficiency due to their rigid conformational structure, which prevents proteolysis (Sheikh et al. 2021).

In peptide-mediated targeting nanoparticle designs, the choice of linker and spacer is crucial (Biscaglia et al. 2019). To achieve high targeting efficiency, cRGD peptides must be linked to plasmonic nanoparticles through a long PEG chain and a short oligolysine spacer. Directly linking cRGD to PEG chains on the nanoparticles may result in a loss of targeting ability (Biscaglia et al. 2019). Additionally, the density of cRGD ligands is important. Moderate targeting cRGD densities (0.2–0.5 ligand nm^{-2}) provide better targeting efficiency due to the appropriate spatial presentation and negligible over-clustering effects of cRGD peptides (Siani et al. 2022). Peptide-mediated targeting nanoparticles can bind not only to receptors but also to other molecules present on cell membranes. For example, it has been reported that the GALA peptide (WEAALAEALAEALAEHLAEALAEALEALAA) specifically binds to sialic acid-terminated sugar chains on the surface of pulmonary endothelial cells (Abd Elwakil et al. 2019; Kusumoto et al. 2013). In related studies, GALA peptides were conjugated to cholesterol, allowing the Cholesteryl-GALA molecules to anchor to the lipid bilayer with the GALA peptide oriented outward on the nanoparticle surface (Kusumoto et al. 2013). By incorporating Cholesteryl-GALA into lipid nanoparticles, the pulmonary accumulation and endothelial cell targeting efficiency were significantly improved both in vitro and in vivo (Hagino et al. 2021).

2.3 *Small Molecule-Mediated Targeting*

Using small molecules as targeting ligands has several advantages, like simplicity of the chemistry for conjugation, high manufacturability, and low cost (Zhao et al. 2020). However, because the binding of small molecules to targets is driven by weak interactions, receptors having deep topographies must be sought to provide the required bonding potential for high-affinity interactions (Srinivasarao and Low 2017). Folic acid (FA), a vitamin that is related to nucleotide synthesis, is the most widely used small molecule for nanoparticle functionalization and specific targeting

(Narmani et al. 2019). The expression of folate receptors (FRs) is low in healthy tissues, but FRα is overexpressed in various cancer cells, while FRβ is expressed on activated macrophages that are involved in a variety of inflammatory and autoimmune diseases (Zhao et al. 2020; Movileanu et al. 2022). In addition, FA has a high affinity for FR ($K_d = 10^{-7}$ mM) and enables efficient intracellular delivery, thus, FA is considered as an ideal targeting ligand in many diseases (Zhao et al. 2020). In the latest research investigating combination therapy efficacy of FOXM1 inhibitor RCM-1 and commercial anticancer drug Vincristine, polymeric nanoparticles with FA functionalization were used for RCM-1 delivery (Donovan et al. 2023). Like other molecules containing carboxyl groups, FA can be conjugated to the primary amine groups on the polymer backbones via EDC/NHS coupling. Compared to the nanoparticle without FA modification, the FA functionalized nanoparticles demonstrated a significantly higher tumor accumulation, which indicated that FA modification can provide a high cancer targeting efficiency (Donovan et al. 2023).

Except FA, some other small molecules also showed their potential to serve as the nanoparticle targeting ligands, for example, anisamide (Goddard et al. 2020; Zhao et al. 2020). Anisamide is a small molecule ligand with high affinity for the sigma receptor that is highly expressed on a variety of human cancer cell lines and rapidly proliferating activated fibroblasts (Luan et al. 2019; Han et al. 2023). To modify the anisamide onto the nanoparticle, the most widely used strategy is using NHS-activated anisic acid. With NHS ester, the anisamide can be easily conjugated to any linkers with a primary amine group for different nanoparticle functionalization. In a study using gold nanoparticles for prostate cancer treatment, the anisamide was coupled with $SH\text{-}PEG_{5000}\text{-}NH_2$ to form PEGylated anisamide for Au nanoparticles surface decoration (Luan et al. 2019). The Au nanoparticles with anisamide significantly increased PC-3 cell uptake (~ 45%) compared to the nanoparticle without functionalization (~ 15%) in vitro, and the in vivo experiments confirmed that the anisamide-Au nanoparticles carried anti-RelA siRNA and paclitaxel is a promising strategy for prostate cancer combination therapy (Luan et al. 2019). For lipid nanoparticles, a recent study reported a one-pot, two-step modular synthetic method to prepare anisamide ligand-tethered lipidoids by using anisoyl-NHS, polyamines and alkyl epoxides (Han et al. 2023). In a preclinical model of liver fibrosis, this anisamide targeted lipid nanoparticle showed a high liver accumulation and led to ~ 65% silencing of HSP47, which was significantly higher than non-targeted lipid nanoparticles and FDA-approved MC3 ionizable lipid (Han et al. 2023).

2.4 Aptamer-Mediated Targeting

Aptamers, which are synthetic single-stranded DNA or RNA oligonucleotides, possess unique three-dimensional conformations that enable them to bind to target molecules with high specificity and affinity (Wu et al. 2021). Typically consisting of around 40–100 nucleotide bases, the 3D structure and binding capabilities of aptamers are closely linked to their sequence (Mignani et al. 2020). Aptamers offer several advantages when used as targeting ligands in biomedical applications, including their small size, ease of synthesis, excellent thermal and chemical stability, low immunogenicity, affordability, and high targeting efficiency (Mignani et al. 2020; Fan et al. 2023). Importantly, aptamers can be produced in large quantities using the Systematic Evolution of Ligands by Exponential Enrichment (SELEX) process (Fan et al. 2023). SELEX involves three main steps: selection, purification, and amplification. The use of the latest cell-SELEX technique allows for effective isolation of aptamers that recognize cell surfaces, without overlooking the target cell's surface molecules. This technique also enables the identification of aptamers capable of entering target cells through receptor-mediated internalization (Fu and Xiang 2020).

Similar to antibodies, aptamers can be conjugated to nanoparticles through covalent or non-covalent methods. Functional groups on the aptamer, such as primary amines or thiol groups, can react with chemical groups on the nanoparticle surface, such as carboxyl, maleimide, or aldehyde groups (Fu and Xiang 2020). For instance, sclerostin, a small protein secreted by osteocytes and a promising therapeutic target in osteoporosis treatment, was targeted using an anti-sclerostin aptamer (Aptscl56)-modified mesoporous silica nanoparticle. This nanomedicine demonstrated high bone targeting efficiency and showcased the clinical potential of this design. The aptamer was conjugated to the PEG linker on the nanoparticle surface through a simple EDC/NHS reaction (Niu et al. 2022). In contrast, non-covalent conjugation strategies rely on affinity interactions or electrostatic interactions between aptamers and the nanoparticle surface coatings (Fu and Xiang 2020). Biotin, a vitamin molecule commonly used for aptamer functionalization, was employed in the synthesis of magnetic nanoparticles for breast cancer testing. Streptavidin was introduced to L-cysteine capped iron oxide nanoparticles, allowing for easy modification by biotin-functionalized MUC-1 binding aptamers and resulting in nanoparticles with high specificity (Kiplagat et al. 2020). Biomimetic camouflage has also proven useful in aptamer conjugation. The SYL3C aptamer, successfully employed in the isolation of circulating tumor cells (CTCs) for early cancer diagnosis, was anchored to iron oxide nanoclusters using DSPE-modified SYL3C aptamers. The nanoclusters were coated with leukocyte membrane fragments in a nickel pattern microfluidic device. This unique design enabled the device to capture over 90% of rare tumor cells from blood samples within 20 min, without experiencing non-specific absorption of leukocytes (Zhang et al. 2019).

3 Nanoparticle Design for Passive Targeting

In contrast to active targeting strategies, passive targeting relies on the physicochemical properties of nanoparticles, eliminating the need for bioactive targeting ligands in nanoparticle designs. While targeting ligands offer excellent cell selectivity, the additional modification process and high costs associated with biomolecules have prompted researchers to explore targeting strategies that do not rely on specific ligands. However, the efficacy of surface ligands in targeting may be hindered by the phenomenon known as "protein corona." Protein corona refers to the absorption of serum proteins from physiological media onto nanoparticle surfaces. The impact of protein corona on the targeting efficiency of antibody-grafted microspheres was investigated by Professor Caruso's group (Dai et al. 2015a). It was observed that in the presence of human serum albumin (HSA) alone, protein coronas had a positive effect on antibody-mediated targeting (Dai et al. 2015a, b). Conversely, in complex conditions with multiple types of serum proteins, a loss of targeting ability in antibody-functionalized nanoparticles was observed (Dai et al. 2015b). The influence of protein corona also depends on the molecular size of the targeting moieties. Larger antibodies may prevent complete shielding of the ligands, while smaller targeting moieties like transferrin or single-domain antibodies on the nanoparticle surface may lose their targeting capability in the presence of protein coronas (Dai et al. 2015a). Similar evidence has shown that protein coronas can diminish the targeting ability of aptamer-functionalized nanoparticles (Ding et al. 2019). Moreover, due to cancer heterogeneity, it is theoretically impossible to find a molecule target that is present at a significant level on all types of cancer cells while being completely absent on normal cells (Han et al. 2017). In cancer early diagnosis and circulating tumor cell (CTC) detection, the most widely used targeting strategy is anti-EpCAM antibody functionalization. However, relying solely on EpCAM-dependent CTC detection may miss CTCs with stem cell-like phenotypes, compromising the accuracy and sensitivity of diagnoses (Deng et al. 2022). Consequently, research efforts have focused on exploring passive targeting strategies that do not rely on biomarkers, reevaluating typical designs and the fundamentals of nanoparticle passive targeting.

3.1 Size-Based Targeting

The hydrodynamic size of nanoparticles plays a crucial role in their in vivo fate and targeting of specific organs or tissues, making it a primary consideration in nanoparticle design. In systemic delivery, particles larger than 200 nm in size are prone to being trapped by the liver and spleen (Nel et al. 2009). Studies have shown that as the size of liposomes/polymeric nanoparticles exceeds 150 nm, more of them are entrapped in these organs (Blanco et al. 2015). Similarly, iron oxide nanoparticles larger than 100 nm can be removed from circulation by the liver and spleen (Kievit and Zhang 2011). Conversely, small nanoparticles (less than 10 nm for iron oxide nanoparticles and less than 5 nm for liposomes/polymeric nanoparticles) can be filtered by the kidneys (Blanco et al. 2015; Kievit and Zhang 2011). Therefore, larger nanoparticles are generally favored for liver or spleen targeting, while smaller nanoparticles are more suitable for kidney delivery. However, determining an optimal size for biodistribution is not sufficient; the tissue structures and cell types must also be considered in size-based targeting nanoparticle design. For instance, nanoparticles targeting Kupffer cells (KCs) or sinusoidal endothelial cells (SECs) in the liver may have a larger size, while nanoparticles targeting hepatocytes are typically designed with a diameter below 100 nm to reach the space of Disse via endothelial fenestrae (Bottger et al. 2020). In the case of lung-targeted nanoparticle design, although large particles (>2000 nm) can accumulate in lung capillaries as well as the liver and spleen (Blanco et al. 2015), such large sizes can lead to rapid clearance and low endocytosis (Huang et al. 2017a; Fan et al. 2020). Therefore, nanoparticles intended for pulmonary delivery must remain small. Researchers focusing on pulmonary vascular diseases gene therapy have found that the size and surface charge of nanoparticles play important roles in targeting pulmonary endothelial cells. The dense microvascular networks in the lungs enable nanoparticles of specific sizes (e.g., 120 nm) to enter and accumulate effectively (Dunn et al. 2018; Deng et al. 2021a).

Size-dependent targeting strategies are also widely used in cancer therapy due to the enhanced permeability and retention (EPR) effect. Tumor blood vessels differ from those in normal tissues, exhibiting heterogeneity, irregular diameter, and leakiness due to endothelial gaps (Kalyane et al. 2019). Tumors also have a poor lymphatic system, resulting in slow drainage and high accumulation of intratumoral components. The EPR effect allows nanoparticles of specific sizes to enter and stay within tumor tissues (Kalyane et al. 2019). Liposome nanoparticles with hydrodynamic sizes between 100–200 nm have demonstrated significantly higher tumor accumulation compared to sizes below 50 nm or above 300 nm (Kalyane et al. 2019). Various studies have highlighted the size effects of different nanoparticles, with the conclusion that nanoparticles in the size range of 20–150 nm exhibit enhanced accumulation in tumor tissues due to the EPR effect (Dolai et al. 2021). It should be noted that the optimal nanoparticle size for the EPR effect varies depending on the nanoparticle type. For example, in a metal–organic frameworks (MOFs) nanoparticle drug delivery system, smaller nanoparticles (60 nm) showed higher tumor accumulation compared to larger ones (130 nm) (Duan et al. 2018). Conversely, in a micelle nanoparticle drug delivery system, 100 nm nanoparticles accumulated 10 to 20 times more in tumors than 30 nm nanoparticles, with the smaller nanoparticles exhibiting greater penetration within the tumor (Wang et al. 2015b). Therefore, when designing nanoparticles for tumor targeting delivery, striking a balance between size for accumulation and penetration is necessary.

3.2 Shape-Based Targeting

Apart from nanoparticle size, the shape of nanoparticles is another crucial parameter that impacts targeting performance (Zhang et al. 2017). While most nanoparticles are typically spherical, bacteria and viruses exhibit various shapes that enhance their infectivity to target cells (Raj et al. 2021). Taking inspiration from natural viruses, Discher's group developed filamentous nanocarriers for delivering anticancer drugs (Geng et al. 2007). The study demonstrated that filomicelles have a longer circulation time and lower systemic clearance, making them more efficient in delivering paclitaxel to tumors compared to spherical nanocarriers (Geng et al. 2007). Similarly, rod-shaped nanoparticles also showed prolonged circulation time and preferential tumor accumulation, attributed to their lower uptake by macrophages and reduced accumulation in the liver (Arnida et al. 2011). Discoidal nanoparticles, on the other hand, were found to be less susceptible to macrophage uptake, resulting in minimal liver concentration (Foster et al. 2017; Jindal 2017). Moreover, discoidal nanoparticles exhibit unique tumbling dynamics and a high propensity for margination, increasing their contact with blood vessel walls and making them ideal for vasculature targeting (Blanco et al. 2015; Foster et al. 2017).

The shape of nanoparticles not only affects their biodistribution but also influences the interaction between nanoparticles and target cells. Studies have shown that gold nanoparticles with different morphologies, such as spherical, rod-like, hollow, and core/shell, exhibit varying interactions with endothelial cells. Spherical and rod-shaped gold nanoparticles were found to have significantly higher interactions with endothelial cells compared to hollow and core/shell nanoparticles (Bartczak et al. 2012). Similarly, rod-shaped particles demonstrated higher cellular uptake and transport across intestinal cells compared to spherical particles (Banerjee et al. 2016). However, it has been reported that cylindrical nanoparticles with extremely low or high aspect ratios may exhibit lower cell uptake, as endocytosis only occurs within a specific range of aspect ratios (Jindal 2017). Simulation studies have shown contradictory results, with some indicating that spherical nanoparticles have the highest uptake rate, while others show different rankings for uptake among different shapes (Li et al. 2015). These variations can be attributed to factors such as membrane bending energy barriers and the specific characteristics of the nanoparticle shapes (Li et al. 2015). In summary, designing nanoparticles with suitable morphologies for specific targeting requires consideration of both biodistribution and cell interaction.

3.3 Surface Charge-Based Targeting

Surface charge of nanoparticles also plays a critical role in specific targeting. This targeting strategy is based on the bioelectricity at the cellular level, which includes the trans-membrane potential and the electrical charges on the cell membrane (Wang et al. 2019). One notable application of surface charge-based targeting is using positively charged nanoparticles to target the negative surface charges of cancer cells. Cancer cells exhibit a metabolic pattern known as aerobic glycolysis, where they take up more glucose and produce lactate even in the presence of oxygen (Warburg 1956; Liberti and Locasale 2016). This metabolic behavior, known as the Warburg effect, results in a net negative charge on the surface of cancer cells due to the abnormal movement of lactate across their membranes.

Studies have shown that cancer cells have a negatively charged cell surface, while normal cells have a neutral or slightly positive charge (Chen et al. 2016). This difference in surface charge enables the targeting of cancer cells using nanoparticles with specific surface charges. Positively charged nanoparticles have been demonstrated to target cancer cells more efficiently in vitro (Han et al. 2017). This bioelectricity-mediated targeting approach has also been applied to isolate circulating tumor cells

(CTCs) using positively charged nanoparticles, effectively separating them from normal blood cells (Wu et al. 2020a, b). Even in the presence of protein coronas, which can hinder targeting efficiency, positively charged nanoparticles have maintained strong electrostatic interactions with cancer cells (Zhao et al. 2018).

Variations in cell membrane composition can also influence the bioelectricity pattern and impact targeting efficiency. For example, endothelial cells lining the blood vessels have a negatively charged surface due to the presence of glycocalyx, an anionic network covering their apical surfaces (Fu et al. 2022). This negative charge facilitates stronger interactions between positively charged nanoparticles and endothelial cells. In the context of pulmonary endothelial cell targeting, positive surface charge has been shown to be important, while reversing the surface charge significantly reduces targeting efficiency. Conversely, rendering nanoparticles with a negative charge can help them avoid endothelial cell uptake and facilitate their passage across cell junctions to reach tissues behind the endothelium (Wang et al. 2018a). Negatively charged nanoparticles have also demonstrated better performance in targeting neurons and inflamed joints in rheumatoid arthritis (Dante et al. 2017; Ren et al. 2019). In these cases, the specific biophysical properties of the targeted cells or the pathological characteristics of the targeted tissues play a crucial role in charge-based nanoparticle targeting design.

In summary, surface charge of nanoparticles is an important parameter in specific targeting. Understanding the bioelectricity patterns and the biophysical properties of targeted cells or tissues is essential for designing nanoparticles with suitable surface charges for efficient targeting.

4 Other Targeting Strategies

Applying external forces is a strategy that can enhance the targeting efficiency of nanoparticles. One example is the use of a magnetic field to guide superparamagnetic nanoparticles to accumulate at specific sites. Superparamagnetism is a unique form of magnetism that occurs only in nanoparticles. Iron oxide-based nanoparticles, which exhibit superparamagnetic properties, have been approved by the FDA and are widely used in biomedical applications such as Magnetic Resonance Imaging (MRI) and anemia treatment (Gavilán et al. 2021). When the iron oxide particles are less than a threshold dimension, their magnetization can randomly flip direction under the influence of temperature (Enriquez-Navas and Garcia-Martin 2012). Superparamagnetism occurs in nanoparticles with a single domain, requiring their diameter to be within the range of 3–50 nm (Marghussian 2015). Consequently, the average magnetization value of these iron oxide nanoparticles is close to zero (Enriquez-Navas and Garcia-Martin 2012). However, they can be magnetized by an external magnetic field, making them useful in applications such as magnetic-guided targeting (Liu et al. 2019b). For instance, in regenerative medicine, human mesenchymal stem cell-derived exosomes have limited organ-targeting ability, which restricts their therapeutic potential (Li et al. 2020). Magnetic targeting can be employed to address this issue. A recent study used iron oxide nanoparticles to label exosomes derived from nanoparticle-treated human mesenchymal stem cells. With magnetic guidance, the accumulation of intravenously injected nanoparticle-labeled exosomes at the injury site was significantly increased (Li et al. 2020).

Another popular strategy to enhance nanoparticle targeting to specific tissues or cells is by utilizing the interaction between nanoparticles and the microenvironment to increase local retention and improve barrier permeability for higher cell uptake at the desired site. One approach is to use nanoparticles that can alter their properties in different microenvironments. For example, the tumor microenvironment is known to be weakly acidic, with a lower pH value compared to normal tissues (Liu et al. 2016). To enhance drug delivery to tumor cells, pH-responsive hollow mesoporous silica nanoparticles have been developed. These nanoparticles are modified with PEG molecules via weak pH-sensitive benzoic-imine bonds (Liu et al. 2016). The tumor microenvironment can break down these bonds and detach the PEG layer, enhancing tumor cell uptake.

Another method involves changing the microenvironment to improve nanoparticle uptake efficiency. In pulmonary epithelial cell targeted delivery through pulmonary administration, a major challenge is the potential trapping of nanoparticles by the mucus layer covering the epithelium. To overcome this barrier, mucolytics have been incorporated into nanoparticle designs. Mucolytics such as disulfide breaking agents (e.g., N-acetylcysteine) and mucolytic enzymes (e.g., papain and bromelain) can decrease mucus viscosity and improve the penetration rate of nanoparticles through the mucus layer (Deng et al. 2021a). By achieving a higher penetration rate, the nanoparticles can avoid mucociliary and macrophage clearance, ensuring efficient delivery to the epithelial cells (Deng et al. 2021a).

5 Combination Targeting Strategies

To achieve maximum targeting efficiency and therapeutic outcomes, researchers are exploring the synergistic combination of multiple targeting strategies. One approach is to utilize two active targeting ligands, which has been shown to enhance targeting efficiency (Jurczyk et al. 2021). For example, Zhang et al. developed gold nanoparticles functionalized with dual multivalent aptamers, Sgc8 and SYL3C, for the recognition of circulating tumor cells (CTCs) in a microfluidic chip (Zhang et al. 2021). These aptamers selectively bind to the biomarker proteins PTK7 and EpCAM expressed on the surface of CTCs, enabling highly efficient and background-free single-CTC recognition in liquid biopsy (Zhang et al. 2021).

Instead of simply adding two targeting ligands, integrating different targeting strategies can lead to synergistic effects. Magnetic fields have a significant influence on the biodistribution of superparamagnetic nanoparticles at the tissue level, but controlling magnetic field guidance to specific cell types is challenging. On the other hand, active targeting using ligands is effective at the cell level. Therefore, researchers are seeking nanoparticles that combine magnetic properties with targeting ligands

(Moradi et al. 2021). For instance, Huang et al. conjugated folic acid (FA) onto iron oxide nanoparticles, enabling dual targeting through magnetic field guidance and active targeting (Huang et al. 2017b). The nanoparticles were injected intravenously into mice, and a permanent magnet was used to guide their accumulation and aggregation at the tumor site. This dual targeting strategy resulted in high nanoparticle concentration in the tumor, making the system suitable for MRI diagnosis (Huang et al. 2017b).

Similarly, active targeting can be combined with passive targeting for optimal targeting efficiency. In a study using $Fe_3O_4@Cu_{2-x}S$ nanoparticles for cancer cell photothermal killing, a novel nanoparticle coating was developed containing cationic amphiphilic polymers (Lauric acid-PEI) for bioelectric targeting and folic acid-conjugated amphiphilic polymers (FA-TPGS) for active targeting (Deng et al. 2021b). The targeting efficiency of negatively charged nanoparticles, positively charged nanoparticles, and dual targeting nanoparticles combining a positive surface charge and folic acid was compared across three cancer cell lines and one normal cell line. The results confirmed that the combination of positive charge and folic acid effectively increased the targeting efficiency in the cancer cell lines without significantly increasing targeting to the normal cell line (Deng et al. 2021b).

Passive targeting strategies, such as controlled size or shape, can also be combined with magnetic field-guided targeting for a synergistic effect (Wang et al. 2018b). For instance, Chrzanowski's group developed a drug nanocarrier system for lung cancer treatment by combining superparamagnetic iron oxide nanoparticles and solid lipid microparticles (Reczynska et al. 2020). They found that particles with diameters ranging from 1 to 5 μm were the most effective for delivery to the lower respiratory tract via inhalation. However, to maintain the superparamagnetic property, it was necessary to keep the iron oxide particles in the nanoscale range (Deng et al. 2021a; Jabbal et al. 2017). Therefore, the group loaded iron oxide nanoparticles into fatty acid microparticles to maintain magnetic mobility for magnetic field-guided targeting and suitable size for inhalational delivery. Another study by Muttil's group developed a nano-in-microparticles system containing superparamagnetic iron oxide nanoparticles for magnetic targeting delivery (Price et al. 2017). Using an external magnet after intratracheal administration in mice, the particles successfully accumulated only in the left lung lobe. Figure 5 illustrates typical combination targeting strategies (Price et al. 2017).

6 Conclusion and Perspectives

The advancements in nanoparticles have opened up vast opportunities for theranostics in life-threatening diseases. Nanoparticles are considered powerful tools in the biomedical field, but their effectiveness relies on specific design considerations. Targeting strategies can be broadly classified into four categories: active targeting, passive targeting, other strategies (such as external forces and changing microenvironment), and combination targeting, which integrates multiple strategies. Successful

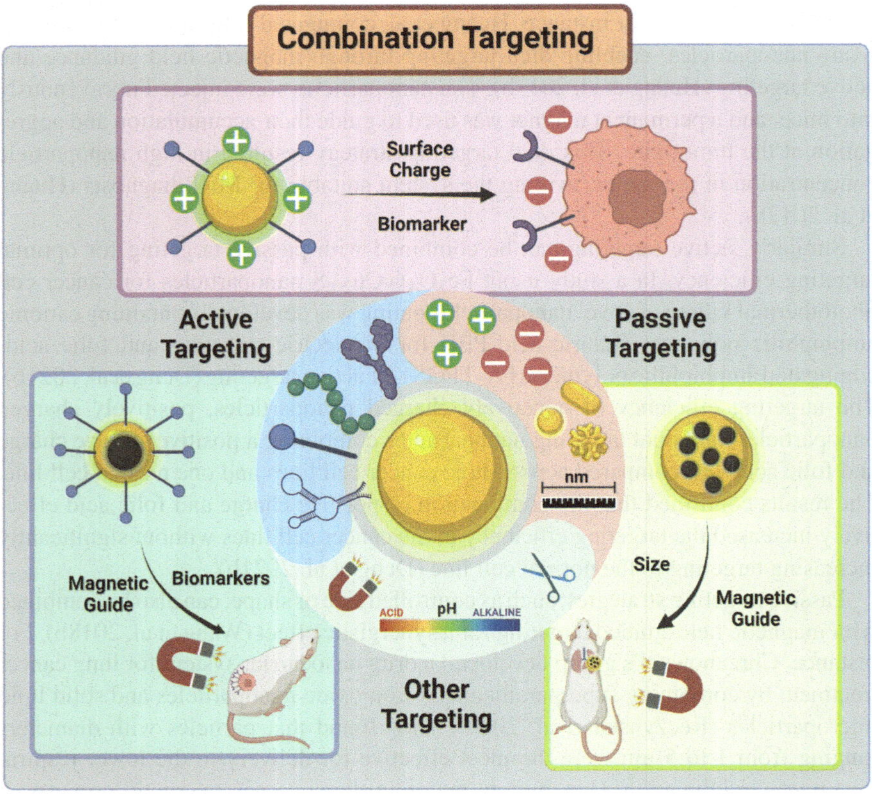

Fig. 5 Typical combination targeting strategies: (1) Combination of the active targeting (biomarkers) and passive targeting (surface charge) to increase the targeting efficiency. (2) Combination of active targeting (biomarkers) and other targeting strategies (magnetic guide) to increase targeting efficiency. (3) Combination of passive targeting (size) and other targeting strategies (magnetic guide) to increase the targeting efficiency. (Created with Biorender.com)

nanoparticle design requires a fundamental understanding of the properties of the nanomaterials and the characterization of the targeted biological entities.

Active targeting is commonly employed when biomarkers on the target cell surface have been well-studied. Nanoparticles are functionalized by targeting ligands that exhibit a strong affinity for specific biomarkers. Passive targeting, on the other hand, can be an excellent option even in the absence of biomarkers or targeting ligands. It relies on leveraging the physicochemical properties of the nanoparticles themselves. Additionally, other designs, such as using magnetic fields or modifying the microenvironment, are employed to enhance nanoparticle accumulation at the target site.

To achieve optimal targeting efficiency, novel designs that combine multiple targeting strategies are being developed. These designs synergistically integrate the advantages of different strategies, making them promising candidates for future precision theranostics research. The choice of a specific nanoparticle design depends on the specific targeting requirements.

Despite recent studies demonstrating nanoparticles with excellent targeting efficiency, only a few have progressed to preclinical and clinical studies. Future research should focus on translating these nanoparticle designs from the laboratory bench to the patient's bedside. Modularization of targeting strategies can be explored to develop "on-demand" nanoparticle targeting systems. This approach would allow clinical physicians to select the most relevant nanoparticle and customize their strategy in precision theranostics. Addressing this challenge will require close collaboration between engineers, chemists, and biomedical researchers.

References

M.M. Abd Elwakil, I.A. Khalil, Y.H.A. Elewa, K. Kusumoto, Y. Sato, N. Shobaki, Y. Kon, H. Harashima, Lung-endothelium-targeted nanoparticles based on a ph-sensitive lipid and the GALA peptide enable robust gene silencing and the regression of metastatic lung cancer. Adv. Funct. Mater. **29**(18), 1807677 (2019)

S.H. Abman, Impaired vascular endothelial growth factor signaling in the pathogenesis of neonatal pulmonary vascular disease. *Advances in Experimental Medicine and Biology* (Humana Press, 2010), pp. 323–335

M. Alvarez-Fernandez, R.H. Medema, Novel functions of FoxM1: from molecular mechanisms to cancer therapy. Front. Oncol. **3**, 30 (2013)

M.M. Arnida, A. Janát-Amsbury, C.M. Ray, H. Peterson, Ghandehari, Geometry and surface characteristics of gold nanoparticles influence their biodistribution and uptake by macrophages. Eur. J. Pharm. Biopharm. **77**(3), 417–423 (2011)

A. Banerjee, J. Qi, R. Gogoi, J. Wong, S. Mitragotri, Role of nanoparticle size, shape and surface chemistry in oral drug delivery. J. Control. Release **238**, 176–185 (2016)

D. Bartczak, O.L. Muskens, S. Nitti, T. Sanchez-Elsner, T.M. Millar, A.G. Kanaras, Interactions of human endothelial cells with gold nanoparticles of different morphologies. Small **8**(1), 122–130 (2012)

S. Behzadi, V. Serpooshan, W. Tao, M.A. Hamaly, M.Y. Alkawareek, E.C. Dreaden, D. Brown, A.M. Alkilany, O.C. Farokhzad, M. Mahmoudi, Cellular uptake of nanoparticles: journey inside the cell. Chem. Soc. Rev. **46**(14), 4218–4244 (2017)

A.I.S. van den Berg, C.O. Yun, R.M. Schiffelers, W.E. Hennink, Polymeric delivery systems for nucleic acid therapeutics: approaching the clinic. J. Controlled Release **331**(December 2020), 121–141 (2021)

F. Bian, Y.-W. Lan, S. Zhao, Z. Deng, S. Shukla, A. Acharya, J. Donovan, T. Le, D. Milewski, M. Bacchetta, A.E. Hozain, Y. Tipograf, Y.-W. Chen, Y. Xu, D. Shi, V.V. Kalinichenko, T.V. Kalin, Lung endothelial cells regulate pulmonary fibrosis through FOXF1/R-Ras signaling. Nat. Commun. **14**(1), 2560 (2023)

F.-C. Bidard, D.J. Peeters, T. Fehm, F. Nolé, R. Gisbert-Criado, D. Mavroudis, S. Grisanti, D. Generali, J.A. Garcia-Saenz, J. Stebbing, C. Caldas, P. Gazzaniga, L. Manso, R. Zamarchi, A.F. de Lascoiti, L. De Mattos-Arruda, M. Ignatiadis, R. Lebofsky, S.J. van Laere, F. Meier-Stiegen, M.-T. Sandri, J. Vidal-Martinez, E. Politaki, F. Consoli, A. Bottini, E. Diaz-Rubio, J. Krell, S.-J. Dawson, C. Raimondi, A. Rutten, W. Janni, E. Munzone, V. Carañana, S. Agelaki, C. Almici, L. Dirix, E.-F. Solomayer, L. Zorzino, H. Johannes, J.S. Reis-Filho, K. Pantel, J.-Y. Pierga, S.

Michiels, Clinical validity of circulating tumour cells in patients with metastatic breast cancer: a pooled analysis of individual patient data. Lancet Oncol. **15**(4), 406–414 (2014)
F. Biscaglia, G. Ripani, S. Rajendran, C. Benna, S. Mocellin, G. Bocchinfuso, M. Meneghetti, A. Palleschi, M. Gobbo, Gold nanoparticle aggregates functionalized with cyclic RGD peptides for targeting and imaging of colorectal cancer cells. ACS Appl. Nano Mater. **2**(10), 6436–6444 (2019)
E. Blanco, H. Shen, M. Ferrari, Principles of nanoparticle design for overcoming biological barriers to drug delivery. Nat. Biotechnol. **33**(9), 941–951 (2015)
C. Bolte, V. Ustiyan, X. Ren, A.W. Dunn, A. Pradhan, G. Wang, O.A. Kolesnichenko, Z. Deng, Y. Zhang, D. Shi, J.M. Greenberg, A.H. Jobe, T.V. Kalin, V.V. Kalinichenko, Nanoparticle delivery of proangiogenic transcription factors into the neonatal circulation inhibits alveolar simplification caused by Hyperoxia. Am. J. Respir. Crit. Care Med. **202**(1), 100–111 (2020)
S. Borhani, A.L. Gartel, FOXM1: a potential therapeutic target in human solid cancers. Expert Opin. Ther. Targets **24**(3), 205–217 (2020)
R. Bottger, G. Pauli, P.H. Chao, N. Al Fayez, L. Hohenwarter, S.D. Li, Lipid-based nanoparticle technologies for liver targeting. Adv. Drug. Deliv. Rev. 154–155 79–101 (2020)
Y. Cai, C. Bolte, T. Le, C. Goda, Y. Xu, T.V. Kalin, V.V. Kalinichenko, FOXF1 maintains endothelial barrier function and prevents edema after lung injury, Science signaling **9**(424), ra40-ra40 (2016)
B. Chen, W. Le, Y. Wang, Z. Li, D. Wang, L. Lin, S. Cui, J.J. Hu, Y. Hu, P. Yang, R.C. Ewing, D. Shi, Z. Cui, Targeting negative surface charges of cancer cells by multifunctional nanoprobes. Theranostics **6**(11), 1887–1898 (2016)
J.S. Choi, W.S. Jang, J.S. Park, Comparison of adsorption and conjugation of Herceptin on poly(lactic-co-glycolic acid) nanoparticles—Effect on cell internalization in breast cancer cells. Mater. Sci. Eng. C Mater Biol. Appl. **92**, 496–507 (2018)
K.L. Clark, E.D. Halay, E. Lai, S.K. Burley, Co-crystal structure of the HNF-3/fork head DNA-recognition motif resembles histone H5. Nature **364**(6436), 412–420 (1993)
Q. Dai, Y. Yan, C.-S. Ang, K. Kempe, M.M.J. Kamphuis, S.J. Dodds, F. Caruso, Monoclonal antibody-functionalized multilayered particles: targeting cancer cells in the presence of protein coronas. ACS Nano **9**(3), 2876–2885 (2015a)
Q. Dai, Y. Yan, J. Guo, M. Björnmalm, J. Cui, H. Sun, F. Caruso, Targeting ability of affibody-functionalized particles is enhanced by albumin but inhibited by serum coronas. ACS Macro Lett. **4**(11), 1259–1263 (2015b)
S. Dante, A. Petrelli, E.M. Petrini, R. Marotta, A. Maccione, A. Alabastri, A. Quarta, F. De Donato, T. Ravasenga, A. Sathya, R. Cingolani, R. Proietti Zaccaria, L. Berdondini, A. Barberis, T. Pellegrino, Selective targeting of neurons with inorganic nanoparticles: revealing the crucial role of nanoparticle surface charge. ACS Nano **11**(7), 6630–6640.
Z. Deng, G.T. Kalin, D. Shi, V.V. Kalinichenko, Nanoparticle delivery systems with cell-specific targeting for pulmonary diseases. Am. J. Respir. Cell Mol. Biol. **64**(3), 292–307 (2021a)
Z. Deng, J. Lin, S.L. Bud'ko, B. Webster, T.V. Kalin, V.V. Kalinichenko, D. Shi, Dual targeting with cell surface electrical charge and folic acid via superparamagnetic Fe_3O_4@Cu_{2}–xS for Photothermal Cancer Cell Killing. Cancers **13**(21), 5275–5275.
Z. Deng, S. Wu, Y. Wang, D. Shi, Circulating tumor cell isolation for cancer diagnosis and prognosis. eBioMedicine **83,** 104237–104237 (2022)
D. Ding, Y. Zhang, E.A. Sykes, L. Chen, Z. Chen, W. Tan, The influence of physiological environment on the targeting effect of aptamer-guided gold nanoparticles. Nano Res. **12**(1), 129–135 (2019)
J. Dolai, K. Mandal, N.R. Jana, Nanoparticle size effects in biomedical applications. ACS Appl. Nano Mater. **4**(7), 6471–6496 (2021)
J. Donovan, Z. Deng, F. Bian, S. Shukla, J. Gomez-Arroyo, D. Shi, V.V. Kalinichenko, T.V. Kalin, Improving anti-tumor efficacy of low-dose Vincristine in rhabdomyosarcoma via the combination therapy with FOXM1 inhibitor RCM1. Front. Oncol. **13**, 1112859 (2023)

D. Duan, H. Liu, M. Xu, M. Chen, Y. Han, Y. Shi, Z. Liu, Size-controlled synthesis of drug-loaded zeolitic imidazolate framework in aqueous solution and size effect on their cancer theranostics in vivo. ACS Appl. Mater. Interfaces **10**(49), 42165–42174 (2018)

A.W. Dunn, V.V. Kalinichenko, D. Shi, Highly efficient in vivo targeting of the pulmonary endothelium using novel modifications of Polyethylenimine: an importance of charge. Adv. Healthcare Mater. **7**(23), 1800876–1800876 (2018)

P.M. Enriquez-Navas, M.L. Garcia-Martin, Application of Inorganic Nanoparticles for Diagnosis Based on MRI, in *Nanobiotechnology* ed. by J.M. de la Fuente, V.B.T.F.o.N. (Grazu Elsevier, 2012), pp. 233–245.

J. Estelrich, M. Antònia Busquets, Iron oxide nanoparticles in photothermal therapy. Molecules **23**(7) (2018)

Z. Fan, P. Zhu, Y. Zhu, K. Wu, C.Y. Li, H. Cheng, Engineering long-circulating nanomaterial delivery systems. Curr. Opin. Biotechnol. **66**, 131–139 (2020)

R. Fan, X. Tao, X. Zhai, Y. Zhu, Y. Li, Y. Chen, D. Dong, S. Yang, L. Lv, Application of aptamer-drug delivery system in the therapy of breast cancer. Biomed. Pharmacother. **161**, 114444 (2023)

J. Fang, H. Nakamura, H. Maeda, The EPR effect: Unique features of tumor blood vessels for drug delivery, factors involved, and limitations and augmentation of the effect. Adv. Drug Deliv. Rev. **63**(3), 136–151 (2011)

C. Foster, A. Watson, J. Kaplinsky, N. Kamaly, *Improved Targeting of Cancers with Nanotherapeutics, Methods in Molecular Biology* (Springer New York, 2017), pp. 13–37.

L. Fu, H.N. Kim, J.D. Sterling, S.M. Baker, M.S. Lord, The role of the cell surface glycocalyx in drug delivery to and through the endothelium. Adv. Drug Del. Rev. **184** (2022)

Z. Fu, J. Xiang, Aptamer-functionalized nanoparticles in targeted delivery and cancer therapy. Int. J. Mol. Sci. **21**(23), 9123 (2020)

H. Gavilán, S.K. Avugadda, T. Fernández-Cabada, N. Soni, M. Cassani, B.T. Mai, R. Chantrell, T. Pellegrino, Magnetic nanoparticles and clusters for magnetic hyperthermia: optimizing their heat performance and developing combinatorial therapies to tackle cancer. Chem. Soc. Rev. **50**(20), 11614–11667 (2021)

Y. Geng, P. Dalhaimer, S. Cai, R. Tsai, M. Tewari, T. Minko, D.E. Discher, Shape effects of filaments versus spherical particles in flow and drug delivery. Nat. Nanotechnol. **2**(4), 249–255 (2007)

Z.R. Goddard, M.J. Marín, D.A. Russell, M. Searcey, Active targeting of gold nanoparticles as cancer therapeutics. Chem. Soc. Rev. **49**(23), 8774–8789 (2020)

A. Goldkorn, B. Ely, D.I. Quinn, C.M. Tangen, L.M. Fink, T. Xu, P. Twardowski, P.J. Van Veldhuizen, N. Agarwal, M.A. Carducci, J.P. Monk, R.H. Datar, M. Garzotto, P.C. Mack, P. Lara, C.S. Higano, M. Hussain, I.M. Thompson, R.J. Cote, N.J. Vogelzang, Circulating tumor cell counts are prognostic of overall survival in SWOG S0421: a phase III trial of docetaxel with or without atrasentan for metastatic castration-resistant prostate cancer. J. Clin. Oncol. **32**(11), 1136–1142 (2014)

Z. Gong, X. Liu, B. Zhou, G. Wang, X. Guan, Y. Xu, J. Zhang, Z. Hong, J. Cao, X. Sun, Z. Gao, H. Lu, X. Pan, J. Bai, Tumor acidic microenvironment-induced drug release of RGD peptide nanoparticles for cellular uptake and cancer therapy. Colloids Surf. B **202**, 111673 (2021)

J.A.C.M. Goos, A. Cho, L.M. Carter, T.R. Dilling, M. Davydova, K. Mandleywala, S. Puttick, A. Gupta, W.S. Price, J.F. Quinn, M.R. Whittaker, J.S. Lewis, T.P. Davis, Delivery of polymeric nanostars for molecular imaging and endoradiotherapy through the enhanced permeability and retention (EPR) effect. Theranostics **10**(2), 567–584 (2020)

Y. Hagino, I.A. Khalil, S. Kimura, K. Kusumoto, H. Harashima, GALA-modified lipid nanoparticles for the targeted delivery of plasmid DNA to the lungs. Mol. Pharm. **18**(3), 878–888 (2021)

X. Han, Z. Deng, Z. Yang, Y. Wang, H. Zhu, B. Chen, Z. Cui, R.C. Ewing, D. Shi, Biomarkerless targeting and photothermal cancer cell killing by surface-electrically-charged superparamagnetic Fe_3O_4 composite nanoparticles. Nanoscale **9**(4), 1457–1465 (2017)

X. Han, N. Gong, L. Xue, M.M. Billingsley, R. El-Mayta, S.J. Shepherd, M.-G. Alameh, D. Weissman, M.J. Mitchell, Ligand-tethered lipid nanoparticles for targeted RNA delivery to treat liver fibrosis. Nat. Commun. **14**(1) (2023)

G. Heller, R. McCormack, T. Kheoh, A. Molina, M.R. Smith, R. Dreicer, F. Saad, R. de Wit, D.T. Aftab, M. Hirmand, A. Limon, K. Fizazi, M. Fleisher, J.S. de Bono, H.I. Scher, Circulating tumor cell number as a response measure of prolonged survival for metastatic castration-resistant prostate cancer: a comparison with prostate-specific antigen across five randomized phase III clinical trials. J. Clin. Oncol. **36**(6), 572–580 (2018)

D. Huang, H. Zhou, X. Gong, J. Gao, Silica sub-microspheres induce autophagy in an endocytosis dependent manner. RSC Adv. **7**(21), 12496–12502 (2017a)

Y. Huang, K. Mao, B. Zhang, Y. Zhao, Superparamagnetic iron oxide nanoparticles conjugated with folic acid for dual target-specific drug delivery and MRI in cancer theranostics. Mater. Sci. Eng. C **70**, 763–771 (2017b)

Y. Huang, J. Wang, K. Jiang, E.J. Chung, Improving kidney targeting: the influence of nanoparticle physicochemical properties on kidney interactions. J. Control. Release **334**, 127–137 (2021)

M. Izci, C. Maksoudian, B.B. Manshian, S.J. Soenen, The use of alternative strategies for enhanced nanoparticle delivery to solid tumors. Chem. Rev. **121**(3), 1746–1803 (2021)

S. Jabbal, G. Poli, B. Lipworth, Does size really matter? Relationship of particle size to lung deposition and exhaled fraction. J. Allergy Clinical Immunol. **139**(6), 2013-2014.e1 (2017)

T. Jamieson, R. Bakhshi, D. Petrova, R. Pocock, M. Imani, A.M. Seifalian, Biological applications of quantum dots. Biomaterials **28**(31), 4717–4732 (2007)

M.H. Jazayeri, H. Amani, A.A. Pourfatollah, H. Pazoki-Toroudi, B. Sedighimoghaddam, Various methods of gold nanoparticles (GNPs) conjugation to antibodies. Sens Bio-Sens Res **9**, 17–22 (2016)

A.B. Jindal, The effect of particle shape on cellular interaction and drug delivery applications of micro- and nanoparticles. Int. J. Pharm. **532**(1), 450–465 (2017)

A. Juan, F.J. Cimas, I. Bravo, A. Pandiella, A. Ocaña, C. Alonso-Moreno, An overview of antibody conjugated polymeric nanoparticles for breast cancer therapy. Pharmaceutics **12**(9), 802 (2020)

M. Jurczyk, K. Jelonek, M. Musiał-Kulik, A. Beberok, D. Wrześniok, J. Kasperczyk, Single-versus dual-targeted nanoparticles with folic acid and biotin for anticancer drug delivery. Pharmaceutics **13**(3), 326 (2021)

D. Kalyane, N. Raval, R. Maheshwari, V. Tambe, K. Kalia, R.K. Tekade, Employment of enhanced permeability and retention effect (EPR): nanoparticle-based precision tools for targeting of therapeutic and diagnostic agent in cancer. Mater. Sci. Eng. C **98**(January), 1252–1276 (2019)

R. Kedmi, N. Veiga, S. Ramishetti, M. Goldsmith, D. Rosenblum, N. Dammes, I. Hazan-Halevy, L. Nahary, S. Leviatan-Ben-Arye, M. Harlev, M. Behlke, I. Benhar, J. Lieberman, D. Peer, A modular platform for targeted RNAi therapeutics. Nat. Nanotechnol. **13**(3), 214–219 (2018)

F.M. Kievit, M. Zhang, Surface engineering of iron oxide nanoparticles for targeted cancer therapy. Acc. Chem. Res. **44**(10), 853–862 (2011)

I.-M. Kim, S. Ramakrishna, G.A. Gusarova, H.M. Yoder, R.H. Costa, V.V. Kalinichenko, The forkhead box m1 transcription factor is essential for embryonic development of pulmonary vasculature. J. Biol. Chem. **280**(23), 22278–22286 (2005)

A. Kiplagat, D.R. Martin, M.O. Onani, M. Meyer, Aptamer-conjugated magnetic nanoparticles for the efficient capture of cancer biomarker proteins. J. Magnet. Magnet. Mater. **497** (2020)

C.Y. Koo, K.W. Muir, E.W. Lam, FOXM1: From cancer initiation to progression and treatment. Biochim. Biophys. Acta **1819**(1), 28–37 (2012)

K. Kusumoto, H. Akita, T. Ishitsuka, Y. Matsumoto, T. Nomoto, R. Furukawa, A. El-Sayed, H. Hatakeyama, K. Kajimoto, Y. Yamada, K. Kataoka, H. Harashima, Lipid envelope-type nanoparticle incorporating a multifunctional peptide for systemic siRNA delivery to the pulmonary endothelium. ACS Nano **7**(9), 7534–7541 (2013)

Y. Li, M. Kröger, W.K. Liu, Shape effect in cellular uptake of PEGylated nanoparticles: comparison between sphere, rod, cube and disk. Nanoscale **7**(40), 16631–16646 (2015)

X. Li, Y. Wang, L. Shi, B. Li, J. Li, Z. Wei, H. Lv, L. Wu, H. Zhang, B. Yang, X. Xu, J. Jiang, Magnetic targeting enhances the cutaneous wound healing effects of human mesenchymal stem cell-derived iron oxide exosomes. J. Nanobiotech. **18**(1) (2020).

G.-B. Liao, X.-Z. Li, S. Zeng, C. Liu, S.-M. Yang, L. Yang, C.-J. Hu, J.-Y. Bai, Regulation of the master regulator FOXM1 in cancer. Cell Commun. Signal. **16**(1) (2018)

M.V. Liberti, J.W. Locasale, The warburg effect: how does it benefit cancer cells? Trends Biochem. Sci. **41**(3), 211–218 (2016)

C.Y. Lim, N.A. Owens, R.D. Wampler, Y. Ying, J.H. Granger, M.D. Porter, M. Takahashi, K. Shimazu, Succinimidyl ester surface chemistry: implications of the competition between aminolysis and hydrolysis on covalent protein immobilization. Langmuir **30**(43), 12868–12878 (2014)

S.B. Lim, C.T. Lim, W.-T. Lim, Single-cell analysis of circulating tumor cells: why heterogeneity matters. Cancers (2019)

M. Liu, B. Dai, S.-H. Kang, K. Ban, F.-J. Huang, F.F. Lang, K.D. Aldape, T.-X. Xie, C.E. Pelloski, K. Xie, R. Sawaya, S. Huang, FoxM1B Is overexpressed in human glioblastomas and critically regulates the tumorigenicity of glioma cells. Can. Res. **66**(7), 3593–3602 (2006)

J. Liu, Z. Luo, J. Zhang, T. Luo, J. Zhou, X. Zhao, K. Cai, Hollow mesoporous silica nanoparticles facilitated drug delivery via cascade pH stimuli in tumor microenvironment for tumor therapy. Biomaterials **83**, 51–65 (2016)

Y.L. Liu, D. Chen, P. Shang, D.C. Yin, A review of magnet systems for targeted drug delivery. J. Control. Release **302**, 90–104 (2019b)

X. Liu, J. Li, B.L. Cadilha, A. Markota, C. Voigt, Z. Huang, P.P. Lin, D.D. Wang, J. Dai, G. Kranz, A. Krandick, D. Libl, H. Zitzelsberger, I. Zagorski, H. Braselmann, M. Pan, S. Zhu, Y. Huang, S. Niedermeyer, C.A. Reichel, B. Uhl, D. Briukhovetska, J. Suárez, S. Kobold, O. Gires, H. Wang, Epithelial-type systemic breast carcinoma cells with a restricted mesenchymal transition are a major source of metastasis. Sci. Adv. **5**(6), eaav4275-eaav4275 (2019)

J. Liu, J. Lian, Y. Chen, X. Zhao, C. Du, Y. Xu, H. Hu, H. Rao, X. Hong, Circulating tumor cells (CTCs): a unique model of cancer metastases and non-invasive biomarkers of therapeutic response. Frontiers in Genetics **12** (2021).

X. Luan, K. Rahme, Z. Cong, L. Wang, Y. Zou, Y. He, H. Yang, J.D. Holmes, C.M. O'Driscoll, J. Guo, Anisamide-targeted PEGylated gold nanoparticles designed to target prostate cancer mediate: Enhanced systemic exposure of siRNA, tumour growth suppression and a synergistic therapeutic response in combination with paclitaxel in mice. Eur. J. Pharm. Biopharm. **137**, 56–67 (2019)

M. Luo, G. Lewik, J.C. Ratcliffe, C.H.J. Choi, E. Mäkilä, W.Y. Tong, N.H. Voelcker, Systematic evaluation of transferrin-modified porous silicon nanoparticles for targeted delivery of doxorubicin to glioblastoma. ACS Appl. Mater. Interfaces **11**(37), 33637–33649 (2019)

V. Marghussian, Magnetic properties of nano-glass ceramics, in *Nano-Glass Ceramics* ed by V.B.T.N.-G.C. Marghussian (Elsevier, Oxford, 2015), pp. 181–223.

A.C. Marques, P.J. Costa, S. Velho, M.H. Amaral, Functionalizing nanoparticles with cancer-targeting antibodies: a comparison of strategies. J. Control. Release **320**, 180–200 (2020)

A.E. Massey, M. Sikander, N. Chauhan, S. Kumari, S. Setua, A.B. Shetty, H. Mandil, V.K. Kashyap, S. Khan, M. Jaggi, M.M. Yallapu, B.B. Hafeez, S.C. Chauhan, Next-generation paclitaxel-nanoparticle formulation for pancreatic cancer treatment, Nanomedicine: Nanotechnology. Biology and Medicine **20**, 102027 (2019)

S. Mignani, X. Shi, V. Ceña, J.-P. Majoral, Dendrimer– and polymeric nanoparticle–aptamer bioconjugates as nonviral delivery systems: a new approach in medicine. Drug Discovery Today **25**(6), 1065–1073 (2020)

J.-M. Montenegro, V. Grazu, A. Sukhanova, S. Agarwal, J.M. de la Fuente, I. Nabiev, A. Greiner, W.J. Parak, Controlled antibody/(bio-) conjugation of inorganic nanoparticles for targeted delivery. Adv. Drug Deliv. Rev. **65**(5), 677–688 (2013)

R. Moradi, R. Mohammadzadeh, A. Akbari, Kappa-carrageenan crosslinked magnetic folic acid-conjugated chitosan nanocomposites for arginase encapsulation, delivery and cancer therapy. Nano LIFE **11**(03), 2140005 (2021)

J. Mosayebi, M. Kiyasatfar, S. Laurent, Synthesis, functionalization, and design of magnetic nanoparticles for theranostic applications. Adv. Healthcare Mater. **6**(23), 1700306 (2017)

J. Mosquera, I. García, L.M. Liz-Marzán, Cellular uptake of nanoparticles versus small molecules: a matter of size. Acc. Chem. Res. **51**(9), 2305–2313 (2018)

C. Movileanu, M. Anghelache, M. Turtoi, G. Voicu, I.A. Neacsu, D. Ficai, R. Trusca, O. Oprea, A. Ficai, E. Andronescu, M. Calin, Folic acid-decorated PEGylated magnetite nanoparticles as efficient drug carriers to tumor cells overexpressing folic acid receptor. Int. J. Pharm. **625**, 122064 (2022)

E. Muntoni, K. Martina, E. Marini, M. Giorgis, L. Lazzarato, I. Salaroglio, C. Riganti, M. Lanotte, L. Battaglia, Methotrexate-loaded solid lipid nanoparticles: protein functionalization to improve brain biodistribution. Pharmaceutics **11**(2), 65 (2019)

S. Nakamura, I. Hirano, K. Okinaka, T. Takemura, D. Yokota, T. Ono, K. Shigeno, K. Shibata, S. Fujisawa, K. Ohnishi, The FOXM1 transcriptional factor promotes the proliferation of leukemia cells through modulation of cell cycle progression in acute myeloid leukemia. Carcinogenesis **31**(11), 2012–2021 (2010)

A. Narmani, M. Rezvani, B. Farhood, P. Darkhor, J. Mohammadnejad, B. Amini, S. Refahi, N. Abdi Goushbolagh, Folic acid functionalized nanoparticles as pharmaceutical carriers in drug delivery systems. Drug Dev. Res. **80**(4), 404–424 (2019)

A.E. Nel, L. Mädler, D. Velegol, T. Xia, E.M.V. Hoek, P. Somasundaran, F. Klaessig, V. Castranova, M. Thompson, Understanding biophysicochemical interactions at the nano–bio interface. Nat. Mater. **8**(7), 543–557 (2009)

Y. Niu, Y. Yang, Z. Yang, X. Wang, P. Zhang, L. Lv, Y. Liu, Y. Liu, Y. Zhou, Aptamer-immobilized bone-targeting nanoparticles in situ reduce sclerostin for osteoporosis treatment. Nano Today **45** (2022)

O. Penon, M.J. Marin, D.A. Russell, L. Perez-Garcia, Water soluble, multifunctional antibody-porphyrin gold nanoparticles for targeted photodynamic therapy. J. Colloid Interface Sci. **496**, 100–110 (2017)

J.L. Perry, K.G. Reuter, M.P. Kai, K.P. Herlihy, S.W. Jones, J.C. Luft, M. Napier, J.E. Bear, J.M. Desimone, PEGylated PRINT nanoparticles: the impact of PEG density on protein binding, macrophage association, biodistribution, and pharmacokinetics. Nano Lett. **12**(10), 5304–5310 (2012)

C. Pilarsky, M. Wenzig, T. Specht, H.D. Saeger, R. Grützmann, Identification and validation of commonly overexpressed genes in solid tumors by comparison of microarray data. Neoplasia **6**(6), 744–750 (2004)

A. Pradhan, A. Dunn, V. Ustiyan, C. Bolte, G. Wang, J.A. Whitsett, Y. Zhang, A. Porollo, Y.-C. Hu, R. Xiao, P. Szafranski, D. Shi, P. Stankiewicz, T.V. Kalin, V.V. Kalinichenko, The S52F FOXF1 mutation Inhibits STAT3 signaling and causes alveolar capillary dysplasia. Am. J. Respir. Crit. Care Med. **200**(8), 1045–1056 (2019a)

A. Pradhan, A. Dunn, V. Ustiyan, C. Bolte, G. Wang, J.A. Whitsett, Y. Zhang, A. Porollo, Y.-C. Hu, R. Xiao, The S52F FOXF1 mutation inhibits STAT3 signaling and causes alveolar capillary dysplasia. Am. J. Respir. Crit. Care Med. **200**(8), 1045–1056 (2019b)

D.N. Price, L.R. Stromberg, N.K. Kunda, P. Muttil, In vivo pulmonary delivery and magnetic-targeting of dry powder nano-in-microparticles. Mol. Pharm. **14**(12), 4741–4750 (2017)

S. Raj, S. Khurana, R. Choudhari, K.K. Kesari, M.A. Kamal, N. Garg, J. Ruokolainen, B.C. Das, D. Kumar, Specific targeting cancer cells with nanoparticles and drug delivery in cancer therapy. Semin. Cancer Biol. **69**, 166–177 (2021)

A. Rasal, N.D. Reddy, Chapter 14 - Nano-pharmacokinetics preclinical to clinical translation, in: N.D. Thorat, N. Kumar (Eds.), Nano-Pharmacokinetics and Theranostics, Academic Press2021, pp. 273–288.

P. Raychaudhuri, H.J. Park, FoxM1: a master regulator of tumor metastasis. Cancer Res. **71**(13), 4329–4333 (2011)

K. Reczynska, P. Marchwica, D. Khanal, T. Borowik, M. Langner, E. Pamula, W. Chrzanowski, Stimuli-sensitive fatty acid-based microparticles for the treatment of lung cancer. Mater Sci Eng C Mater Biol Appl **111**, 110801 (2020)

H. Ren, Y. He, J. Liang, Z. Cheng, M. Zhang, Y. Zhu, C. Hong, J. Qin, X. Xu, J. Wang, Role of liposome size, surface charge, and PEGylation on rheumatoid arthritis targeting therapy. ACS Appl. Mater. Interfaces **11**(22), 20304–20315 (2019)

D.A. Richards, A. Maruani, V. Chudasama, Antibody fragments as nanoparticle targeting ligands: a step in the right direction. Chem. Sci. **8**(1), 63–77 (2016)

D. Rosenblum, A. Gutkin, R. Kedmi, S. Ramishetti, N. Veiga, A.M. Jacobi, M.S. Schubert, D. Friedmann-Morvinski, Z.R. Cohen, M.A. Behlke, J. Lieberman, D. Peer, CRISPR-Cas9 genome editing using targeted lipid nanoparticles for cancer therapy. Sci. Adv. **6**(47), eabc9450, (2020)

E. Ruoslahti, Peptides as targeting elements and tissue penetration devices for nanoparticles. Adv. Mater. **24**(28), 3747–3756 (2012)

S. Sharma, R. Zhuang, M. Long, M. Pavlovic, Y. Kang, A. Ilyas, W. Asghar, Circulating tumor cell isolation, culture, and downstream molecular analysis. Biotechnol. Adv. **36**(4), 1063–1078 (2018)

A. Sheikh, S. Md, P. Kesharwani, RGD engineered dendrimer nanotherapeutic as an emerging targeted approach in cancer therapy. J. Control. Release **340**, 221–242 (2021)

D. Shi, Cancer cell surface negative charges: a bio-physical manifestation of the Warburg effect, NAno LIFE 07(03n04) (2017) 1771001–1771001.

A. Shiriny, M. Bayareh, Inertial focusing of CTCs in a novel spiral microchannel. Chem. Eng. Sci. **229**, 116102–116102 (2021)

S. Shukla, D. Milewski, A. Pradhan, N. Rama, K. Rice, T. Le, M.J. Flick, S. Vaz, X. Zhao, K.D. Setchell, E. Logarinho, V.V. Kalinichenko, T.V. Kalin, The FOXM1 inhibitor RCM-1 decreases carcinogenesis and nuclear beta-catenin. Mol. Cancer Ther. **18**(7), 1217–1229 (2019)

P. Siani, G. Frigerio, E. Donadoni, C. Di Valentin, Molecular dynamics simulations of cRGD-conjugated PEGylated TiO_2 nanoparticles for targeted photodynamic therapy. J. Colloid Interface Sci. **627**, 126–141 (2022)

E. Sinkala, E. Sollier-Christen, C. Renier, E. Rosàs-Canyelles, J. Che, K. Heirich, T.A. Duncombe, J. Vlassakis, K.A. Yamauchi, H. Huang, S.S. Jeffrey, A.E. Herr, Profiling protein expression in circulating tumour cells using microfluidic western blotting. Nat. Commun. **8**(1), 14622–14622 (2017)

Y. Song, Z. Zhu, Y. An, W. Zhang, H. Zhang, D. Liu, C. Yu, W. Duan, C.J. Yang, Selection of DNA aptamers against epithelial cell adhesion molecule for cancer cell imaging and circulating tumor cell capture. Anal. Chem. **85**(8), 4141–4149 (2013)

M. Srinivasarao, P.S. Low, Ligand-targeted drug delivery. Chem. Rev. **117**(19), 12133–12164 (2017)

S. Sun, Y. Wang, R. Zhou, Z. Deng, Y. Han, X. Han, W. Tao, Z. Yang, C. Shi, D. Hong, J. Li, D. Shi, Z. Zhang, Targeting and regulating of an oncogene via nanovector delivery of MicroRNA using patient-derived tumor xenografts. Theranostics **7**(3), 677–693 (2017b)

L. Sun, X. Ren, I.-C. Wang, A. Pradhan, Y. Zhang, H.M. Flood, B. Han, J.A. Whitsett, T.V. Kalin, V.V. Kalinichenko, The FOXM1 inhibitor RCM-1 suppresses goblet cell metaplasia and prevents IL-13 and STAT6 signaling in allergen-exposed mice, Science Signaling **10**(475) (2017) eaai8583.

Y. Tang, X. Wang, J. Li, Y. Nie, G. Liao, Y. Yu, C. Li, Overcoming the reticuloendothelial system barrier to drug delivery with a "Don't-Eat-Us" strategy. ACS Nano **13**(11), 13015–13026 (2019)

M.-T. Teh, S.-T. Wong, G.W. Neill, L.R. Ghali, M.P. Philpott, A.G. Quinn, FOXM1 Is a downstream target of Gli1 in basal cell carcinomas1. Can. Res. **62**(16), 4773–4780 (2002)

B. Thapa, R. Narain, Mechanism, current challenges and new approaches for non viral gene delivery, in: *Polymers and Nanomaterials for Gene Therapy* ed. by R.B.T.P. Narain, T. Nanomaterials for Gene (Elsevier, 2016), pp. 1–27.

V. Torchilin, Intracellular delivery of protein and peptide therapeutics. Drug Discov. Today Technol. **5**(2–3), e95–e103 (2008)

E. Truzzi, T.L. Nascimento, V. Iannuccelli, L. Costantino, E.M. Lima, E. Leo, C. Siligardi, M.L. Gualtieri, E. Maretti, In Vivo biodistribution of respirable solid lipid nanoparticles surface-decorated with a mannose-based surfactant: a promising tool for pulmonary tuberculosis treatment? Nanomaterials (2020)

A.M. Wagner, J.M. Knipe, G. Orive, N.A. Peppas, Quantum dots in biomedical applications. Acta Biomater. **94**, 44–63 (2019)

J. Wang, B. Zhang, L. Wang, M. Wang, F. Gao, One-pot synthesis of water-soluble superparamagnetic iron oxide nanoparticles and their MRI contrast effects in the mouse brains. Mater. Sci. Eng. C **48**, 416–423 (2015a)

J. Wang, W. Mao, L.L. Lock, J. Tang, M. Sui, W. Sun, H. Cui, D. Xu, Y. Shen, The role of micelle size in tumor accumulation. Penetrat. Treatment, ACS Nano **9**(7), 7195–7206 (2015b)

J. Wang, L. Zhang, F. Peng, X. Shi, D.T. Leong, Targeting endothelial cell junctions with negatively charged gold nanoparticles. Chem. Mater. **30**(11), 3759–3767 (2018a)

Z. Wang, Z. Chang, M. Lu, D. Shao, J. Yue, D. Yang, X. Zheng, M. Li, K. He, M. Zhang, L. Chen, W.F. Dong, Shape-controlled magnetic mesoporous silica nanoparticles for magnetically-mediated suicide gene therapy of hepatocellular carcinoma. Biomaterials **154**, 147–157 (2018b)

Y. Wang, X. Han, Z. Cui, D. Shi, Bioelectricity, Its Fundamentals, Characterization Methodology, and Applications in Nano-Bioprobing and Cancer Diagnosis. Adv. Biosys. **3**(10), 1900101–1900101 (2019)

O. Warburg, On the Origin of Cancer Cells. Science **123**(3191), 309–314 (1956)

Y. Wei, X. Gu, Y. Sun, F. Meng, G. Storm, Z. Zhong, Transferrin-binding peptide functionalized polymersomes mediate targeted doxorubicin delivery to colorectal cancer in vivo. J. Control. Release **319**, 407–415 (2020)

S. Wu, L. Gu, J. Qin, L. Zhang, F. Sun, Z. Liu, Y. Wang, D. Shi, Rapid label-free isolation of circulating tumor cells from patients' peripheral blood using electrically charged Fe_3O_4 nanoparticles. ACS Appl. Mater. Interfaces **12**(4), 4193–4203 (2020a)

S. Wu, Y. Wang, D. Shi, Positively charged magnetic nanoparticles for capture of circulating tumor cells from clinical blood samples. Nano LIFE **10**(03), 1971001–1971001 (2020b)

L. Wu, Y. Wang, X. Xu, Y. Liu, B. Lin, M. Zhang, J. Zhang, S. Wan, C. Yang, W. Tan, Aptamer-Based Detection of Circulating Targets for Precision Medicine. Chem. Rev. **121**(19), 12035–12105 (2021)

J. Wu, The enhanced permeability and retention (EPR) effect: the significance of the concept and methods to enhance its application. J. Personal. Med. (2021)

B. Yadav, M. Chauhan, S. Shekhar, A. Kumar, A.K. Mehata, A.K. Nayak, R. Dutt, V. Garg, V. Kailashiya, M.S. Muthu, Sonali, R.P. Singh, RGD-decorated PLGA nanoparticles improved effectiveness and safety of cisplatin for lung cancer therapy. Int. J. Pharmaceut. **633** (2023) 122587.

S. Yang, D. Yao, Y. Wang, W. Yang, B. Zhang, D. Wang, Enzyme-triggered self-assembly of gold nanoparticles for enhanced retention effects and photothermal therapy of prostate cancer. Chem. Commun. **54**(70), 9841–9844 (2018)

N.J. Yang, M.J. Hinner, Getting across the cell membrane: an overview for small molecules, peptides, and proteins, Site-specific protein labeling, pp. 29–53 (2015)

J. Zhang, H. Tang, Z. Liu, B. Chen, Effects of major parameters of nanoparticles on their physical and chemical properties and recent application of nanodrug delivery system in targeted chemotherapy. Int. J. Nanomed. **12**, 8483–8493 (2017)

F. Zhang, L. Wu, W. Nie, L. Huang, J. Zhang, F. Li, H.-Y. Xie, Biomimetic microfluidic system for fast and specific detection of circulating tumor cells. Anal. Chem. **91**(24), 15726–15731 (2019)

X. Zhang, X. Wei, X. Men, C.-X. Wu, J.-J. Bai, W.-T. Li, T. Yang, M.-L. Chen, J.-H. Wang, Dual-multivalent-aptamer-conjugated nanoprobes for superefficient discerning of single circulating tumor cells in a microfluidic chip with inductively coupled plasma mass spectrometry detection. ACS Appl. Mater. Interfaces **13**(36), 43668–43675 (2021)

J. Zhao, S. Wu, J. Qin, D. Shi, Y. Wang, Electrical-charge-mediated cancer cell targeting via protein corona-decorated superparamagnetic nanoparticles in a simulated physiological environment. ACS Appl. Mater. Interfaces **10**(49), 41986–41998 (2018)

Z. Zhao, A. Ukidve, J. Kim, S. Mitragotri, Targeting strategies for tissue-specific drug delivery. Cell **181**(1), 151–167 (2020)

Development of Hybrid Biomaterials Able to Achieve both Hyperthermia and Bone Repair

Toshiki Miyazaki

Abstract Hyperthermia is attracting attention as a treatment with less invasiveness and side effects. Examples of the thermoseeds include ferromagnetic or ferrimagnetic metal oxides such as magnetite and ferrite. If these thermoseeds show ability of bone bonding, they are useful for repair of bone tumor. In this chapter, development of hybrid biomaterials able to achieve both hyperthermia and bone repair has been reviewed, especially focusing on hybrids of apatite and magnetic nanoparticles.

Keywords Hyperthermia · Magnetite · Bone-bonding · Apatite · Hybrid materials · Bone cement

1 The Need for Biomaterials Able to Combine Hyperthermia and Bone Repair

Cancer is the number one cause of death in Japan and the second in the United States, and there is an urgent need to improve cancer treatment methods. The main cancer treatment methods are surgery and chemotherapy, but the problems are that the function of the resected area does not sometimes recover and there are serious side effects. On the other hand, hyperthermia is attracting attention as a treatment with less invasiveness and side effects. Cancer cells are in lower pH environment compared to normal cells, so they are highly sensitive to heat, and heating hardly changes blood flow and may rather decrease it (Song 1984). Due to these factors, cancer cells are killed at a lower temperature than normal cells. In hyperthermia, these properties are utilized by implanting magnetic thermoseeds into the body and irradiating the tumor with an alternating magnetic field from the outside to heat the tumor at 42—43 °C for 30—60 min. Examples of the thermoseeds include ferromagnetic or ferrimagnetic metal oxides such as magnetite (Fe_3O_4) and ferrite.

T. Miyazaki (✉)
Graduate School of Life Science and Systems Engineering, Kyushu Institute of Technology, Hibikino, Wakamatsu-ku, Kitakyushu, Japan
e-mail: tmiya@life.kyutech.ac.jp

R. Narayan (ed.), *Nanostructured Biomaterials and Their Applications*,
https://doi.org/10.1007/978-3-032-16316-5_18

On the other hand, in the case of bone tumors, there is concern that deterioration of bone quality may impair motor function. Therefore, in parallel with tumor treatment, it is also necessary to promote bone repair and regeneration. Some calcium phosphate and silicate ceramics can bond to bone without foreign body reaction to and promote bone regeneration, and are used clinically in orthopedics, neurosurgery, dentistry, and other fields for the purpose of bone repair and regeneration (Hench 1998). It is expected that a novel biomaterial with the multiple functions of hyperthermia, bone repair, and regeneration can be developed by combining iron oxide ceramics, which act as a thermoseed, with bone-bonding ceramics. In addition, Fe_3O_4 has been reported to exhibit antibacterial properties by generating reactive oxygen species (Behera et al. 2012), so it is expected to be used as a highly functional biomaterial. Apatite, a kind of calcium phosphate, has different electric charge states depending on the crystalline surface. Therefore, the apatite can well adsorb biomolecules such as proteins and nucleic acid (Aizawa et al. 2013). On the other hand, Fe_3O_4 is easily attracted to magnetism, so Fe_3O_4-apatite hybrids are also attracting attention as a material for separating and recovering biomolecules.

2 Properties of Magnetic Nanoparticles

When magnetic particles such as Fe_3O_4 and ferrite are reduced in size from the submicron order, they transition from a multi-domain structure to a single-domain structure, and when they are further reduced in size, the single-domain structure becomes unstable due to thermal disturbance and no longer exhibits coercivity. This state is called superparamagnetism. When ferromagnetic or ferrimagnetic materials are exposed to an alternating magnetic field, they achieve heat generation due to magnetic hysteresis loss, but superparamagnetic materials generate heat through a different mechanism, Néel relaxation or Brownian relaxation. It is known that the heat generation characteristics of nanoparticles depend on their particle size, with particles of around 12 nm being most likely to achieve heat generation (Jeyadevan 2010).

Fe_3O_4 nanoparticles can be easily synthesized under conditions of 100 °C or less by an aqueous solution process. Attempts are being made to control the crystalline structure of Fe_3O_4 by allowing organic molecules to coexist in the synthesis process, and the effects of functional groups in side chain, complex formation constants with iron ions, and molecular weight have been reported (Yu et al. 2010; Oaki et al. 2012; Kuwahara et al. 2014; Kuwahara et al. 2016; Miyazaki et al. 2020). The author has found that when Fe^{2+} ions form strong complexes with organic molecules and are easily oxidized by air, iron oxides other than Fe_3O_4 such as iron oxide hydroxide are formed (Table 1).

PEG: Polyethylene glycol

PSS: Poly (styrene sulfonic acid)

PEI: Polyethylenimine (Fig. 1)

Table 1 Behavior of iron oxide formation with coexistence of organic polymers with different chemical structure and molecular weight (Miyazaki et al. 2020)

Added polymer	Molecular weight	Electric charge	Crystallite size/nm	Crystalline phase
None	None	None	21.3	Fe_3O_4
PEG	600	Neutral	13.8	Fe_3O_4
PEG	6000	Neutral	11.0	Fe_3O_4
PSS	300,000	Anionic	18.3	Fe_3O_4, γ-FeOOH
PSS	500,000	Anionic	14.4	Fe_3O_4
PEI	600	Cationic	19.3	Fe_3O_4
PEI	10,000	Cationic	Not measured	α-FeOOH, Fe_3O_4

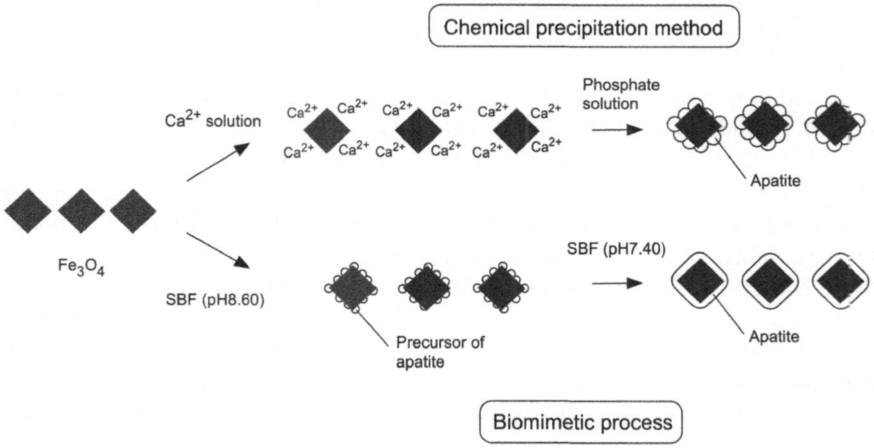

Fig. 1 Schematic representation of Fe_3O_4-apatite hybrids by aqueous process (Biedrzycka et al. 2021; Yabutsuka and Yao 2011)

3 Preparation Method of Fe_3O_4-Apatite Hybrids

When Fe_3O_4 is heated at high temperature, it may be oxidized and lose its magnetism, or the excellent heat generating properties of the nanoparticles may be lost due to aggregation or sintering. Therefore, aqueous solution processes that do not use high temperatures are widely used to prepare Fe_3O_4-apatite hybrids. For example, apatite can be coated by reacting previously prepared Fe_3O_4 or ferrite with Ca^{2+} and phosphate ions to form a precipitate (Biedrzycka et al. 2021). Yabutsuka et al. have presented a biomimetic process for coating the apatite on the surface of Fe_3O_4 (Yabutsuka and Yao 2011). This method uses simulated body fluid (SBF) that is supersaturated with respect to the apatite. Namely, Fe_3O_4 microparticles are placed in SBF with pH 8.60, and calcium phosphate nanoparticles, which act as a precursor of the apatite, are attached to the surface and grown in SBF at pH 7.40. Furthermore, such hybrid can be obtained by hydrothermal treatment of the mixture of Fe_3O_4 and α-tricalcium phosphate (Murakami et al. 2008).

4 Hybrids of Fe_3O_4 and Different Materials with Apatite-Forming Ability

Several materials bond to bone through the apatite layer with similar composition and structure to inorganic phase of natural bone formed by chemical reaction with body fluid. Calcium silicate is a representative example of the bone-bonding ceramics. In order to provide functions of hyperthermia and bone bonding, iron oxide is added to the calcium silicate system, and glass ceramics precipitated with Fe_3O_4 or ferrite have been prepared by heat treatment at controlled atmosphere (Ebisawa et al. 1997; Omidian et al. 2022).

In addition to Si–OH, various functional groups such as Ti–OH (Li et al. 1994), Zr–OH (Uchida et al. 2003), TaOH (Miyazaki et al. 2001a), Nb–OH (Miyazaki et al. 2001b), COOH (Tanahashi and Matsuda 1997; Miyazaki et al. 2003a) and phosphate groups (Tanahashi and Matsuda 1997) are known to have apatite-forming ability in a body fluid environment. Based on the knowledge that COOH has apatite-forming ability, it has been reported that nanohybrids consisting of reduced graphene oxide and Fe_3O_4 show the apatite formation in SBF (Miyazaki et al. 2019). The apatite-forming ability of the hybrids rather decreased as the amount of graphene in the hybrids increased. This was thought to be because the negatively charged graphene strongly attracted Ca^{2+} and inhibited the subsequent binding of phosphate ions. Interestingly, the apatite formation was also observed in pure Fe_3O_4 that did not contain graphene. The apatite-forming ability of iron oxides with different crystalline structures was comprehensively investigated by Kato et al. (Kato et al. 2015). As a result, Fe_3O_4 and α-Fe_2O_3 formed calcium phosphates, although they were not identified as the apatite by X-ray diffraction. Recently, Mg–Ti ferrite has been found to form the apatite in SBF (Miyazaki et al. 2025). These results suggest that even iron oxide alone can exhibit bone-bonding properties if its microstructure is appropriately controlled.

5 Application to Injectable Bone Cement

Bone paste made of calcium phosphate is converted to apatite in vivo after setting, and is therefore clinically used as bone-repairing materials that can be injected to treat complex-shaped bone defects. Matsumine et al. attempted to use the bone paste containing Fe_3O_4 microparticles for hyperthermia of bone tumor patients (Matsumine et al. 2007). As a result, the group that underwent hyperthermia showed a significant difference in the radiographic outcome compared to the group that only underwent palliative care, although there was no significant difference between the group that received both palliative care and radiotherapy.

Polymethylmethacrylate (PMMA)-based bone cement is often used to fix artificial joints in bone. In the cement, PMMA powder and liquid made of methylmethacrylate monomer are mixed with a polymerization initiator to form a paste, which is then set in vivo. Recently, it has also been used in spinal treatments such as percutaneous vertebroplasty. Attempts have been made to add the apatite (Dalby et al. 2002), calcium silicate components (Shinzato et al. 2000; Miyazaki et al. 2003b), and TiO_2 (Goto et al. 2005) to impart bone-bonding properties. Kubota et al. found that the simultaneous addition of TiO_2 and Fe_3O_4 caused heat generation in an alternating magnetic field and the formation of apatite in SBF (Kubota et al. 2021). Furthermore, it has been found that a multifunctional bulk hybrid material that exhibits antibacterial properties can be obtained by adding apatite, zinc ferrite, and ZnO to PMMA (Bakina et al. 2023).

6 Conclusions

Novel biomaterials with both cancer hyperthermia and functions of bone repair and regeneration can be obtained by hybridizing iron oxide magnetic materials with bone-bonding materials. They are expected to be used not only in medicine but also in a wide range of fields such as purification and separation of biological molecules and environmental purification.

Acknowledgments This study was financially supported by the Research Center for Biomedical Engineering and JSPS KAKENHI Grant Number 24K01163.

References

C.W. Song, Effect of local hyperthermia on blood flow and microenvironment: a review. Cancer Res. **44**, 4721s–4730s (1984)

L.L. Hench, Bioceramics. J. Am. Ceram. Soc. **81**, 1705–1728 (1998)

S. Behera, J. Patra, K. Pramanik, N. Panda, H. Thatoi, Characterization and evaluation of antibacterial activities of chemically synthesized iron oxide nanoparticles. World J. Nano Sci. Eng. **2**, 196–200 (2012)

M. Aizawa, T. Matsuura, Z. Zhuang, Syntheses of single-crystal apatite particles with preferred orientation to the a- and c-axes as models of hard tissue and their applications. Biol. Pharm. Bull. **36**, 1654–1661 (2013)

B. Jeyadevan, Present status and prospects of magnetite nanoparticles-based hyperthermia. J. Ceram. Soc. Jpn. **118**, 391–401 (2010)

C.J. Yu, C.Y. Lin, C.H. Liu, T.L. Cheng, W.L. Tseng, Synthesis of poly(diallyldimethylammonium chloride)-coated Fe_3O_4 nanoparticles for colorimetric sensing of glucose and selective extraction of thiol. Biosens. Bioelectron. **26**, 913–917 (2010)

Y. Oaki, N. Yagita, H. Imai, One-pot aqueous solution syntheses of iron oxide nanostructures with controlled crystal phases through a microbial-mineralization-inspired approach. Chem. Eur. J. **18**, 110–116 (2012)

Y. Kuwahara, T. Miyazaki, Y. Shirosaki, M. Kawashita, Effects of organic polymer addition in magnetite synthesis on its crystalline structure. RSC Adv. **4**, 23359–23363 (2014)

Y. Kuwahara, T. Miyazaki, Y. Shirosaki, G. Liu, M. Kawashita, Structures of organic additives modified magnetite nanoparticles. Ceram. Int. **42**, 6000–6004 (2016)

T. Miyazaki, T. Tange, M. Kawashita, B. Jeyadevan, Structural control of magnetite nanoparticles for hyperthermia by modification with organic polymers: Effect of molecular weight. RSC Adv. **10**, 26374–26380 (2020)

A. Biedrzycka, E. Skwarek, U.M. Hanna, Hydroxyapatite with magnetic core: Synthesis methods, properties, adsorption and medical applications. Adv. Colloid Interf. Sci. **291**, 102401 (2021)

T. Yabutsuka, T. Yao, Preparation of encapsulated magnetite microparticles with hydroxyapatite. Energy Procedia **9**, 532–538 (2011)

S. Murakami, T. Hosono, B. Jeyadevan, M. Kamitakahara, K. Ioku, Hydrothermal synthesis of magnetite/hydroxyapatite composite material for hyperthermia therapy for bone cancer. J. Ceram. Soc. Jpn. **116**, 950–954 (2008)

Y. Ebisawa, F. Miyaji, T. Kokubo, K. Ohura, T. Nakamura, Bioactivity of ferrimagnetic glass-ceramics in the system $FeO–Fe_2O_3–CaO–SiO_2$. Biomaterials **18**, 1277–1284 (1997)

S. Omidian, M.H. Nazarpak, Z. Bagher, F. Moztarzadeh, The effect of vanadium ferrite doping on the bioactivity of mesoporous bioactive glass-ceramics. RSC Adv. **12**, 25639–25653 (2022)

P. Li, C. Ohtsuki, T. Kokubo, K. Nakanishi, N. Soga, K. de Groot, The role of hydrated silica, titania and alumina in inducing apatite on implants. J. Biomed. Mater. Res. **28**, 7–15 (1994)

M. Uchida, H.M. Kim, T. Kokubo, S. Fujibayashi, T. Nakamura, Structural dependence of apatite formation on titania gels in a simulated body fluid. J. Biomed. Mater. Res. A **64**, 164–170 (2003)

T. Miyazaki, H.M. Kim, T. Kokubo, H. Kato, T. Nakamura, Induction and acceleration of bonelike apatite formation on tantalum oxide gel in simulated body fluid. J. Sol-gel Sci. Tech. **21**, 83–88 (2001a)

T. Miyazaki, H.M. Kim, T. Kokubo, C. Ohtsuki, T. Nakamura, Bonelike apatite formation induced on niobium oxide gels in simulated body fluid. J. Ceram Soc. Japan **109**, 934–938 (2001b)

M. Tanahashi, T. Matsuda, Surface functional group dependence on apatite formation on self-assembled monolayers in a simulated body fluid. J. Biomed. Mater. Res. **34**, 305–315 (1997)

T. Miyazaki, C. Ohtsuki, Y. Akioka, M. Tanihara, J. Nakao, Y. Sakaguchi, S. Konagaya, Apatite deposition on polyamide films containing carboxyl group in a biomimetic solution. J. Mater. Sci. Mater. Med. **14**, 569–574 (2003a)

T. Miyazaki, J. Akaike, M. Kawashita, H.N. Lim, In vitro apatite mineralization and heat generation of magnetite-reduced graphene oxide nanocomposites for hyperthermia treatment. Mater. Sci. Eng. C **99**, 68–72 (2019)

Y. Kato, T. Yokoi, E. Shin, I.Y. Kim, M. Kawashita, K. Kikuta, C. Ohtsuki, J. Asian Ceramic Soc. **3**, 44–49 (2015)

T. Miyazaki, J. Miyamoto, J. Nakamura, S. Usuki, T. Yokoi, M. Kawashita, Magnetic properties, heat generation, and apatite formation ability of Mg-Ti ferrite particles synthesized by solid-state reaction and polymerized complex methods. Adv. Eng. Mater. **27**, 2401803 (2025)

A. Matsumine, K. Kusuzaki, T. Matsubara, K. Shintani, H. Satonaka, T. Wakabayashi, S. Miyazaki, K. Morita, K. Takegami, A. Uchida, Novel hyperthermia for metastatic bone tumors with magnetic materials by generating an alternating electromagnetic field. Clin. Exp. Metastasis **24**, 191–200 (2007)

M.J. Dalby, L. Di Silvio, E.J. Harper, W. Bonfield, Increasing hydroxyapatite incorporation into poly(methylmethacrylate) cement increases osteoblast adhesion and response. Biomaterials **23**, 569–576 (2002)

S. Shinzato, M. Kobayashi, W.F. Mousa, M. Kamimura, M. Neo, Y. Kitamura, T. Kokubo, T. Nakamura, Bioactive polymethyl methacrylate-based bone cement: Comparison of glass beads, apatite-and wollastonite-containing glass-ceramic, and hydroxyapatite fillers on mechanical and biological properties. J. Biomed. Mater. Res. **51**, 258–272 (2000)

T. Miyazaki, C. Ohtsuki, M. Kyomoto, M. Tanihara, A. Mori, K. Kuramoto, Bioactive PMMA bone cement prepared by modification with Methacryloxypropyltrimethoxysilane and calcium chloride. J. Biomed. Mater. Res. **67A**, 1417–1423 (2003b)

K. Goto, J. Tamura, S. Shinzato, S. Fujibayashi, M. Hashimoto, M. Kawashita, T. Kokubo, T. Nakamura, Bioactive bone cements containing nano-sized titania particles for use as bone substitutes. Biomaterials **26**, 6496–6505 (2005)

M. Kubota, T. Yokoi, T. Ogawa, S. Saito, M. Furuya, K. Yokota, H. Kanetaka, B. Jeyadevan, M. Kawashita, In-vitro heat-generating and apatite-forming abilities of PMMA bone cement containing TiO_2 and Fe_3O_4. Ceram. Int. **47**, 12292–12299 (2021)

O. Bakina, N. Svarovskaya, L. Ivanova, E. Glazkova, N. Rodkevich, V. Evstigneev, M. Evstigneev, A. Mosunov, M. Lerner, New PMMA-based hydroxyapatite/$ZnFe_2O_4$/ZnO composite with antibacterial performance and low toxicity. Biomimetics **8**, 488 (2023)

Silver Nanoparticles in Dental Adhesives: Antibacterial Mechanisms, Incorporation Strategies, and Clinical Applications

Vivek Aggarwal and Saranjit Singh Bhasin

Abstract In recent decades, dental restorative materials have evolved significantly, shifting from conventional amalgam-based systems to more sophisticated and aesthetic composite resin materials. Dental adhesives, which create a strong bond between composite materials and tooth structures, are fundamental to the success of restorative treatments. However, secondary caries remain a persistent issue despite advances in adhesive dentistry. The most common cause of secondary caries is bacterial infiltration at the tooth-restoration interface, often due to Streptococcus mutans' biofilm-forming capabilities.

1 Introduction

In recent decades, dental restorative materials have evolved significantly, shifting from conventional amalgam-based systems to more sophisticated and aesthetic composite resin materials. Dental adhesives, which create a strong bond between composite materials and tooth structures, are fundamental to the success of restorative treatments. However, secondary caries remain a persistent issue despite advances in adhesive dentistry. The most common cause of secondary caries is bacterial infiltration at the tooth-restoration interface, often due to Streptococcus mutans' biofilm-forming capabilities.

To address this issue, researchers have explored the incorporation of antibacterial agents into dental adhesives. One of the most promising developments in this regard is the inclusion of silver nanoparticles (AgNPs) into dental adhesive systems. AgNPs possess broad-spectrum antimicrobial properties, making them highly effective in inhibiting the growth of cariogenic bacteria like *Streptococcus mutans*. Additionally, their nanoscale size allows for excellent dispersion in adhesive matrices without compromising the mechanical integrity of the materials.

This chapter provides a comprehensive review of the role of silver nanoparticles in dental adhesives. We will explore their antibacterial mechanisms, the various

V. Aggarwal · S. S. Bhasin (✉)
Faculty of Dentistry, Jamia Millia Islamia, New Delhi, India
e-mail: drsmyle@yahoo.com

R. Narayan (ed.), *Nanostructured Biomaterials and Their Applications*,
https://doi.org/10.1007/978-3-032-16316-5_19

methods of incorporating AgNPs into adhesive systems, their impact on adhesives' physical and mechanical properties, and their clinical implications. By understanding the current advancements and challenges associated with silver nanoparticles in dental adhesives, we can envision future innovations that may further improve the longevity and efficacy of composite restorations.

2 Background on Silver Nanoparticles

Silver has been valued for its antimicrobial properties for thousands of years. Historically, silver coins were dropped into water containers to preserve water quality, and silver nitrate was used in medical and dental applications as an antiseptic. In the early twentieth century, silver nitrate was commonly applied to carious lesions in paediatric dentistry to arrest decay, though its use declined due to aesthetic concerns such as tooth staining.

The advent of nanotechnology has reintroduced silver into dental materials in the form of silver nanoparticles (AgNPs). Nanoparticles, defined as particles smaller than 100 nm, possess unique physical and chemical properties due to their high surface area-to-volume ratio. This allows nanoparticles to interact more effectively with bacterial cells compared to larger silver particles, enhancing their antimicrobial efficacy.

AgNPs are particularly promising in the context of dental adhesives because of their ability to prevent bacterial colonization and biofilm formation on the surface of composite restorations. Biofilms, which are communities of bacteria that adhere to surfaces and secrete an extracellular matrix, are a significant contributor to secondary caries. *Streptococcus mutans* is one of the primary bacteria involved in biofilm formation on dental restorations, and its presence at the tooth-restoration interface can lead to recurrent decay and restoration failure.

Incorporating AgNPs into dental adhesives provides a dual function: they act as a bonding agent and offer long-term antibacterial protection. This dual functionality addresses one of the key limitations of traditional adhesives, which do not possess inherent antimicrobial properties. The development of AgNP-containing adhesives represents a significant advancement in the field of restorative dentistry, offering the potential for improved restoration longevity and reduced incidence of secondary caries.

3 Properties and Antibacterial Mechanisms of Silver Nanoparticles

Silver nanoparticles exhibit potent antibacterial activity due to their unique interactions with bacterial cells. The small size of AgNPs allows them to penetrate bacterial cell membranes, where they can disrupt cellular processes and induce cell death. The antibacterial effects of silver nanoparticles are driven by several mechanisms:

1. Disruption of Cell Membranes: Silver nanoparticles interact with bacterial cell membranes, causing structural changes that increase membrane permeability. This leads to the leakage of essential cellular components, which ultimately results in cell death. The nanoscale size of AgNPs enables them to embed within the bacterial cell wall and disrupt its integrity.
2. Generation of Reactive Oxygen Species (ROS): AgNPs can generate reactive oxygen species (ROS), such as hydrogen peroxide and superoxide radicals, which induce oxidative stress within bacterial cells. ROS are highly reactive molecules that can damage bacterial proteins, lipids, and nucleic acids. This oxidative stress overwhelms the bacterial cell's repair mechanisms, leading to cell death.
3. Silver Ion Release: In aqueous environments, AgNPs release silver ions (Ag+), which are highly toxic to bacterial cells. Silver ions can interact with thiol groups in bacterial proteins, inhibiting enzymatic activity and disrupting essential cellular processes, such as respiration and DNA replication. The continuous release of silver ions from AgNPs provides long-term antibacterial effects, even after the initial exposure to the nanoparticles.
4. Interruption of Biofilm Formation: Biofilms are protective structures that bacteria produce to shield themselves from external threats, including antimicrobial agents. Silver nanoparticles have been shown to inhibit biofilm formation by preventing bacterial adhesion to surfaces and disrupting the extracellular matrix of existing biofilms. This makes AgNPs particularly useful in dental applications, where biofilm formation is a leading cause of secondary caries.

Due to these multifaceted antibacterial mechanisms, AgNPs are effective against a broad range of bacterial species, including both gram-positive and gram-negative bacteria. In dentistry, their effectiveness against *Streptococcus mutans* makes them an ideal candidate for incorporation into dental adhesives, where preventing bacterial colonization at the tooth-restoration interface is critical.

4 Incorporation Methods of Silver Nanoparticles into Dental Adhesives

The method by which silver nanoparticles (AgNPs) are incorporated into dental adhesives plays a critical role in determining both the antibacterial efficacy and the physical properties of the adhesive. The size, dispersion, and stability of the AgNPs within the adhesive matrix can significantly affect the adhesive's performance. Two primary methods of incorporating AgNPs into dental adhesives are direct incorporation and in situ fabrication. Each method has distinct advantages and challenges, which are outlined below.

4.1 Direct Incorporation of Silver Nanoparticles

The direct incorporation method involves adding pre-synthesized, commercially available silver nanoparticles into the adhesive matrix. This process is relatively straightforward and involves blending the nanoparticles into the adhesive solution before the material is applied or polymerized. Silver nanoparticles used for this purpose typically range from 20 to 100 nm in size and are readily available from suppliers in various forms, including as colloidal suspensions or powders (Fig. 1).

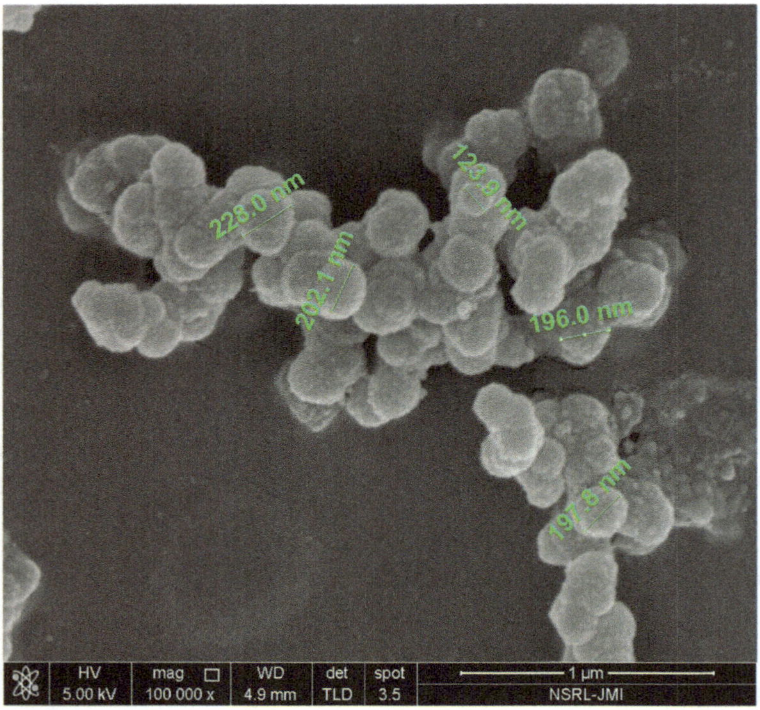

Fig. 1 SEM image of silver nanoparticles in dental adhesive prepared by direct incorporation. This image shows silver nanoparticles directly incorporated into the dental adhesive. The particle size is relatively large, ranging from approximately **123.9–228.0 nm**. The aggregation of nanoparticles is visible, indicating uneven dispersion. Magnification is **100,000×**, and the scale bar represents **1 μm**

Advantages of Direct Incorporation

Ease of Use: This method is simpler to implement than in situ fabrication. Commercially available AgNPs can be directly mixed into the adhesive formulation, reducing the time and expertise required to synthesize nanoparticles.

Customizable Concentrations: The concentration of AgNPs in the adhesive can be easily controlled by adjusting the amount of nanoparticles added to the mixture. This allows for flexibility in determining the optimal concentration for antibacterial efficacy while maintaining the mechanical properties of the adhesive.

Rapid Implementation: Since this method relies on pre-synthesized nanoparticles, it can be readily adopted in commercial dental adhesive formulations. No additional chemical reactions or processes are required during the incorporation.

Challenges of Direct Incorporation

Nanoparticle Aggregation: One of the main drawbacks of direct incorporation is the tendency for silver nanoparticles to aggregate or clump together within the adhesive matrix. This occurs due to the high surface energy and Van der Waals forces between nanoparticles, which causes them to cluster. Aggregation reduces the surface area of the nanoparticles that are exposed to bacterial cells, thereby diminishing their antibacterial efficacy.

Aggregates of nanoparticles can also disrupt the homogeneity of the adhesive, leading to uneven distribution of mechanical stresses during bonding. This can weaken the bond strength between the adhesive and the tooth structure.

Limited Control over Particle Size and Dispersion: While commercially available AgNPs come in a range of sizes, the direct incorporation method provides limited control over their distribution within the adhesive matrix. Poorly dispersed nanoparticles can lead to inconsistent antibacterial effects and negatively impact the adhesive's mechanical performance.

Potential for Reduced Bond Strength: Research has shown that the addition of silver nanoparticles via direct incorporation can reduce the shear bond strength of dental adhesives, particularly when nanoparticle aggregation occurs. Large clusters of nanoparticles can create weak points within the adhesive layer, leading to reduced bonding between the tooth and the restorative material.

Impact on Antibacterial Properties

Despite the challenges associated with nanoparticle aggregation, directly incorporated silver nanoparticles have been shown to exhibit significant antibacterial properties, particularly at the resin-dentin interface. Studies have demonstrated that even low concentrations of directly incorporated AgNPs (around 0.05–0.1%) can inhibit the growth of *Streptococcus mutans* and other cariogenic bacteria. However, higher concentrations of AgNPs may be needed to achieve optimal antibacterial effects, but this could further compromise the physical properties of the adhesive.

The antibacterial effect is primarily contact-based, with the nanoparticles embedded in the adhesive matrix acting to inhibit bacterial colonization and biofilm formation. The release of silver ions from the nanoparticles provides long-term antibacterial effects, although the efficacy may decrease over time as the release of ions diminishes.

4.2 *In Situ Fabrication of Silver Nanoparticles*

In contrast to direct incorporation, the in situ fabrication method involves synthesizing silver nanoparticles directly within the adhesive matrix. This is typically achieved by mixing silver precursors (such as silver salts) into the adhesive formulation, followed by a chemical reaction that reduces the silver ions to form nanoparticles in situ. This method allows for more precise control over the size, shape, and dispersion of the nanoparticles within the adhesive matrix (Figs. 2, 3 and 4).

Advantages of In Situ Fabrication

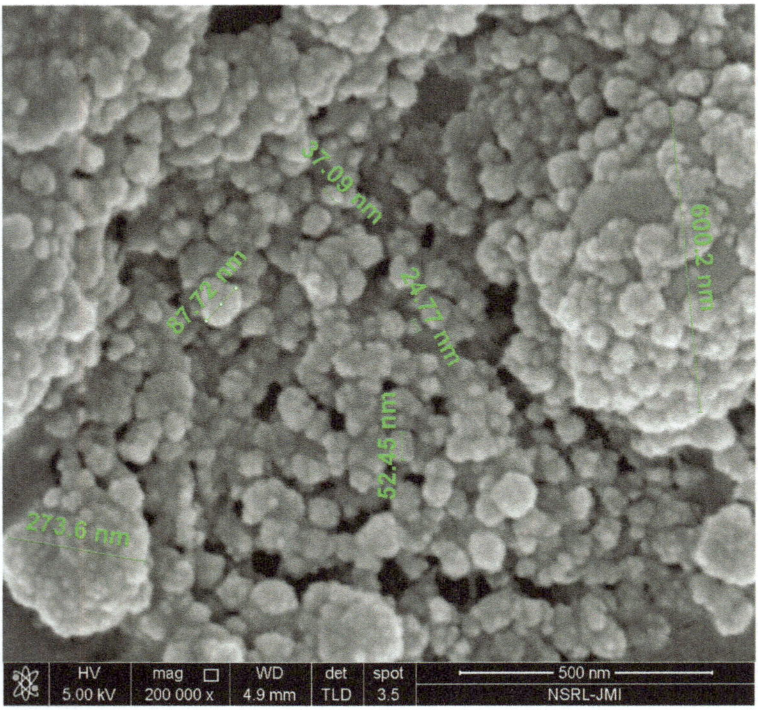

Fig. 2 SEM image of silver nanoparticles fabricated in situ within dental adhesive. This image highlights in situ fabrication of silver nanoparticles within the dental adhesive. The particle sizes are significantly smaller compared to direct incorporation, with a range between **24.17 and 87.72 nm**. The uniform dispersion and smaller size suggest better integration into the adhesive matrix. Magnification is **200,000×**, and the scale bar is **500 nm**

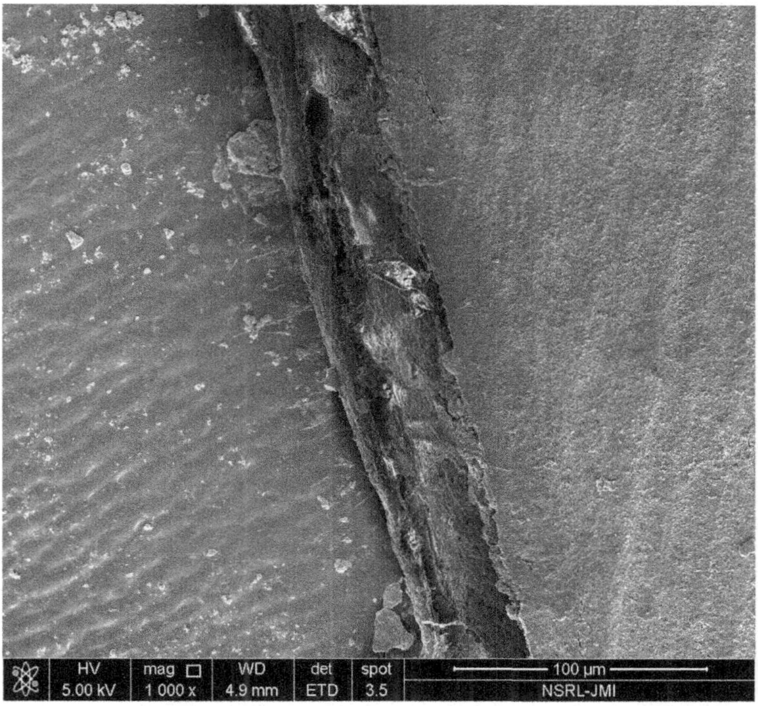

Fig. 3 SEM image of the hybrid dental adhesive layer containing silver nanoparticles. This image presents the intact hybrid layer of dental adhesive with silver nanoparticles. The hybrid layer is smooth and continuous, showing no visible gaps or defects. This indicates effective adhesive bonding to the tooth substrate. Magnification is **1000×**, and the scale bar represents **100 μm**

Improved Dispersion: Since the silver nanoparticles are formed within the adhesive matrix, they are more evenly dispersed compared to those introduced through direct incorporation. This uniform dispersion enhances the adhesive's antibacterial efficacy, as a larger proportion of the nanoparticles is available to interact with bacterial cells.

The even distribution of nanoparticles also contributes to better mechanical performance, as some fewer weak points or clusters could compromise bond strength.

Smaller Particle Size: In situ fabrication typically produces smaller nanoparticles (often in the range of 5–20 nm) compared to pre-synthesized commercial AgNPs. Smaller nanoparticles have a higher surface area-to-volume ratio, which enhances their interaction with bacteria and increases their antibacterial effectiveness.

Greater Stability: The nanoparticles produced via in situ fabrication are often more stable within the adhesive matrix, as they are chemically integrated into the adhesive formulation. This reduces the likelihood of nanoparticle aggregation and ensures that the antibacterial properties are maintained over a longer period.

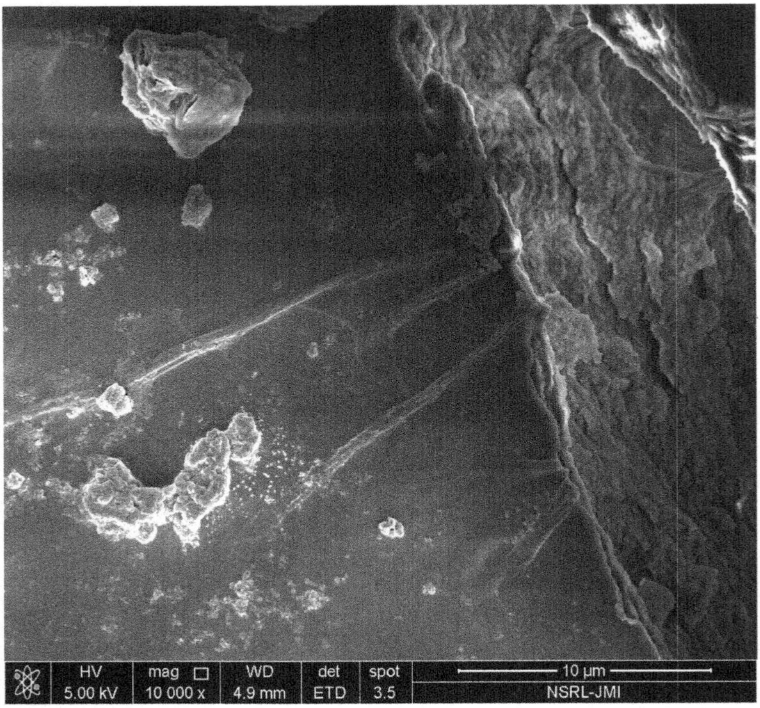

Fig. 4 SEM image showing silver nanoparticles dispersed inside the hybrid dental adhesive layer. This image reveals the presence of silver nanoparticles dispersed within the hybrid layer. The nanoparticles are integrated within the adhesive matrix, confirming deep penetration. Magnification is **10,000×**, and the scale bar is **10 μm**

Challenges of In Situ Fabrication

Complexity of the Process: In situ fabrication is a more complex process than direct incorporation. It requires precise control of the chemical reactions involved in nanoparticle synthesis, as well as careful selection of the silver precursor and reducing agent. The reaction conditions, such as temperature and pH, must be optimized to ensure the formation of nanoparticles with the desired size and properties.

Potential Interference with Polymerization: The in situ formation of silver nanoparticles occurs simultaneously with the polymerization of the dental adhesive. In some cases, the presence of silver precursors or reducing agents can interfere with the polymerization process, affecting the degree of conversion of the adhesive. This can result in a lower degree of cross-linking within the adhesive matrix, which may weaken the bond strength or reduce the durability of the restoration.

Cost and Scalability: The additional steps involved in synthesizing nanoparticles in situ may increase the cost of producing AgNP-containing adhesives. Furthermore, scaling up the in situ fabrication process for commercial production can be challenging, as it requires precise control over chemical reactions on a larger scale.

Impact on Antibacterial Properties

In situ, fabricated silver nanoparticles exhibit superior antibacterial properties compared to directly incorporated nanoparticles. The smaller size and even distribution of nanoparticles ensure a greater surface area for interaction with bacteria, resulting in enhanced bacterial inhibition. Additionally, the stable integration of the nanoparticles within the adhesive matrix ensures that the antibacterial effects are maintained over time.

Studies have shown that dental adhesives containing in situ fabricated silver nanoparticles can significantly reduce the growth of *Streptococcus mutans* and prevent biofilm formation on composite restorations. The continuous release of silver ions from these nanoparticles provides long-lasting antibacterial protection, making in situ fabrication a highly effective method for enhancing the antibacterial properties of dental adhesives.

4.3 Comparative Analysis of Incorporation Methods

The choice between direct incorporation and in situ fabrication depends on several factors, including the desired balance between antibacterial efficacy and mechanical properties, the ease of manufacturing, and cost considerations.

Table 1 summarizes the key differences between the two methods.

Overall, in situ fabrication tends to offer superior antibacterial properties and better retention of mechanical properties, but at the cost of increased complexity and potential challenges with scalability. Direct incorporation, on the other hand, offers ease of implementation but may require optimization to prevent nanoparticle aggregation and its associated effects on bond strength.

Table 1 Comparison of incorporation methods for silver nanoparticles in dental adhesives

Feature	Direct incorporation	In situ fabrication
Ease of use	Simple and cost-effective	More complex; requires precise control
Nanoparticle size	Larger, prone to aggregation	Smaller, more uniform
Nanoparticle dispersion	Uneven, prone to clustering	Even, well-dispersed
Antibacterial efficacy	Moderate	High
Impact on bond strength	Can reduce bond strength due to clusters	Less impact due to better dispersion
Stability	Prone to aggregation over time	More stable, integrated into the matrix
Scalability	Easy to scale commercially	More challenging to scale

5 Clinical Relevance of Silver Nanoparticles in Dental Adhesives

The inclusion of silver nanoparticles (AgNPs) in dental adhesives offers several clinical advantages that directly address key issues in restorative dentistry, particularly the prevention of secondary caries and the improvement of restoration longevity. Secondary caries is one of the leading causes of restoration failure, especially with composite resin restorations. By inhibiting bacterial colonization and biofilm formation at the resin-dentin interface AgNP-containing adhesives provide both preventive and therapeutic benefits. This section will discuss the primary clinical applications and relevance of AgNPs in dental adhesives, focusing on their role in preventing secondary caries, enhancing restoration longevity, and their potential in minimally invasive high-risk cases.

5.1 Prevention of Secondary Caries

One of the primary clinical applications of AgNP-containing dental adhesives is in the prevention of secondary caries, which is the most common cause of failure in dental composite restorations. Secondary caries occurs when cariogenic bacteria such as *Streptococcus mutans* colonize the margins of the restoration, leading to decay beneath the restoration. Once this process begins, the restoration becomes compromised, often necessitating replacement.

Antibacterial Action Against *Streptococcus mutans*

AgNPs are particularly effective against *Streptococcus mutans*, the primary bacterium responsible for caries formation. The ability of silver nanoparticles to disrupt bacterial cell membranes, generate reactive oxygen species (ROS), and release silver ions creates an inhospitable environment for *S. mutans* at the tooth restoration on interface. As *S. mutans* is highly adept at forming biofilms on composite surfaces, its inhibition through AgNP-containing adhesives is critical for reducing the risk of secondary caries.

Several studies have demonstrated the ability of silver nanoparticles to significantly reduce bacterial colonization when integrated into dental adhesives. By maintaining an antibacterial environment around the restoration margins, AgNPs help ensure that bacteria cannot proliferate in these vulnerable areas, thus prolonging the lifespan of the restoration and reducing the frequency of replacement.

Biofilm Prevention

Biofilms are complex communities of bacteria that adhere to surfaces and secrete a protective extracellular matrix, making them more resistant to antibacterial agents and the body's immune response. Once established, biofilms are challenging to remove and serve as reservoirs for bacteria that can lead to recurrent decay.

The unique properties of silver nanoparticles allow them to prevent the initial formation of biofilms at the tooth-restoration interface. The nanoparticles interfere with bacterial adhesion, a critical first step in biofilm development. Additionally, AgNPs can penetrate existing biofilms and disrupt their structure by interfering with the extracellular matrix. This dual action makes AgNP-containing adhesives a valuable tool in preventing the development of biofilms that can lead to secondary caries.

5.2 *Enhanced Longevity of Restorations*

The longevity of dental restorations is a key concern in restorative dentistry, as patients and clinicians alike seek materials and techniques that offer durable, long-lasting results. Composite restorations, while popular for their aesthetics and versatility, are often prone to failure due to issues such as marginal leakage, bacterial infiltration, and recurrent caries.

Marginal Integrity and Sealing Ability

The marginal integrity of a restoration refers to the continuity of the seal between the tooth and the restorative material. If the seal is compromised, bacteria can infiltrate the restoration margins, leading to secondary caries and eventual failure of the restoration. AgNP-containing adhesives can enhance marginal integrity by providing an additional line of defence against bacterial invasion.

Although the primary role of the adhesive is to bond the composite material to the tooth, the antibacterial properties of AgNPs ensure that the interface remains inhospitable to bacterial colonization. This helps to maintain a tighter seal between the restoration and the tooth, reducing the likelihood of marginal breakdown and bacterial infiltration.

Reduction in Frequency of Restoration Replacement

By preventing secondary caries and maintaining better marginal integrity, AgNP-containing adhesives can significantly reduce the need for restoration replacement. In clinical practice, replacing a failed restoration is often more invasive and costly than the original procedure. The ability of silver nanoparticles to extend the life of a restoration, particularly in high-risk patients with poor oral hygiene or a history of recurrent decay, can improve patient outcomes and reduce long-term costs.

In many cases, the decision to replace a restoration is driven by the presence of caries around the margins, which often goes unnoticed until the decay has progressed significantly. The use of AgNP-containing adhesives in patients prone to high caries risk can act as a preventive measure, reducing the likelihood of recurrent decay and the associated need for frequent replacement.

5.3 Application in Minimally Invasive Dentistry

The concept of minimally invasive dentistry (MID) emphasizes the preservation of as much healthy tooth structure as possible while treating decay or restoring damaged teeth. In line with this philosophy, AgNP-containing adhesives can play an important role in providing antibacterial protection in cases where traditional caries removal methods are limited.

Protection in Deep Cavity Preparations

In minimally invasive procedures, especially in deep carious lesions, complete removal of infected dentin may not always be possible. This leaves behind potentially active bacteria, particularly in areas close to the pulp where aggressive excavation may cause unnecessary damage to the tooth structure. In such cases, the use of an adhesive with incorporated AgNPs can offer a way to kill or inhibit the growth of any remaining bacteria without further excavation. The long-lasting release of silver ions can suppress bacterial activity within the deeper layers of the tooth, improving the prognosis of the restoration.

AgNP-containing adhesives are also advantageous when performing selective caries removal or stepwise excavation, where a portion of the affected dentin is intentionally left to preserve tooth structure. The antibacterial properties of silver nanoparticles can help control bacterial activity and prevent the progression of caries in these areas.

5.4 Application in High-Risk Patients

Certain populations, such as those with high caries risk, compromised immune systems, or limited ability to maintain proper oral hygiene, stand to benefit greatly from the use of AgNP-containing adhesives. These patients often face a greater risk of developing secondary caries, recurrent decay, and restoration failure due to their predisposition to bacterial colonization and biofilm formation.

Elderly Patients and Those with Xerostomia

Elderly patients, particularly those suffering from xerostomia (dry mouth), are prone to increased rates of dental decay. Xerostomia, often caused by medication or systemic conditions, reduces saliva production, which is crucial for neutralizing acids and providing natural antibacterial protection. For these patients, the antibacterial properties of AgNP-containing adhesives can offer an additional safeguard against the rapid development of caries around restorations.

In clinical practice, AgNP-containing adhesives can be used as part of a comprehensive preventive strategy for elderly patients with xerostomia. By providing long-lasting antibacterial effects at the restoration margins, these adhesives can reduce the incidence of secondary caries and the need for frequent dental interventions.

Paediatric Patients

Children, particularly those with high caries risk or poor oral hygiene habits, are also prime candidates for AgNP-containing adhesives. In paediatric dentistry, managing dental decay and ensuring the longevity of restorations are critical to maintaining overall oral health. The antibacterial properties of AgNP-containing adhesives can be particularly beneficial in preventing recurrent decay in primary teeth or during the transition to permanent dentition.

Additionally, in cases where dental caries is already present, the use of an adhesive that can inhibit bacterial growth and protect the tooth-restoration interface can help delay the progression of caries, providing time for the child to adopt better oral hygiene practices.

5.5 Use in Adhesive Systems for Post-endodontic Restorations

Post-endodontic restorations, especially in teeth with significant structural loss, are vulnerable to bacterial contamination. In these cases, the use of AgNP-containing adhesives provides an additional level of protection. After endodontic treatment, there may still be residual bacteria in the root canal system or the remaining tooth structure, which can lead to reinfection or post-treatment disease.

Incorporating silver nanoparticles into the adhesive used for post-endodontic restorations can inhibit bacterial growth within the coronal portion of the tooth and prevent reinfection of the root canal system. This is particularly relevant in cases where the tooth is restored with adhesive-based restorations like fibre posts or composite build-ups, as the antibacterial properties of AgNPs can help maintain the integrity of the restoration over time.

6 Challenges and Limitations of Silver Nanoparticles in Dental Adhesives

While silver nanoparticles (AgNPs) offer significant advantages in terms of antibacterial efficacy and preventing secondary caries, their incorporation into dental adhesives is not without challenges. These limitations, which need to be addressed for widespread clinical adoption, primarily revolve around issues of cytotoxicity, nanoparticle stability, potential compromise of mechanical properties, and the cost effectiveness of AgNP-containing adhesives. This section will provide a detailed discussion of these challenges, highlighting areas where future research is needed to optimize the use of AgNPs in dental adhesives.

6.1 Cytotoxicity Concerns

One of the most pressing challenges associated with the use of silver nanoparticles in dental materials, including adhesives, is their potential cytotoxicity. While silver nanoparticles are effective in inhibiting bacterial growth, they can also have toxic effects on human cells, particularly at higher concentrations. This duality poses a significant challenge, as the concentration of AgNPs that is optimal for antibacterial effects may also negatively impact the surrounding tissue.

Impact on Human Cells

Studies have demonstrated that silver nanoparticles, particularly in higher concentrations, can be cytotoxic to various human cell types, including fibroblasts, keratinocytes, and pulp cells. Cytotoxicity occurs due to the same mechanisms that make silver nanoparticles effective against bacteria—disruption of cell membranes, generation of reactive oxygen species (ROS), and interference with cellular processes. Unfortunately, these effects are not limited to bacterial cells and can also damage human cells that come into contact with the adhesive.

For dental adhesives, the proximity to vital tooth structures, such as the pulp, increases the likelihood of cytotoxic effects. If the adhesive penetrates too deeply into the dentinal tubules or is applied in large quantities, there is a risk that silver nanoparticles will reach the dental pulp, where they can cause inflammatory reactions or even cell death. This is particularly relevant in deep cavity preparations, where the remaining dentin layer is thin.

Balancing Antibacterial Efficacy and Cytotoxicity

A critical area of research focuses on finding the balance between maximizing the antibacterial properties of AgNPs while minimizing their cytotoxic effects. Lower concentrations of silver nanoparticles have been shown to be effective at inhibiting bacterial growth without significantly affecting human cell viability. For example, concentrations of AgNPs as low as 0.05% have been shown to provide substantial antibacterial activity while posing minimal risk to surrounding tissues.

However, the relationship between nanoparticle size, concentration, and cytotoxicity is complex. Smaller nanoparticles may exhibit greater antibacterial efficacy due to their higher surface area, but they may also be more cytotoxic because they can more easily penetrate human cells. This balance must be carefully considered in the design of AgNP-containing adhesives to ensure both safety and efficacy.

6.2 Long-Term Stability of Silver Nanoparticles

Another significant challenge is the long-term stability of silver nanoparticles within dental adhesives. Over time, silver nanoparticles may undergo changes that reduce their effectiveness, such as agglomeration, loss of surface activity, or changes in the rate of silver ion release. These changes can impact both the antibacterial properties of the adhesive and its physical performance.

Nanoparticle Agglomeration

Agglomeration refers to the tendency of nanoparticles to clump together, which is a common issue with silver nanoparticles due to their high surface energy. When nanoparticles aggregate, their surface area decreases, which reduces their ability to interact with bacterial cells and diminishes their antibacterial efficacy.

In the context of dental adhesives, agglomeration can also impact the mechanical properties of the material. Aggregates of silver nanoparticles can disrupt the homogeneity of the adhesive matrix, leading to weak spots that may reduce bond strength and affect the long-term durability of the restoration. This is particularly an issue in adhesives where nanoparticles are directly incorporated, as discussed in the earlier section on incorporation methods.

Loss of Antibacterial Activity

The antibacterial properties of AgNPs are largely due to the release of silver ions, which can interact with bacterial cells and disrupt their functions. However, over time, the rate of silver ion release may decrease as the nanoparticles become embedded within the adhesive matrix or as the outer layers of the nanoparticles are consumed. This gradual reduction in ion release can lead to a loss of antibacterial activity, which may allow bacteria to colonize the tooth-restoration interface after the initial protective effects have diminished.

To address this issue, researchers are exploring ways to control the release of silver ions over time, ensuring that the antibacterial properties of the adhesive are maintained for the duration of the restoration's lifespan. Controlled release systems or the use of coating materials that slow the rate of silver ion release are potential solutions, but these approaches are still in the experimental stages.

6.3 Impact on Mechanical Properties

The addition of silver nanoparticles to dental adhesives can have both positive and negative effects on the mechanical properties of the material. While the antibacterial benefits of AgNPs are well documented, their impact on key mechanical properties such as bond strength, elastic modulus, and marginal adaptation must be carefully considered to ensure that the adhesive performs effectively in clinical applications.

Shear Bond Strength

As mentioned in earlier sections, one of the main concerns with AgNP-containing adhesives is their potential to reduce the shear bond strength between the composite restoration and the tooth structure. This issue is particularly pronounced when silver nanoparticles are incorporated in high concentrations or when they aggregate within the adhesive matrix.

A reduction in shear bond strength can compromise the longevity of the restoration, as the bond between the adhesive and the tooth may fail under mechanical stresses, leading to restoration failure or debonding. Studies have shown that while low concentrations of AgNPs (e.g. 0.05%) may not significantly affect bond strength, higher concentrations can lead to a notable reduction in bond strength, particularly if the nanoparticles are not well dispersed.

Marginal Adaptation

The marginal adaptation of a restoration is critical for preventing bacterial infiltration at the restoration margins. Poor marginal adaptation can result in the formation of gaps between the tooth and the restoration, which can serve as entry points for bacteria, leading to secondary caries.

Silver nanoparticles, particularly when poorly dispersed or aggregated, can negatively impact the flow properties of the adhesive, leading to compromised marginal adaptation. Aggregates of nanoparticles may interfere with the adhesive's ability to flow into and seal the microgaps at the restoration margins, increasing the risk of bacterial infiltration.

To mitigate these issues, adhesive formulations with silver nanoparticles must be carefully optimized to ensure that the nanoparticles do not interfere with the adhesive's ability to form a tight seal with the tooth structure. In situ fabrication methods, which produce smaller, better dispersed nanoparticles, may help improve marginal adaptation compared to direct incorporation methods.

6.4 Cost Effectiveness and Scalability

The incorporation of silver nanoparticles into dental adhesives introduces additional costs related to the synthesis, incorporation, and quality control of the nanoparticles. While the cost of silver as a raw material is relatively low, the production of nanoparticles and the technology required to stabilize and integrate them into dental materials can be expensive. This presents a challenge for widespread clinical adoption, particularly in cost-sensitive markets.

Manufacturing Challenges

Scaling up the production of AgNP-containing adhesives for commercial use presents several challenges, particularly with regard to maintaining consistent nanoparticle size, dispersion, and stability. The in situ fabrication method, while effective for producing well-dispersed nanoparticles, is more complex and costly than direct incorporation methods. The need for precise control over chemical reactions during nanoparticle synthesis adds to the production cost, and ensuring the consistent quality of nanoparticles across large production batches can be difficult.

Cost Versus Clinical Benefits

While the clinical benefits of AgNP-containing adhesives are clear, particularly in preventing secondary caries and reducing restoration failure, the cost effectiveness of these materials must be carefully considered. In high-risk patients or cases where restoration longevity is a critical concern, the additional cost of using AgNP-containing adhesives may be justified by the reduced need for restoration replacement and the prevention of recurrent decay. However, in lower-risk cases, the added cost may be less easily justified, particularly if conventional adhesives can provide satisfactory performance at a lower price point.

To make AgNP-containing adhesives more accessible, future research should focus on reducing production costs, improving manufacturing scalability, and ensuring that the added benefits of these materials outweigh their additional costs.

6.5 Environmental and Ethical Considerations

As the use of nanoparticles in medical and dental materials becomes more widespread, concerns have been raised about their potential environmental impact. Silver nanoparticles, like other nanomaterials, can enter the environment through various pathways, including wastewater from dental offices or manufacturing facilities. Once in the environment, nanoparticles may accumulate in aquatic ecosystems, where they can have toxic effects on marine life and potentially disrupt ecological balance.

Environmental Impact of Silver Nanoparticles

Research on the environmental impact of silver nanoparticles is still in its early stages, but studies suggest that AgNPs can be toxic to aquatic organisms, particularly when they accumulate in high concentrations. The release of silver ions from nanoparticles can interfere with biological processes in fish, algae, and other aquatic species, leading to concerns about the long-term environmental consequences of widespread nanoparticle use.

Ethical Considerations in Nanotechnology

From an ethical standpoint, the use of nanotechnology in medical and dental materials raises questions about patient safety, informed consent, and the potential long-term effects of exposure to nanoparticles. While silver nanoparticles have been shown to be safe in many applications, their potential risks, particularly in terms of cytotoxicity and environmental impact, must be carefully weighed against their benefits. Dental professionals and researchers have a responsibility to ensure that the use of nanotechnology is based on sound scientific evidence and that patients are fully informed of the potential risks and benefits of these materials.

7 Future Directions in Silver Nanoparticles for Dental Adhesives

While silver nanoparticles (AgNPs) have already shown significant promise in improving the antibacterial properties of dental adhesives, there is still considerable room for innovation and optimization. The following future directions highlight key areas of research and development that could enhance the effectiveness, safety, and accessibility of AgNP-containing adhesives in clinical practice.

7.1 Development of Hybrid Nanocomposites

One of the most promising areas of research involves the development of hybrid nanocomposites that combine silver nanoparticles with other bioactive materials. For example:

Calcium Phosphate and Fluoride-Based Nanoparticles: Combining AgNPs with calcium phosphate or fluoride nanoparticles can create a dual action adhesive with both antibacterial properties and remineralization potential. Such materials could actively promote the repair of demineralized tooth structure while preventing bacterial colonization.

Antioxidant-Enhanced Nanocomposites: Incorporating antioxidants into AgNP-containing adhesives could help mitigate the oxidative stress caused by reactive oxygen species (ROS) generated by silver nanoparticles. This could reduce potential cytotoxic effects on surrounding tissues while maintaining the antibacterial efficacy of the adhesive.

These hybrid materials could address multiple clinical concerns simultaneously, making them highly versatile for use in a wide range of restorative procedures.

7.2 Controlled Release Systems for Silver Ions

The long-term antibacterial efficacy of AgNP-containing adhesives depends on the sustained release of silver ions over time. Research into controlled release systems aims to develop adhesives that can release silver ions at a steady rate, ensuring prolonged antibacterial activity without compromising the material's mechanical properties. Potential strategies include:

Encapsulation of Silver Nanoparticles: Encapsulating AgNPs in biocompatible polymers or coatings could slow the release of silver ions, extending the duration of antibacterial effects while preventing rapid ion depletion.

Layered Nanostructures: Creating layered nanostructures within the adhesive matrix could allow for staged release of silver ions, providing antibacterial protection at critical time points during the restoration's lifespan.

Controlled release systems represent a significant step toward enhancing the durability and efficacy of AgNP-containing adhesives, particularly in high-risk clinical cases.

7.3 *Personalized Dentistry Applications*

Advancements in personalized medicine and dentistry offer exciting possibilities for tailoring dental materials to individual patients' needs. For example:

Patient-Specific Formulations: AgNP-containing adhesives could be customized based on a patient's caries risk profile, oral microbiome composition, and medical history. Patients with high caries risk or compromised immune systems might benefit from adhesives with higher concentrations of silver nanoparticles, while lower-risk patients could use formulations with reduced nanoparticle content.

Smart Adhesive Systems: The integration of smart technologies into dental adhesives could enable dynamic responses to environmental conditions. For instance, adhesives could release silver ions in response to bacterial activity, providing targeted antibacterial effects when needed.

Such personalized approaches could improve patient outcomes while minimizing unnecessary exposure to silver nanoparticles in low-risk cases.

7.4 *Innovations in Nanoparticle Synthesis and Stability*

Improving the synthesis and stability of silver nanoparticles is a critical area of focus for future research. Innovations in this field could address issues such as aggregation, variability in particle size, and long-term stability within the adhesive matrix. Specific advancements may include:

Green Synthesis Methods: Developing environmentally friendly methods for synthesizing silver nanoparticles using natural reducing agents, such as plant extracts or enzymes, could reduce the environmental impact of nanoparticle production and enhance biocompatibility.

Surface Functionalization: Modifying the surface of silver nanoparticles with stabilizing agents or functional groups could improve their dispersion within the adhesive matrix and reduce the risk of aggregation. Functionalized nanoparticles may also exhibit enhanced antibacterial properties or reduced cytotoxicity.

These advancements could make AgNP-containing adhesives more reliable and scalable for widespread clinical use.

7.5 Addressing Environmental Concerns

As the use of nanoparticles in dental materials becomes more prevalent, it is essential to address their potential environmental impact. Research into biodegradable or environmentally friendly nanoparticle systems could help mitigate concerns about the accumulation of silver nanoparticles in aquatic ecosystems. Additionally, implementing waste management protocols in dental practices and manufacturing facilities could minimize nanoparticle release into the environment.

8 Conclusion

Silver nanoparticles have revolutionized the field of dental adhesives, offering a powerful tool for preventing secondary caries and improving the longevity of restorations. By inhibiting bacterial colonization and biofilm formation at the tooth-restoration interface, AgNP-containing adhesives address one of the most significant challenges in restorative dentistry. However, their adoption in clinical practice is not without challenges, including concerns about cytotoxicity, long-term stability, and cost effectiveness.

Future research and innovation will play a critical role in overcoming these challenges. Advances in hybrid nanocomposites, controlled release systems, and personalized dentistry hold the potential to enhance the safety, efficacy, and accessibility of AgNP-containing adhesives. By addressing environmental and ethical considerations, the dental community can ensure that these materials are used responsibly and sustainably.

As the field of nanotechnology continues to evolve, the integration of silver nanoparticles into dental adhesives represents a significant step towards more durable, effective, and patient-centred restorative materials. With continued research and collaboration, AgNP-containing adhesives could become a cornerstone of modern restorative dentistry, benefiting clinicians and patients alike.

Index

R. Narayan (ed.), *Nanostructured Biomaterials and Their Applications*,
https://doi.org/10.1007/978-3-032-16316-5

The manufacturer's authorised representative in the EU is Springer Nature Customer Service Centre GmbH, Europaplatz 3, 69115 Heidelberg, Germany. If you have any concerns regarding our products, please contact ProductSafety@springernature.com

Printed and bound by CPI Group (UK) Ltd, Croydon, CR0 4YY
19/09/2026
02219437-0002